Dermatology and Solid Organ Transplantation

Series in Dermatological Treatment

Published in association with the *Journal of Dermatological Treatment*, the *Series in Dermatological Treatment* keeps readers up to date with the latest clinical therapies to improve problems with the skin, hair, and nails. Each volume in the series is prepared separately and typically focuses on a topical theme. Volumes are published on an occasional basis, depending on the emergence of new developments.

About the Series

Techniques in the Evaluation and Management of Hair Disease
Rubina Alves and Juan Grimalt

Retinoids in Dermatology
Ayse Serap Karadag, Berna Aksoy, and Lawrence Charles Parish

Facial Skin Disorders
Ronald Marks

Dermatologic Reactions to Cancer Therapies
Gabriella Fabbrocini, Mario E. Lacouture, and Antonella Tosti

Acne Scars: Classification and Treatment, Second Edition
Antonella Tosti, Maria Pia De Padova, Gabriella Fabbrocini, and Kenneth Beer

Phototherapy Treatment Protocols, Third Edition
Steven R. Feldman and Michael D. Zanolli

Dermatoscopy in Clinical Practice: Beyond Pigmented Lesions, Second Edition
Giuseppe Micali and Francesco Lacarrubba

Nail Surgery
Bertrand Richert, Niton Di Chiacchio, and Eckart Haneke

Abdominal Stomas and Their Skin Disorders, Second Edition
Callum C. Lyon and Amanda Smith

Textbook of Atopic Dermatitis
Sakari Reitamo, Thomas A. Luger, and Martin Steinhoff

For more information about this series please visit: *www.crcpress.com/Series-in-Dermatological-Treatment/book-series/CRCSERDERTRE*

Dermatology and Solid Organ Transplantation

Edited by
Nathalie C. Zeitouni, MDCM, FRCPC
Mohs and Reconstructive Surgery
Medical Dermatology Specialists
Professor of Dermatology, University of Arizona College of Medicine – Phoenix
Phoenix, AZ
Adjunct Professor of Oncology
Roswell Park Comprehensive Cancer Center
Buffalo, NY, USA

Faramarz H. Samie, MD, PhD
J. Lowry Miller Professor of Dermatology
Vice-Chair, Clinical Affairs
Director, Mohs Micrographic Surgery
Director, Micrographic Surgery and Dermatologic Oncology Fellowship
Department of Dermatology, Columbia University Irving Medical Center
New York, NY, USA

CRC Press
Taylor & Francis Group
Boca Raton London New York

CRC Press is an imprint of the Taylor & Francis Group, an **informa** business

First edition published 2022
by CRC Press
6000 Broken Sound Parkway NW, Suite 300, Boca Raton, FL 33487–2742

and by Taylor & Francis Group
2 Park Square, Milton Park, Abingdon, Oxon, OX14 4RN

Library of Congress Cataloging-in-Publication Data

Names: Zeitouni, Nathalie C., editor. | Samie, Faramarz H., editor.
Title: Dermatology and solid organ transplantation / edited by Nathalie C. Zeitouni, Faramarz H. Samie.
Other titles: Series in dermatological treatment.
Description: First edition. | Boca Raton : CRC Press, 2022. | Series: Series in dermatological treatment | Includes bibliographical references and index. | Summary: "This textbook brings together experts in the field of transplant dermatology to review both state of the art and practical knowledge regarding the clinical presentation and management of the various cutaneous diseases seen in patients with solid organ transplant"— Provided by publisher.
Identifiers: LCCN 2021011672 (print) | LCCN 2021011673 (ebook) | ISBN 9780367431464 (hardback) | ISBN 9781032044910 (paperback) | ISBN 9781003001461 (ebook)
Subjects: MESH: Skin Neoplasms—etiology | Skin Neoplasms—therapy | Organ Transplantation—adverse effects | Immunosuppressive Agents—adverse effects
Classification: LCC RC280.S5 (print) | LCC RC280.S5 (ebook) | NLM WR 650 | DDC 616.99/477—dc23
LC record available at https://lccn.loc.gov/2021011672
LC ebook record available at https://lccn.loc.gov/2021011673

ISBN: 978-0-367-43146-4 (hbk)
ISBN: 978-1-032-04491-0 (pbk)
ISBN: 978-1-003-00146-1 (ebk)

DOI: 10.1201/9781003001461

Typeset in Times
by Apex CoVantage, LLC

This textbook is dedicated in memory of our friend and colleague,
Oscar R. Colegio, MD, PhD (1972–2020).

To Zoe, Camille, and Matthew—you mean the world to me.
—NCZ

To my family Mahnaz, Iraj, Farzaneh, and Lily.
—FHS

To all our patients, for your trust and inspiration, to our wonderful colleagues, our mentors and trainees for your support, patience, and constant encouragement.
—NCZ and FHS

Contents

Foreword ix
Preface x
List of Contributors xi

1 History of Transplant Dermatology and Current Epidemiologic Trends in Posttransplant Skin Cancer **1**
Deniz Seçkin and Megan H. Trager

2 Immunosuppressive Therapy for Solid Organ Transplantation **23**
Ethan P. Marin, Elizabeth Cohen, and Divyanshu Malhotra

3 Dermatologic Imaging for Immunosuppressed Patients **36**
Shenara Musthaq, Aditi Sahu, and Veronica Rotemberg

4 Skin Cancer Prevention, Chemoprevention, and Revision of Immunosuppression **51**
Tom Kovitwanichkanont and Alvin H. Chong

5 Topical and Intralesional Modalities for Actinic Keratoses and Nonmelanoma Skin Cancer in Transplant Recipients **62**
Stacy McMurray, Lee Wheless, and Allison Hanlon

6 Advances in Photodynamic Therapy for the Treatment of Actinic Keratoses and Nonmelanoma Skin Cancer in Solid Organ Transplant Recipients **82**
Jonathan Alvarez, Michael T. Olson, and Nathalie C. Zeitouni

7 Pediatric Transplant Dermatology **99**
Carrie C. Coughlin, James Lancaster, and Shivani Tripathi

8 Melanoma in Solid Organ Transplant Recipients **118**
Alexandra Gosh, Mohammed Almashali, Susan Pei, and Gyorgy Paragh

9 Cutaneous Squamous Cell Carcinoma in Solid Organ Transplant Recipients **139**
Ali Rajabi-Estarabadi, Caiwei Zheng, Courtney J. Ensslin, and Ally-Khan Somani

10 Management of Squamous Cell Carcinoma in Solid Organ Transplant Recipients **150**
Courtney J. Ensslin and Faramarz H. Samie

11 Merkel Cell Carcinoma in Solid Organ Transplant Recipients **172**
Liang Ding, Nathalie C. Zeitouni, and Michael Bax

12 Rare Skin Cancers: Kaposi's Sarcoma, Sebaceous Carcinoma, Atypical Fibroxanthoma, and Dermatofibrosarcoma Protuberans **188**
Kimberly L. Brady

13 Immunotherapy in Organ Transplant Recipients **204**
Maressa C. Criscito and John A. Carucci

14 Bacterial, Fungal, and Viral Skin Infections in Organ Transplant Recipients **217**
Alexandra Geusau

15 Direct Dermatologic Side Effects of Immunosuppressive Therapy in Solid Organ Transplant Recipients **247**
Margaret Dowd, Nico Shary, Mike Wang, and Oscar R. Colegio

16 Nail Disease and Nail Surgery in Solid Organ Transplant Recipients **261**
Aleksandar L. Krunic and Severin Laeuchli

17 How to Build a Transplant Dermatology Clinic **293**
Amarachi Eseonu, Kristin Bibee, and Manisha Loss

Index 301

Foreword

Advances in surgical technique, pharmacology, and medical practice have enabled solid organ transplantation to transform organ failure from a universally terminal event to a treatable chronic disease. Acute and chronic skin diseases, ranging from infections to malignancies, have accompanied this dramatic increase in patient survival and unfortunately weigh heavily on the quality of life during these extended years. As the measurement of transplant success moved from months to decades of extended life expectancy, transplant specialists and dermatologists recognized this burden of skin disease. Nowhere in modern medicine is the balance between life-sustaining therapy and undesirable consequences more vividly demonstrated. The immunosuppressive drugs that allow for graft and patient survival also directly and indirectly enable the development of infections and neoplasms. Understanding not only the skin conditions associated with transplantation but also the complex interactions between all elements of this intricate dance which leads to high-quality survival is essential in caring for transplant recipients.

Dermatology and Solid Organ Transplantation builds on the foundation established by previous investigators of transplant skin disease. It provides insights from an international assembly of experts in transplant dermatology. Each chapter concisely summarizes the current knowledge regarding individual aspects of how the skin is affected by transplantation and long-term immunosuppression and then dives in deeply to explore advances in our understanding of etiology, prevention, and treatment of these conditions. Detailed attention is provided to the basics of transplant immunosuppression and its relationship to skin disease. Essential to the reader, cutaneous infections and the common development of cutaneous neoplasms, troubling and at times life-threatening conditions, are explored from proposed mechanisms of development to detection, diagnosis, treatment, and prevention. This book goes further to describe and explore less common, but fundamental, topics in transplant dermatology. Pediatric patients are a small subset of transplant recipients but are among those with the longest potential increase in life span. Early, preventative care in this population may yield great dividends. Nail changes in transplant patients have only been touched upon in the literature but are described in depth. The evolving utility of imaging, optical to ultrasound, available to aid in the skin care of transplant patients is detailed. Even the mechanisms of establishing effective methods of delivery of dermatologic care to transplant patients are elucidated. In short, the editors and authors have provided a text that succeeds in uniting basic science and the nuts and bolts of patient care while weaving a tapestry that illustrates the complex interactions of immunosuppression and the skin. This text will help today's clinicians while providing the building blocks for the next generation of patient care and investigation.

This book comes after the loss of one of our outstanding colleagues in transplant dermatology, Oscar Colegio. Before his untimely death, Oscar contributed to the chapter on the direct dermatologic side effects of immunosuppressive therapy in solid organ transplant recipients. He was a friend and inspiration to all in the dermatology transplant community. We miss him as a brother and grieve the loss of advances in our understanding of transplant dermatology he would have surely given us.

Transplant patients are a special population; however, basically they are just like all other humans with a desire to live a fulfilling life not completely dominated by their illness. The goal of this book is to improve the lives of the inspiring transplant recipients we have the honor to know and care for.

Thomas Stasko, MD

Preface

Over the past seven decades, solid organ transplantation has become a widely performed life-saving procedure throughout the globe. With better surgical techniques, understanding of immunology, immunosuppressive medications, and clinical care, the life span of these patients has increased dramatically over time. As the consequence of prolonged survival of solid organ transplant recipients, dermatologists are now commonly involved in their care, as these patients develop a myriad of inflammatory and infectious diseases and cutaneous malignancies over time.

This book focuses on diseases that are the result of the organ transplantation or more commonly the result of the required immunosuppression for maintenance of the transplanted organ. It is intended to give the reader a thorough clinical understanding of diseases that are seen in a transplant dermatology clinic and serve as a guide for their latest management. It also provides clinicians and trainees with a practical approach to managing difficult dermatologic diseases and guidance on setting up a clinic focused on transplant patients.

It is important to recognize that this work would not be possible without the early and ongoing contributions of dedicated clinicians who recognized the unique medical challenges faced by this cohort of patients. It was through their efforts that the high incidences of malignancies in transplant recipients were recognized, which led to the creation of tumor registries that exist to this day and form the foundation of the data that is presented in the following chapters. Subsequently, with ever-increasing recognition of the high incidence of cutaneous squamous cell carcinoma and other dermatologic disorders in solid organ transplant recipients, organizations such as Skin Care in Organ Transplant Patients, Europe (SCOPE) and The International Immunosuppression and Transplant Skin Cancer Collaborative (ITSCC) were created to improve the care of these patients and educate the medical community and wider society on the special needs of this population. We wish to thank all those pioneering individuals who created this field and educated, guided, and inspired us and so many others to continue the work.

Finally, the idea for this textbook was developed based on some of the topics presented at the transplant dermatology session of the 2019 American Academy of Dermatology Annual Meeting. As we refined our thoughts about the book, we were delighted that Oscar Colagio, MD, PhD, agreed to join us as well in this endeavor. His enthusiasm and experience with this topic are well-known. Sadly, Oscar passed away in June of 2020, and he did not have the opportunity to review the content set forth. We wish to sincerely acknowledge his support and thoughtful contributions to the planning phase of this book.

Faramarz H. Samie, MD, PhD
Nathalie C. Zeitouni, MDCM

Contributors

Mohammed Almashali
Departments of Dermatology and Cell Stress Biology, Roswell Park Comprehensive Cancer Center, Buffalo, NY, USA
Department of Dermatology, College of Medicine, Al Imam Mohammad Ibn Saud Islamic University, Riyadh, Saudi Arabia

Jonathan Alvarez
University of Arizona College of Medicine
Tucson, AZ, USA

Michael Bax
Department of Dermatology
Roswell Park Comprehensive Cancer Center
Buffalo, NY, USA

Kristin Bibee
Department of Dermatology
Johns Hopkins School of Medicine
Baltimore, MD, USA

Kimberly L. Brady
Department of Dermatology
Roswell Park Comprehensive Cancer Center
Buffalo, NY, USA

John A. Carucci
The Ronald O. Perelman Department of Dermatology
New York University Grossman School of Medicine
New York, NY, USA

Alvin H. Chong
Skin and Cancer Foundation and St Vincent's Hospital
Melbourne, Victoria, Australia

Elizabeth Cohen
Yale New Haven Transplant Center
Yale New Haven Hospital
New Haven, CT, USA

†Oscar R. Colegio
Department of Dermatology, Roswell Park Comprehensive Cancer Center
Buffalo, NY, USA

Carrie C. Coughlin
Division of Dermatology
Departments of Medicine and Pediatrics
Washington University School of Medicine in St. Louis
St. Louis, MO, USA

Maressa C. Criscito
The Ronald O. Perelman Department of Dermatology
New York University Grossman School of Medicine
New York, NY, USA

Liang Ding
Department of Pathology
Roswell Park Comprehensive Cancer Center
Buffalo, NY, USA

Margaret Dowd
Department of Dermatology
Columbia University Irving Medical Center
New York, NY, USA

Courtney J. Ensslin
Department of Dermatology
Columbia University Irving Medical Center
New York, NY, USA

Amarachi Eseonu
Department of Dermatology
Johns Hopkins School of Medicine
Baltimore, MD, USA

Alexandra Geusau
Department of Dermatology
Medical University of Vienna
and
Department of Dermatology
General Hospital Vienna
Vienna, Austria

Alexandra Gosh
Departments of Dermatology and Cell Stress Biology
Roswell Park Comprehensive Cancer Center
Buffalo, NY, USA

Allison Hanlon
Department of Dermatology
Vanderbilt University School of Medicine
Nashville, TN, USA

Tom Kovitwanichkanont
Faculty of Medicine, Nursing and Health Sciences, Monash University
Melbourne, Victoria, Australia

Aleksandar L. Krunic
Department of Dermatology
Northwestern University Feinberg School of Medicine
Chicago, IL, USA

Severin Laeuchli
Department of Dermatology
University Hospital
Zurich, Switzerland

James Lancaster
Washington University School of Medicine in St. Louis
St. Louis, MO, USA

Manisha Loss
Department of Dermatology
Johns Hopkins School of Medicine
Baltimore, MD, USA

Divyanshu Malhotra
Department of Medicine — Nephrology
Yale School of Medicine
New Haven, CT, USA

Ethan P. Marin
Department of Medicine — Nephrology
Yale School of Medicine
New Haven, CT, USA

Stacy McMurray
Department of Dermatology
Hospital of the University of Pennsylvania
Philadelphia, PA, USA

Shenara Musthaq
Dermatology, Memorial Sloan Kettering Cancer Center
New York, NY, USA

Michael T. Olson
University of Arizona College of Medicine—Phoenix Campus
Phoenix, AZ, USA

Gyorgy Paragh
Departments of Dermatology and Cell Stress Biology
Roswell Park Comprehensive Cancer Center
Buffalo, NY, USA

Susan Pei
Departments of Pathology and Dermatology
Roswell Park Comprehensive Cancer Center
Buffalo, NY, USA

Ali Rajabi-Estarabadi
Dr. Phillip Frost Department of Dermatology and Cutaneous Surgery
University of Miami Miller School of Medicine
Miami, FL, USA

Veronica Rotemberg
Department of Dermatology
Memorial Sloan Kettering Cancer Center
New York, NY, USA

Aditi Sahu
Department of Dermatology
Memorial Sloan Kettering Cancer Center
New York, NY, USA

Faramarz H. Samie
Department of Dermatology
Columbia University Irving Medical Center
New York, NY, USA

Deniz Seçkin
Department of Dermatology
Başkent University Faculty of Medicine
Ankara, Turkey

Nico Shary
State University of New York at Buffalo School of Medicine and Biomedical Sciences
Buffalo, NY, USA

Ally-Khan Somani
Divison of Dermatologic Surgery and Cutaneous Oncology
Department of Dermatology
Indiana University School of Medicine
Indianapolis, IN, USA

Megan H. Trager
Department of Dermatology
Columbia University Irving Medical Center
New York, NY, USA

Shivani Tripathi
Division of Dermatology
Department of Medicine
Washington University School of Medicine in St. Louis
St. Louis, MO, USA

Mike Wang
Department of Dermatology
Yale New Haven Hospital
Yale School of Medicine
New Haven, CT, USA

Lee Wheless
Department of Dermatology
Vanderbilt University School of Medicine
Nashville, TN, USA

Nathalie C. Zeitouni
Medical Dermatology Specialists
University of Arizona College of Medicine
Phoenix, AZ, USA
Roswell Park Comprehensive Cancer Center
Buffalo, NY, USA

Caiwei Zheng
Dr. Phillip Frost Department of Dermatology and Cutaneous Surgery
University of Miami Miller School of Medicine
Miami, FL, USA

History of Transplant Dermatology and Current Epidemiologic Trends in Posttransplant Skin Cancer

1

Deniz Seçkin and Megan H. Trager

INTRODUCTION

Over the years, solid organ transplantation has provided the opportunity for a new life to many people all over the world who suffer from the physical and psychological burdens of various failing organs. Early attempts at organ transplantation failed in terms of both allograft and recipient survival. The first successful renal transplantation was performed in 1954 in Boston between monozygotic twins.[1] In 1962, the first long-term successful cadaveric renal transplantation was accomplished in the United States (U.S.).[2,3] The other organs (lungs, pancreas, liver, intestines, heart, and bone) were successfully transplanted in the following few years.[2] *The dark days of transplantation* were over once it became clear that the transplanted organs, especially the allograft ones, failed because of *biological* rather than surgical factors,[4] and immunosuppression was needed to prevent the graft rejection, an immunologic event. Initially, total body irradiation, and then chemical immunosuppression with 6-mercaptopurine were introduced in 1959.[2] Over the following years, use of systemic corticosteroids and azathioprine either alone or in combination, and the introduction of cyclosporine, a calcineurin inhibitor (CNI), in 1983 led to a marked improvement of graft survival.[2,3] Combination of the immunosuppressive drugs, and more recently the use of tacrolimus, mTOR inhibitors (mTORi; sirolimus, everolimus), and other immunosuppression methods have resulted in even better success rates.

DOI: 10.1201/9781003001461-1

ADVANCES IN SOLID ORGAN TRANSPLANTATION

In the early transplantation era, prognosis after solid organ transplantation was highly variable. Over the past 60 years, significant advances in the field of solid organ transplantation,[5] including improvements in antimicrobial treatments, surgical techniques, medical diagnosis, selection of organ transplant recipients (OTRs), and posttransplant immunosuppression have contributed to increased survival of recipients.[6] A review of liver transplant recipients (LTRs) in Colorado found that between 1963 and 1977, 28% of patients had an overall survival of at least 1 year.[7] The reasons for the high mortality rate included graft rejection as well as technical or mechanical issues during surgery, such as complications from biliary duct reconstruction.[7] When these issues were identified and addressed in 1976, patient prognosis was reevaluated and drastically improved; 50% of patients survived at least 1 year in the Colorado cohort.[7] Today, survival is significantly longer, and renal transplantation is one of the most successful organ transplant procedures.[7] The median survival of renal transplant recipients (RTRs) is 12.4 years, and over 50% of liver and heart transplant recipients have a survival of >7 years posttransplant.[8] Establishment of legal definitions of brain and cardiac death as well as advances in organ preservation led to an increase in the use of cadaveric organs in the 1980s and a rise in the number of transplants performed. According to the Global Observatory on Donation and Transplantation, the number of transplants performed worldwide is continuing to increase (www.transplant-observatory.org/data-charts-and-tables/).[6] Between 2018 and 2019, the rate of transplant per million population rose dramatically from 19.31 to 29.33. In 2019, a total of 143,146 transplants were performed (65% kidney, 23% liver, 5.8% heart, 4.4% lung, 1.5% pancreas, 0.09% small bowel). Figure 1.1 shows the number of transplants in 2019 broken down by geographic region and solid organ.

SOLID ORGAN TRANSPLANTATION AND CANCER

With the prolonged lifespan and the increased number of OTRs over the years, medical complications secondary to long-term immunosuppression have been identified including various infections and malignancies. Cutaneous malignancies, especially cutaneous squamous cell carcinoma (SCC), are increasingly recognized as patients live longer posttransplant, and the incidence of cutaneous malignancy rises with time from transplantation.[9] Early diagnosis and management of these cancers is of utmost importance as they are recognized as the second leading cause of death in solid OTRs.[10]

In 1969, Israel Penn and his colleagues from the University of Colorado were the first to recognize the relationship between organ transplantation and malignant disease by reporting the development of lymphomas in five RTRs.[11] They proposed that this was "an indirect complication of organ transplantation or the measures taken to prevent rejection." By 1971, Schneck and Penn reported a series of 11 posttransplant brain neoplasms in 184 OTRs.[12] Dr. Penn started an informal registry (the Denver Transplant Tumor Registry), and after he moved to Cincinnati, Ohio, this registry became known as the Cincinnati Transplant Tumor Registry, which has tracked data on more than 15,000 posttransplant malignancies. After Dr. Penn passed away in 1999, the registry was renamed as the Israel Penn International Transplant Tumor Registry (https://ipittr.uc.edu/registry).[2] This database showed that the frequencies of cancers that are common in the general population (e.g., lung, prostate, breast, and colon) were not increased in OTRs. Instead, other malignancies (e.g., lymphomas, SCC of the lip, Kaposi's sarcoma [KS], carcinomas of the vulva, kidney, and liver) were more frequent in the OTRs.

In their 1971 *Lancet* article, Walder et al.[13] reported a 14% increase in skin cancer in OTRs along with a reversal of the ratio of SCC to basal cell carcinoma (BCC) from 1 to 5 in the general population to 1.8 to 1 in transplant recipients. Since then, the relationship between organ transplantation and increased risk of

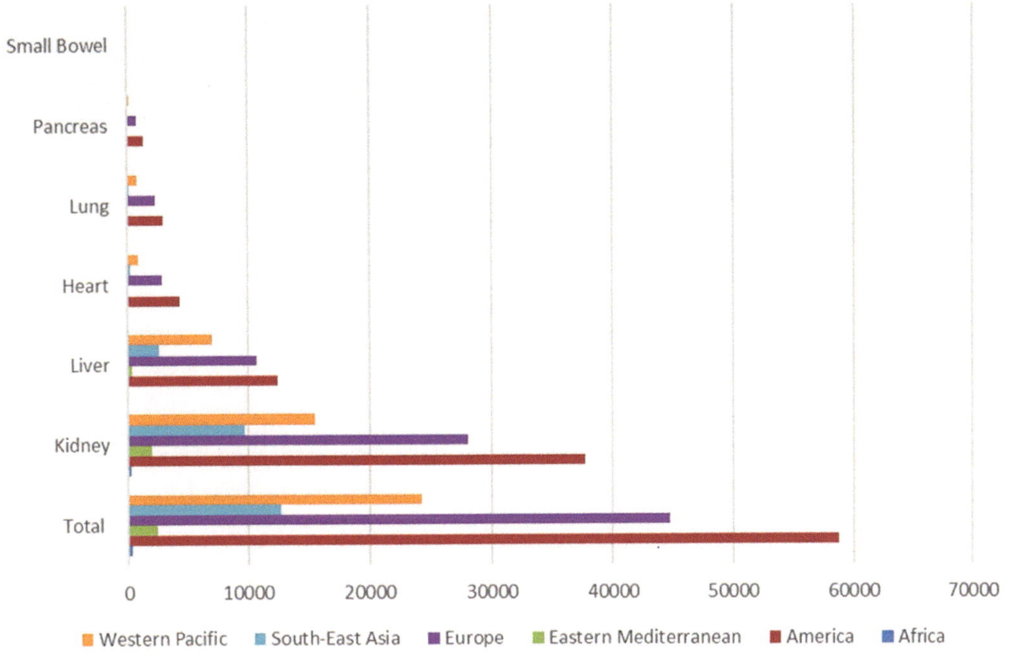

FIGURE 1.1 Data showing the number of solid organ transplants divided by region and organ in 2019. Of the total 143,146 transplants performed in 2019, the majority were in America (58,804) followed by Europe (44,750). The majority of total organs transplanted were renal (65%) followed by liver (23%), heart (5.8%), lung (4.4%), pancreas (1.5%), and small bowel (0.09%). Western Pacific: Mongolia, Japan, Malaysia, New Zealand, Australia, China; South-East Asia: India; Europe: Serbia, Turkey, Austria, Belgium, Bulgaria, Croatia, Cyprus, Czech Republic, Denmark, Estonia, Finland, Germany, Greece, France, Hungary, Ireland, Italy, Latvia, Lithuania, Luxembourg, Malta, Netherlands, Poland, Portugal, Spain, Slovakia, Sweden, United Kingdom, Slovenia, Romania, Switzerland; Eastern Mediterranean: Qatar, Sudan, Syrian Arab Republic, Kuwait, Saudi Arabia, United Arab Emirates; America: Argentina, Brazil, Chile, Colombia, Costa Rica, Cuba, Dominican Republic, Ecuador, Mexico, Panama, Paraguay, Peru, Uruguay, United States, Guatemala, Nicaragua, Venezuela; Africa: Algeria. (Data from the Global Observatory on Donation and Transplantation: www.transplant-observatory.org.[6])

various skin cancers (SCC, BCC, melanoma, KS, and Merkel cell carcinoma [MCC]) has been confirmed by other publications from different transplant centers.[14–18] Those skin cancers are more prone to local recurrence and metastasis compared with those in the immunocompetent population.[19] Studies have also documented that OTRs often develop multiple skin cancers, especially SCC.[20,21]

HISTORY OF TRANSPLANT DERMATOLOGY

Early information regarding the increased incidence of skin cancers in OTRs was mostly reported by transplant surgeons. However, when the number of transplantations, and OTRs with skin cancers, cutaneous infections, as well as mucocutaneous side effects of immunosuppressive medications increased, dermatologists became involved in transplant medicine. Dermatologists seeing OTRs thought that it was important to understand the magnitude of the skin cancers, to investigate the etiopathogenesis and the risk factors, and to apply the best preventive and therapeutic approaches. In 1977, Hoxtell et al.[22] reported that the risk of skin cancer in the Minnesota renal transplant cohort was 7.1 times higher than expected, which was due primarily to SCCs. A CME review in the *Journal of the American Academy of Dermatology (JAAD)* underlined the importance of posttransplant skin cancers, cutaneous manifestations of opportunistic infections, and immunosuppressive drug-related changes.[23] Coordinated by Euvrard, Kanitakis, and Claudy, the first book on transplant dermatology entitled *Skin Diseases After Organ Transplantation*[24] was published in 1998. This book reflected the pioneering work performed by those three dermatologists from Lyon, France, and aimed to help the physicians to manage their OTRs with practical aspects of dermatologic care and to provide some important guidelines for treatment. Another 2002 CME article provided an update on the epidemiology, pathogenesis, and management of posttransplant skin cancers.[25]

Because skin cancers, especially SCC, constituted an important part of all posttransplant *de novo* cancers and caused higher mortality compared with their counterparts in the general population, titles on posttransplant cutaneous oncology appeared in the scientific programs of congresses. Moreover, there was a need for a more systematic approach requiring a collaborative effort by transplant surgeons, dermatologists and basic scientists. Two international groups were founded to improve prevention and treatment of posttransplant skin cancers. Initiated by Dr. Eggert Stockfleth, the Skin Care in Organ Transplant Patients, Europe (SCOPE) was established in Berlin, Germany, in 2000 by transplant dermatologists, transplant physicians, and basic researchers to provide an internet-based database of posttransplant skin cancer. This expanded to include research into treatment of OTRs with skin cancers and their transplant-related other skin issues. The SCOPE Network (www.scopenetwork.org) subsequently expanded to include many European countries and now collaborates with its sister organization, the International immunosuppression and Transplant Skin Cancer Collaborative (ITSCC). Aiming to define the clinical course of posttransplant metastatic SCC, in 2000, the initiative of Dr. Clark Otley and Dr. Juan Carlos Martinez led to the establishment of a multiinstitutional group of dermatologists with similar interests. The participants, under the guidance of Dr. Clark Otley and Dr. Stuart J. Salasche, had their first meeting in October 2001, in conjunction with the American Society of Dermatologic Surgery and the American College of Mohs Micrographic Surgery and Cutaneous Oncology combined annual meeting in Dallas, Texas, which resulted in the foundation of the North American Transplant-Skin Cancer Collaborative. As physicians and researchers from Central and South America, Australia, and other countries also gradually became members, the name was changed to ITSCC (www.itscc.org). Dr Stuart J. Salasche played a key role in bringing ITSCC and SCOPE together. Both networks also provide education for nontransplant dermatologists, OTRs, and primary care doctors both independently and under the umbrella of the European Academy of Dermatology and Venereology (EADV) and the American Academy of Dermatology (AAD). ITSCC collaborated with the International Transplant Nurses Society to establish the After Transplant-Reduce the Incidence of Skin Cancer (AT-RISC) Alliance. To educate physicians, nurses, transplant coordinators, and patients about the risks of posttransplant skin cancers, sun protection, and the signs and symptoms for early recognition of skin cancers, AT-RISC has developed downloadable educational materials (www.at-risc.org).

SCOPE and ITSCC have organized joint scientific meetings every year and every other year, respectively, since their establishment until 2020 to address problematic issues relating especially to skin cancers. Both groups have organized virtual meetings in 2020 and 2021 due to the COVID-19 pandemic. A number of workshops and symposiums as part of EADV, European Academy of Dermato-Oncology, and AAD meetings have been organized to highlight the importance of transplant-related skin cancers and other diseases. SCOPE also organized several fostering courses for dermatology residents. Apart from SCOPE and ITSCC, national European networks such as the British Society for Skin Care in Immunosuppressed Individuals and Skin and Organ Transplantation Group of the French Society of Dermatology have also been active.

Over the years, joint efforts of SCOPE and ITSCC resulted in the publication of several textbooks, namely *Skin Disease in Organ Transplantation*,[26] *Skin Cancer after Organ Transplantation*,[27] *Advances in Transplant Dermatology: Clinical and Practical Implications*,[28] and *Skin Diseases in the Immunosuppressed*.[29]

The dedicated work of both SCOPE and ITSCC has resulted in the establishment of specialty dermatology clinics in most transplant centers. These clinics provide effective care to OTRs both before and after the organ transplantation including education on self-examination of the skin and sun-protective behaviors, and at least annual in-office skin examination to diagnose and efficiently treat skin cancers and other skin diseases. There are three types of clinics: *multidisciplinary transplant clinics* where a dermatology transplant subspecialty clinic is within a multidisciplinary clinic (e.g., Mayo Clinic, Rochester, MN, USA), *designated dermatology transplant subspecialty clinics* (e.g., Charité University Hospital in Berlin as the largest and one of the early clinics), and *integration of transplant recipient care within an existing medical and/or surgical dermatology clinic.* [30] Over the years, it became clear that the collaboration of transplant surgeons with transplant dermatologists was of great importance, and the dermatologists should play an active role in the best care of OTRs.

CURRENT EPIDEMIOLOGIC TRENDS IN POSTTRANSPLANT SKIN CANCER

Squamous Cell Carcinoma

The earliest report of increased cutaneous SCC in OTRs came from Australia, which described seven patients with SCC in a group of 51 RTRs.[13] Keratinocyte carcinomas (KC), namely SCC and BCC, account for over 90% of all posttransplant skin cancers. SCC is the most frequent posttransplant skin cancer, and the ratio of 1:4 for SCC to BCC in the general population is reversed in OTRs.[31] Development of multiple and aggressive posttransplantation KCs, especially SCC, is associated with significant morbidity and mortality.[31] To date, the highest risk of SCC, with a standardized incidence ratio (SIR) of 253, was reported in Dutch RTRs.[15] Of note, the cancer registries in most countries document the first skin cancers and do not record the subsequent skin cancers, which may lead to underestimation of the overall disease burden in OTRs who often develop multiple skin cancers.[32]

A recent retrospective cohort study from the U.S. reported that the incidence ratio (IR) for posttransplant SCC was 25-fold increased compared with the IR in the general population.[33] The IR for posttransplant skin cancer overall was 1437 per 100,000 person-years, and the specific subtype rate for SCC was 812 per 100,000 person-years, followed by rates for melanoma and MCC (75 and 2 per 100,000 person-years, respectively).[33]

Solid OTRs have also a markedly elevated risk of lip cancer, which are primarily SCCs.[34–37] A recent population-based U.S. study found elevated risks of both invasive and *in situ* lip cancers (SIRs of 15.3 and 26.2, respectively).[37]

Temporal Trends in Incidence

Incidence rates of KC have been rising in the general population worldwide (www.skincancer.org). Interestingly, although the risk of SCC in OTRs is still much higher than that in the general population, some of the recent population-based studies have revealed a reduction[32,38–40] or no change[41,42] in the risk of posttransplant SCC in the current transplantation era.

A recent population-based Norwegian study[38] found an overall SIR of 51.9 for SCC in all OTRs. In those who underwent transplantation between 1983 and 1987, the unadjusted SIR for SCC was 102.7 and declined to 21.6 in those transplanted between 2003 and 2007. After adjusting for age at transplantation, sex, graft type, follow-up time, and increasing incidence of SCC in the background population,[43] a significant decline (but still elevated compared with that in the general population) over time still existed in the risk of cutaneous SCC.[38] The overall SIR for SCC in OTRs in this study was similar to SIRs reported in other Northern European studies.[14,15,36,42,44–49]

Another recent nationwide study from Ireland including all solid OTRs transplanted between 1994 and 2014 reported an overall SIR of 19.7 for SCC.[32] This study also showed a progressive and dramatic fall in SIRs for SCC from peak SIR in the 1994–1996 period of 26.4 to 6.3 in the 2012–2014 period and also confirmed a halving of the risk of SCC since the beginning of the century.[32]

In a recent Nordic population-based cohort study of adult LTRs, the SIR for nonmelanoma skin cancer, presumably mostly SCC, also declined significantly over 3 decades (1982–2013), from 80.0 to 10.4.[40] Furthermore, this was observed across sex, age, and transplant indication groups.

A Dutch study also reported a significant decline in the incidence of SCC among RTRs; although the frequency of SCC was 48% between 1976 and 1985, it dropped to 2.3% between 1996 and 2006.[39]

A Canadian population-based study[50] including adult OTRs from 1994 to 2012 showed an incidence rate of 2.63 per 100 patient-years for KC and found a 6.6-fold increased risk of KC in OTRs compared with that in the general population. The incidence of posttransplant KC also tended to be lower in those who had undergone transplantation in recent years, although SCC and BCC were not examined separately.[50]

Although the incidence of posttransplant skin cancers is low among Asian OTRs,[51,52] the risk of skin cancer in OTRs is still considerably higher than that in the Korean general population.[51] Another study from Korea[53] also showed that the relative SIRs for SCC were lower in 2009–2018 than those in 1990–2008. The SIR for SCC *in situ* increased in the last decade, indicating that over the last decade, SCC has been diagnosed earlier.[53]

Incidence of posttransplant lip cancer also declined across calendar periods of transplantation.[37]

The trend of decline in the incidence of posttransplant skin cancer reported in all those previously mentioned studies coincided with temporal changes in the immunosuppressive drug protocols.[32,37–40,50,53] Thus, less aggressive and more individualized immunosuppressive treatment (i.e., replacing azathioprine with mycophenolate mofetil [MMF] and cyclosporine with other immunosuppressive drugs, using lower doses, or using mTORi), regular dermatologic follow-ups, and effective sun protection habits could be the possible explanations.[32,38]

A recent population-based Swedish cohort study of OTRs transplanted from 1970–2008 found a SIR of 121 for SCC, and when only the first SCC was considered, risk estimates were elevated 69-fold in heart/lung transplanted patients.[36] During follow-up, risk of all cancer types excluding SCC remained stable while the risk of SCC quadrupled over 20 years,[36] in contrast to the previously mentioned studies.[32,37–40,50,53] In this study, however, OTRs were grouped according to decade of transplantation, which led to inclusion of OTRs taking and not taking cyclosporine-based immunosuppressive therapy in the same group.[36] This suboptimal stratification may have masked a possible difference in the risk of posttransplant SCC between those two groups, and a subsequent decline over time.

Like in most countries, OTRs in the United Kingdom transplanted before 1984 received azathioprine and corticosteroids as a standard immunosuppressive protocol, and after this date cyclosporine was introduced. In the late 1990s, azathioprine was widely replaced by MMF, and tacrolimus was also used. Nevertheless, a 22-year prospective British study found no significant time of transplantation difference between pre-1985 and 1985–2000 periods,[42] again in contrast to the studies that showed a decline in the risk of posttransplant SCC over time.[32,37–40,50,53] However, possible temporal changes within the 1985–2000 period were not mentioned.[42]

A U.S. cohort study also showed that patients transplanted in 2008 vs. 2003 had a higher IR of skin cancer, which could be related to improved overall survival because of newer immunosuppressive agents and more aggressive immediate posttransplant immunosuppression in the more recent era. However, this study had no data on background population risk.[33]

A recent French epidemiological study also reported a similar prevalence of SCC from 1991–2015.[41]

Risk Factors

Long-term immunosuppression to prevent graft rejection is the major causal factor for development of posttransplant KC by resulting in both a decreased immune response and an exposure to potentially carcinogenic drugs.[54,55]

More details on the risk factors are included in Table 1.1. Major risk factors include the type of organ transplanted (heart/lung > renal/liver because of higher levels of immunosuppression),[32,33,36–38,47] male

TABLE 1.1 Risk Factors Identified for Posttransplant Squamous Cell Carcinoma

RISK FACTORS	PUBLICATION	STUDY POPULATION (N)	COUNTRY	RESULTS	SUMMARY
Sex[32,33,36–38]	Menzies et al. 2019	3580	Ireland	Male sex was not found to be a risk factor for posttransplant SCC	Male sex is accepted to be a risk factor for development of posttransplant SCC in the majority of studies
	Garrett et al. 2017	10,649	U.S.	Male sex was associated with an increased HR for development of SCC (1.67)	
	Krynitz et al. 2013	10,476	Sweden	Male sex was associated with higher IRR for first posttransplant SCC	
	Laprise et al. 2018	261,500	U.S.	Increased IRR (2.01) of lip SCC in males	
	Rizvi et al. 2017	8026	Norway	Increased HR for males compared with females (1.58)	
Organ Transplanted[32,33,36–38,47]	Menzies et al. 2019	3580	Ireland	Lung transplant associated with highest IRR (1.46)	Heart or lung transplant recipients have the highest risk for SCC whereas liver transplant recipients have the lowest risk
	Garrett et al. 2017	10,649	U.S.	Thoracic transplant (compared with abdominal) was associated with a higher risk (1.51)	
	Krynitz et al. 2013	10,476	Sweden	Highest SIR in heart and lung transplants up to 19 years post transplant	
	Laprise et al. 2018	261,500	U.S.	Increased IR for lung transplant (3.07)	
	Rizvi et al. 2017	8026	Norway	Increased HR in heart and lung transplant (1.59 and 1.53, respectively). Lowest in liver (0.37)	
	Jensen et al. 2010	5279	Denmark	SIR for SCC is highest among heart transplants (SIR = 113), then renal (SIR = 81), lung (SIR = 65), and liver (SIR = 60) recipients	
Age at Transplantation[33,37,50,53]	Garrett et al. 2017	10,649	U.S.	Increased HR in those ≥ 50 (2.77)	Increased age at transplantation is associated with increased risk for development of posttransplant SCC in three of the four studies
	Laprise et al. 2018	261,500	U.S.	No significant difference between those < 20 years and ≥20 years	
	Park et al. 2019	10,198	Canada	Highest 10-year cumulative incidence was highest in those > 50 years at transplant (adjusted HR: 9.27)	
	Kim et al. 2020	13,469	Korea	Patients ≥ 45 years (HR = 6.74) and ≥ 55 years (HR = 24.8) were at higher risk	

(Continued)

TABLE 1.1 Risk Factors Identified for Posttransplant Squamous Cell Carcinoma (Continued)

RISK FACTORS	*PUBLICATION*	*STUDY POPULATION (N)*	*COUNTRY*	*RESULTS*	*SUMMARY*
Race[33,37,50,54]	Garrett et al. 2017	10,649	U.S.	White race was associated with increased HR (8.18)	White race and light skin are associated with increased risk for posttransplant SCC
	Laprise et al. 2018	261,500	U.S.	White, non-Hispanic had the highest Lower adjusted IRR for other race/ethnicity (0.09)	
	Park et al. 2019	10,198	Canada	Increased HR in those of white vs. black race (8.50)	
	Madeleine et al. 2017	NA	NA	Geographical differences suggest that dark pigmented skin is protective	
Pretransplant skin cancers[33,50]	Garrett et al. 2017	10,649	U.S.	Pretransplant skin cancer was associated with an increased HR for development of posttransplant SCC (4.69)	History of pretransplant skin cancer is a risk factor for posttransplant SCC
	Park et al. 2019	10,198	Canada	Increased HR in those with pretransplant invasive skin cancer (4.30)	
Medication use[53,59,60,64,66,67,69]	Kim et al. 2020	13,469	Korea	Treatment with two or more immunosuppressive agents associated with higher risk	Immunosuppressive medications and voriconazole may confer higher risk of SCC
	Jiyad et al. 2016	NA	NA	Increased risk for SCC in OTRs on azathioprine	
	Coghill et al. 2016	170	U.S.	Patients treated with azathioprine more than twice as likely to develop SCC. Not seen in patients on MMF and tacrolimus No difference between tacrolimus and cyclosporine	mTORi may confer a protective effect on the development of SCCs. More details are included in the text
	Euvrard et al. 2012	129	France	Switching from CNIs to an mTORi, sirolimus, led to an antitumoral effect among RTRs	
	Murray et al. 2020	4930	Ireland	Lower incidence of skin cancers on mTORi compared with CNIs	
	Asgari et al. 2015	3539	U.S.	No reduction in posttransplant SCC risk with sirolimus	
	D'Arcy et al. 2020	9793	U.S.	Increased risk of SCC with voriconazole in lung transplant	

Note: Immunosuppressive medications are another risk factor that are discussed more extensively in the text.

Abbreviations: CNIs, calcineurin inhibitors; HR, hazard ratio; IR, incidence ratio; IRR, incidence rate ratio; MMF, mycophenolate mofetil; mTORi, mammalian target of rapamycin inhibitor; NA, not applicable; n, number; RTRs, renal transplant recipients; SCC, squamous cell carcinoma; SIR, standardized incidence ratio; U.S., United States.

sex,[33,36–38] older age at transplantation[50] (especially >50,[33] >55,[53] and >60[38]), white race,[33,37,50,54] history of pretransplant skin cancer,[50] posttransplant precancerous skin lesions,[50] and high sun exposure.[58] The number of previous SCCs strongly predicted the occurrence of additional SCCs.[36] Geographical location was also a factor as higher rates of KC were reported among Australian OTRs compared with rates in European or North American OTRs, and the lowest rates were seen in Africa, East Asia, and India.[51,52,54]

Treatment with more than two immunosuppressive agents[53] and subsequent transplants causing a surge in immunosuppressant exposure[50] are known risk factors for new posttransplant skin cancers. However, some immunosuppressive medications may confer additional risk for SCC whereas others may be protective. For example, azathioprine is associated with an increased risk that is not seen with MMF or tacrolimus.[59,60] In fact, MMF was associated with a decreased risk, which persisted after adjustment for simultaneous use of tacrolimus.[60] In terms of SCC risk, there was no difference between tacrolimus and cyclosporine.[60] A recent study was also unable to verify the association between CNIs and skin cancer, probably because of a progressive decrease in trough level targets over time.[40] There is, however, some evidence that cyclosporine may confer a dose-dependent risk of SCC.[14,61] Finally, two recent reviews found inconclusive evidence of increased risk of skin cancer with use of a CNI.[62,63] There is also controversy whether prednisone is associated with an increased skin cancer risk.[63]

Switching from CNIs to sirolimus, a mTORi known for its antioncogenic effects, caused an antitumoral effect among RTRs with previous SCC and provided longer SCC-free survival when compared with that with CNI use.[64] A systematic review of 29 trials[65] and a recent study[66] confirmed the lower incidence of skin cancers in OTRs on mTORi compared with that of those on CNIs. In contrast, a large cohort study found that sirolimus use did not cause a reduction in posttransplantation SCC risk.[67] A limitation of this study was that it did not include data on exposure to CNIs and voriconazole, which might have been confounding factors.

A recent systematic review and meta-analysis found an increased risk of SCC associated with voriconazole use in lung transplant recipients.[68] The most recent U.S. population-based cohort study confirmed this association.[69] Itraconazole exposure was also associated with increased SCC risk.[69]

Metastasis and Mortality

Immunosuppression in OTRs does not seem to increase the risk of metastasis in a single cutaneous SCC but could be an overall risk factor for metastasis because of the multiplicity of cutaneous SCC in OTRs.[70] A recent European multicenter case series of 51 OTRs with aggressive SCC (defined by nodal or distant metastasis or death by local progression of primary SCC) found that the 5-year overall survival rate was 23% and the 5-year disease-specific survival was 30.5%.[71] In a large single-center study in France that followed 188 OTRs, 10 developed metastatic SCC and seven died of disease.[20]

A recent U.S. population-based study found that the overall and skin cancer-specific posttransplantation mortalities were 5308 and 35.27 per 100,000 person-years, respectively. The mortality of skin cancer in the OTR cohort was nearly 9 times higher than that reported for the general population.[72] The SCC-specific mortality rate in that OTR cohort was 4.9 per 100,000 person-years.[72] A United Kingdom-based study reported that 27% of all OTRs with >10 diagnosed skin cancers succumbed to disease.[42] Age >50 years, thoracic versus abdominal transplantation, male sex, white race, and a more recent date of transplantation from 1987 to 2013 were the risk factors for skin cancer mortality.[72]

Basal Cell Carcinoma

Earlier studies revealed a 2- to 10-fold risk of BCC among OTRs.[15,73,74] Population-based studies show that the risk of BCC after transplantation is increased between 6-fold and 16-fold.[14,46,47] A recent population-based Swedish study found that the cumulative incidence of first BCC was 6.7% at 5 years posttransplantation among RTRs, and a 6-fold increased risk of BCC compared with that in the general population.[75]

BCC developed earlier after transplantation compared with SCC,[75] a finding contrasting with that of another study that reported similar cumulative incidences for first SCC and BCC <5 years posttransplantation.[42] However, beyond 5 years posttransplantation, the cumulative incidence of SCC was higher than that of BCC. In a large French OTR cohort, 0.34% developed basosquamous cell carcinoma (BSCC) after a mean duration of 13.2 years, later than other skin carcinomas.[76]

Temporal Trends in Incidence

An Irish population-based study showed that the overall SIR for BCC was 7.0, and there was a progressive fall in the SIR for BCC from a peak value of 9.1 in the 1994–1996 transplant period to 3.2 in the 2012–2014 transplant period.[32] The ratio of posttransplant SCC to BCC has remained relatively stable at 3:1 during the last two decades, indicating that both cancers are decreasing at a similar rate.[32]

A Korean population-based study also showed that the relative SIR for BCC declined over time (SIR of 1990–2008 vs. SIR of 2009–2018).[53]

However, a recent single-center epidemiological study reported that the prevalence of BCC remained unchanged between 1991 and 2015.[41]

Risk Factors

Risk factors for development of posttransplant BCC include male sex,[32,75] type of transplant received (heart and lung > liver),[32,47,75] age at transplantation (risk increases with older age),[32,46,75] time since transplantation,[47,75] history of prior nonmelanoma skin cancers (NMSCs),[21,42,75] and posttransplant immunosuppression.[21,69] Detailed information on these risk factors is included in Table 1.2.

Metastasis and Mortality

Population-based estimates of metastasis and mortality because of posttransplant BCC are lacking because of a lack of reliable registration in most countries, and because BCCs and SCCs are often grouped under the umbrella terms: NMSC and KC. A single-center cohort study reported that out of 12 OTRs with BSCC, only two developed lymph node metastases, indicating that BSCCs do not seem to behave more aggressively than other NMSCs.[76]

Melanoma

A recent systematic review and meta-analysis disclosed the pooled relative risk (pRR) of 2.71 for melanoma in OTRs.[77] The recent population-based Norwegian[38] and Canadian[78] cohort studies also reported 2.4- and 2.3-fold increased risks, respectively. A large U.S. cohort study reported an overall prevalence of 0.47% for posttransplant melanoma, with RTRs at 4.9-times increased risk for developing melanoma than the Surveillance, Epidemiology, and End Results (SEER) database patients.[79] A large retrospective U.S. study of 2017 showed an incidence rate of 125 per 100,000 person-years for posttransplant melanoma.[33]

Another U.S. population-based study of 2015 found lower incidence rates of 74.0 and 27.1 per 100 000 person-years for invasive and *in situ* melanoma, respectively, and the SIRs for invasive melanoma and *in situ* melanoma were 2.20 and 1.47, respectively.[80] Although most patients (76%) had localized melanomas and melanoma in OTRs were elevated across tumor stages, the greatest increase in risk (SIR = 4.11) was detected for regional stage melanoma.[80]

A population-based Swedish study found that superficial spreading melanoma was the most common type and the trunk was the most common site.[81]

TABLE 1.2 Risk Factors Identified for Posttransplant Basal Cell Carcinoma

RISK FACTORS	*PUBLICATION*	*STUDY POPULATION (N)*	*COUNTRY*	*RESULTS*	*SUMMARY*
Sex[32,75]	Menzies et al. 2019	3580	Ireland	26% lower SIR for females	Higher risk of posttransplant BCC in males
	Krynitz et al. 2016	4023	Sweden	62% posttransplant BCCs in males; similar SIR for males and females (6.0 vs. 6.3)	
Organ transplanted[32,47,75]	Menzies et al. 2019	3580	Ireland	Lower SIR for liver vs. renal; higher SIR for lung and heart but not statistically significant	LTRs may have the lowest risk of BCC Higher risk of BCC in especially heart and lung recipients
	Jensen et al. 2010	5279	Denmark	No difference in SIR among organ types	
	Krynitz et al. 2016	4023	Sweden	SIR higher in kidney and heart/lung compared with LTRs	
Age at transplantation[32,46,75]	Menzies et al. 2019	3580	Ireland	Lower SIR >50 years compared with those <30 years at transplant	BCC risk tends to increase with age
	Moloney et al. 2006	1755	Ireland	Rate of skin cancer increased with age (38% in 50–59 years). BCC comprised 27% of NMSC	
	Krynitz et al. 2016	4023	Sweden	Highest SIR in age group 55–64 years (7.2), lower in those ≥65 years (4.3) and <45 years (5.3)	
Time since transplantation[47,75]	Jensen et al. 2010	5279	Denmark	Highest risk 5 to 10 years posttransplant	Risk of BCC increases over time
	Krynitz et al. 2016	4023	Sweden	Increased relative risk with follow-up time	

(Continued)

TABLE 1.2 Risk Factors Identified for Posttransplant Basal Cell Carcinoma (Continued)

RISK FACTORS	PUBLICATION	STUDY POPULATION (N)	COUNTRY	RESULTS	SUMMARY
Prior skin cancer[21,42,75]	Wisgerhof et al. 2010	1906	Netherlands	Initial BCC was associated with subsequent BCC development	Increased risk of BCC in patients with a prior SCC
	Harwood et al. 2012	931	United Kingdom	9 patients with a history of pretransplant skin cancer had shorter time to first posttransplant cancer (71.0 months versus 104.9 months for those without pretransplant skin cancer	Patients who developed one BCC after transplant were at risk for additional BCC development
	Krynitz et al. 2016	4023	Sweden	55-fold increased risk in OTRs with a history of prior SCC; no risk associated with history of non-SCC malignancies	Pretransplant SCC increases the risk of developing posttransplant BCC
Medication use[21,69]	Wisgerhof et al. 2010	1906	Netherlands	Immunosuppression with azathioprine and prednisone associated with SCC not BCC development	BCC risk is associated with antifungal use
	D'Arcy et al. 2020	9599	U.S.	Increased risk of BCC with itraconazole and posaconazole in lung transplant recipients	

Abbreviations: BCC, basal cell carcinoma; LTRs, liver transplant recipients; n, number; NMSC, nonmelanoma skin cancer; OTRs, organ transplant recipients; SCC, squamous cell carcinoma; SIR, standardized incidence ratio; U.S., United States.

Temporal Trends in Prevalence

A retrospective epidemiological study showed that there was a 3.9-fold increase in the prevalence of posttransplant melanoma after 2000 compared with that between 1991 and 2000.[41]

Risk Factors

Risk factors for the development of posttransplant melanoma are detailed in Table 1.3. The major risk factors include male sex,[79–81] white race,[33,79] increased age,[33,79,81] type of transplanted organ (majority renal transplant),[33,79–82] and immunosuppressive agents received.[79,80] Although the overall risk is higher in patients of white race, among African American RTRs, the annual incidence of melanoma was 17.2-times greater than the reported rate for African Americans in the general population.[83]

In the Swedish nationwide cohort study, reassessment of histologic slides revealed a melanoma-adjacent melanocytic nevus in 73% of the posttransplantation melanomas. Those nevi were primarily atypical/dysplastic nevi on trunk location.[81] A retrospective cohort study showed that seven of 11 posttransplant melanomas (64%) arose *de novo*.[84]

Metastasis and Mortality

Some population-based studies reported that posttransplant melanoma was more advanced at diagnosis than melanoma in the general population.[78,81,85,86] However, only 2 of 11 melanomas were >1 mm in Breslow thickness at diagnosis in an Australian OTR cohort.[84] Posttransplant melanoma had a higher risk of metastasis compared with that in the normal population.[81,86] Melanoma-specific mortality was increased (1.9-,[78] 3-,[80,81], and 4.3-fold[86]) in OTRs compared with that in the nontransplant population. Two multicenter studies in Europe[87] and the U.S.[88] reported that outcome for melanoma in OTRs was significantly worse for thicker tumors. In contrast, other studies found worse survival also for thin tumors,[78,80,81] (but not for tumors 1 mm or thinner[81]), or only for tumors of 1 mm or thinner.[86] Robbins et al.[80] showed that posttransplant melanoma-specific mortality was strongest for localized stage melanoma followed by regional stage melanoma whereas it was not elevated for distant stage.

Median time from melanoma diagnosis to melanoma-specific death was 1.6 years compared with 3.2 years in the general population.[81]

Posttransplant skin cancer-specific mortality was highest for melanoma (11.48 per 100,000 person-years). White patients, males, thoracic transplant recipients, and patients aged 50 years or older were at particularly high risk of dying from melanoma.[72,79] Sirolimus and cyclosporine were also associated with worse survival.[79]

Kaposi's Sarcoma

Due to their immunosuppressive state, OTRs have an increased risk for KS. The prevalence of KS after organ transplantation parallels the overall prevalence of human herpesvirus 8 (HHV-8) in different countries.[89]

A recent nationwide Norwegian cohort study showed that the overall SIR for KS in OTRs was 54.9, even higher than the risk for SCC.[38] Although KS is one of the common posttransplant cancers, this high SIR might reflect the low incidence of KS among nonimmunosuppressed Norwegian individuals.[38] A Swedish nationwide study reported a SIR of 39 for KS in OTRs.[36] Recent multicenter Italian cohort studies including RTRs and LTRs found SIRs of 135[90] and 54,[91] respectively, for KS. The incidence rates for KS in Italian RTR and LTR cohorts were 16-times[90] or 6.3-times[91] higher, respectively, than those reported in a population-based U.S. study,[92] which likely reflects the much higher prevalence of HHV-8 infection in Italy than in the U.S. In a 22-year prospective study from England, 15 of 931 OTRs developed KS, 11 of whom were of African or African Caribbean origin.[42]

TABLE 1.3 Risk Factors Identified for Posttransplant Melanoma

RISK FACTORS	PUBLICATION	STUDY POPULATION (N)	COUNTRY	RESULTS	SUMMARY
Sex[33,79–81]	Garrett et al. 2017	10,649	U.S.	No significant difference between males and females	Overall, data suggests that posttransplant melanoma risk is greater for males
	Ascha et al. 2017	105,174	U.S.	Male sex associated with development of melanoma (71.5% males vs. 60.7% males in those without melanoma, $P<.001$)	
	Robbins et al. 2015	139,991	U.S.	Increased IRR of localized and regional/distant stage melanoma for men (1.64 and 1.89, respectively)	
	Krynitz et al. 2015	22,545	Sweden	Majority of patients with posttransplant melanoma were men (71%)	
Organ Transplanted[77,79–81]	Green et al. 2015	NA	NA	The risk of melanoma for liver and heart transplant recipients was over 5 times higher than the risk of melanoma among the general population, and even higher than in RTRs	Majority of the data showed that posttransplant melanoma develop predominantly in RTRs
	Ascha et al. 2017	105,174	U.S.	RTRs had greater risk of developing melanoma compared with their non-renal transplant counterparts	
	Robbins et al. 2015	139,991	U.S.	Higher IRR for posttransplant melanoma in RTRs	
	Krynitz et al. 2015	22,545	Sweden	Majority of posttransplant melanomas diagnosed in RTRs (84%)	
Age of recipient[33,79,81]	Garrett et al. 2017	10,649	U.S.	Increased HR in those $\geq$ 50 years ($P = .03$)	Increased risk of melanoma with increasing age
	Ascha et al. 2017	105,174	U.S.	Older age associated with development of melanoma (mean, 60.5 years vs. 49.7 years in those who did not develop melanoma, $P<.001$)	
	Krynitz et al. 2015	22,545	Sweden	Higher proportion of posttransplant melanoma diagnosed in 60–69-year-old range	
Age of organ donor[79]	Ascha et al. 2017	105,174	U.S.	Older age among donors associated with risk of developing melanoma (42.6 vs. 39.2 years, $P<.001$)	One study looked at risk of melanoma based on donor age and found increased risk with older age

Race[33,79]	Garrett et al. 2017 Ascha et al. 2017	10,649 105,174	U.S. U.S.	Increased HR in those of white race (7.21) White race is more common among RTRs with melanoma (96.1% vs. 66.5% among those with no melanoma, *P*<.001)	Increased risk of posttransplant melanoma in OTRs with white race
Time since transplantation[80]	Robbins et al. 2015	139,991	U.S.	Risk of regional and distant stage melanoma peaked (up to 6-fold for regional melanoma) within 4 years posttransplantation and steadily declined thereafter; risk of *in situ* and localized melanoma stayed elevated (1.5- to 2-fold) which probably reflected the occurrence of *de novo* tumors	Incidence of localized melanoma not affected by time since transplantation. Regional and distant melanoma increased in 4 years posttransplant.
Prior skin cancer[33]	Garrett et al. 2017	10,649	U.S.	Increased HR with pretransplant skin cancer (7.15)	Patients who had pretransplant skin cancer had increased risk of developing posttransplant melanoma
HLA type[79]	Ascha et al. 2017	105,174	U.S.	Less than 4 HLA mismatches associated with increased posttransplant melanoma (44.9 vs. 37.1%, *P* = .001)	Less than 4 HLA mismatches found to be associated with increased posttransplant melanoma in one study
Medication use[79,80]	Ascha et al. 2017 Robbins et al. 2015	105,174 139,991	U.S. U.S.	Sirolimus (HR 1.54) and cyclosporine (HR 1.93) associated with worse survival and are risk factors for developing melanoma Azathioprine associated with increased IRR of posttransplant localized melanoma (1.35) Regional/distant melanoma associated with polyclonal antibody induction therapy (IRR = 1.65)	Sirolimus, cyclosporine, azathioprine, and polyclonal antibody induction have all been associated with increased posttransplant melanoma risk

Abbreviations: HLA, human leukocyte antigen; HR, hazard ratio; IRR, incidence rate ratio; n, number; NA, not applicable; OTRs, organ transplant recipients; RTRs, renal transplant recipients; U.S., United States.

Temporal Trends in Incidence

A population-based U.S. study of OTRs followed up for 27 years (1987–2014) found a significant decline in the incidence of KS, which could reflect optimized dosing of immunosuppressive drugs.[92] A decreasing trend in KS incidence was evident, especially for the nonusers of mTORi, mostly within the first 3-years posttransplant.[93]

A Korean cohort study of 2020 also showed that the relative SIR for KS was lower in 2009–2018 compared with that in 1990–2008.[53]

Risk Factors

Several studies have been conducted examining risk factors associated with posttransplant KS. These included HHV-8 prevalence in the region,[89] male sex,[92,94] organ transplanted (lung and kidney),[92,94] older age at transplantation,[92] time since transplantation (within 1 year is associated with highest risk),[92] and history of prior skin cancer.[92] Detailed information on these risk factors is included in Table 1.4.

Systemic Involvement and Mortality

A multicenter European cohort study of 145 OTRs with KS diagnosed between 1985 and 2011 disclosed that 51% of patients had visceral KS, and those treated with chemotherapy or switched to an mTORi, interestingly, were more likely to have visceral KS.[94] Overall survival was 82% at 5 years and 64% at 10 years and was not related to extent of disease at the time of diagnosis.[94]

SUMMARY OF KEY POINTS

- Lifelong immunosuppression is usually required in OTRs to prevent organ rejection. As a result, development of various posttransplant infections and several malignancies, especially skin cancers, is a serious problem in these patients as they cause both high morbidity and mortality.
- Dermatologists should play an active role in the treatment of solid OTRs in order to provide optimal care for skin-related comorbidities. Besides providing early and best treatment modalities, prevention of the posttransplant skin cancers is also of utmost importance.
- Communication and networking with other dermatologists, transplant surgeons, and pathologists through international networks, i.e., SCOPE and ITSCC, or national groups, and establishment of specialist dermatology clinics are helpful in dealing with the skin cancers and other cutaneous issues in OTRs.
- Several recent population-based studies show a significant reduction in the incidence of skin cancers, especially SCC, BCC, and KS following solid organ transplantation over time especially in the last two decades, which is probably related to less aggressive and more individualized immunosuppressive treatment, more frequent dermatologic follow-up, and effective sun protection habits.
- Despite these promising observations, the risk of various posttransplant skin cancers is still higher in OTRs than that in the general population. Thus, skin cancer still remains an important problem in OTRs.
- As the life span of OTRs increases with recent advances, primary and secondary preventive measures will continue to be of utmost importance in this high-risk population.

TABLE 1.4 Risk Factors Identified for Posttransplant Kaposi's Sarcoma

RISK FACTORS	*PUBLICATION*	*STUDY POPULATION (N)*	*COUNTRY*	*RESULTS*	*SUMMARY*
Sex[92,94]	Cahoon et al. 2018	264,624	U.S.	163 OTRs had KS. IR is higher in males than in females (15.3 vs. 8.0), IRR (1.87)	Posttransplant KS appears to be more common in males
	Delyon et al. 2019	145	European	The majority of transplant recipients with KS were males (76%)	
Organ transplanted[92,94]	Cahoon et al. 2018	264,624	U.S.	Increased IRR (2.22) of posttransplant KS in lung transplant recipients	One study showed lung transplant has the most increased risk, while the other found highest prevalence in kidney recipients
	Delyon et al. 2019	145	European	The majority of posttransplant KS patients had received kidney transplants (89%)	
Age at transplantation[92]	Cahoon et al. 2018	264,624	U.S.	Increase in posttransplant KS in patients of older age at time of transplantation (IRR 6.24 for patients 65+ at transplantation)	There is an increased risk of posttransplant KS in patients who are older when they receive the transplant
Time since transplantation[92]	Cahoon et al. 2018	264,624	U.S.	Highest rate of posttransplant KS was at <1 year post transplant	The highest KS incidence was within 1 year of transplantation highlighting the effect of intense immunosuppression in first months
Race[92]	Cahoon et al. 2018	264,624	U.S.	Increased incidence rate in non-white race (19.7 vs. 8.6 per 10^5 person-years) and increased IRR in non-white (2.67)	There is an increased rate of posttransplant KS in non-white patients
Citizenship[92]	Cahoon et al. 2018	264,624	U.S.	Increased incidence rate in non-U.S. citizens (30.1 vs. 11.7 per 10^5 person-years) and increased IRR (2.10)	There is an increased rate of posttransplant KS in non-U.S. citizens

(*Continued*)

TABLE 1.4 Risk Factors Identified for Posttransplant Kaposi's Sarcoma (Continued)

RISK FACTORS	*PUBLICATION*	*STUDY POPULATION (N)*	*COUNTRY*	*RESULTS*	*SUMMARY*
HHV-8[89]	Lebbé et al. 2008	NA	NA	Prevalence of posttransplant KS is highest in countries with high HHV-8 prevalence (e.g., Italy)	Posttransplant KS is most common in countries with high HHV-8 prevalence
Non-KS skin cancer[92]	Cahoon et al. 2018	264,624	U.S.	Posttransplant KS associated with diagnosis of SCC (OR = 4.83). No significant relationship with melanoma or BCC	OTRs with SCC may also be at higher risk of KS
Medication use[92–94]	Cahoon et al. 2018	264,624	U.S.	Immunosuppressive medications or induction therapy did not affect the risk of KS mTORi did not reduce risk of KS	Controversial evidence on risk of posttransplant KS with immunosuppressives used
	Piselli et al. 2019	11,624	Italy	mTORi users had a significantly decreased KS risk initially, but no differences observed after 3 years of posttransplantation	It is possible that mTORi use might reduce KS incidence due to reduction of total burden of immunosuppression rather than due to its antitumor effect
	Delyon et al. 2019	145	European	81% of patients with posttransplant KS had a history of induction therapy Patients switched to mTORi were more likely to have visceral KS	

Abbreviations: BCC, basal cell carcinoma; HHV-8, human herpesvirus-8; IRR, incidence rate ratio; KS, Kaposi's sarcoma; mTORi, mammalian target of rapamycin inhibitor; n, number; NA, not applicable; OR, odds ratio; OTRs, organ transplant recipients; SCC squamous cell carcinoma; U.S., United States.

REFERENCES

1. Murray JE, Merrill JP, Harrison JH. Renal homotransplantation in identical twins. Surg Forum. 1955;6:432–6.
2. Randle HW. The historical link between solid-organ transplantation, immunosuppression, and skin cancer. Dermatol Surg. 2004;30:595–7.
3. Eedy DJ. Summary of inaugural meeting of the skin care in organ recipients group, UK, held at the royal society of medicine, 7 October 2004. Br J Dermatol. 2005;153:6–10.
4. Morrissey PE, Madras PN, Monaco AP. History of solid organ transplant. In: Kuo PC, Shcroeder RA, Johnson LB, editors. Clinical management of the transplant patient. London: Arnold; 2001. p. 1–26.
5. Linden PK. History of solid organ transplantation and organ donation. Crit Care Clin. 2009;25:165–84.
6. Global Observatory on Donation and Transplantation. 2016. Available from: www.transplant-observatory.org/data-charts-and-tables/.
7. Starzl TE, Koep LJ, Halgrimson CG, Hood J, Schroter GP, Porter KA et al. Fifteen years of clinical liver transplantation. Gastroenterol. 1979;77:375–88.
8. Rana A, Godfrey EL. Outcomes in solid-organ transplantation: success and stagnation. Tex Heart Inst J. 2019;46:75–6.
9. Bouwes Bavinck JN, Hardie DR, Green A, Cutmore S, MacNaught A, O'Sullivan B et al. The risk of skin cancer in renal transplant recipients in Queensland, Australia: a follow-up study. Transplant. 1996;61:715–21.
10. Acuna SA, Fernandes KA, Daly C, Hicks LK, Sutradhar R, Kim SJ et al. Cancer mortality among recipients of solid-organ transplantation in Ontario, Canada. JAMA Oncol. 2016;2:463–9.
11. Penn I, Hammond W, Brettschneider L, Starzl TE. Malignant lymphomas in transplantation patients. Transplant Proc. 1969;1:106–12.
12. Schneck SA, Penn I. De-novo brain tumours in renal-transplant recipients. Lancet. 1971;297:983–4.
13. Walder BK, Robertson MR, Jeremy D. Skin cancer and immunosuppression. Lancet. 1971;2:1282–3.
14. Jensen P, Hansen S, Moller B et al. Skin cancer in kidney and heart transplant recipients and different long-term immunosuppressive therapy regimens. J Am Acad Dermatol. 1999;40:177–86.
15. Hartevelt MM, Bavinck JN, Kootte AM et al. Incidence of skin cancer after renal transplantation in the Netherlands. Transplant. 1990;49:506–9.
16. Penn I. Malignant melanoma in organ allograft recipients. Transplant. 1996;61:274–8.
17. Ong CS, Keogh AM, Kossard S, Macdonald PS, Spratt PM. Skin cancer in Australian heart transplant recipients. J Am Acad Dermatol. 1999;40:27–34.
18. Penn I, First MR. Merkel's cell carcinoma in organ recipients: report of 41 cases. Transplantation. 1999;68:1717–21.
19. Genders RE, Weijns ME, Dekkers OM, Plasmeijer EI. Metastasis of cutaneous squamous cell carcinoma in organ transplant recipients and the immunocompetent population: is there a difference? A systematic review and meta-analysis. J Eur Acad Dermatol Venereol. 2019;33:828–41.
20. Euvrard S, Kanitakis J, Decullier E et al. Subsequent skin cancers in kidney and heart transplant recipients after the first squamous cell carcinoma. Transplant. 2006;81:1093–100.
21. Wisgerhof HC, Edelbroek JR, de Fijter JW et al. Subsequent squamous- and basal-cell carcinomas in kidney-transplant recipients after the first skin cancer: cumulative incidence and risk factors. Transplant. 2010;89:1231–8.
22. Hoxtell EO, Mandel JS, Murray SS et al. Incidence of skin carcinoma after renal transplantation. Arch Dermatol. 1977;113:436–8.
23. Abel EA. Cutaneous manifestations of immunosuppression in organ transplant recipients. J Am Acad Dermatol. 1989;21(2 Pt 1):167–79.
24. Euvrard S, Kanitakis J, Claudy A. Skin diseases after organ transplantation. 1st ed. Paris: John Libbey Eurotext; 1998.
25. Berg D, Otley CC. Skin cancer in organ transplant recipients: epidemiology, pathogenesis, and management. J Am Acad Dermatol. 2002;47:1–17.
26. Otley CC, Stasko T, Griffin MD, Murphy GM, Hirose R, Chong AH, editors. Skin disease in organ transplantation. 1st ed. New York, NY: Cambridge University Press; 2008.
27. Stockfeth E, Ulrich C, Euvrard S, Proby C, Bouwes Bavinck JN, Geissler EK, editors. Skin cancer after organ transplantation. 1st ed. New York, NY: Springer; 2009.
28. Zwald F, Brown MD, editors. Advances in transplant dermatology: clinical and practical implications. 1st ed. New York, NY: Springer; 2015.

29. Colegio OR, editor. Skin diseases in the immunosuppressed. 1st ed. Cham, Switzerland: Springer International Publishing; 2018.
30. Christenson LJ, Geusau A, Ferrandiz C et al. Specialty clinics for the dermatologic care of solid-organ transplant recipients. Dermatol Surg. 2004;30:598–603.
31. Euvrard S, Kanitakis J, Claudy A. Skin cancers after organ transplantation. N Engl J Med. 2003;348:1681–91.
32. Menzies S, O'Leary E, Callaghan G et al. Declining incidence of keratinocyte carcinoma in organ transplant recipients. Br J Dermatol. 2019;181:983–91.
33. Garrett GL, Blanc PD, Boscardin J et al. Incidence of and risk factors for skin cancer in organ transplant recipients in the United States. JAMA Dermatol. 2017;153:296–303.
34. Engels EA, Pfeiffer RM, Fraumeni JF. et al. Spectrum of cancer risk among US solid organ transplant recipients. JAMA Dermatol. 2011;306:1891–901.
35. Piselli P, Serraino D, Segoloni GP et al. Risk of de novo cancers after transplantation: results from a cohort of 7217 kidney transplant recipients, Italy 1997–2009. Eur J Cancer. 2013;49:336–44.
36. Krynitz B, Edgren G, Lindelöf B et al. Risk of skin cancer and other malignancies in kidney, liver, heart and lung transplant recipients 1970 to 2008-a Swedish population-based study. Int J Cancer. 2013;132:1429–38.
37. Laprise C, Cahoon EK, Lynch CF et al. Risk of lip cancer after solid organ transplantation in the United States. Am J Transplant. 2019;19:227–37.
38. Rizvi SMH, Aagnes B, Holdaas H et al. Long-term change in the risk of skin cancer after organ transplantation. A population-based nationwide cohort study. JAMA Dermatol. 2017;153:1270–7.
39. Wisgerhof HC, Wolterbeek R, de Fijter JW et al. Kidney transplant recipients with cutaneous squamous cell carcinoma have an increased risk of internal malignancy. J Invest Dermatol. 2012;132:2176–83.
40. Nordin A, Åberg F, Pukkala E et al. Decreasing incidence of cancer after liver transplantation: a Nordic population-based study over 3 decades. Am J Transplant. 2018;18:952–63.
41. Fattouh K, Ducroux E, Decullier E et al. Increasing incidence of melanoma after solid organ transplantation: a retrospective epidemiological study. Transplant Int. 2017;30:1172–80.
42. Harwood CA, Mesher D, McGregor JM et al. A surveillance model for skin cancer in organ transplant recipients: a 22-year prospective study in an ethnically diverse population. Am J Transplant. 2013;13:119–29.
43. Robsahm TE, Helsing P, Veierød MB. Cutaneous squamous cell carcinoma in Norway 1963–2011: increasing incidence and stable mortality. Cancer Med. 2015;4:472–80.
44. Lindelöf B, Sigurgeirsson B, Gäbel H, Stern RS. Incidence of skin cancer in 5356 patients following organ transplantation. Br J Dermatol. 2000;143:513–19.
45. Adami J, Gäbel H, Lindelöf B et al. Cancer risk following organ transplantation: a nationwide cohort study in Sweden. Br J Cancer. 2003;89:1221–7.
46. Moloney FJ, Comber H, O'Lorcain P et al. A population-based study of skin cancer incidence and prevalence in renal transplant recipients. Br J Dermatol. 2006;154:498–504.
47. Jensen AO, Svaerke C, Farkas D et al. Skin cancer risk among solid organ recipients: a nationwide cohort study in Denmark. Acta Derm Venereol. 2010;90:474–9.
48. Wisgerhof HC, van der Geest LG, de Fijter JW et al. Incidence of cancer in kidney-transplant recipients: a long-term cohort study in a single center. Cancer Epidemiol. 2011;35:105–11.
49. Hortlund M, Arroyo Mühr LS, Storm H et al. Cancer risks after solid organ transplantation and after long-term dialysis. Int J Cancer. 2017;140:1091–101.
50. Park CK, Fung K, Austin PC et al. Incidence and risk factors of keratinocyte carcinoma after first solid organ transplant in Ontario, Canada. JAMA Dermatol. 2019;155:1041–8.
51. Park GH, Chang SE, Won CH et al. Incidence of primary skin cancer after organ transplantation: an 18-year single-center experience in Korea. J Am Acad Dermatol. 2014;70:465–72.
52. Ishikawa N, Tanabe K, Tokumoto T et al. Clinical study of malignancies after renal transplantation and impact of routine screening for early detection: a single-center experience. Transplant Proc. 2000;32:1907–10.
53. Kim YJ, Jung CJ, Park GH et al. Twenty-eight-year incidence and characteristics of post-transplant skin cancers: comparative analysis of past and recent 10-year experience. J Dermatol. 2020;47:1131–40.
54. Madeleine MM, Patel NS, Plasmeijer EI et al. Epidemiology of keratinocyte carcinomas after organ transplantation. Br J Dermatol. 2017;177:1208–16.
55. Kuschal C, Thoms KM, Schubert S et al. Skin cancer in organ transplant recipients: effects of immunosuppressive medications on DNA repair. Exp Dermatol. 2012;21:2–6.
56. Åberg F, Isoniemi H, Pukkala E et al. Cancer after liver transplantation in children and young adults: a population-based study from 4 Nordic countries. Liver Transpl. 2018;24:1252–9.
57. Foo SH, Nightingale PG, Gazzani P et al. A 10-year longitudinal follow-up study of a U.K. paediatric transplant population to assess for skin cancer. Br J Dermatol. 2018;179:1368–75.

58. Bernat García J, Morales Suárez-Varela M, Vilata JJ et al. Risk factors for non-melanoma skin cancer in kidney transplant patients in a Spanish population in the Mediterranean region. Acta Derm Venereol. 2013;93:422–7.
59. Jiyad Z, Olsen CM, Burke MT et al. Azathioprine and risk of skin cancer in organ transplant recipients: systematic review and meta-analysis. Am J Transplant. 2016;16:3490–503.
60. Coghill AE, Johnson LG, Berg D et al. Immunosuppressive medications and squamous cell skin carcinoma: nested case-control study within the skin cancer after organ transplant (SCOT) cohort. Am J Transplant. 2016;16:565–73.
61. Jensen P, Hansen S, Møller B et al. Are renal transplant recipients on CsA-based immunosuppressive regimens more likely to develop skin cancer than those on azathioprine and prednisolone? Transpl Proc. 1999;31:1120.
62. Howard MD, Su JC, Chong AH. Skin cancer following solid organ transplantation: a review of risk factors and models of care. Am J Clin Dermatol. 2018;19:585–97.
63. Plasmeijer EI, Sachse MM, Gebhardt C et al. Cutaneous squamous cell carcinoma (cSCC) and immunosurveillance: the impact of immunosuppression on frequency of cSCC. J Eur Acad Dermatol Venereol. 2019;33(Suppl 8):33–7.
64. Euvrard S, Morelon E, Rostaing L et al. Sirolimus and secondary skin-cancer prevention in kidney transplantation. N Engl J Med. 2012;367:329–39.
65. Lim WH, Eris J, Kanellis J et al. A systematic review of conversion from calcineurin inhibitor to mammalian target of rapamycin inhibitors for maintenance immunosuppression in kidney transplant recipients. Am J Transpl. 2014;14:2106–19.
66. Murray SL, Daly FE, O'Kelly P et al. The impact of switching to mTOR inhibitor-based immunosuppression on long-term non-melanoma skin cancer incidence and renal function in kidney and liver transplant recipients. Ren Fail. 2020;42:607–12.
67. Asgari MM, Arron ST, Warton EM et al. Sirolimus use and risk of cutaneous squamous cell carcinoma (SCC) in solid organ transplant recipients (SOTRs). J Am Acad Dermatol. 2015;73:444–50.
68. Tang H, Shi W, Song Y, Han J. Voriconazole exposure and risk of cutaneous squamous cell carcinoma among lung or hematopoietic cell transplant patients: a systematic review and meta-analysis. J Am Acad Dermatol. 2019;80:500–7.
69. D'Arcy ME, Pfeiffer RM, Rivera DR et al. Voriconazole and the risk of keratinocyte carcinomas among lung transplant recipients in the United States. JAMA Dermatol. 2020;156:1–9.
70. Genders RE, Weijns ME, Dekkers OM, Plasmeijer EI. Metastasis of cutaneous squamous cell carcinoma in organ transplant recipients and the immunocompetent population: is there a difference? a systematic review and meta-analysis. J Eur Acad Dermatol Venereol. 2019;33:828–41.
71. Lanz J, Bouwes Bavinck JN, Westhuis M et al. Aggressive squamous cell carcinoma in organ transplant recipients. JAMA Dermatol. 2019;155:66–71.
72. Garrett GL, Lowenstein SE, Singer JP et al. Trends of skin cancer mortality after transplantation in the United States: 1987 to 2013. J Am Acad Dermatol. 2016;75:106–12.
73. Hardie IR, Strong RW, Hartley LC et al. Skin cancer in Caucasian renal allograft recipients living in a subtropical climate. Surgery. 1980;87:177–83.
74. Cohen EB, Komorowski RA, Clowry LJ. Cutaneous complications in renal transplant recipients. Am J Clin Pathol. 1987;88:32–7.
75. Krynitz B, Olsson H, Lundh Rozell B et al. Risk of basal cell carcinoma in Swedish organ transplant recipients: a population-based study. Br J Dermatol. 2016;174:95–103.
76. Mougel F, Kanitakis J, Faure M, Euvrard S. Basosquamous cell carcinoma in organ transplant patients: a clinicopathologic study. J Am Acad Dermatol. 2012;66:e151–e157.
77. Green AC, Olsen CM. Increased risk of melanoma in organ transplant recipients: systematic review and meta-analysis of cohort studies. Acta Derm Venereol. 2015;95:923–7.
78. Park CK, Dahlke EJ, Fung K et al. Melanoma incidence, stage, and survival after solid organ transplant: a population-based cohort study in Ontario, Canada. J Am Acad Dermatol. 2020;83:754–61.
79. Ascha M, Ascha MS, Tanenbaum J, Bordeaux JS. Risk factors for melanoma in renal transplant recipients. JAMA Dermatol. 2017;153:1130–6.
80. Robbins HA, Clarke CA, Arron ST et al. Melanoma risk and survival among organ transplant recipients. J Invest Dermatol. 2015;135:2657–65.
81. Krynitz B, Rozell BL, Lyth J et al. Cutaneous malignant melanoma in the Swedish organ transplantation cohort: a study of clinicopathological characteristics and mortality. J Am Acad Dermatol. 2015;73:106–13.
82. Farrugia D, Mahboob S, Cheshire J et al. Malignancy-related mortality following kidney transplantation is common. Kidney Int. 2014;85:1395–403.
83. Hollenbeak CS, Todd MM, Billingsley EM et al. Increased incidence of melanoma in renal transplantation recipients. Cancer. 2005;104:1962–7.

84. Maor D, Vajdic CM, Cumming S et al. Melanoma in a cohort of organ transplant recipients: experience from a dedicated transplant dermatology clinic in Victoria, Australia. J Am Acad Dermatol. 2020;83:773–9.
85. Miao Y, Everly JJ, Gross TG et al. De novo cancers arising in organ transplant recipients are associated with adverse outcomes compared with the general population. Transplantation. 2009;87:1347–59.
86. Vajdic CM, Chong AH, Kelly PJ et al. Survival after cutaneous melanoma in kidney transplant recipients: a population-based matched cohort study. Am J Transplant. 2014;14:1368–75.
87. Matin RN, Mesher D, Proby CM et al. Melanoma in organ transplant recipients: clinicopathological features and outcome in 100 cases. Am J Transplant. 2008;8:1891–900.
88. Brewer JD, Christenson LJ, Weaver AL et al. Malignant melanoma in solid transplant recipients: collection of database cases and comparison with surveillance, epidemiology, and end results data for outcome analysis. Arch Dermatol. 2011;147:790–6.
89. Lebbé C, Legendre C, Francès C. Kaposi sarcoma in transplantation. Transplant Rev (Orlando). 2008;22:252–61.
90. Piselli P, Serraino D, Segoloni GP et al. Risk of de novo cancers after transplantation: results from a cohort of 7217 kidney transplant recipients, Italy 1997–2009. Eur J Cancer. 2013;49:336–44.
91. Taborelli M, Piselli P, Ettorre GM et al. Risk of virus and non-virus related malignancies following immunosuppression in a cohort of liver transplant recipients. Italy, 1985–2014. Int J Cancer. 2018;143:1588–94.
92. Cahoon EK, Linet MS, Clarke CA et al. Risk of Kaposi sarcoma after solid organ transplantation in the United States. Int J Cancer. 2018;143:2741–8.
93. Piselli P, Taborelli M, Cimaglia C et al. Decreased incidence of Kaposi sarcoma after kidney transplant in Italy and role of mTOR-inhibitors: 1997–2016. Int J Cancer. 2019;145:597–8.
94. Delyon J, Rabate C, Euvrard S et al. Management of Kaposi sarcoma after solid organ transplantation: a European retrospective study. J Am Acad Dermatol. 2019;81:448–55.

Immunosuppressive Therapy for Solid Organ Transplantation

2

Ethan P. Marin, Elizabeth Cohen, and Divyanshu Malhotra

ABBREVIATIONS

APC, antigen presenting cell; ATG, anti-thymocyte globulin; CNI, calcineurin inhibitor; CMV, cytomegalovirus; EBV, Epstein-Barr virus; IL-2R, interleukin 2 receptor; MHC, major histocompatibility complex; MPA, mycophenolic acid; mTOR, mammalian target of rapamycin; NFAT, nuclear factor of activated T cells; SOT, solid organ transplant; TCR, T cell receptor

INTRODUCTION

Solid organ transplantation (SOT) has become a mainstay of therapy for patients with end-stage failure of liver, heart, kidneys, lungs, and intestines. Even in the case of end-stage kidney disease, in which dialysis can provide lifesaving therapy, transplantation is the preferred treatment option. Pharmacologic suppression of the host immune system is necessary to avoid rejection, the immunological attack and destruction of the allograft. The development of a suite of medications that can effectively prevent rejection has been the seminal advance in allowing for the successful growth in SOT over the last several decades. This chapter will provide an overview of the key drugs in common usage in the current era of SOT. Sections in this chapter will: 1) review the molecular basis of T lymphocyte activation with a focus on the events targeted by drugs; 2) review the classes of immunosuppressive medication used in SOT, with a focus on their mechanisms of action and their adverse effects; and 3) review the clinical situations in which each drug may be used with a review of key clinical data. Clinical usage and supporting data vary among different transplanted organs. Herein, we have used kidney transplant as the model system as the kidney is by far the most common solid organ transplanted in the U.S.

DOI: 10.1201/9781003001461-2

MECHANISM OF T CELL ACTIVATION

The key cellular mediator of rejection in modern SOT is the T lymphocyte. T cells can attack and destroy allografts directly by a process known as cellular rejection. They may also facilitate the activation and maturation of B lymphocytes into antibody-producing plasma cells, which then elaborate donor-specific antibodies that mediate the humoral rejection of the allograft. Hyperacute rejection caused by preformed antibodies against the graft, though an issue in the past, is rarely encountered because of modern techniques for the detection of such antibodies and avoidance of performing transplants in their presence.

Immunosuppressive drugs work primarily by disrupting key pathways in the activation of T cells by antigen-presenting cells (APCs) (Figure 2.1).[1] The first signal pathway is initiated by interaction of the T cell receptor (TCR) on the T cells with the major histocompatibility complex (MHC) molecule on the surface of the APC. This interaction triggers downstream signaling mediated by calcineurin, a phosphatase that dephosphorylates NFAT (nuclear factor of activated T cells). Subsequently, dephosphorylated NFAT translocates to the nucleus, where it mediates expression of multiple activating cytokines, including interleukin 2 (IL-2). Signaling by the TCR–MHC binding requires a second set of molecular interactions, termed co-stimulation, which involves the cell-surface molecule CD28 on the T cell and CD80 and CD86 on the APC. In the absence of co-stimulatory signals, TCR–MHC signaling does not activate the T cell.[2]

IL-2 produced because of the nuclear translocation of NFAT is secreted and acts in an autocrine and a paracrine fashion to trigger signaling via IL-2 receptors (IL-2R) on T cells. IL-2R activation induces pathways involving the mammalian target of rapamycin (mTOR), which triggers cellular proliferation. Cellular proliferation requires the synthesis of nucleic acids to support the necessary DNA synthesis.

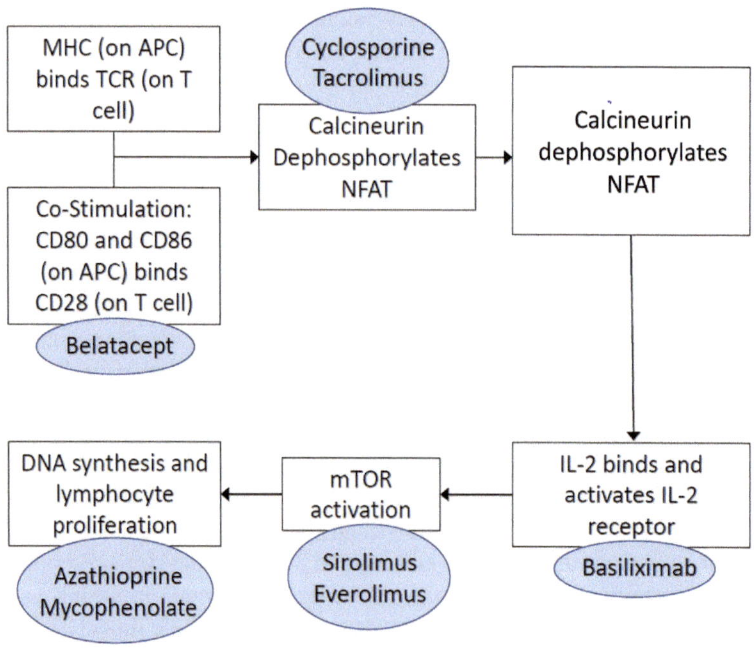

FIGURE 2.1 Overview of immunosuppressive drugs in SOT. The steps in T cell activation are shown in rectangles. The sites of action of the drugs commonly used in transplantation are shown in ovals. Drugs not shown include ATGs and alemtuzumab, which trigger lymphocyte depletion, and corticosteroids, which have multiple mechanisms of action. See text for additional details.

Different immunosuppressive agents interfere with each of the steps in T cell activation outlined prior. Additional agents work via triggered destruction of lymphocytes. Some agents used in treatment of antibody-mediated rejection target not T cells, but rather B cells and plasma cells; they are described following ("Treatment of Humoral Rejection").

PHARMACOLOGY OF DRUGS USED IN SOLID ORGAN TRANSPLANTATION

Calcineurin inhibitors (CNIs) are amongst the most commonly used agents in solid organ transplant recipients. These drugs, which include tacrolimus and cyclosporine, function by inhibiting calcineurin. Inhibition of calcineurin depends on the binding of the CNI to a receptor protein (FKBP in the case of tacrolimus and cyclophilin in the case of cyclosporine). Inhibition of calcineurin blocks the dephosphorylation and activation of the transcription factor NFAT thus preventing transcription of IL-2.

Cyclosporine, approved by the FDA in 1983, is one of the oldest drugs used in transplantation and is available in several preparations, including an unmodified version (Sandimmune) and an emulsified preparation (Neoral) that exhibits more consistent absorption.[3]

Tacrolimus, approved in 1994 by the FDA, is available in both immediate-release formulations (Prograf) as well as extended-release versions (Astagraf XL; Envarsus XR). The immediate-release versions of tacrolimus and cyclosporine are generally dosed every 12 hours, whereas extended-release tacrolimus may be dosed once daily. Both CNIs exhibit a narrow therapeutic index coupled with absorption and metabolism kinetics that lead to both intrapatient and interpatient variability depending on genetics, bowel function, and other factors. CNIs are metabolized by the cytochrome P450 system, and thus drug levels are affected by inducers and inhibitors of P450 activity. As a result, monitoring of therapeutic drug levels is necessary with CNIs. Levels are typically measured as troughs, immediately prior to the next dose. Frequent adjustment of drug doses is commonly required, especially when these drugs are first started.[4]

CNIs exhibit significant toxicities, which often correlate with drug levels. Of note, as a class, immunosuppressive agents generally entail increased risk of infectious diseases as well as of malignancies, especially those associated with viral triggers.[5] In particular, immunosuppression increases the risk of nonmelanoma skin cancer 50-fold or more.[6] Common toxicities specific to both tacrolimus and cyclosporine include neurotoxicity, which may manifest as tremor, peripheral nerve irritation, and/or cognitive impairment. CNIs also cause vasoconstriction, which can manifest as hypertension and acute kidney injury in the short term. With chronic use, renal injury characterized by striped fibrosis and vascular hyalinosis may develop. CNI nephrotoxicity is a leading cause of renal failure amongst recipients of nonrenal SOTs and may also damage kidney allografts. CNIs commonly exhibit metabolic side effects including hypertension and hyperlipidemia. Additionally, CNIs can cause electrolyte disturbances, such as hyperkalemia and hypomagnesemia. A serious but less common side effect is thrombotic microangiopathy, which can damage the allograft and often necessitates cessation of the CNI. Tacrolimus may cause hair loss, whereas cyclosporine is associated with hirsutism and gingival hyperplasia.[7]

Costimulatory signaling between CD28 on T cells and CD80 and CD86 on APCs is the target of belatacept (Nulojix). Belatacept is a soluble fusion protein between the IgG Fc domain and CTLA4; the latter domain binds CD80 and CD86 and blocks costimulatory signaling by these molecules thereby inhibiting T cell activation. Belatacept is given monthly by IV infusion and thus requires access to an infusion facility or home infusion. Belatacept does not require therapeutic drug monitoring. Adverse effects of belatacept include posttransplant lymphoproliferative disorders which are commonly caused by Epstein-Barr virus (EBV) infection; it should only be used in patients who are IgG-positive for EBV. Progressive multifocal leukoencephalopathy caused by JC virus is another viral disease associated with belatacept. Both toxicities are very rare, but potentially life threatening.[8]

Activation of IL-2 receptors can be blocked by biologic agents that bind to the receptor and prevent its activation. The agent in current usage is basiliximab (Simulect); it is a recombinant IgG targeted against the alpha chain of the IL-2 receptor (CD25). Used primarily for induction of immunosuppression (see following), it is delivered as two sequential infusions given 4 days apart, with the initial dose typically infused intraoperatively just before reperfusion of the allograft. The duration of action is 4–6 weeks, and apart from occasional infusion reactions, the side effects are generally minimal.

Signaling downstream of the activated IL-2R involves signaling via the mTOR pathway, which may be blocked by mTOR inhibitors such as sirolimus or everolimus. Both drugs successfully limit T cell proliferation. Sirolimus is typically dosed once a day, whereas everolimus is dosed every 12 hours. Both require therapeutic drug monitoring to achieve appropriate serum levels. The mTOR inhibitors are associated with significant adverse effects including hyperlipidemia (which can be severe), edema, oral ulcers, proteinuria, impaired wound healing, and a potentially severe pulmonary toxicity.

Proliferation of T cells that occurs downstream of the mTOR pathway requires synthesis of new nucleotides to support the required DNA production. Two drugs, azathioprine (Imuran) and mycophenolic acid (MPA), are known as antimetabolites and inhibit nucleotide synthesis and thus limit T cell activation. Azathioprine is converted to the active metabolite 6-mercaptopurine and reduces purine synthesis. Azathioprine may cause bone marrow suppression and/or liver toxicity. Measurement of drug levels is not routinely required, but the levels of the azathioprine metabolites may be useful in adjusting the doses in the case of suspected toxicity. Of note, a small percentage of the population harbors genetic polymorphisms in the gene encoding thiopurine methyltransferase that lead to very slow rates of azathioprine metabolism. Genetic testing for these polymorphisms is recommended before initiating therapy,[9] so that significant toxicities may be avoided.

MPA may be given as mycophenolate mofetil (Cellcept) or as mycophenolate sodium (Myfortic). Both preparations are dosed every 12 hours and neither requires routine serum level monitoring. The most common and bothersome side effect of MPA is gastrointestinal (GI) irritation, manifesting as nausea, vomiting, dyspepsia, diarrhea, and/or colitis. MPA can also cause bone marrow suppression and teratogenic effects. Mycophenolate sodium is prepared with enteric coating and is generally used in patients with GI intolerance to mycophenolate mofetil, especially upper GI tract issues.

Corticosteroids cause immunosuppression via a variety of mechanisms. They act by binding and activating intracellular steroid receptors, which inhibit expression of activating cytokines. In addition, they can downregulate the expression of activating molecules on the surface of T lymphocytes. Commonly used corticosteroids include oral prednisone and IV methylprednisolone. Therapeutic drug level monitoring is not required. Adverse effects associated with long-term steroid use in SOT include glucose intolerance, dyslipidemia, impaired wound healing, osteoporosis, skin atrophy, and many others.

Several biologic drugs are used in SOT and work not by inhibiting T cell activation but rather by triggering destruction of lymphocytes directly. These agents, which are lymphodepleting, cause long-lasting immunosuppression as recovery of lymphocyte counts typically takes months. Amongst these agents is rabbit anti-thymocyte globulin (ATG; thymoglobulin), which is a polyclonal antibody preparation derived from immunizing rabbits with human thymocytes. (A similar drug prepared in horses is also available but used less commonly in SOT). The preparation includes antibodies that target an array of T cell antigens. ATG is typically dosed at 3.0–7.5 mg/kg, delivered in divided doses of 1.5 mg/kg on consecutive days. ATG may trigger an infusion reaction characterized by cytokine release and associated fever, hypotension, headache, and urticaria. It can also cause leukopenia and thrombocytopenia. Alemtuzumab (Campath) is a humanized rat antibody against CD52, which is found on T lymphocytes as well as on natural killer cells, B lymphocytes, monocytes, and other immune cells. It is approved by the FDA for the treatment of multiple sclerosis but is commonly used in SOT. It leads to widespread destruction of components of the cellular immune system. It is typically delivered as a single subcutaneous injection of 30 mg. Alemtuzumab may cause bone marrow suppression characterized by leukopenia, which may persist for months.

CLINICAL USAGE OF IMMUNOSUPPRESSION DRUGS IN SOT

The treatment of the SOT recipient generally involves several phases characterized by different immunosuppressive drugs (Figure 2.2). At the time of allograft implantation, patients are commonly treated with aggressive immunosuppression known as induction therapy. The goal of induction therapy is to mitigate the initial allorecognition that occurs at the time of organ reperfusion, reduce the rate of early rejection, and extend the life of the graft. Maintenance therapy refers to the drug or drug combinations used chronically to maintain sufficient immunosuppression to avoid rejection. Maintenance therapy is initiated shortly after implantation of the allograft and is continued for the life of the graft. Finally, rejection therapies are to reverse rejection.

Drugs Used in Induction Therapy

Induction therapy refers to aggressive immunosuppression given at the time of allograft implantation (Table 2.1). Its use varies by the type of organ transplanted and by physician preference according to the perceived immunological risk of the recipient. In the U.S., nearly 90% of kidney transplants are performed with induction therapy because of evidence showing reduced rates of rejection as compared with those with no induction.[10] Clinical practice guidelines for kidney transplant strongly endorse the use of induction therapy based on multiple studies.[11] Induction generally involves high-dose methylprednisolone pulse, typically given as 500 mg IV daily for 3 days. In addition, induction therapy includes lymphocyte-depleting or nondepleting biological therapies.

Nondepleting therapy is given to patients at low or moderate immunological risk, and generally involves basiliximab, which functions by blocking IL-2 receptor (see prior). Basiliximab was approved by the FDA in 1998 based on four key studies that compared it with placebo.[12–15] The majority of the studies showed statistically significant reductions in a composite end point of death, graft loss, or acute rejection in the first year after transplant. A subsequent review from the Cochrane Library group published in 2010 examined 32 studies involving 5854 patients.[16] This meta-analysis showed that compared with placebo, basiliximab induction therapy was associated with ~25% reduction in graft loss at 6 and 12 months. Biopsy proven rejection was also reduced by ~28% at 12 months.

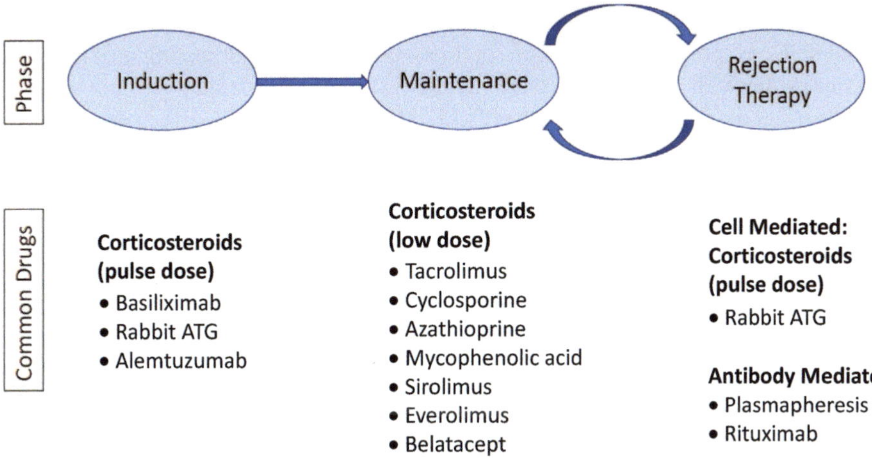

FIGURE 2.2 Phases of immunosuppression in SOT.

TABLE 2.1 Induction Agents Commonly Used in Transplantation

AGENT	CLASS	MECHANISM	ADVERSE EFFECTS
Basiliximab	Lymphocyte non-depleting	Blocks IL-2 receptor	Minimal
Rabbit anti-thymocyte globulin	Lymphocyte depleting	Polyclonal rabbit antisera; destroys T lymphocytes by targeting multiple antigens	Infections, bone marrow suppression, infusion reactions
Alemtuzumab	Lymphocyte depleting	Humanized rat monoclonal antibody; destroys T lymphocytes and other immune cells by targeting CD-52	Infections, bone marrow suppression

For patients at moderate to high immunologic risk, lymphocyte-depleting agents are generally used, such as rabbit ATG (thymoglobulin) or alemtuzumab (Campath). These agents are more aggressive and lead to more profound and longer-lived immunosuppression because of destruction of lymphocytes. Rabbit ATG was approved by the FDA based on two studies comparing it with IL2 receptor antagonists in high-risk patients.[17,18] Rabbit ATG-treated patients displayed lower rates of rejection in the first year, although no significant improvement in graft and patient survival at 12 months.

A subsequent Cochrane Library meta-analysis compared ATGs with placebo/no induction and to IL2RA in multiple studies.[19] The bulk of the data showed that ATGs (different preparations) reduced rejections compared with placebo or IL2RA, but did not clearly affect graft or patient survival. Of note, ATG use was associated with higher rates of hematologic and infectious complications.

Alemtuzumab (Campath) is a humanized rat anti-CD52 IgG that causes destruction of a variety of immune cell lineages. It has not been approved for use in transplantation by the FDA but is nonetheless commonly employed off-label as induction therapy. A meta-analysis of studies comparing alemtuzumab with ATGs showed similar results with regard to graft survival and rejection.[19]

Drugs Used in Maintenance Immunosuppression

Maintenance immunosuppression (Table 2.2) is usually started immediately after an organ transplant and is continued throughout the life of a graft unless there are specific reasons that dictate either reduction or discontinuation. Conventional maintenance regimens consist of a combination of immunosuppressive agents that differ by mechanisms of action and side effect profiles. This strategy minimizes the morbidity and mortality associated with each class of agent while maximizing overall effectiveness. Such regimens may vary by patient, transplant center, and geographic area. The most commonly used regimens in the U.S. are usually a combination of a CNI, antimetabolite, and prednisone. An mTOR inhibitor and belatacept may be used under certain conditions. There is no one clear optimal regimen for every patient, and the choice is based on a variety of factors including tolerability, side effect profile, immunologic risk, infectious risk, cost, and other considerations.

Calcineurin Inhibitors

CNIs are considered the backbone of maintenance immunosuppression regimens and are used by >90% of kidney recipients in the U.S.[20,21] Cyclosporine and tacrolimus are the two drugs in this class with the former being approved more than a decade earlier and being touted as a game changer in the world of transplantation. A large meta-analysis of 30 trials (4102 patients) comparing these two agents favored tacrolimus for multiple end points.[22] Graft loss and acute rejection rates were reduced (by 44% and 31%, respectively) thus resulting in a lower serum creatinine level in the groups treated with tacrolimus. In contrast, several adverse effects were found to be more pronounced with tacrolimus including tremor,

TABLE 2.2 Drugs Commonly Used in Maintenance Immunosuppression

DRUG	*CLASS MECHANISM*	*USAGE*	*ADVERSE EFFECTS*	*SPECIAL NOTES*
Tacrolimus	CNI	Used in most combination regimens for maintenance immunosuppression	Neurotoxicity that includes tremor and memory loss, nephrotoxicity, increased incidence of DM	Part of >90% regimens in the US. Also available as a long-acting formulation now
Cyclosporine	CNI	Limited use in maintenance immunosuppression	Hirsutism, gingival enlargement, nephrotoxicity	Was approved more than a decade before tacrolimus but is now primarily used in patients who are intolerant to tacrolimus
Mycophenolic acid	Antimetabolite	In combination with tacrolimus, makes up more >90% of maintenance immunosuppression regimens	GI side effects including nausea, vomiting, and diarrhea; bone marrow suppression	Contraindicated in pregnancy
Azathioprine	Antimetabolite	Used in combination with CNI in rare conditions	Bone marrow suppression, hepatotoxicity	Useful in pregnancy and in case of intolerable side effects to MPA. Genetic polymorphisms exist that alter metabolism
Prednisone	Corticosteroid	Used in about 70% of maintenance immunosuppression regimens	Metabolic side effects, osteoporosis, weight gain	Can be used as part of induction, maintenance, and rejection treatment regimens
Sirolimus	mTOR inhibitor	Used rarely either in combination with CNI or other agents	Hyperlipidemia, lymphedema, bone marrow suppression, lung injury, oral ulcers, proteinuria, impaired wound healing	Useful in special circumstances like skin cancer and certain viral infections like BK and CMV
Everolimus	mTOR inhibitor	Used rarely either in combinations with CNI or other agents	Hyperlipidemia, lymphedema, bone marrow suppression, lung injury, oral ulcers, impaired wound healing	Useful in special circumstances like skin cancer and certain viral infections like BK and CMV. Newer agent compared with sirolimus and its use is increasing slowly
Belatacept	CTLA-4 Ig fusion; works as co-stimulation blockade to selectively halt T-cell activation	Used as part of maintenance immunosuppression in patients who cannot tolerate CNI; de novo use is rare	Infusion reactions, bone marrow suppression, diarrhea	Black box warning in EBV-seronegative patients because of increased risk of PTLD. Use is increasing because of much less nephrotoxicity. Cost remains a major issue

Abbreviations: BK, BK polyoma virus; CMV, cytomegalovirus; CTLA-4, cytotoxic T-lymphocyte-associated protein 4; CNI, calcineurin inhibitor; DM, diabetes mellitus; EBV, Epstein-Barr virus; GI, gastrointestinal; MPA, mycophenolic acid; mTOR, mammalian target of rapamycin; PTLD, posttransplant lymphoproliferative disorder.

headache, GI disturbances, and hypomagnesemia. The rate of new-onset diabetes (DM) was higher with tacrolimus and sustained over a 3-year follow-up period. Cyclosporine use was associated with more constipation and cosmetic side effects including hirsutism, hypertrichosis, and gingival enlargement. No difference in infection or malignancy was noted between tacrolimus and cyclosporine. Similar findings have also been found in the liver transplant literature.[23] Given these findings, tacrolimus has largely replaced cyclosporine as the drug of choice for long-term immunosuppression regimens.

Antimetabolites

Antimetabolites are a usual part of combined maintenance immunosuppression regimens in transplant centers across the country. The most frequently used antimetabolites are MPA or azathioprine. MPA was approved by the FDA for the prevention of rejection in kidney transplants in 1995. This was based on the results of three randomized controlled trials (RCTs), in which a total of 1493 patients in North America, Europe, and Australia, were enrolled.[24] In all three studies, MPA showed superior ability to prevent acute rejection within the first 6 months after transplantation. A meta-analysis of 23 studies that included a total of 3301 patients was recently published.[24] The studies all used CNIs, with variation in the induction agents. The aggregate analyses showed that MPA was superior to azathioprine with regard to graft loss (relative risk [RR] 0.82), death-censored graft loss (RR 0.78), and acute rejection (RR 0.65). There was no statistically significant difference in mortality or kidney function between treatments. Tissue-invasive cytomegalovirus (CMV) disease and GI symptoms were higher with MPA. Based on these findings, MPA has largely replaced azathioprine as a first-line antimetabolite agent in primary immunosuppression. As of 2016, >95% of patients used MPA as compared with <5% using azathioprine.[10] Azathioprine is used commonly in patients who have intolerable adverse effects with MPA or those who want to become pregnant, as MPA is teratogenic.

Steroids

Steroids are the grand old drugs in transplantation and remain a fundamental part of most maintenance immunosuppression regimens. They are usually tapered to very low doses (e.g., 5–10 mg of prednisone daily) for this purpose. However, because of the concern regarding metabolic and other adverse effects, the focus shifted towards evaluation of various strategies to avoid or withdraw steroids without increasing the risk of rejection or graft loss. A recent meta-analysis evaluated 48 studies that included a total of 7803 patients in which two different strategies for reducing steroid use were evaluated: steroid avoidance (discontinuation within 14 days of transplantation) or withdrawal (discontinuation later).[25] Overall, acute rejection within 1 year was increased (RR 1.77; 95% confidence interval [CI] 1.2–2.6) in early steroid withdrawal; however, mortality and graft loss were not statistically different between the various comparison groups. There was no difference in the occurrence of DM, cardiovascular events, infection, CMV infection, and malignancy between groups up to 5 years after transplantation. Confidence in these data is tempered by the low to moderate quality of the studies involved, which frequently were unblinded and/or observed relatively few numbers of events. Multiple similar, but smaller, reviews in the past have also shown an increased risk of acute rejection in the steroid-free groups; however, no definitive trends in long-term mortality, graft loss, and side effects could be established.[26,27] Thus, steroid-free maintenance regimens remain controversial and are used variably at different centers. Overall, steroids are used in approximately 70% of adult kidney transplant recipients in the U.S. at 1 year following transplant.[10]

mTOR Inhibitors

mTOR inhibitors are usually not the first-line maintenance immunosuppression agents and are primarily used for certain specific indications. The two mTOR inhibitors, sirolimus and everolimus, have been evaluated in four different primary immunosuppressive algorithms; as replacement for

CNIs and for antimetabolites, in combination with a CNI at low and high dose and with a variable dose of CNI. This evaluation was summarized in a large meta-analysis encompassing 33 trials of mTOR inhibitors in different contexts involving 7114 patients.[28] In general, these agents have been found to be equivalent to comparator drugs with regard to patient and graft survival. Although they do have certain favorable outcomes like higher glomerular filtration rate (GFR) and lower rates of rejection, they are associated with significant adverse effects including higher rates of dyslipidemia, lymphedema, wound complications, and bone marrow suppression that limit their tolerability. Evidence of antiviral and anti-malignancy effects exists and thus mTORi are often used in patients with skin cancers and specific viral infections.[29–31] Overall, use of mTOR inhibitors in U.S. kidney transplant recipients is rare with only 1.9% of recipients using them at the time of transplant and 4.3% at 1 year.[10]

Belatacept

Although CNIs remain the cornerstone of immunosuppression, they are nephrotoxic and exacerbate cardiovascular and metabolic risk factors that can limit graft and patient survival.[8,32] This has led to further research for alternative agents. Belatacept is a first-in-class co-stimulation blocker that selectively blocks T-cell activation. It was approved by the FDA in 2011 for use in kidney transplant recipients to prevent rejection and prolong graft survival. This was based on two landmark randomized controlled trials that compared a couple of regimens of belatacept with cyclosporine in recipients of standard criteria or living-donor kidneys[8] or extended criteria kidneys. Both studies had comparable induction and additional maintenance immunosuppression regimens. Both reported that renal function was similar or better in patients receiving belatacept at 12 months and also at long-term follow-up for up to 7 years.[32–34] The rate and severity of acute rejection was higher in the belatacept patients who received living or standard criteria donor kidneys; however, this did not have any significant impact on patient or graft survival with long-term follow-up.[33] Unfortunately, the rate of posttransplant lymphoproliferative disorder was higher in the belatacept cohort with a clear increased risk in the EBV seronegative group, and thus there is a black box warning against the use of this drug in this population of patients. Subsequent meta-analyses of five studies that compared belatacept and CNIs (1535 patients) have reported similar rates of death, renal allograft survival, and acute rejection after the first 3 years of transplant. There is evidence of better GFR, better lipid profiles, lower blood pressure, less new-onset DM, and less chronic kidney scarring on biopsy in patients on belatacept as compared with those on CNIs.[17,35]

Studies of conversion from CNIs to belatacept have also shown similar trends.[36] Belatacept use has been limited by greater cost, delays in production, and logistical issues related to the requirement for IV infusions.

Drugs Used in the Treatment of Rejection

One of the major factors that limits the survival of the transplanted organ is immunological rejection, which can manifest as cellular rejection, mediated by T cells, or humoral rejection, mediated by B cells and antibodies against the allograft. There are several risk factors for rejection including human leukocyte antigen (HLA) mismatches, donor and recipient characteristics, and immunosuppression nonadherence.[37,38] Definitive diagnosis of transplant rejection typically requires organ dysfunction along with a tissue biopsy graded based on the Banff Criteria for each organ.[39] Treatment of rejection includes increases in maintenance therapy (see previously) in addition to targeted therapy based on the type of rejection (Table 2.3). Of note, acute rejections which occur in the first few months after transplant are generally much more amenable to successful treatment than chronic rejections which occur years after transplant.

TABLE 2.3 Drugs Used to Treat Rejection

DRUG	MECHANISM OF ACTION	TYPE OF REJECTION
Methylprednisolone	T cell apoptosis	Cellular
ATG	Lymphocyte depletion	Cellular
Rituximab	Anti-CD20, monoclonal antibody	Antibody
Eculizumab	Complement inhibitor, monoclonal antibody for C5	Antibody
Bortezomib	Reversible proteasome inhibitor	Antibody
Carfilzomib	Irreversible proteasome inhibitor	Antibody

Treatment of Cellular Rejection

Corticosteroids are the mainstay of treatment for cellular rejection. Although not fully understood, it is hypothesized that by binding to glucocorticoid receptors there is inhibition of NFκ B and DNA transcription thus leading to decreased T cell proliferation and increased T cell apoptosis.[40] This mechanism lends them well for induction of immunosuppression at the time of transplant (see previously) in addition to treatment of rejection. For rejection, steroids are typically administered as a "pulse" dose and may be tapered over a period of weeks to months depending on the severity of the rejection and the organ.

Alternatively, data demonstrate that many cases of acute cellular rejection are resistant to corticosteroids and require additional antibody therapy with rabbit ATG as discussed previously. Meta-analyses have demonstrated that antibody therapy is likely superior to corticosteroids at reversing and preventing additional episodes of acute cellular rejection and graft loss in kidney transplant.[41] This likely holds true for other organs, but the risks and benefits of therapy need to be considered including infections and malignancy.

Treatment of Humoral Rejection

There are many more options for the treatment of humoral rejection; however, data demonstrating any clear benefit of one therapy over another are limited. The mainstay of treatment is plasmapheresis and the removal of circulating antibodies. Patients typically require 5–10 sessions to remove all antibodies from the circulation.

In addition to removing antibodies, several therapies may be used that target B cells or the antibody-producing plasma cells, in order to prevent additional antibodies from forming. Rituximab is an anti-CD20 monoclonal antibody that targets B cells, leading to complement-mediated and antibody-dependent apoptosis. Data are mixed with regard to outcomes with some studies showing favorable results when used in addition to plasmapheresis.[42]

Humoral rejection resistant to plasmapheresis and rituximab may require alternative salvage therapy. An alternative pathway for humoral rejection treatment is to prevent complement-mediated cell lysis of the transplanted organ, especially when there is significant complement deposition in biopsy samples. Eculizumab is a monoclonal antibody for C5, which ultimately prevents the formation of the membrane attack complex. Results from using eculizumab in humoral rejection are mixed, but positive data are emerging when used early in treatment.[43]

The proteasome inhibitors, bortezomib and carfilzomib, induce apoptosis of plasma cells thus reducing antibodies. Bortezomib binds reversibly to the 26S proteasome whereas carfilzomib binds irreversibly to the 20S proteasome. However, there is limited data, primarily in case studies and case series, regarding their use, and it is not a standard of care.[44]

Ultimately, humoral rejection is difficult to treat; treatment depends on the time from diagnosis and specific patient characteristics that may respond to specific treatment.

CONCLUSION

Immunosuppressive drugs that prevent rejection of the allograft are indispensable to the practice of SOT. A variety of drugs have been developed over the last several decades that work by different mechanisms and thus may synergize with one another. Different drugs are used at different phases in the transplantation process. A comprehensive understanding of the mechanisms and adverse effects of these drugs allows the transplant specialist to elicit prolonged allograft function with a minimum of adverse effects.

SUMMARY OF KEY POINTS

- Immunosuppressive medications are required for successful allotransplantation of solid organs.
- The primary mechanism of immunosuppression is inhibition of T cell activation pathways.
- Multiple drug classes are used synergistically to suppress T cell function including calcineurin inhibitors, antimetabolites, corticosteroids, co-stimulation blockers, IL2-receptor blockers, and lymphocyte-depleting agents.
- Different agents are used for distinct phases of transplantation, including induction, maintenance, and treatment of rejection.
- A thorough knowledge of the mechanism of action, the efficacy, and the adverse effects of each immunosuppressive agent is critical to successful care of the transplant patient.

REFERENCES

1. Halloran PF. Immunosuppressive drugs for kidney transplantation. N Engl J Med. 2004 Dec 24;351(26):2715–29.
2. Maltzman JS, Turka LA. T-cell costimulatory blockade in organ transplantation. Cold Spring Harb Perspect Med. 2013 Dec 4;3(12):a015537. PubMed PMID:24296352; PubMed Central PMCID:PMCPMC3839597.
3. Ritschel WA. Microemulsion technology in the reformulation of cyclosporine: the reason behind the pharmacokinetic properties of neoral. Clin Transplant. 1996 Aug 1;10(4):364–73. PubMed PMID:8884110.
4. Thervet E, Loriot MA, Barbier S, Buchler M, Ficheux M, Choukroun G et al. Optimization of initial tacrolimus dose using pharmacogenetic testing. Clin Pharmacol Ther. 2010 Apr 16;87(6):721–6. PubMed PMID:20393454.
5. Geissler EK. Post-transplantation malignancies: here today, gone tomorrow? Nat Rev Clin Oncol. 2015 Oct 21;12(12):705–17. PubMed PMID:26483298.
6. Mittal A, Colegio OR. Skin cancers in organ transplant recipients. Am J Transplant. 2017 May 31;17(10):2509–30. PubMed PMID:28556451.
7. Ilyas M, Colegio OR, Kaplan B, Sharma A. Cutaneous toxicities from transplantation-related medications. Am J Transplant. 2017 Apr 30;17(11):2782–9. PubMed PMID:28452165.
8. Vincenti F, Charpentier B, Vanrenterghem Y, Rostaing L, Bresnahan B, Darji P et al. A phase III study of belatacept-based immunosuppression regimens versus cyclosporine in renal transplant recipients (BENEFIT study). Am J Transplant. 2010 Apr 27;10(3):535–46. PubMed PMID:20415897.
9. Hindorf U, Appell ML. Genotyping should be considered the primary choice for pre-treatment evaluation of thiopurine methyltransferase function. J Crohns Colitis. 2012 Mar 9;6(6):655–9. PubMed PMID:22398041.
10. Hart A, Smith JM, Skeans MA, Gustafson SK, Wilk AR, Robinson A et al. OPTN/SRTR 2016 annual data report: kidney. Am J Transplant. 2018 Jan 3;18(Suppl 1):18–113. PubMed PMID:29292608; PubMed Central PMCID:PMCPMC5772947.

11. Kidney disease: improving global outcomes transplant work G. KDIGO clinical practice guideline for the care of kidney transplant recipients. Am J Transplant. 2009 Oct 23;9(Suppl 3):S1–155. PubMed PMID:19845597.
12. Nashan B, Moore R, Amlot P, Schmidt AG, Abeywickrama K, Soulillou JP. Randomised trial of basiliximab versus placebo for control of acute cellular rejection in renal allograft recipients. CHIB 201 International Study Group. Lancet. 1997 Jul 4;350(9086):1193–8. PubMed PMID:9652559.
13. Kahan BD, Rajagopalan PR, Hall M. Reduction of the occurrence of acute cellular rejection among renal allograft recipients treated with basiliximab, a chimeric anti-interleukin-2-receptor monoclonal antibody. United States Simulect Renal Study Group. Transplant. 1999 Feb 12;67(2):276–84. PubMed PMID:10075594.
14. Ponticelli C, Yussim A, Cambi V, Legendre C, Rizzo G, Salvadori M et al. A randomized, double-blind trial of basiliximab immunoprophylaxis plus triple therapy in kidney transplant recipients. Transplant. 2001 Oct 17;72(7):1261–7. PubMed PMID:11602853.
15. Lawen JG, Davies EA, Mourad G, Oppenheimer F, Molina MG, Rostaing L et al. Randomized double-blind study of immunoprophylaxis with basiliximab, a chimeric anti-interleukin-2 receptor monoclonal antibody, in combination with mycophenolate mofetil-containing triple therapy in renal transplantation. Transplant. 2003 Jan 25;75(1):37–43. PubMed PMID:12544868.
16. Webster AC, Playford EG, Higgins G, Chapman JR, Craig J. Interleukin 2 receptor antagonists for kidney transplant recipients. Cochrane Database Syst Rev. 2010 Feb 20(1):CD003897. PubMed PMID:14974043.
17. Brennan DC, Daller JA, Lake KD, Cibrik D, Del Castillo D, Thymoglobulin induction study G. Rabbit anti-thymocyte globulin versus basiliximab in renal transplantation. N Engl J Med. 2006 Nov 10;355(19):1967–77. PubMed PMID:17093248.
18. Noel C, Abramowicz D, Durand D, Mourad G, Lang P, Kessler M et al. Daclizumab versus antithymocyte globulin in high-immunological-risk renal transplant recipients. J Am Soc Nephrol. 2009;20(6):1385–92. PubMed PMID:WOS:000266617200031.
19. Hill P, Cross NB, Barnett AN, Palmer SC, Webster AC. Polyclonal and monoclonal antibodies for induction therapy in kidney transplant recipients. Cochrane Database Syst Rev. 2017 Jan 11;1:CD004759. PubMed PMID:28073178.
20. Hart A, Smith JM, Skeans MA, Gustafson SK, Wilk AR, Castro S et al. OPTN/SRTR 2017 annual data report: kidney. Am J Transplant. 2019 Feb 28;19(Suppl 2):19–123. PubMed PMID:30811893.
21. Hart A, Smith JM, Skeans MA, Gustafson SK, Wilk AR, Castro S et al. OPTN/SRTR 2018 annual data report: kidney. Am J Transplant. 2020;20(Suppl 1):20–130. PubMed PMID:31898417.
22. Webster A, Woodroffe RC, Taylor RS, Chapman JR, Craig JC. Tacrolimus versus cyclosporin as primary immunosuppression for kidney transplant recipients. Cochrane Database Syst Rev. 2005 Oct 20(4):CD003961. PubMed PMID:16235347.
23. Haddad EM, McAlister VC, Renouf E, Malthaner R, Kjaer MS, Gluud LL. Cyclosporin versus tacrolimus for liver transplanted patients. Cochrane Database Syst Rev. 2006 Oct 21(4):CD005161. PubMed PMID:17054241.
24. Wagner M, Earley AK, Webster AC, Schmid CH, Balk EM, Uhlig K. Mycophenolic acid versus azathioprine as primary immunosuppression for kidney transplant recipients. Cochrane Database Syst Rev. 2015 Dec 4(12):CD007746. PubMed PMID:26633102.
25. Haller MC, Royuela A, Nagler EV, Pascual J, Webster AC. Steroid avoidance or withdrawal for kidney transplant recipients. Cochrane Database Syst Rev. 2016 Aug 23(8):CD005632. PubMed PMID:27546100.
26. Hricik DE, O'Toole MA, Schulak JA, Herson J. Steroid-free immunosuppression in cyclosporine-treated renal transplant recipients: a meta-analysis. J Am Soc Nephrol. 1993;4(6):1300–5. PubMed PMID:8130356.
27. Pascual J, Royuela A, Galeano C, Crespo M, Zamora J. Very early steroid withdrawal or complete avoidance for kidney transplant recipients: a systematic review. Nephrol Dial Transplant. 2012 Jul 22;27(2):825–32. PubMed PMID:21785040.
28. Webster AC, Lee VW, Chapman JR, Craig JC. Target of rapamycin inhibitors (TOR-I; sirolimus and everolimus) for primary immunosuppression in kidney transplant recipients. Cochrane Database Syst Rev. 2006 Apr 21;2:CD004290. PubMed PMID:16625599.
29. Geissler EK. Skin cancer in solid organ transplant recipients: are mTOR inhibitors a game changer? Transplant Res. 2015 Feb 24;4:1. PubMed PMID:25699174; PubMed Central PMCID:PMCPMC4332735.
30. Dantal J, Morelon E, Rostaing L, Goffin E, Brocard A, Tromme I et al. Sirolimus for secondary prevention of skin cancer in kidney transplant recipients: 5-year results. J Clin Oncol. 2018 Jul 17;36(25):2612–20. PubMed PMID:30016177.
31. Pascual J, Berger SP, Witzke O, Tedesco H, Mulgaonkar S, Qazi Y et al. Everolimus with reduced calcineurin inhibitor exposure in renal transplantation. J Am Soc Nephrol. 2018 May 13;29(7):1979–91. PubMed PMID:29752413.

32. Durrbach A, Pestana JM, Pearson T, Vincenti F, Garcia VD, Campistol J et al. A phase III study of belatacept versus cyclosporine in kidney transplants from extended criteria donors (BENEFIT-EXT study). Am J Transplant. 2010 Apr 27;10(3):547–57. PubMed PMID:20415898.
33. Vincenti F, Rostaing L, Grinyo J, Rice K, Steinberg S, Gaite L et al. Belatacept and long-term outcomes in kidney transplantation. N Engl J Med. 2016;374(4):333–43. PubMed PMID:26816011.
34. Durrbach A, Pestana JM, Florman S, Del Carmen Rial M, Rostaing L, Kuypers D et al. Long-term outcomes in belatacept- versus cyclosporine-treated recipients of extended criteria donor kidneys: final results from BENEFIT-EXT, a phase III randomized study. Am J Transplant. 2016 Jun 9;16(11):3192–201. PubMed PMID:27130868; PubMed Central PMCID:PMCPMC5516151.
35. Masson P, Henderson L, Chapman JR, Craig JC, Webster AC. Belatacept for kidney transplant recipients. Cochrane Database Syst Rev. 2014 Nov 25;11:CD010699. PubMed PMID:25416857.
36. Rostaing L, Massari P, Garcia VD, Mancilla-Urrea E, Nainan G, del Carmen Rial M et al. Switching from calcineurin inhibitor-based regimens to a belatacept-based regimen in renal transplant recipients: a randomized phase II study. Clin J Am Soc Nephrol. 2011 Nov 6;6(2):430–9. PubMed PMID:21051752; PubMed Central PMCID:PMCPMC3052236.
37. Cippà PE, Schiesser M, Ekberg H, van Gelder T, Mueller NJ, Cao CA et al. Risk stratification for rejection and infection after kidney transplantation. Clin J Am Soc Nephrol. 2015 Oct 1;10(12):2213–20. PubMed PMID:26430088; PubMed Central PMCID:PMCPMC4670759.
38. Nevins TE, Robiner WN, Thomas W. Predictive patterns of early medication adherence in renal transplantation. Transplant. 2014;98(8):878–84. PubMed PMID:24831921; PubMed Central PMCID:PMCPMC4199876.
39. Haas M, Loupy A, Lefaucheur C, Roufosse C, Glotz D, Seron D et al. The Banff 2017 kidney meeting report: revised diagnostic criteria for chronic active T cell-mediated rejection, antibody-mediated rejection, and prospects for integrative endpoints for next-generation clinical trials. Am J Transplant. 2018 Dec 16;18(2):293–307. PubMed PMID:29243394.
40. De Lucena DD, Rangel É. Glucocorticoids use in kidney transplant setting. Expert Opin Drug Metab Toxicol. 2018 Oct 5;14(10):1023–41. PubMed PMID:30265586.
41. Webster AC, Wu S, Tallapragada K, Park MY, Chapman JR, Carr SJ. Polyclonal and monoclonal antibodies for treating acute rejection episodes in kidney transplant recipients. Cochrane Database Syst Rev. 2017 Jul 22;7:CD004756. PubMed PMID:28731207.
42. Kaposztas Z, Podder H, Mauiyyedi S, Illoh O, Kerman R, Reyes M et al. Impact of rituximab therapy for treatment of acute humoral rejection. Clin Transplant. 2009;23(1):63–73. PubMed PMID:19200217.
43. Tan EK, Bentall A, Dean PG, Shaheen MF, Stegall MD, Schinstock CA. Use of eculizumab for active antibody-mediated rejection that occurs early post-kidney transplantation: a consecutive series of 15 cases. Transplantation. 2019;103(11):2397–404. PubMed PMID:30801549; PubMed Central PMCID:PMCPMC6699919.
44. Ejaz NS, Alloway RR, Halleck F, Dürr M, Budde K, Woodle ES. Review of bortezomib treatment of antibody-mediated rejection in renal transplantation. Antioxid Redox Signal. 2014 Apr 28;21(17):2401–18. PubMed PMID:24635140.

Dermatologic Imaging for Immunosuppressed Patients

3

Shenara Musthaq, Aditi Sahu, and Veronica Rotemberg

INTRODUCTION

Dermatologic diagnosis has strongly relied on the human sense of visual perception. Although the trained human eye still remains the cornerstone of a dermatologic assessment, technological advances have expanded the capabilities of the field immensely, allowing for subsurface visualization and *in vivo* assessment without a biopsy. Skin cancer is the most common cancer in patients who have received solid organ transplants, who have an increased risk for developing both melanoma and nonmelanoma skin cancers.[1–4]

No specific guidelines have been developed for image-based screening and monitoring of organ transplant patients or those on immunosuppressive agents; however, through extrapolation of efficacious screening and diagnostic methods in other high-risk dermatologic patients, recommendations for this population can be set forth. We outline noninvasive imaging modalities used in dermatology, their utilization in monitoring and diagnosing skin cancer or other dermatologic conditions in organ transplant cases, and image-based management considerations after diagnosis.

TOTAL BODY PHOTOGRAPHY

Total body photography (TBP) refers to the use of standardized photography of a patient's entire body to monitor changes in a patient's lesions over time. TBP is used in conjunction with the clinicians' total body skin exam as a reference to compare the skin to a previous time point with or without dermoscopic images.[5–8] Photographs can be used by patients for self-exams. Traditionally photos of the skin have been obtained in the flat, or two-dimensional (2D) form; however, the conversion of the three-dimensional (3D)

 DOI: 10.1201/9781003001461-3

TABLE 3.1 Sensitivity and Specificity of Imaging Modalities in Detection of Different Skin Cancers

	BCC		SCC		MELANOMA	
	SENSITIVITY	SPECIFICITY	SENSITIVITY	SPECIFICITY	SENSITIVITY	SPECIFICITY
Dermoscopy	40–97%[10]	50–100%[10]	79%[11]	87%[11]	94.4%[6,9]	75.5%[6,9]
RCM	87–95%[12,13]	94–96%[12,13]	63%[13]	–	90–95%[12]	76–81%[12]
Ultrasound	0–91%[14]	3–52%[14]	–	–	83.5;	33–75%[15]
OCT	90.8–98.4%[16]	65.2–83.6%[16]	–	–	–	–
MelaFind®	–	–	–	–	82.5%[17]	52.4%[17]
Verisante AuraTM	–	–	–	–	21.4%[17]	86.2%[17]
FotoFinder® Moleanalyzer Pro	–	–	–	–	88.1%[17]	78.8%[17]

surface of the skin into a 2D image compromised the accuracy of the image, specifically with respect to quantitative assessment of a flat projection. Additionally, many photos were needed to visualize all aspects of the skin with the missing areas. In recent years, advances in photography have introduced 3D TBP imaging systems able to create 360-degree rotatable images to view all areas of the body, including curved surfaces that would be distorted or missed in 2D imaging.[9] To date, several systems are clinically available and commonly used for total body monitoring including those from FotoFinder®, MetaOptima®, and Canfield Scientific® (Table 3.1).

Melanoma

TBP has been used in patients with atypical moles and has been shown to improve detection of new or changing lesions and aid in earlier detection of melanoma. A survey of 38 dermatologists with an interest in skin cancer in transplant patients found 54% performed dermoscopic pictures of dermoscopically suspicious nevi, 37% performed close-up photography of clinically suspicious nevi, 34% performed TBP at baseline, whereas 19.5% performed all three photography methods together.[18] The combination of TBP and dermoscopy for monitoring has led to increased melanoma detection rates compared with those of TBP alone or dermoscopy alone.[8] Excision of lesions suspected to be melanoma in high-risk patients was triggered by clinicians detecting them with the aid of TBP. No lesions were noted by patients with the aid of TBP suggesting that this is a tool better used in clinical practice than for self-examination.[19]

DERMOSCOPY

Dermoscopy is an in vivo technique used for examination of skin lesions. Often likened to a dermatologists' stethoscope, dermatoscopes are simple hand-held tools used for performing dermoscopic imaging. This modality allows for the visualization of subsurface structures in the epidermis, the dermo-epidermal junction, and the papillary dermis.[20] Because of the high reflective index of the stratum corneum compared with that of air (1.55 vs. 1.0), under normal conditions most light is reflected by the skin surface. Dermoscopy reduces this reflection through the use of media with reflective indices closer to that of the stratum corneum.[20]

Dermatoscopes contain trans illuminating polarized and unpolarized light sources, allowing for multiple methods of visualization:

- Unpolarized light, contact
- Polarized light, contact
- Polarized light, noncontact

Contact denotes the connection of a glass plate with the skin using an immersion fluid such as water, alcohols, water-soluble gels or oils that have a reflective index matched to that of the stratum corneum. Polarized light dermoscopy utilizes cross-polarization with orthogonally placed filters. Light reflected by the skin surface maintains its polarization and is blocked by the filter. Light that enters deeper portions of the skin is scattered upon reflection, losing its original angle of polarization and is able to pass through the filter to be visualized by the viewer.[20,21] Devices are also capable of magnification ranging from 6–100×. The diagnosis of lesions and the risk of malignancy are assessed based on the presence or absence of certain architectural characteristics as well as on the morphology of vascular configurations.[22]

Dermoscopy is relatively easy to learn and integrate into practice compared with other imaging modalities. However, there are limitations; although there is the ability to visualize into the subsurface, there is no histology available. Additionally, certain dermatologic features can overlap between benign and malignant melanocytic lesions and other pigmented lesions; therefore, training and level of expertise is important.

Melanoma

Dermoscopy enhances the early diagnosis of melanoma by increasing the specificity. With an algorithmic approach, such as the 2-step dermoscopy algorithm, physicians can be guided in the decision-making process whether or not to biopsy. Melanocytic lesions are first differentiated from non-melanocytic lesions through identification of specific architectural and vascular features that research comparisons have shown to be more common in melanocytic lesions. The second step evaluates the melanocytic lesions to differentiate benign neoplasms from melanoma. There are multiple methods that can be utilized for the second step, including pattern analysis, the ABCD scoring method, the 7-point checklist, and the Menzies method.[23,24] Use of dermoscopy by those properly trained can reduce the number of excisions by 40%–70% without sacrificing sensitivity.[25]

A small study of European clinicians who treat transplant patients showed 70.7% of the surveyed clinicians performed dermoscopy of clinically suspicious nevi, whereas 53.6% performed dermoscopic photography of the suspicious nevi and 24.4% conducted dermoscopy of all nevi.[18] The authors suggested the use of sequential digital dermatoscopic imaging may be beneficial in the transplant population.[6] There have been few studies of the differences in dermoscopy of lesions in transplant patients. One study found no differences in the distribution of features in melanomas in organ transplant recipients (OTRs) compared to non-OTRs.[26] However, dermoscopic features of nevi in patients receiving immunosuppression and biologics showed significant change over time in a 12-month period in comparison with results in control groups. Changes were minor, consisting mostly of symmetric structural or color changes and a maximum growth of 2 mm. The lesions with dermoscopic changes were subsequently excised and found to be benign, suggesting that those showing minimal change can be monitored.[27]

Nonmelanoma Skin Cancer

Identification of actinic keratoses (AKs) or squamous cell carcinoma (SCC) can be performed with dermoscopy. Nonpigmented AKs typically show erythema, a pink-red pseudo network, perifollicular wavy vessels, and targetoid hair follicles. With polarized light, AKs can display the rosette sign.[28] Pigmented AKs show evident follicles, white circles, and gray rhomboidal structure. SCC in situ or Bowen's disease can be diagnosed with 98% probability when there is the simultaneous finding of surface scale and clusters of glomerular vessels.[29] The dermoscopic features of invasive SCC show a central keratin mass and ulceration that clinically corresponds to scale and crusting, and additionally hairpin vessels, linear-irregular vessels, and targetoid hair follicles.[30] Dermoscopic features of AKs and SCCs are highlighted in Figure 3.1.

Dermoscopic features of nonpigmented basal cell carcinoma (BCC) include featureless areas, white-red structureless background, atypical red vessels, arborizing vessels, comma vessels, and telangiectatic vessels. Because of the inclusion of pigmented BCC in the differential diagnosis of melanoma, dermoscopic features have been well-outlined and include ulceration, maple leaf-like areas, large gray-blue ovoid nests, multiple gray-blue globules, spoke wheel areas, and arborizing telangiectasias. The addition of dermoscopy to visual inspection increases the diagnostic odds by 7.5–8.2 times.[10] An example of a pigmented BCC is shown in Figure 3.1c.

REFLECTANCE CONFOCAL MICROSCOPY

Reflectance confocal microscopy (RCM) allows for *in vivo* imaging of the skin. Considered an in vivo biopsy, commercially available confocal microscopes are able to create histologically detailed images. A near infrared light (830 nm) is emitted from a diode laser to optically section layers of the skin in a horizontal plane. As light passes between cellular structures with different refractive indexes, it is reflected, captured, and rendered into 2D gray scale images. The skin is visualized in an en face manner to a depth of 150–200 µm or the level of the superficial dermis.[22] Vertical stacks of en face images can be made of horizonal sections for a 3D-like reconstruction of the skin.[22]

RCM significantly improves the diagnostic accuracy and early detection of both melanocytic and nonmelanocytic skin cancers compared with both clinical and/or dermoscopic imaging alone.[32–34] At present, RCM is used in conjunction with other examination tactics as the clinical history and dermoscopy can narrow the differential diagnosis and increase the diagnostic accuracy.

The depth of imaging reaches 300 µm; however, the imaging resolution decreases after 100–150 µm. This prevents detection of tumor invasion or deep tumor margins, and results in decreased accuracy when evaluating nodular lesions or those with epidermal thickening, ulceration, or hyperkeratosis.[35,36] Diagnostic inaccuracy is sometimes not attributable to the functionality of the modality, underlining the importance of the user expertise level. The average RCM session requires at least 5 minutes to perform, which cumulatively may add significant time to the clinic flow. Additionally, the required training time for a physician to reach what is considered "acceptable" diagnostic accuracy and expertise is 4–6 months.[37]

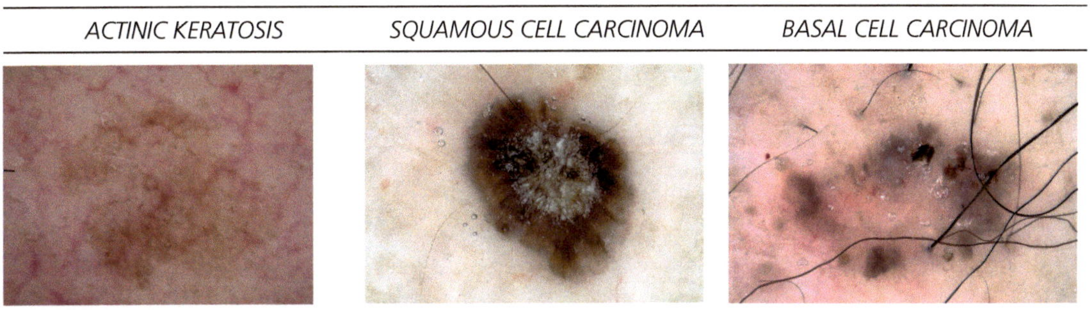

FIGURE 3.1 Classic dermoscopic features of actinic keratosis (pink pseudonetwork and white circles), squamous cell carcinoma (central keratin mass and ulceration), and basal cell carcinoma (gray-blue ovoid nests and globules).[31]

Melanoma

Melanosomes and melanin are strong sources of contrast in RCM, meaning that melanocytic cells stand out using this technique. The RCM features of different melanocytic lesions have been outlined; however, in order to first differentiate melanocytic from non-melanocytic lesions, there must be four features present: cobble stoning of the epidermal layers, pagetoid spread, a mesh appearance of the dermo-epidermal junction, and dermal nests. Secondly, the presence of roundish suprabasal cells and dermal cells with nuclear atypia were associated with melanoma.[38]

Lentigo maligna often has evidence of subclinical spread and unclear borders. The use of RCM can identify the areas most likely to show the greatest histologic atypia, which will provide the best histologic diagnosis and reduce the need for scouting biopsies by showing the extent of the atypia.[39] A range of 5%–29% of lentigo maligna lesions were found to have an invasive portion on surgical removal.[40] Use of RCM can aid in management by determining the appropriateness of topical treatment or mapping borders for surgical excision. Excisions guided by RCM lead to smaller potential surgical defects than when guided by Woods's light and dermoscopy.[39] Studies have attempted to use RCM to evaluate the efficacy of noninvasive treatments to avoid the need for a clearance confirmation biopsy; however, because of the limited depth of visualization, one must take caution to avoid missing residual deeper cells.[38]

Nonmelanoma Skin Cancer

Preliminary studies suggested that nonmelanoma skin cancers in OTRs may be amenable to diagnosis using RCM.[41] In a small cohort of OTRs, BCCs were diagnosed with 100% sensitivity and 80% specificity. For more hyperkeratotic lesions, RCM was more challenging because of the penetration difficulty but still performed well on a small number of lesions with two readers.

In general, BCC has distinctive RCM features. At the epidermal level, there is alteration in the normal honeycombed pattern of the epidermal layers. At the level of the dermo-epidermal junction, aggregates of tightly packed cells are seen with palisading cells at the periphery of the tumor correlating with tumor islands. The packed cells form cordlike structures that are surrounded by non-refractile spaces, which are mucin deposits on histology. The stroma displays low refraction whereas the tumor cells have high refractivity.[38]

The diagnostic algorithm with the highest sensitivity and specificity for diagnosis of BCC was outlined by Guiterra et al.[42] It relies on identification of four positive RCM features and three negative features.

Basal cell subtypes can be differentiated via RCM to aid in management consideration. Nodular BCC has been associated with larger tumor nests, increased clefting, and larger vessel caliber. Infiltrative BCCs show the presence of dark silhouettes and abundant bright compact collagen.[38]

Squamous Cell Carcinoma

AK, the precursor of squamous cell carcinoma (SCC), has been shown to have the following RCM features: stratum corneum disruption, parakeratosis, individual corneocytes, exocytosis, and architectural disarray at the granular and spinous layers.

SCC can be difficult to differentiate clinically from AKs and other precursor lesions.[43,44] Although AKs and SCC can be differentiated through RCM based on these statistically significant differences, studies have found poor interobserver agreement. This suggests that it is difficult to have the level of experience necessary to differentiate between the two with this imaging modality, despite the differences in appearance.[45]

RCM may also be useful in clinical management once the diagnosis has been made. In studies in nontransplant populations, the margin assessment of lentigo maligna and nonmelanoma skin cancer have been useful prior to definitive surgery and may also be useful for nonsurgical management.[32,34,46–50]

OPTICAL COHERENCE TOMOGRAPHY

Optical coherence tomography (OCT) is an imaging technique that produces cross-sectional images of tissue microstructure and was adapted from use in the field of ophthalmology. Using infrared light and interferometric methods, reflected light from the tissue is sensed to create an image. OCT provides both cross-sectional and en face images to skin depths of 0.4–2.0 mm into the reticular dermis even with resolutions as low as 1–3 μm. Although OCT does not image histologic morphology, lesional architecture is able to be assessed as shown in Figure 3.2.

Melanoma

OCT findings in melanoma have been defined in comparison with benign nevi. Melanoma displays more architectural chaos with atypical melanocytes seen in the upper part of the epidermis on the cross-sectional view. Melanocytes in melanoma lesions are large, often twice the size of adjacent keratinocytes, and have abundant reflective cytoplasm. The architecture of the dermo-epidermal junction is irregular with broadened rete ridges. In the en face mode, a cobble-stoning pattern was predominant in the epidermis.[51] Atypical melanocytes are initially seen in the epidermis and expand towards the dermo-epidermal junction.[52] Combining the two modes showed the loss of cellular maturation with melanocytes in the deep dermis indistinguishable from those in the papillary dermis.[51]

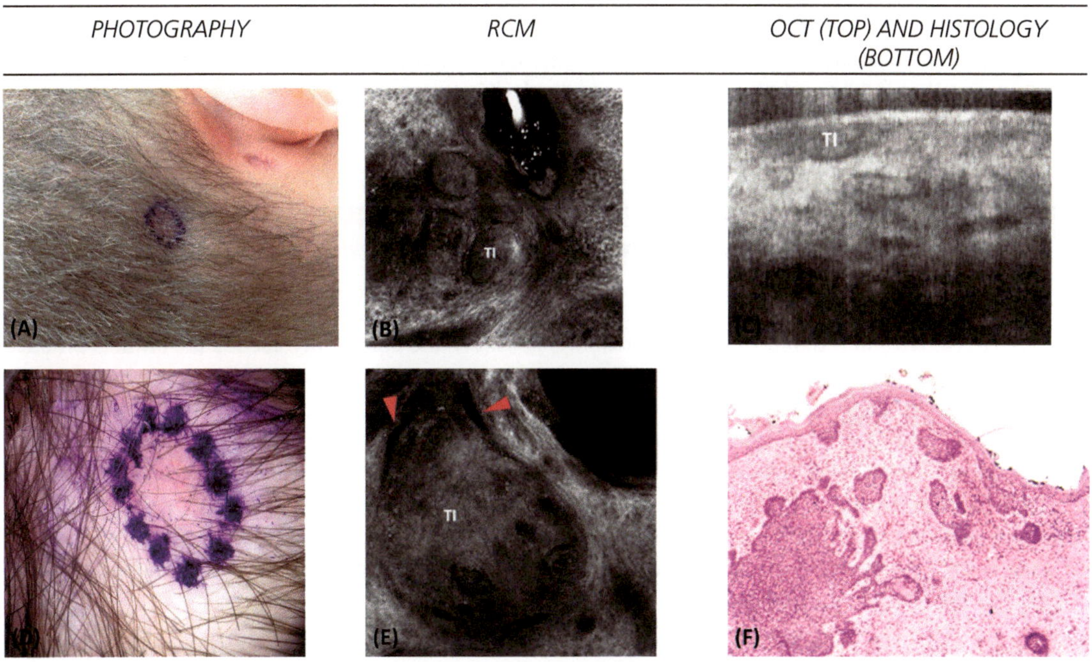

FIGURE 3.2 Clinical photographs **(a)** and dermoscopy **(d)** of a basal cell carcinoma. Reflectance confocal microscopy (RCM) of basal cell carcinoma highlighting tumor islands (TI) **(b)** and peripheral clefting (red arrowheads) **(e)**. Tumor islands highlighted as visible on optical coherence tomography **(c)** and histopathology **(f)**.

Nonmelanoma Skin Cancer

OCT has been used in the diagnosis of BCC and the differentiation of BCC subtypes. Features suggestive of a BCC were the absence of well-defined layering and dark lobules. Superficial tumor nests and superficial dermal tumor nests can be visualized and are delineated by a darker shadow. There is high accuracy in diagnosing superficial BCC with OCT with the best predictive feature being "clefting."

The limitation of OCT in imaging of BCC is depth. Structures were less visible at the level of the reticular dermis, and histological correlates of depth were best when the lesion was ≤1 mm. Use of OCT could reduce biopsy rates by 40% with a 4% margin of error in those lesions that were not biopsied.[53] Experience was not a significant factor when looking at interobserver agreement.

OCT has limited efficacy in visualization of AKs because of the hyperkeratotic nature of the disease blurring visualization. In comparison with normal skin, a thickened epidermis with alternating hypertrophy and atrophy is suggestive of AK, with increased thickness associated with worse disease severity. The epidermis will show evidence of a disrupted layer with hyperreflective streaks and dots that suggest inflammation or acantholysis. Differentiating AKs from SCC is possible by the loss of a clearly defined dermo-epidermal junction, pronounced differentiation in hypertrophy, and increased intralesional acantholysis seen in SCC.[54] Determining the presence of an outlined dermo-epidermal junction on cross-sectional imaging is considered a discriminatory step of differentiating SCC from both AK and normal skin. Using the en face mode, the presence of an atypical honeycomb pattern differentiates AK from normal skin.[55]

With the increased use of topical agents for the treatment of skin cancer, noninvasive imaging can be used to establish management options and treatment success without the need for re-biopsy. Superficial BCCs may be more likely to respond to imiquimod treatment than other subtypes because of the depth of penetration, which suggests that pretreatment depth analysis could be useful.[56] OCT has been used to monitor imiquimod treatment and treatment success of BCCs and AKs. Although inflammation during the treatment process obscured the imaging quality, a decrease in epidermal thickness could be visualized before and after treatment of AKs and the disappearance of tumor islands and their replacement with hyperechoic rimmed cysts was seen in the treatment of BCC.

OCT has demonstrated clinical utility in a transplant recipient receiving vismodegib and imiquimod 5% cream together.[57] Although this report tracked one BCC, it suggested that OTRs, especially those who are severely affected by BCCs, may be amenable to longitudinal monitoring with OCT.

ULTRASOUND

Although a relatively new diagnostic tool, ultrasound is widely and commonly used in the clinical practice of many medical fields such as radiology and cardiology. The use of ultrasound in dermatology is more recent; originally used as a method to measure skin thickness, it has expanded to diagnostic and therapeutic purposes.[58] In ultrasonic imaging, there is a direct trade-off between depth of penetration and resolution, such that cutaneous malignancy-level resolution cannot penetrate into the skin deeper than 1–2 cm. Higher frequency ultrasound (20–100 MHz) allows for high resolution study of the superficial skin and structures such as hair follicles and sebaceous glands.[59] In addition to classic B-mode ultrasound, doppler imaging at high frequency can assess tumor vasculature. Limitations of ultrasound include visualization of only the epidermis and of the lack of differentiation of pigment.

Melanoma

Superficial spreading melanoma is seen as hypoechoic (dark), thin structures with a depth of 0.75–1.34 mm. Thin ovoid, hypoechoic structures are located beneath the level of the papillary dermis. This is associated with histologic results showing atypical singular melanocytic cells or nests throughout the epidermis, as well as deep tumor cells between lymphocytes.

Nodular melanomas were assessed by ultrasound, which identified hypoechoic structures in the dermis with a mean depth of 1.06 mm.[59] High-frequency ultrasound was able to detect tumoral vessels in 40% of cutaneous melanomas; 40 of the 43 lesions were over 2 mm thick. Increased vascularity in lesions correlated with other features of advanced disease such as Breslow thickness and lymph node status and was shown to be an adverse prognostic feature.[60,61]

Ultrasound-derived lesion depth was found initially to be an overestimate in nodular melanoma and an underestimate in superficial spreading melanoma. However, depth can be corrected to reach high correlation with the histologic stage.[59] Although diagnosis using ultrasound is difficult, assessment of tumor thickness can aid in planning surgical excision margins, as current recommendations suggest that melanoma in situ can be excised with 0.5 cm margins, whereas invasive melanomas, such as those from 1.01–2 mm in depth, should be excised with larger margins of 1–2 cm.[62]

Ultrasound can be used to detect local and regional spread. Satellite metastases, found 2–3 cm from the tumor along the lymphatic course, can be detected via ultrasound, appearing as subcutaneous hypoechoic nodules.

Basal Cell Carcinoma

Ultrasound performed on nodular BCC showed hypoechoic, highly vascular structures located at the dermal level. Basal cells typically have hyperechoic spots described as “cotton flower-like” and lacking posterior shadowing, which is a useful sign to differentiate the tumor from other skin cancers.[63] Removing superficial scale, clinicians were able to identify the tumor depth; no statistically significant difference was seen between the ultrasound determined and histologically determined depth. Similar to nodular melanoma, the depth of nodular BCC was overestimated by high-frequency ultrasound.[59]

Features visible on ultrasound can direct the choice of treatment and surgery and subsequent monitoring. Ultrasound can be used in areas like the nose and ear to determine the lesional involvement of the cartilage. Knowing the extent of the cartilage invasion can help dermatologists plan for the extent of surgery and the techniques that may need to be employed.[64] It can aid additionally in monitoring as hyperechoic spots seen within a lesion on ultrasound were found to correlate with histologic subtypes that had a higher likelihood of recurrence. The presence of ≥7 hyperechoic spots predicted a high risk of recurrence subtype with a sensitivity of 79%[65] (Table 3.2).

OTHER

National Comprehensive Cancer Network (NCCN) guidelines for cutaneous SCC indicate imaging studies for tumors that present with the suspicion of more extensive disease such as bone involvement, perineural spread, or deep soft tissue involvement. Radiologic imaging of patients decreased disease-related outcomes regarding local recurrence, nodal metastasis, and death compared with outcomes in high-risk, nonimaged patients, with imaging changing the management course in 33% of patients.[66]

SCC in organ transplant patients was associated with a more aggressive disease course leading to higher incidences of metastasis and death.[67,68] A study of five European centers with a transplant center showed that men who had kidney transplants were the most likely to develop an aggressive SCC. Features of aggressive behavior in a tumor included location on the face, followed by the scalp and upper extremities, histology showing poor differentiation, a tumor thickness >2 mm, and perineural invasion. Perineural invasion is relatively rare for primary SCC in the general population with an incidence of

TABLE 3.2 Imaging Tool and Associated Advantages and Disadvantages

IMAGING TOOL	*ADVANTAGES*	*DISADVANTAGES*
Dermoscopy	Easy to learn to use Inexpensive Hand-held device Magnifies lesions Increases sensitivity of melanoma diagnosis	User dependent Non-histologic assessment Overlap of features between pigmented lesions
Reflectance Confocal Microscopy	Allows for horizontal, new face imaging Histological level of imaging High sensitivity in detection of melanoma, basal cell carcinoma, benign nevi, and seborrheic keratoses	Expensive Learning of the diagnostic features is needed Experience with the tool is needed for good imaging Increased exam time Poor-quality images produced because of make-up, air bubbles, obstruction from hair, movement of the patient Increased depth affects image quality
Optical Coherence Tomography	Can visualize the architecture of the lesion En face and vertical sectioning Increased depth of visualization	Cannot differentiate between basal cell and actinic keratoses Sensitive to artifacts Images show variation from person to person or different sites within one individual Cannot visualize pigment No histologic assessment
Ultrasound	High-resolution imaging Increased depth of visualization Familiarity in the medical field, increased ease of use Can visualize blood flow	High-resolution ultrasounds are less common No visualization of histology No visualization of pigment
Total Body Photography	Early detection of melanoma Reduction in patient and physician anxiety	Hypopigmented lesion detection is less reliable IT management and data storage are expensive Higher biopsy rates in younger patients

2.5%–5%; however, it is associated with an increased risk of nodal metastasis and local recurrence. Tumor local recurrence was seen in 45% of aggressive lesions. The 5-year overall survival was 23% with a decrease to 11.3% at 10 years.[69]

Perineural spread in SCC can be monitored through the use of magnetic resonance imaging (MRI) because of the superior soft tissue contrast. With the typically used imaging method of contrast-enhanced T1-weighted MRI with fat suppression, the features suggestive of perineural invasion include nerve enhancement and increase in diameter. Disruption of the blood–nerve barrier results in increased permeability of the endoneural capillaries, allowing for nerve enhancement with contrast agents, whereas proliferation of tumor cells along the nerve increases the diameter. Secondary features may include atrophy of the muscles enervated by the invaded nerve in the acute phase (within 4 weeks of denervation), which will read as edema and hyperintense signaling on T2-weighted imaging.[70] Computed tomography (CT) evidence of bony invasion includes destruction or increased lucency of the bone underlying the lesion.

Ultrasound has been used for lymph node evaluation in different specialties. In regard to melanoma, tumors that measure ≥1 mm in thickness indicate the need for a sentinel lymph node procedure. Sonography can be utilized to help locate the sentinel lymph node and guide cytologic procedures through identifying signs of a malignant lymph node in the draining lymph node basin. Signs that can indicate malignancy in a lymph node include: round shape, loss of difference in echogenicity between the cortex and medulla, cortical hypoechoic nodules or asymmetric thickness of the cortex, diffuse hypoechogenicity in the lymph node, increased echogenicity in the hypodermis surrounding the lymph node, size >1 cm, and diffuse or prominent cortical flow associated with irregular vessels.[64] Doppler flow typically slows the loss of normal central vascularization and instead multiple penetrating capsular vessels spread inwards.[71] Use of ultrasound with fine needle aspiration can aid in staging and reduce the number of sentinel lymph node biopsies.[72]

For patients with high-risk cutaneous SCC, imaging can be a useful tool to identify nodal metastases earlier than with simple clinical monitoring.[66] Although ultrasound for this purpose has not yet been prospectively demonstrated in cutaneous SCCs, it is widely used to guide fine-needle aspiration for other types of head and neck cancers and may be a useful adjunct in this setting.[73]

ARTIFICIAL INTELLIGENCE

Artificial intelligence (AI) is ever expanding in the medical field. The computational accuracy of cutaneous lesions has reached that of a dermatologist for diagnosis of melanoma.[74,75] Translation to the clinical setting has been slow, however, because of concerns over the "black box" nature of automated diagnoses. The improvement of AI means that it is likely to be introduced in an approved fashion to smartphone cameras or imaging systems over the next 10 years. Efforts to improve interpretability can be introduced to the clinical setting through methods such as content-based image retrieval (CBIR), in which the system is able to pull "similar" images and diagnoses for the clinician's consideration.

TELEDERMATOLOGY

Teledermatology is allowing increased access to health care delivery while reducing health care costs and improving the quality of care. The main platforms of teledermatology include synchronous, in which there is real-time evaluation between the dermatologist and the patient with live video; asynchronous, in which the dermatologist obtains images and can review the clinical history; or a hybrid. The use of noninvasive imaging, such as dermoscopic, RCM, OCT, or ultrasound photos can aid remote diagnosis and management when a clinician is not able to fully examine a lesion with palpation and other examination tools; this was especially noted after the expansion of teledermatology during the coronavirus disease 2019 (COVID-19) pandemic. Overall diagnostic accuracy reached the mid—high 70th percentile, which is comparable to face-to-face in clinic care. Interobserver agreement between teledermatology and clinic-based evaluations reaches 70%–90%, indicating relative non-inferiority.[76] The majority (86%–100%) of physicians involved in the teledermatology care of transplant patients desired face-to-face consultations following receipt of a referral letter with a clinical history, even when accompanied by electronic photographs. A provisional diagnosis could be made when there were accompanying photographs with 81% accuracy after final biopsy.[77] The use of teledermatology can be extremely useful to transplant patients living in areas with limited access to dermatologists. Because of the change in the growth patterns of lesions such as melanoma, or the aggressive nature of other disease etiologies such as SCC, having access to a dermatologist when questions or new lesions arise is crucial.

Guidelines for Imaging in Organ Transplant Patients

Transplant patients are at high risk for the development of locally or systemically aggressive cutaneous skin malignancy or other cutaneous skin manifestations. Currently there are no guidelines set forth for the treatment of OTRs.

Based on previous studies in other high-risk patient populations such as xeroderma pigmentosum, we recommend a three-fold approach of total skin exam, TBP, and dermoscopy, with the consideration of RCM and dermoscopy for difficult lesions when trained expertise is available.[78] The combination of identifying suspicious lesions via dermoscopy and following with in vivo RCM has the potential in certain patient populations to decrease excisions by 35%.[79]

The combined use of different noninvasive imaging modalities to aid in monitoring, diagnosis, and treatment can be extremely useful in the transplant population to avoid the extraneous surgeries in a patient population that will almost inevitably need multiple procedures over the course of their care. A dermatologist should be included in the management team of transplant patients even before operation to first establish care, and to overview the risks of skin cancer and the preventative measures that can be taken. Teledermatology is a reasonable method of establishing care and following patients who have limited access to dermatologic services, especially as AI algorithms improve for remote monitoring; however, in person visits, especially for confirming the diagnosis of suspicious lesions, will be necessary as well.

SUMMARY OF KEY POINTS

- RCM allows for histologic en face and vertical imaging of the skin, and it can differentiate between subtypes of melanoma, BCC, and SCC but is associated with a learning curve in using the machine and interpreting the results.
- OCT can potentially reduce biopsies by 40% and can guide management and determine treatment success with topical therapy.
- Ultrasound allows for visualization of anatomical structures of lesions with blood flow in some cases.

Melanoma:

- TBP and Dermoscopy are useful for monitoring and will improve the clinician's ability to identify melanomas.
- RCM, in expert hands, can be used to aid diagnosis of melanoma but will not provide information about the depth of invasion.

Basal Cell Carcinoma

- Dermoscopy is useful for diagnosis.
- RCM, in tandem with OCT, can provide enhanced diagnostic information and BCC subtyping for consideration of treatment options, especially in superficial BCC.

Squamous Cell Carcinoma

- Dermoscopy can aid diagnosis and monitoring.
- RCM may be useful in select cases, but hyperkeratosis, especially in OTRs, may limit diagnostic utility

Lymph Node Monitoring

- Ultrasound may be useful in expert hands for monitoring lymph nodes in patients with melanoma and with high-risk SCC.

REFERENCES

1. Jensen P, Hansen S, Møller B et al. Skin cancer in kidney and heart transplant recipients and different long-term immunosuppressive therapy regimens. J Am Acad Dermatol. 1999;40(2 Pt 1):177–86.
2. Jemec GB, Holm EA. Nonmelanoma skin cancer in organ transplant patients. Transplantation. 2003;75(3):253–7.
3. Howard MD, Su JC, Chong AH. Skin cancer following solid organ transplantation: a review of risk factors and models of care. Am J Clin Dermatol. 2018;19(4):585–97.
4. Mittal A, Colegio OR. Skin cancers in organ transplant recipients. Am J Transplant: Off J Am Soc Transplant Surg. 2017;17(10):2509–30.
5. Hibler BP, Qi Q, Rossi AM. Current state of imaging in dermatology. Semin Cutan Med Surg. 2016;35(1):2–8.
6. Petersen BW, Higgins HW. Chapter 27 — use of total body photography and serial digital dermoscopy in dermatology. In: Hamblin MR, Avci P, Gupta GK, editors. Imaging in dermatology. Boston: Academic Press; 2016. p. 387–93.
7. Quigley EA, Tokay BA, Jewell ST, Marchetti MA, Halpern AC. Technology and technique standards for camera-acquired digital dermatologic images: a systematic review. JAMA Dermatol. 2015;151(8):883–90.
8. Salerni G, Carrera C, Lovatto L et al. Benefits of total body photography and digital dermatoscopy ("two-step method of digital follow-up") in the early diagnosis of melanoma in patients at high risk for melanoma. J Am Acad Dermatol. 2012;67(1):e17–27.
9. Rayner JE, Laino AM, Nufer KL et al. Clinical perspective of 3D total body photography for early detection and screening of melanoma. Front Med. 2018;5:152–2.
10. Dinnes J, Deeks JJ, Chuchu N et al. Visual inspection and dermoscopy, alone or in combination, for diagnosing keratinocyte skin cancers in adults. Cochrane Database Syst Rev. 2018;12(12):CD011901.
11. Kato J, Horimoto K, Sato S, Minowa T, Uhara H. Dermoscopy of melanoma and non-melanoma skin cancers. Front Med (Lausanne). 2019;6:180.
12. Xiong YD, Ma S, Li X, Zhong X, Duan C, Chen Q. A meta-analysis of reflectance confocal microscopy for the diagnosis of malignant skin tumours. J Eur Acad Dermatol Venereol. 2016;30(8):1295–302.
13. Pellacani G, Scope A, Gonzalez S et al. Reflectance confocal microscopy made easy: the 4 must-know key features for the diagnosis of melanoma and nonmelanoma skin cancers. J Am Acad Dermatol. 2019;81(2):520–6.
14. Dinnes J, Bamber J, Chuchu N et al. High-frequency ultrasound for diagnosing skin cancer in adults. Cochrane Database Syst Rev. 2018;12.
15. Dinnes J, Bamber J, Chuchu N et al. High-frequency ultrasound for diagnosing skin cancer in adults. Cochrane Database Syst Rev. 2018;12(12):CD013188.
16. Ulrich M, von Braunmuehl T, Kurzen H et al. The sensitivity and specificity of optical coherence tomography for the assisted diagnosis of nonpigmented basal cell carcinoma: an observational study. Br J Dermatol. 2015;173(2):428–35.
17. MacLellan AN, Price EL, Publicover-Brouwer P et al. The use of non-invasive imaging techniques in the diagnosis of melanoma: a prospective diagnostic accuracy study. J Am Acad Dermatol. 2020.
18. Özcan D, Seçkin D, Haberal M. A multicenter survey: how do transplant dermatologists monitor organ transplant recipients with nevi? Exp Clin Transplant. 2018;16(Suppl 1):198–202.

19. Moloney FJ, Guitera P, Coates E et al. Detection of primary melanoma in individuals at extreme high risk: a prospective 5-year follow-up study. JAMA Dermatol. 2014;150(8):819–27.
20. Marghoob AA, Swindle LD, Moricz CZM et al. Instruments and new technologies for the in vivo diagnosis of melanoma. J Am Acad Dermatol. 2003;49(5):777–99.
21. Lake A, Jones B. Dermoscopy: to cross-polarize, or not to cross-polarize, that is the question. J Vis Comm Medi. 2015;38(1–2):36–50.
22. Wassef C, Rao BK. Uses of non-invasive imaging in the diagnosis of skin cancer: an overview of the currently available modalities. Int J Dermatol. 2013;52(12):1481–9.
23. Chen LL, Dusza SW, Jaimes N, Marghoob AA. Performance of the first step of the 2-step dermoscopy algorithm. JAMA Dermatol. 2015;151(7):715–21.
24. Weber P, Tschandl P, Sinz C, Kittler H. Dermatoscopy of neoplastic skin lesions: recent advances, updates, and revisions. Curr Treat Options Oncol. 2018;19(11):56.
25. van der Rhee JI, Bergman W, Kukutsch NA. Impact of dermoscopy on the management of high-risk patients from melanoma families: a prospective study. Acta Derm Venereol. 2011;91(4):428–31.
26. Polesie S, Gillstedt M, Zaar O, Osmancevic A, Paoli J. Dermoscopic features of melanomas in organ transplant recipients. Acta Derm Venereol. 2019;99(12):1180–1.
27. Koseoglu G, Akay BN, Kucuksahin O, Erdem C. Dermoscopic changes in melanocytic nevi in patients receiving immunosuppressive and biologic treatments: results of a prospective case-control study. J Am Acad Dermatol. 2015;73(4):623–9.
28. Zalaudek I, Giacomel J, Argenziano G et al. Dermoscopy of facial nonpigmented actinic keratosis. Br J Dermatol. 2006;155(5):951–6.
29. Rosendahl C, Cameron A, Argenziano G, Zalaudek I, Tschandl P, Kittler H. Dermoscopy of squamous cell carcinoma and keratoacanthoma. Arch Dermatol. 2012;148(12):1386–92.
30. Zalaudek I, Giacomel J, Schmid K et al. Dermatoscopy of facial actinic keratosis, intraepidermal carcinoma, and invasive squamous cell carcinoma: a progression model. J Am Acad Dermatol. 2012;66(4):589–97.
31. Tschandl P, Rosendahl C, Kittler H. The HAM10000 dataset: a large collection of multi-source dermatoscopic images of common pigmented skin lesions. Scientific Data. 2018;5 (Archive I. ISIC. ISIC Archive—Literature. 2017. Available from: http://isic-archive.com/).
32. Guitera P, Pellacani G, Crotty KA et al. The impact of in vivo reflectance confocal microscopy on the diagnostic accuracy of lentigo maligna and equivocal pigmented and nonpigmented macules of the face. J Investig Dermatol. 2010;130(8):2080–91.
33. Iftimia N, Yélamos O, Chen CSJ et al. Handheld optical coherence tomography-reflectance confocal microscopy probe for detection of basal cell carcinoma and delineation of margins. J Biomed Opt. 2017;22(7):76006.
34. Menge TD, Hibler BP, Cordova MA, Nehal KS, Rossi AM. Concordance of handheld reflectance confocal microscopy (RCM) with histopathology in the diagnosis of lentigo maligna (LM): a prospective study. J Am Acad Dermatol. 2016;74(6):1114–20.
35. Cinotti E, Labeille B, Debarbieux S et al. Dermoscopy vs. reflectance confocal microscopy for the diagnosis of lentigo maligna. 2018;32(8):1284–91.
36. Guo A, Chen J, Yang C, Ding Y, Zeng Q, Tan L. The challenge of diagnosing seborrheic keratosis by reflectance confocal microscopy. Skin Res Technol. 2018;24(4):663–6.
37. Levine A, Markowitz O. Introduction to reflectance confocal microscopy and its use in clinical practice. JAAD Case Rep. 2018;4(10):1014–23.
38. Alarcon I, Longo C, González S. Chapter 15: in vivo reflectance confocal microscopy in dermatology. In: Hamblin MR, Avci P, Gupta GK, editors. Imaging in dermatology. Boston: Academic Press; 2016. p. 169–86.
39. Yélamos O, Cordova M, Blank N et al. Correlation of handheld reflectance confocal microscopy with radial video mosaicing for margin mapping of lentigo maligna and lentigo maligna melanoma. JAMA Dermatol. 2017;153(12):1278–84.
40. Higgins HW, Lee KC, Galan A, Leffell DJ. Melanoma in situ: part II. histopathology, treatment, and clinical management. J Am Acad Dermatol. 2015;73(2):193–203.
41. Rueter L, Ramadori P, Ulrich M, Jung S, Kardorff B, Lademann J. Reflectance confocal microscopy for noninvasive examination of nonmelanocytic tumors and virus-associated skin lesions in organ transplant recipients. Skin Res Technol. 2020;26(3):376–89.
42. Guitera P, Menzies SW, Longo C, Cesinaro AM, Scolyer RA, Pellacani G. In vivo confocal microscopy for diagnosis of melanoma and basal cell carcinoma using a two-step method: analysis of 710 consecutive clinically equivocal cases. J Investig Dermatol. 2012;132(10):2386–94.
43. Moy RL. Clinical presentation of actinic keratoses and squamous cell carcinoma. J Am Acad Dermatol. 2000;42(1 Pt 2):8–10.

44. Wheller L, Soyer HP. Clinical features of actinic keratoses and early squamous cell carcinoma. Curr Probl Dermatol. 2015;46:58–63.
45. Peppelman M, Nguyen KP, Hoogedoorn L, van Erp PE, Gerritsen MJ. Reflectance confocal microscopy: non-invasive distinction between actinic keratosis and squamous cell carcinoma. J Eur Acad Dermatol Venereol. 2015;29(7):1302–9.
46. Chen CSJ, Elias M, Busam K, Rajadhyaksha M, Marghoob AA. Multimodal in vivo optical imaging, including confocal microscopy, facilitates presurgical margin mapping for clinically complex lentigo maligna melanoma. Br J Dermatol. 2005;153(5):1031–6.
47. Guitera P, Moloney FJ, Menzies SW et al. Improving management and patient care in lentigo maligna by mapping with in vivo confocal microscopyconfocal microscopy mapping in lentigo maligna. JAMA Dermatol. 2013;149(6):692–8.
48. Nadiminti H, Scope A, Marghoob AA, Busam K, Nehal KS. Use of reflectance confocal microscopy to monitor response of lentigo maligna to nonsurgical treatment. Dermatol Surg. 2010;36(2):177–84.
49. Yélamos O, Cordova M, Blank N et al. Correlation of handheld reflectance confocal microscopy with radial video mosaicing for margin mapping of lentigo maligna and lentigo maligna melanomamargin mapping of lentigo maligna and lentigo maligna melanoma with HRCM-RV margin. JAMA Dermatol. 2017;153(12):1278–84.
50. Flores E, Yélamos O, Cordova M et al. Peri-operative delineation of non-melanoma skin cancer margins in vivo with handheld reflectance confocal microscopy and video-mosaicking. J Euro Acad Dermatol Venereol. 2019;33(6):1084–91.
51. Boone MA, Norrenberg S, Jemec GB, Del Marmol V. High-definition optical coherence tomography imaging of melanocytic lesions: a pilot study. Arch Dermatol Res. 2014;306(1):11–26.
52. Mogensen M, Thrane L, Jørgensen TM, Andersen PE, Jemec GBE. OCT imaging of skin cancer and other dermatological diseases. J Biophotonics. 2009;2(6–7):442–51.
53. Cheng HM, Lo S, Scolyer R, Meekings A, Carlos G, Guitera P. Accuracy of optical coherence tomography for the diagnosis of superficial basal cell carcinoma: a prospective, consecutive, cohort study of 168 cases. Br J Dermatol. 2016;175(6):1290–300.
54. Themstrup L, Jemec GBE. Chapter 6: optical coherence tomography for skin cancer and actinic keratosis. In: Hamblin MR, Avci P, Gupta GK, editors. Imaging in dermatology. Boston: Academic Press; 2016:59–67.
55. Boone MA, Marneffe A, Suppa M et al. High-definition optical coherence tomography algorithm for the discrimination of actinic keratosis from normal skin and from squamous cell carcinoma. J Eur Acad Dermatol Venereol. 2015;29(8):1606–15.
56. Shumack S, Robinson J, Kossard S et al. Efficacy of topical 5% imiquimod cream for the treatment of nodular basal cell carcinoma: comparison of dosing regimens. Arch Dermatol. 2002;138(9):1165–71.
57. Markowitz O, Schwartz M. The use of noninvasive optical coherence tomography to monitor the treatment progress of vismodegib and imiquimod 5% cream in a transplant patient with advanced basal cell carcinoma of the nose. J Clin Aesth Dermatol. 2016;9(8):37–41.
58. Kleinerman R, Whang TB, Bard RL, Marmur ES. Ultrasound in dermatology: principles and applications. J Am Acad Dermatol. 2012;67(3):478–87.
59. Crisan M, Crisan D, Sannino G, Lupsor M, Badea R, Amzica F. Ultrasonographic staging of cutaneous malignant tumors: an ultrasonographic depth index. Arch Dermatol Res. 2013;305(4):305–13.
60. Uren RF, Sanki A, Thompson JF. The utility of ultrasound in patients with melanoma. Expert Review of Anticancer Therapy. 2007;7(11):1633–42.
61. Lassau N, Lamuraglia M, Koscielny S et al. Prognostic value of angiogenesis evaluated with high-frequency and colour Doppler sonography for preoperative assessment of primary cutaneous melanomas: correlation with recurrence after a 5 year follow-up period. Cancer Imaging. 2006;6(1):24–9.
62. Leilabadi SN, Chen A, Tsai S, Soundararajan V, Silberman H, Wong AK. Update and review on the surgical management of primary cutaneous melanoma. Healthcare (Basel). 2014;2(2):234–49.
63. Wortsman X. Sonography of facial cutaneous basal cell carcinoma: a first-line imaging technique. J Ultrasound Med. 2013;32(4):567–72.
64. Wortsman X. Ultrasound of Skin Cancer. 2018. Available from: https://link.springer.com/article/10.1007/s40477-019-00379-0
65. Wortsman X, Vergara P, Castro A et al. Ultrasound as predictor of histologic subtypes linked to recurrence in basal cell carcinoma of the skin. J Eur Acad Dermatol Venereol. 2015;29(4):702–7.
66. Ruiz ES, Karia PS, Morgan FC, Schmults CD. The positive impact of radiologic imaging on high-stage cutaneous squamous cell carcinoma management. J Am Acad Dermatol. 2017;76(2):217–25.
67. Strong Rodrigues K, Oliveira-Ribeiro C, de Abreu Fiuza Gomes S, Knobler R. Cutaneous graft-versus-host disease: diagnosis and treatment. Am J Clin Dermatol. 2018;19(1):33–50.

68. Lott DG, Manz R, Koch C, Lorenz RR. Aggressive behavior of nonmelanotic skin cancers in solid organ transplant recipients. Transplant. 2010;90(6):683–7.
69. Lanz J, Bouwes Bavinck JN, Westhuis M et al. Aggressive squamous cell carcinoma in organ transplant recipients. JAMA Dermatol. 2019;155(1):66–71.
70. Ong CK, Chong VFH. Imaging of perineural spread in head and neck tumours. Cancer Imag. 2010;10 Spec no A(1A):S92–8.
71. Catalano O, Caraco C, Mozzillo N, Siani A. Locoregional spread of cutaneous melanoma: sonography findings. AJR Am J Roentgenol. 2010;194(3):735–45.
72. Rossi CR, Mocellin S, Scagnet B et al. The role of preoperative ultrasound scan in detecting lymph node metastasis before sentinel node biopsy in melanoma patients. J Surg Oncol. 2003;83(2):80–4.
73. Ying M, Bhatia KSS, Lee YP, Yuen HY, Ahuja AT. Review of ultrasonography of malignant neck nodes: greyscale, Doppler, contrast enhancement and elastography. Cancer Imag. 2014;13(4):658–69.
74. Tschandl P, Codella N, Akay BN et al. Comparison of the accuracy of human readers versus machine-learning algorithms for pigmented skin lesion classification: an open, web-based, international, diagnostic study. Lancet Oncol. 2019;20(7):938–47.
75. Tschandl P, Rinner C, Apalla Z et al. Human—computer collaboration for skin cancer recognition. Nat Med. 2020;26(8).
76. Lee JJ, English JC. Teledermatology: a review and update. Am J Clin Dermatol. 2018;19(2):253–60.
77. Hasan Z-U, Mokbel R, Goiriz R et al. Teledermatology as a tool for triaging dermatology referrals in organ transplant recipients. Austr J Dermatol. 2019;60(4):e355–7.
78. Green WH, Wang SQ, Cognetta AB, Jr. Total-body cutaneous examination, total-body photography, and dermoscopy in the care of a patient with xeroderma pigmentosum and multiple melanomas. Arch Dermatol. 2009;145(8):910–15.
79. Rocha L, Ferreira PS, Avancini J et al. In vivo confocal microscopy of dermoscopic suspicious lesions in patients with xeroderma pigmentosum: a cross-sectional study. J Am Acad Dermatol. 2019;83(6).

Skin Cancer Prevention, Chemoprevention, and Revision of Immunosuppression

4

Tom Kovitwanichkanont and Alvin H. Chong

INTRODUCTION

Organ transplant recipients (OTRs) have an estimated 65- to 100-fold increased risk of cutaneous squamous cell carcinoma (SCC) and 10-fold increased risk of basal cell carcinoma (BCC).[1] SCCs are frequently multiple and also tend to behave more aggressively in OTRs, with reported rates of metastases of up to 8% compared with 1% in the immunocompetent population.[2,3] In this chapter, we summarize currently available methods of skin cancer prevention, including photoprotection, chemoprevention, and revision of immunosuppression.

PHOTOPROTECTION AND EDUCATION

Photoprotection refers to the avoidance of harmful effects of ultraviolet (UV) radiation on the skin. UV radiation is an important modifiable environmental risk factor for SCC development in OTRs. Patients should be encouraged to use a combination of protective measures and advised not to rely on only one form of protection. These measures include use of protective clothing, hat, and sunglasses, application of broad-spectrum sunscreen with a sun protection factor (SPF) of at least 30, and avoidance of sun exposure especially during the period between 10 am and 3 pm. The World Health Organization (WHO) recommends that photoprotection be applied whenever the UV level is 3 or above.[4]

DOI: 10.1201/9781003001461-4

Sunscreens

A case-control study of 120 immunosuppressed OTRs found that sunscreen application of 5–6 times weekly over a 24-month period was associated with a significant reduction in the number of actinic keratoses and invasive SCCs.[5] Although sunscreen can be effective when used correctly, the efficacy of sunscreen is often limited by its suboptimal application. Studies found that people commonly apply less sunscreen than the recommended amount, resulting in inadequate photoprotection.[6,7] Sunscreen application is also often missed on some crucial areas, such as the ears and posterior neck. Moreover, people tend to forget to reapply sunscreen every 2 hours, rendering it less effective because of sunscreen film evaporation.[8]

Sun Safety Education

Despite the carcinogenic effect of cumulative sun exposure, studies found that many OTRs were poorly adherent to photoprotection measures.[9–13] Older and/or male OTRs were found to be less likely to wear sunscreen than younger and/or female individuals.[9] Reasons for not wearing sunscreen included cosmetic unacceptability, cost of sunscreens, lack of knowledge about the harmful effect of UV, and forgetting to apply sunscreen.[9,14] There appears to be a correlation between sun safety awareness and photoprotection habits[15,16]; therefore, several education strategies to improve OTRs' adherence to photoprotection have been suggested. A British transplant center found a significant improvement in adherence following the use of written information sheets in the clinic waiting rooms and regularly revisiting the issue of photoprotection and self-monitoring.[17] A simple 5-minute education video shown to OTRs within 2 months of transplantation was demonstrated to increase patient knowledge and positively influence sun protective behaviours.[18] In fact, a US study found that an educational video was more effective and appealing than the use of a pamphlet.[19] A multicenter Australian study found that OTRs were more likely to use protective clothing and sunscreen than the nonimmunosuppressed control group; these positive behaviors were attributed to the intensive education of OTRs about photoprotection.[20] Similarly, another Australian study found that the use of multiple sun protection behaviors increased among OTRs even after participation in a research study that did not incorporate any specific education intervention.[21] This finding was attributed to the preventative educational advantages provided by dermatologists and elevated patient awareness of skin cancer risk. These observations were supported by the results of a systematic review, which found that photoprotection education appears to be effective in inducing a behavioral change.[22] However, there have been no studies examining the direct impact of educational interventions on the skin cancer incidence. In addition, optimal timing of education in OTRs is unknown. No studies have yet compared the effectiveness of education in the pre- and posttransplantation periods. By taking lessons from the comprehensive literature on health education in alcohol cessation, maintaining a behavioral change may prove to be as difficult as initiation of the change.[23] Brief multi-contact interventions were found to have the greatest durability in terms of sustaining alcohol abstinence.[23] By extending this logic, it is possible that frequent sun safety education and brief reminders may be a better approach than a single education session.

Although sun-safety education is important, a high level of skin cancer awareness may not necessarily translate into appropriate sun protection behaviours.[24] A European online-based study of 200 OTRs demonstrated that although 90% of the participants were well informed about the risk of skin cancer, most patients continued having exposure to moderate sun intensity at least monthly and only about a quarter of them self-monitored their skin.[24] Therefore, an appropriate prevention strategy needs to be tailored based on the patient's preferences. For example, this study found that younger patients were more inclined to use a cosmetically attractive cream-based approach whereas older patients preferred an oral formulation approach for skin cancer prevention.

CHEMOPREVENTION

Chemoprevention or chemoprophylaxis is defined as oral or topical use of pharmacological or dietary agents to prevent cancer development.[25] In OTRs who have had multiple SCCs, several evidence-based chemopreventive therapies, including acitretin, nicotinamide, topical 5-fluorouracil, and photodynamic therapy, can be offered to reduce the number of new keratinocytes or cancer development. Notably, chemoprevention does not obviate the need for surgical management of malignant lesions, and regular dermatological surveillance is still indispensable.

Acitretin

Three randomized controlled trials demonstrated that acitretin is an effective therapy to significantly reduce the number of actinic keratoses and/or new SCCs in OTRs with a previous history of keratinocyte cancer.[26–28] Following a 6-month treatment with acitretin 30 mg daily, Bavinck et al.[26] demonstrated an absolute risk reduction in the number of keratoses of 41.6% ($P = .008$) and an absolute risk reduction in the cumulative new skin cancers of 84% ($P = .009$). De Sevaux et al.[28] studied the effect of 1 year of treatment with acitretin starting at either 0.4 mg/kg/day or 0.4 mg/kg/day during the first 3 months followed by 0.2 mg/kg/day for the remaining 9 months. They found an absolute risk reduction in the number of keratoses of 50% ($P < .001$) but found no significant reduction in the incidence of SCCs.[28] In a randomized crossover trial, George et al.[27] found an increased risk of SCC in the drug-free period compared with the acitretin period (relative risk 1.44, $P = .002$). The beneficial prophylactic effects of acitretin appeared to be limited to the duration of therapy as significant relapses of skin cancer were reported following discontinuation of acitretin.[26–28] In general, acitretin therapy would need to be continued long-term to achieve effectiveness. The main side effects of acitretin were mucocutaneous dryness, cheilitis, teratogenicity, liver function test abnormalities, and hyperlipidemia. Both beneficial and adverse effects were mostly dose-dependent; therefore, gradual dose escalation starting at 10 mg daily is a practical way to facilitate tolerance of adverse effects.[29] The optimal maintenance dose needs to be personalized depending on the patient's response and adverse effects. In practice, the usual maintenance dosage ranges from 10 mg alternating with 20 mg daily to a dosage of 25 mg daily.[29] As acitretin is highly teratogenic and its metabolite has a very prolonged elimination half-life, pregnancy must be avoided for at least 3 years following treatment discontinuation.[30] Consequently, acitretin is generally avoided in females of childbearing potential.

The following indications have been suggested for starting acitretin chemoprophylaxis in OTRs: multiple keratinocyte cancers (>5 per year), innumerable actinic keratoses and multiple keratinocyte cancers, development of keratinocyte cancers in high-risk areas, high-risk keratinocyte cancer (>20% risk of metastasis), acceleration in the frequency of keratinocyte cancer occurrence, eruptive keratoacanthomas, metastatic keratinocyte cancer, and OTRs with a history of leukemia or lymphoma and keratinocyte cancer.[31–33]

Field-Based Therapy

Actinic keratoses are indicative of photo-damage and have the potential to progress to an invasive SCC, providing a rationale for therapy.[34] In OTRs, actinic keratoses are more common and may undergo an accelerated progression to SCC.[35] Management of actinic keratoses can be either lesion-directed or field-directed. Field cancerization refers to the influence of an environmental carcinogen (UV) on large areas of the skin surface leading to simultaneous actinic damage of epithelial cells, and thus the entire exposed skin surface becomes at risk of malignant transformation.[36] Ultimately, pro-tumorigenic genetic mutations lead to the development of skin cancer within a contiguous field of premalignant cells. For patients with multiple actinic keratoses or field cancerization, field therapy is indicated to reduce the risk of SCC development. The main options for field therapy include topical 5-fluorouracil, topical imiquimod, topical diclofenac, and photodynamic therapy (PDT). A network meta-analysis and a randomized controlled trial comparing field therapies found topical 5% fluorouracil to be the most effective intervention for the treatment of actinic keratoses in nonimmunosuppressed patients.[37,38]

Among the limited literature on field therapy in immunosuppressed OTRs, PDT has been well-studied and demonstrated to reduce the number of new keratotic lesions.[39–43] A split-site randomized controlled trial of 25 renal transplant recipients with clinically normal skin found that prophylactic PDT applied at 6-month intervals for 5 years was effective in the primary prevention of actinic keratoses.[39] At the 3-year follow-up, the number of actinic keratoses was significantly lower in PDT-treated skin compared with that in untreated skin (28% vs. 63%, $P = .005$).[39] An uncontrolled study of 12 OTRs demonstrated a potential prophylactic effect of cyclic PDT applied at 4- to 8-week intervals for 2 years in reducing the incidence of SCC in high-risk OTRs. The median reductions in SCC incidence at 12- and 24-months posttreatment were 79% and 95%, respectively, from the pretreatment counts ($P < .001$).[42] However, a meta-analysis of three randomized trials found that PDT had uncertain effects for prevention of keratinocyte cancer and, although generally well-tolerated, might cause pain at the treatment site during illumination and occasionally for a few days following the procedure.[44] There is currently no head-to-head trial comparing the efficacy of PDT applied at different intervals.

In small studies, topical imiquimod was deemed safe for use in the treatment of superficial BCC, SCC in situ (off-label use), and actinic keratoses in OTRs when applied appropriately.[45–48] In treating actinic keratoses, imiquimod cream is applied three times per week for up to 16 weeks to a limited area of 60–100 cm^2; the clearance rates were reported to be 36%–62.1%.[48,49] It should be used with caution because of a small possible risk of systemic immune activation and organ rejection.[50] In one case report, a 44-year-old renal transplant recipient used topical imiquimod once every 2 days for treatment-resistant viral warts over the arms, hands, and face. He developed biopsy-proven acute tubular necrosis 42 days following the topical application.[50] In general, topical imiquimod is considered safe in OTRs when used in limited areas, and there were no other reported detrimental effects on allograft function.

A case-series study of topical 5% 5-fluorouracil in a small group of OTRs found it to be well-tolerated and efficacious for treatment of actinic keratoses on the face.[51] Topical 5% 5-fluorouracil was applied twice daily for 3 weeks, and the side effects were mild, including erythema, scaling, and pruritus.[51] Interestingly, a small randomized trial showed that a 4-day course of 0.005% calcipotriol ointment combined with 5% 5-fluorouracil was more effective than 5% 5-fluorouracil alone in the treatment of actinic keratoses in immunocompetent patients.[52] In addition, fewer patients in the combined topical group developed an SCC on their treated scalp and face (hazard ratio 0.22, 95% confidence interval [CI] 0.05–0.97).[52] Further research is required to replicate this finding in the OTR population.

A randomized controlled trial of topical diclofenac 3% gel twice daily for 16 weeks demonstrated a greater clearance rate of actinic keratoses compared with that of placebo (41% vs. 0%).[53] Side effects of diclofenac gel were reported to be mild, including erythema and swelling; no graft rejections were detected.[53] A direct head-to-head comparison trial in a transplant cohort is still needed to determine the best treatment for actinic field damage in OTRs.

Nicotinamide

Nicotinamide is a water-soluble vitamin B3 derivative that is found in food, such as meat, fish, nuts, and grains.[54] Nicotinamide was found to enhance deoxyribonucleic acid (DNA) repair and decrease UV-induced immune suppression in human skin.[55] In a cohort of immunocompetent patients with a history of at least two keratinocyte cancers, a randomized controlled trial of nicotinamide 500 mg twice daily vs. placebo found an 11%, 20%, and 30% reduction in the number of actinic keratoses, new BCCs, and SCCs, respectively.[56] The effect of nicotinamide in reducing keratinocyte cancer was not maintained at 6-month follow-up after drug discontinuation.[56] Thus, continuous administration of nicotinamide is required for an ongoing chemoprevention effect. There were no clinically significant differences in the adverse effects between the nicotinamide and placebo groups.

A case-control study of 38 OTRs demonstrated that 88% of OTRs taking nicotinamide 250 mg three times daily had a significant reduction in the size of actinic keratoses.[57] Conversely, 91% of the control group had an increase in the size of actinic keratoses and/or developed new actinic keratoses.[57] A phase II pilot study of nicotinamide 500 mg twice daily in 22 immunosuppressed renal transplant recipients demonstrated a statistically nonsignificant reduction in the number of new keratinocyte cancers (35%) and actinic keratoses (16%).[58] Greater reduction was seen in patients with a previous history of keratinocyte cancer. Phase III trials are currently underway to determine the effectiveness of nicotinamide for keratinocyte cancer prevention in OTRs.[59]

Nicotinamide has a good safety profile and was well tolerated at pharmacological doses of up to 3 g daily over many years.[60] Another form of vitamin B3 is nicotinic acid, also known as niacin. Nicotinic acid is known for its use in cardiology because of its lipid-lowering effect. Although it has the same vitamin actions as nicotinamide, nicotinic acid can cause a vasodilatory effect, including flushing, hypotension, and headache.[61] Misunderstanding between nicotinamide and nicotinic acid may occur, as demonstrated by a case of new-onset flushing following unintentional substitution of nicotinic acid for nicotinamide by a pharmacist.[62] Therefore, it is important to understand the differences between these two forms of vitamin B3 to ensure that our patients take the correct medication.

As there have not yet been any large phase III trials to assess the safety and efficacy of nicotinamide in the transplant population, there is currently no consensus recommendation on when nicotinamide should be started in OTRs. Our approach is to offer nicotinamide 500 mg twice daily to high-risk patients with a history of multiple SCCs, while explaining that its efficacy is not yet proven in the OTR populations.

Capecitabine

Capecitabine is an oral 5-fluorouracil precursor chemotherapeutic agent that has been observed to reduce cutaneous SCC development in OTRs in three retrospective case series.[63–65] Low-dose capecitabine has been used for chemoprevention in OTRs who developed > 2 cutaneous SCCs over a 6-month period. In a case series of 10 OTRs, low-dose capecitabine (0.5–1.5 g/m^2 per day) resulted in a mean reduction of new SCCs of 68% ($P < .005$) during the first 12 months of treatment.[64] Common adverse effects were fatigue, hand-foot-and-mouth syndrome, nausea, reduced renal function, and gout. Moderate-to-severe adverse effects led to dose adjustment in 7 of 10 patients, and 2 of these discontinued treatment because of the adverse effects.

REVISION OF IMMUNOSUPPRESSION

Certain immunosuppressive agents are known to be associated with a higher risk of keratinocyte cancer development. Accordingly, revision of immunosuppression is an important strategy as part of a multidisciplinary approach to curtail the skin cancer morbidity and mortality in OTRs. The early traditional immunosuppressive medications, azathioprine and cyclosporine, have mostly been replaced by newer agents, including mycophenolate mofetil and tacrolimus, as well as sirolimus and everolimus.[66] The risk of cutaneous SCC development appears to be decreasing, which may be partially related to the application of modern immunosuppressive regimens.[66]

Reduction of Immunosuppression

Evidence from a few observational studies suggested that reduction of immunosuppression can decrease the rates of skin cancer development.[67,68] Reduction of immunosuppression may be considered as a neoadjuvant/adjuvant therapeutic strategy in transplant recipients who confront a life-threatening skin cancer or multiple skin cancers with significant morbidity from frequent surgeries.[69] Although no robust prospective data are available on the effectiveness of this strategy, an expert consensus document was developed as a general guidance to physicians who regularly face these difficult clinical dilemmas.[70] This document was based on the consensus opinion of an expert panel who reviewed 13 hypothetical patient scenarios with varying morbidity and mortality risks and subsequently made recommendations on the degree of reduction of systemic immunosuppression (mild, moderate, and severe). Progressively more aggressive reduction of immunosuppression corresponded with greater risks of morbidity and mortality from skin cancer and associated allograft rejection. Because immunosuppressant minimization may be associated with worsened graft survival, this strategy is more practical in renal transplant recipients than in hepatic, pulmonary, or cardiac allograft recipients, as graft rejection is typically not fatal in renal transplant recipients as they may return to dialysis. Considering the potential for graft rejection, the risk-benefit assessment of reducing immunosuppression needs to be carefully carried out in close collaboration with the transplant physician and involve patients in the shared decision-making.

mTOR Inhibitor

Mammalian target of rapamycin (mTOR) is a protein kinase that is involved in the regulation of growth factors and angiogenesis.[71] It is now apparent that many human cancers occur because of dysregulation of the mTOR signaling pathway. The antineoplastic mechanisms of mTOR inhibitors in OTRs are thought to be related to the inhibition of tumor vascularization more so than the direct inhibition of tumor mTOR activation.[72] mTOR inhibitors have been used not only as a therapy in oncology but also as immunosuppression in the transplant population. Therefore, it is unsurprising that interest in mTOR inhibitors has grown enormously with the hope that their properties can be harnessed to prevent allograft rejection and simultaneously reduce skin cancer development in OTRs.

Two meta-analyses found that sirolimus was associated with a 40%–50% reduction in the incidence of keratinocyte cancers compared with controls.[73,74] Evidence suggests that the greatest benefit is seen when the conversion to an mTOR inhibitor-based regimen occurs early.[75–77] Although sirolimus was shown to also be protective against renal cancer, the protective effect was not observed with many other cancer types.[73,74] Sirolimus was associated with an increased risk of mortality, which was mainly because of cardiovascular and infection-related causes, rather than death secondary to graft loss.[74] Subgroup analyses discovered that this elevated mortality risk occurred in patients receiving high-dose sirolimus and induction therapy.[74] When the analysis was limited to low-dose sirolimus trials, the mortality was no longer statistically significant but the skin cancer preventive effect was maintained.[74]

In a 5-year extension randomized trial comparing conversion to sirolimus vs. continuation of calcineurin inhibitor (CNI)-based therapy, there was a significant reduction of keratinocyte cancers that was maintained at 5 years.[76] Reassuringly, there was no significant difference in the mortality rates and graft survival and function between the two groups. The question whether the skin cancer prophylactic effect was because of the introduction of sirolimus or the withdrawal of the CNI is difficult to evaluate. The cessation of CNI likely made an important contribution, as CNIs are known to be carcinogenic through mechanisms such as alteration of DNA repair, inhibition of TP53 expression, and promotion of angiogenesis.[78] Nevertheless, data from the registries found that combination therapy with sirolimus and a CNI could also decrease the incidence of new cancer, suggesting that the effect does not stem from the CNI withdrawal alone. A direct comparison study between sirolimus and combination sirolimus/CNI is still required to clarify this issue.[79,80]

Everolimus is another mTOR inhibitor that has been used as a posttransplantation immunosuppressant. There is currently less data relating to the switch to everolimus than there is for sirolimus.[81] There is limited evidence from case series and case reports demonstrating a low rate of keratinocyte cancer recurrence after introduction of everolimus.[81] However, data from cohort study and national registry showed that de novo or early switch to everolimus did not reduce the risk of keratinocyte cancers.[82,83] Prospective trials are needed.

In clinical practice, the use of an mTOR inhibitor is still limited by a substantial adverse effect profile, causing treatment discontinuation in approximately 40% of sirolimus users.[75,77] There is evidence to suggest that mTOR inhibitors may be associated with a higher incidence of postoperative wound complications.[84,85] In addition, sirolimus was associated with proteinuria and posttransplant glomerulonephritis, which occurs most commonly in OTRs who were converted from a CNI to sirolimus.[86–89] Although an mTOR inhibitor may not be considered a standard first-line immunosuppressive agent, it may be valuable for certain groups of OTRs, such as those with aggressive SCC, in whom the potential benefits outweigh the adverse effects. Future studies are required to develop a risk-benefit model to inform practice and improve decision-making surrounding appropriateness of conversion to an mTOR inhibitor.

Belatacept

Belatacept is a biological immunosuppressive agent approved for use in renal transplant recipients (RTRs). Belatacept is a cytotoxic T-lymphocyte-associated antigen 4 (CTLA-4) fusion antibody that selectively inhibits T-cell activation through costimulation blockade by binding to CD80 and CD81 (B7 protein) and inhibiting CD28 mediated co-stimulation. A retrospective cohort study of 154 RTRs demonstrated that switching from a CNI to belatacept was associated with increased survival free of additional SCC, but not BCC.[90] Other earlier studies found equivocal rates of skin cancers among the belatacept- and CNI-treated RTRs.[91,92]

Reassuringly though, a long-term, phase III randomized trial showed that belatacept was associated with a 38%–45% reduction in the risk of death or graft loss as compared with CNI-based therapy; this effect was sustained at 7 years.[93]

When considering belatacept-based immunosuppression, it is important to note that belatacept is contraindicated in OTRs who are Epstein-Barr virus (EBV) seronegative because of an increased risk of developing posttransplant lymphoproliferative disorder (PTLD).[94] Belatacept is also not recommended in liver transplant recipients because of a higher risk of mortality and graft loss.[95] Although belatacept has the potential to replace CNI as a first-line immunosuppressive therapy, more prospective data is required to assess its favorable skin safety profile.[94]

SUMMARY OF KEY POINTS

- Photoprotection is necessary when the UV level is 3 or above. This advice applies to all people but is particularly important for OTRs given the magnitude of the skin cancer risk.
- Sun safety education should highlight the need to rely on more than one form of photoprotective measures, including correct application of sunscreen, use of protective clothing, and avoidance of UV exposure when possible.
- Acitretin is an effective chemoprophylaxis agent against skin cancer development; the “start low, go slow” approach to dosing can help to improve its tolerability.
- For patients with multiple actinic keratoses or field cancerization, field-directed therapy is indicated.
- Revision of immunosuppression can be a useful neoadjuvant/adjuvant strategy in a multidisciplinary setting to reduce skin cancer morbidity and mortality in OTRs with frequent skin cancers.

REFERENCES

1. Krynitz B, Edgren G, Lindelof B, Baecklund E, Brattstrom C, Wilczek H et al. Risk of skin cancer and other malignancies in kidney, liver, heart and lung transplant recipients 1970 to 2008: a Swedish population-based study. Int J Cancer. 2013;132(6):1429–38.
2. Euvrard S, Kanitakis J, Claudy A. Skin cancers after organ transplantation. N Engl J Med. 2003;348(17):1681–91.
3. Karia PS, Han J, Schmults CD. Cutaneous squamous cell carcinoma: estimated incidence of disease, nodal metastasis, and deaths from disease in the United States, 2012. J Am Acad Dermatol. 2013;68(6):957–66.
4. World Health Organization. The global UV project: a guide and compendium. Nairobi: WHO; 2003.
5. Ulrich C, Jurgensen JS, Degen A, Hackethal M, Ulrich M, Patel MJ et al. Prevention of non-melanoma skin cancer in organ transplant patients by regular use of a sunscreen: a 24 months, prospective, case-control study. Br J Dermatol. 2009;161(Suppl 3):78–84.
6. Neale R, Williams G, Green A. Application patterns among participants randomized to daily sunscreen use in a skin cancer prevention trial. Arch Dermatol. 2002;138(10):1319–25.
7. Stokes R, Diffey B. How well are sunscreen users protected? Photodermatol Photoimmunol Photomed. 1997;13(5–6):186–8.
8. Petersen B, Wulf HC. Application of sunscreen: theory and reality. Photodermatol Photoimmunol Photomed. 2014;30(2–3):96–101.
9. Moloney FJ, Almarzouqi E, O'Kelly P, Conlon P, Murphy GM. Sunscreen use before and after transplantation and assessment of risk factors associated with skin cancer development in renal transplant recipients. Arch Dermatol. 2005;141(8):978–82.
10. Ramsay HM, Fryer AA, Hawley CM, Smith AG, Harden PN. Non-melanoma skin cancer risk in the Queensland renal transplant population. Br J Dermatol. 2002;147(5):950–6.
11. Robinson JK, Rigel DS. Sun protection attitudes and behaviors of solid-organ transplant recipients. Dermatol Surg. 2004;30(4 Pt 2):610–15.
12. Gellen E, Papp BG, Janka EA, Gall T, Paragh G, Emri G et al. Comparison of pre- and post-transplant sun-safe behavior of kidney transplant recipients: what is needed to improve? Photodermatol Photoimmunol Photomed. 2018;34(5):322–9.
13. Mahe E, Morelon E, Fermanian J, Lechaton S, Pruvost C, Ducasse MF et al. Renal-transplant recipients and sun protection. Transplantation. 2004;78(5):741–4.
14. Traboulsi D, Potok OV, Ruzycki SM, Surmanowicz P, Hardin J, Khokhar B et al. Skin cancer knowledge and photoprotective practices of organ transplant recipients. Clin Transplant. 2019;33(5):e13524.
15. Borghi A, Corazza M, Battaglia Y, Maietti E, Minghetti S, Virgili A. What is the key to improving renal transplant recipients' awareness of skin cancer risk? Dermatol. 2016;232(6):715–20.
16. Tuncer Vural A, Karatas Togral A, Kirnap M, Gulec AT, Haberal M. Skin cancer risk awareness and sun-protective behavior among solid-organ transplant recipients. Exp Clin Transplant. 2018;16(Suppl 1):203–7.
17. Rose RF, Moniem K, Seukeran DC, Stables GI, Newstead CG. Compliance of renal transplant recipients with advice about sun protection measures: completing the audit cycle. Transplant Proc. 2005;37(10):4320–2.
18. Patel PH, Bibee K, Lim G, Malik SM, Wu C, Pugliano-Mauro M. Evaluating retention of skin cancer education in kidney transplant recipients reveals a window of opportunity for re-education. Transplant Proc. 2017;49(6):1318–24.
19. Trinh N, Novice K, Lekakh O, Means A, Tung R. Use of a brief educational video administered by a portable video device to improve skin cancer knowledge in the outpatient transplant population. Dermatol Surg. 2014;40(11):1233–9.
20. Leung VKY, Dobbinson SJ, Goodman DJ, Kanellis J, Chong AH. Skin cancer history, sun-related attitudes, behaviour and sunburn among renal transplant recipients versus general population. Australas J Dermatol. 2018;59(2):e106–13.
21. Hartman RI, Green AC, Gordon LG. Sun protection among organ transplant recipients after participation in a skin cancer research study. JAMA Dermatol. 2018;154(7):842–4.
22. Wu SZ, Jiang P, DeCaro JE, Bordeaux JS. A qualitative systematic review of the efficacy of sun protection education in organ transplant recipients. J Am Acad Dermatol. 2016;75(6):1238–44, e5.
23. Jonas DE, Garbutt JC, Amick HR, Brown JM, Brownley KA, Council CL et al. Behavioral counseling after screening for alcohol misuse in primary care: a systematic review and meta-analysis for the U.S. preventive services task force. Ann Intern Med. 2012;157(9):645–54.

24. Basset Seguin N, Malvehy J, Nadal F, Creancier L, Rauly-Lestienne I, Beauchamp R et al. Risk behaviour and patient preferences for an improved non-melanoma skin cancer prevention modality for organ-transplanted patients: a European, multi-country, online patient community study. Eur J Dermatol. 2019;29(5):518–23.
25. Wright TI, Spencer JM, Flowers FP. Chemoprevention of nonmelanoma skin cancer. J Am Acad Dermatol. 2006;54(6):933–46; quiz 47–50.
26. Bavinck JN, Tieben LM, Van der Woude FJ, Tegzess AM, Hermans J, ter Schegget J et al. Prevention of skin cancer and reduction of keratotic skin lesions during acitretin therapy in renal transplant recipients: a double-blind, placebo-controlled study. J Clin Oncol. 1995;13(8):1933–8.
27. George R, Weightman W, Russ GR, Bannister KM, Mathew TH. Acitretin for chemoprevention of non-melanoma skin cancers in renal transplant recipients. Australas J Dermatol. 2002;43(4):269–73.
28. de Sevaux RG, Smit JV, de Jong EM, van de Kerkhof PC, Hoitsma AJ. Acitretin treatment of premalignant and malignant skin disorders in renal transplant recipients: clinical effects of a randomized trial comparing two doses of acitretin. J Am Acad Dermatol. 2003;49(3):407–12.
29. Otley CC, Stasko T, Tope WD, Lebwohl M. Chemoprevention of nonmelanoma skin cancer with systemic retinoids: practical dosing and management of adverse effects. Dermatol Surg. 2006;32(4):562–8.
30. Malka I, Ziv M. Safety of common medications for treating dermatology disorders in pregnant women. Cur Dermatol Rep. 2013;2(4):249–57.
31. Herold M, Good AJ, Nielson CB, Longo MI. Use of topical and systemic retinoids in solid organ transplant recipients: update and review of the current literature. Dermatol Surg. 2019;45(12):1442–9.
32. Perez HC, Benavides X, Perez JS, Pabon MA, Tschen J, Maradei-Anaya SJ et al. Basic aspects of the pathogenesis and prevention of non-melanoma skin cancer in solid organ transplant recipients: a review. Int J Dermatol. 2017;56(4):370–8.
33. O'Reilly Zwald F, Brown M. Skin cancer in solid organ transplant recipients: advances in therapy and management: part II. management of skin cancer in solid organ transplant recipients. J Am Acad Dermatol. 2011;65(2):263–79.
34. Ackerman AB, Mones JM. Solar (actinic) keratosis is squamous cell carcinoma. Br J Dermatol. 2006;155(1):9–22.
35. Johnson TM, Rowe DE, Nelson BR, Swanson NA. Squamous cell carcinoma of the skin (excluding lip and oral mucosa). J Am Acad Dermatol. 1992;26(3 Pt 2):467–84.
36. Kaufmann R. The concept of field cancerization. Melanoma Res. 2010;20:e13–14.
37. Jansen MHE, Kessels J, Nelemans PJ, Kouloubis N, Arits A, van Pelt HPA et al. Randomized trial of four treatment approaches for actinic keratosis. N Engl J Med. 2019;380(10):935–46.
38. Gupta AK, Paquet M. Network meta-analysis of the outcome 'participant complete clearance' in nonimmunosuppressed participants of eight interventions for actinic keratosis: a follow-up on a Cochrane review. Br J Dermatol. 2013;169(2):250–9.
39. Togsverd-Bo K, Omland SH, Wulf HC, Sørensen SS, Hædersdal M. Primary prevention of skin dysplasia in renal transplant recipients with photodynamic therapy: a randomized controlled trial. Am J Transplant. 2015;15(11):2986–90.
40. Wulf HC, Pavel S, Stender I, Bakker-Wensveen CA. Topical photodynamic therapy for prevention of new skin lesions in renal transplant recipients. Acta Derm Venereol. 2006;86(1):25–8.
41. de Graaf YG, Kennedy C, Wolterbeek R, Collen AF, Willemze R, Bouwes Bavinck JN. Photodynamic therapy does not prevent cutaneous squamous-cell carcinoma in organ-transplant recipients: results of a randomized-controlled trial. J Invest Dermatol. 2006;126(3):569–74.
42. Willey A, Mehta S, Lee PK. Reduction in the incidence of squamous cell carcinoma in solid organ transplant recipients treated with cyclic photodynamic therapy. Dermatol Surg. 2010;36(5):652–8.
43. Dragieva G, Prinz BM, Hafner J, Dummer R, Burg G, Binswanger U et al. A randomized controlled clinical trial of topical photodynamic therapy with methyl aminolaevulinate in the treatment of actinic keratoses in transplant recipients. Br J Dermatol. 2004;151(1):196–200.
44. Chung EYM, Palmer SC, Strippoli GFM. Interventions to prevent nonmelanoma skin cancers in recipients of a solid organ transplant: systematic review of randomized controlled trials. Transplant. 2019;103(6): 1206–15.
45. Kovach BT, Stasko T. Use of topical immunomodulators in organ transplant recipients. Dermatol Ther. 2005;18(1):19–27.
46. Das G, Tan B, Nicholls K. Safety and efficacy of a novel short occlusive regimen of imiquimod for selected non-melanotic skin lesions in renal transplant patients. Intern Med J. 2016;46(3):352–5.
47. Ben M'barek L, Mebazaa A, Euvrard S, Frances C, Thervet E, Morel P et al. 5% topical imiquimod tolerance in transplant recipients. Dermatol. 2007;215(2):130–3.

48. Ulrich C, Bichel J, Euvrard S, Guidi B, Proby CM, van de Kerkhof PC et al. Topical immunomodulation under systemic immunosuppression: results of a multicentre, randomized, placebo-controlled safety and efficacy study of imiquimod 5% cream for the treatment of actinic keratoses in kidney, heart, and liver transplant patients. Br J Dermatol. 2007;157(Suppl 2):25–31.
49. Brown VL, Atkins CL, Ghali L, Cerio R, Harwood CA, Proby CM. Safety and efficacy of 5% imiquimod cream for the treatment of skin dysplasia in high-risk renal transplant recipients: randomized, double-blind, placebo-controlled trial. Arch Dermatol. 2005;141(8):985–93.
50. Santos-Juanes J, Esteve A, Mas-Vidal A, Coto-Segura P, Salgueiro E, Gomez E et al. Acute renal failure caused by imiquimod 5% cream in a renal transplant patient: review of the literature on side effects of imiquimod. Dermatol. 2011;222(2):109–12.
51. Ingham AI, Weightman W. The efficacy and safety of topical 5% 5-fluorouracil in renal transplant recipients for the treatment of actinic keratoses. Australas J Dermatol. 2014;55(3):204–8.
52. Cunningham TJ, Tabacchi M, Eliane JP, Tuchayi SM, Manivasagam S, Mirzaalian H et al. Randomized trial of calcipotriol combined with 5-fluorouracil for skin cancer precursor immunotherapy. J Clin Invest. 2017;127(1):106–16.
53. Ulrich C, Johannsen A, Röwert-Huber J, Ulrich M, Sterry W, Stockfleth E. Results of a randomized, placebo-controlled safety and efficacy study of topical diclofenac 3% gel in organ transplant patients with multiple actinic keratoses. Eur J Dermatol. 2010;20(4):482–8.
54. Snaidr VA, Damian DL, Halliday GM. Nicotinamide for photoprotection and skin cancer chemoprevention: a review of efficacy and safety. Exp Dermatol. 2019;28(Suppl 1):15–22.
55. Yiasemides E, Sivapirabu G, Halliday GM, Park J, Damian DL. Oral nicotinamide protects against ultraviolet radiation-induced immunosuppression in humans. Carcinogenesis. 2009;30(1):101–5.
56. Chen AC, Martin AJ, Choy B, Fernandez-Penas P, Dalziell RA, McKenzie CA et al. A phase 3 randomized trial of nicotinamide for skin-cancer chemoprevention. N Engl J Med. 2015;373(17):1618–26.
57. Drago F, Ciccarese G, Parodi A. Nicotinamide for skin-cancer chemoprevention. N Engl J Med. 2016;374(8):789–90.
58. Chen AC, Martin AJ, Dalziell RA, McKenzie CA, Lowe PM, Eris JM et al. A phase II randomized controlled trial of nicotinamide for skin cancer chemoprevention in renal transplant recipients. B J Dermatol. 2016;175(5):1073–5.
59. Gollins CE, Shah A, Sinha K, Khan S, Paul N, Meeajun B et al. Feasibility of a trial to evaluate nicotinamide for chemoprevention of skin cancers in organ transplant recipients in the UK. Br J Dermatol. 2020;183(2).
60. Knip M, Douek IF, Moore WP, Gillmor HA, McLean AE, Bingley PJ et al. Safety of high-dose nicotinamide: a review. Diabetologia. 2000;43(11):1337–45.
61. Chen AC, Damian DL. Nicotinamide and the skin. Australas J Dermatol. 2014;55(3):169–75.
62. Kademian M, Bechtel M, Zirwas M. Case reports: new onset flushing due to unauthorized substitution of niacin for nicotinamide. J Drugs Dermatol. 2007;6(12):1220–1.
63. Jirakulaporn T, Endrizzi B, Lindgren B, Mathew J, Lee PK, Dudek AZ. Capecitabine for skin cancer prevention in solid organ transplant recipients. Clin Transplant. 2011;25(4):541–8.
64. Endrizzi B, Ahmed RL, Ray T, Dudek A, Lee P. Capecitabine to reduce nonmelanoma skin carcinoma burden in solid organ transplant recipients. Dermatol Surg. 2013;39(4):634–45.
65. Endrizzi BT, Lee PK. Management of carcinoma of the skin in solid organ transplant recipients with oral capecitabine. Dermatol Surg. 2009;35(10):1567–72.
66. Plasmeijer EI, Sachse MM, Gebhardt C, Geusau A, Bouwes Bavinck JN. Cutaneous squamous cell carcinoma (cSCC) and immunosurveillance—the impact of immunosuppression on frequency of cSCC. J Eur Acad Dermatol Venereol. 2019;33(Suppl 8):33–7.
67. Dantal J, Hourmant M, Cantarovich D, Giral M, Blancho G, Dreno B et al. Effect of long-term immunosuppression in kidney-graft recipients on cancer incidence: randomised comparison of two cyclosporin regimens. Lancet. 1998;351(9103):623–8.
68. Otley CC, Coldiron BM, Stasko T, Goldman GD. Decreased skin cancer after cessation of therapy with transplant-associated immunosuppressants. Arch Dermatol. 2001;137(4):459–63.
69. Otley CC, Maragh SL. Reduction of immunosuppression for transplant-associated skin cancer: rationale and evidence of efficacy. Dermatol Surg. 2005;31(2):163–8.
70. Otley CC, Berg D, Ulrich C, Stasko T, Murphy GM, Salasche SJ et al. Reduction of immunosuppression for transplant-associated skin cancer: expert consensus survey. Br J Dermatol. 2006;154(3):395–400.
71. de Fijter JW. Cancer and mTOR inhibitors in transplant recipients. Transplant. 2017;101(1):45–55.
72. Geissler EK, Schlitt HJ, Thomas G. mTOR, cancer and transplantation. Am J Transplant. 2008;8(11):2212–18.
73. Yanik EL, Siddiqui K, Engels EA. Sirolimus effects on cancer incidence after kidney transplantation: a meta-analysis. Cancer Med. 2015;4(9):1448–59.

74. Knoll GA, Kokolo MB, Mallick R, Beck A, Buenaventura CD, Ducharme R et al. Effect of sirolimus on malignancy and survival after kidney transplantation: systematic review and meta-analysis of individual patient data. BMJ. 2014;349:g6679.
75. Campbell SB, Walker R, Tai SS, Jiang Q, Russ GR. Randomized controlled trial of sirolimus for renal transplant recipients at high risk for nonmelanoma skin cancer. Am J Transplant. 2012;12(5):1146–56.
76. Dantal J, Morelon E, Rostaing L, Goffin E, Brocard A, Tromme I et al. Sirolimus for secondary prevention of skin cancer in kidney transplant recipients: 5-year results. J Clin Oncol. 2018;36(25):2612–20.
77. Hoogendijk-van den Akker JM, Harden PN, Hoitsma AJ, Proby CM, Wolterbeek R, Bouwes Bavinck JN et al. Two-year randomized controlled prospective trial converting treatment of stable renal transplant recipients with cutaneous invasive squamous cell carcinomas to sirolimus. J Clin Oncol. 2013;31(10):1317–23.
78. Hojo M, Morimoto T, Maluccio M, Asano T, Morimoto K, Lagman M et al. Cyclosporine induces cancer progression by a cell-autonomous mechanism. Nature. 1999;397(6719):530–4.
79. Lim WH, Russ GR, Wong G, Pilmore H, Kanellis J, Chadban SJ. The risk of cancer in kidney transplant recipients may be reduced in those maintained on everolimus and reduced cyclosporine. Kidney Int. 2017;91(4):954–63.
80. Kauffman HM, Cherikh WS, Cheng Y, Hanto DW, Kahan BD. Maintenance immunosuppression with target-of-rapamycin inhibitors is associated with a reduced incidence of de novo malignancies. Transplant. 2005;80(7):883–9.
81. Holdaas H, De Simone P, Zuckermann A. Everolimus and malignancy after solid organ transplantation: a clinical update. J Transplant. 2016:4369574.
82. Gräger N, Leffler M, Gottlieb J, Fuge J, Warnecke G, Gutzmer R et al. Risk factors for developing nonmelanoma skin cancer after lung transplantation. J Skin Cancer. 2019:7089482.
83. Ying T, Wong G, Lim W, Kanellis J, Pilmore H, Campbell S et al. De novo or early conversion to everolimus and long-term cancer outcomes in kidney transplant recipients: a trial-based linkage study. Am J Transplant. 2018;18(12):2977–86.
84. Dean PG, Lund WJ, Larson TS, Prieto M, Nyberg SL, Ishitani MB et al. Wound-healing complications after kidney transplantation: a prospective, randomized comparison of sirolimus and tacrolimus. Transplant. 2004;77(10):1555–61.
85. Kuppahally S, Al-Khaldi A, Weisshaar D, Valantine HA, Oyer P, Robbins RC et al. Wound healing complications with de novo sirolimus versus mycophenolate mofetil-based regimen in cardiac transplant recipients. Am J Transplant. 2006;6(5 Pt 1):986–92.
86. Dittrich E, Schmaldienst S, Soleiman A, Hörl WH, Pohanka E. Rapamycin-associated post-transplantation glomerulonephritis and its remission after reintroduction of calcineurin-inhibitor therapy. Transpl Int. 2004;17(4):215–20.
87. Izzedine H, Brocheriou I, Frances C. Post-transplantation proteinuria and sirolimus. N Engl J Med. 2005;353(19):2088–9.
88. Letavernier E, Pe'raldi MN, Pariente A, Morelon E, Legendre C. Proteinuria following a switch from calcineurin inhibitors to sirolimus. Transplant. 2005;80(9):1198–203.
89. Aliabadi AZ, Pohanka E, Seebacher G, Dunkler D, Kammerstätter D, Wolner E et al. Development of proteinuria after switch to sirolimus-based immunosuppression in long-term cardiac transplant patients. Am J Transplant. 2008;8(4):854–61.
90. Wang M, Mittal A, Colegio OR. Belatacept reduces skin cancer risk in kidney transplant recipients. J Am Acad Dermatol. 2019;82.
91. Durrbach A, Pestana JM, Florman S, Del Carmen Rial M, Rostaing L, Kuypers D et al. Long-term outcomes in belatacept- versus cyclosporine-treated recipients of extended criteria donor kidneys: final results from BENEFIT-EXT, a phase III randomized study. Am J Transplant. 2016;16(11):3192–201.
92. Grinyo JM, Del Carmen Rial M, Alberu J, Steinberg SM, Manfro RC, Nainan G et al. Safety and efficacy outcomes 3 years after switching to belatacept from a calcineurin inhibitor in kidney transplant recipients: results from a phase 2 randomized trial. Am J Kidney Dis. 2017;69(5):587–94.
93. Vincenti F, Rostaing L, Grinyo J, Rice K, Steinberg S, Gaite L et al. Belatacept and long-term outcomes in kidney transplantation. N Engl J Med. 2016;374(4):333–43.
94. Sam T, Gabardi S, Tichy EM. Risk evaluation and mitigation strategies: a focus on belatacept. Prog Transplant. 2013;23(1):64–70.
95. Klintmalm GB, Feng S, Lake JR, Vargas HE, Wekerle T, Agnes S et al. Belatacept-based immunosuppression in de novo liver transplant recipients: 1-year experience from a phase II randomized study. Am J Transplant. 2014;14(8):1817–27.

Topical and Intralesional Modalities for Actinic Keratoses and Nonmelanoma Skin Cancer in Transplant Recipients

5

Stacy McMurray, Lee Wheless, and Allison Hanlon

INTRODUCTION

Solid organ transplant recipients (SOTR) have a markedly increased risk of developing actinic keratoses (AK) and nonmelanoma skin cancers (NMSC) when compared with the general population secondary to long-term immunosuppression and impaired deoxyribonucleic acid (DNA) repair mechanisms.[1–3] Precursor lesions like AK have an increased risk of progression to malignancy and a lower likelihood of spontaneous regression.[4,5] Although surgical treatment is ideal for many NMSC given pathological margin control, SOTR often have areas of field cancerization (diffuse AK and NMSC) that necessitate treatment tailored to large anatomical areas.

There is a relative paucity of high-quality randomized controlled trials (RCTs) for topical and intralesional therapy of keratinocyte carcinomas and AK. Limited evidence for specific therapeutic regimens in SOTR presents a therapeutic challenge, and the safety profiles and efficacy of individual treatments may vary when compared with those in the immunocompetent population. This chapter outlines the topical and intralesional treatment options for AK and NMSC in the transplant population. The goals of therapy are similar to those of immunocompetent patients, to prevent invasive disease and optimize patient quality of life.

 DOI: 10.1201/9781003001461-5

SUNSCREEN

The role of photoprotection must not be underestimated as a prevention strategy. A prospective case-control study by Ulrich et al.[6] demonstrated the impact of sunscreen use and education in SOTR. The control group developed new AK and eight new invasive squamous cell carcinomas (SCC) compared with the sunscreen group, who remained free of new SCC. Despite the evidence for photoprotection as a preventative strategy, compliance with sun protection in SOTR has been shown to be poor, partly due to limited education, cost, and practicality.[7,8]

Recent evidence suggests that sun protective behaviors in the transplant population may be improving. A questionnaire-based follow-up study showed a significant increase in the proportion of renal transplant recipients taking appropriate precautions over a 6-year period.[9] Additionally, participation in a skin cancer research study was linked to an increase in multiple sun protection behaviors among organ transplant recipients.[10] It is worth noting the possibility for recall and response bias in these studies. However, given the potential impact of photoprotection on the continued development of AK and NMSC, patient counseling on photoprotective strategies should be an integral part of the transplant dermatology practice.

ACTINIC KERATOSES/FIELD CANCERIZATION

The combination of chronic immunosuppression and protracted exposure to a carcinogen such as ultraviolet light often leads to field cancerization (Figure 5.1). Cutaneous field cancerization is a term used to describe the group of alterations observed in chronically photodamaged skin with multiple foci of non-melanocytic cutaneous neoplasms.[11] Clinically, this manifests as diffuse AK and NMSC. The goals of treatment include clearing the background damage to assess for higher risk lesions such as invasive SCC and decreasing the burden of actinic damage, which may be uncomfortable and even disfiguring for patients.

Evidence for the treatment of AK stems largely from RCTs and treatment guidelines developed in immunocompetent patients. Thus, it can be difficult to determine the optimal treatment regimen in SOTR. Although destructive modalities such as cryotherapy may be effective for individual lesions, they poorly address diffuse disease and may be impractical as a treatment option for larger areas.[12–14] Field treatments studied in SOTR include topical 5-fluorouracil (5-FU), imiquimod, cyclooxygenase (COX) inhibitors, ingenol mebutate, and photodynamic therapy (PDT). Figure 5.2 outlines treatment options for AK in SOTR.

CRYOTHERAPY

Cryotherapy with liquid nitrogen is an effective treatment modality for individual or limited numbers of AK and some early, low-risk NMSC (i.e., small, diameter <1 cm, SCC in situ [SCCis] or superficial basal cell carcinoma [sBCC] on the trunk or extremities) with reported short-term clearance rates up to 90% in immunocompetent patients for select BCC.[15] One study of AK in SOTR showed comparable clearance rates with methyl aminolevulinate (MAL)-PDT versus cryotherapy (77% vs. 74%, respectively) at 3 months, but field clearance and complete clearance were not assessed.[13] Therefore, although cryotherapy is an effective focal treatment modality, it should be used in conjunction with field-directed therapy to adequately address diffuse disease such as that often seen in SOTR. Thicker,

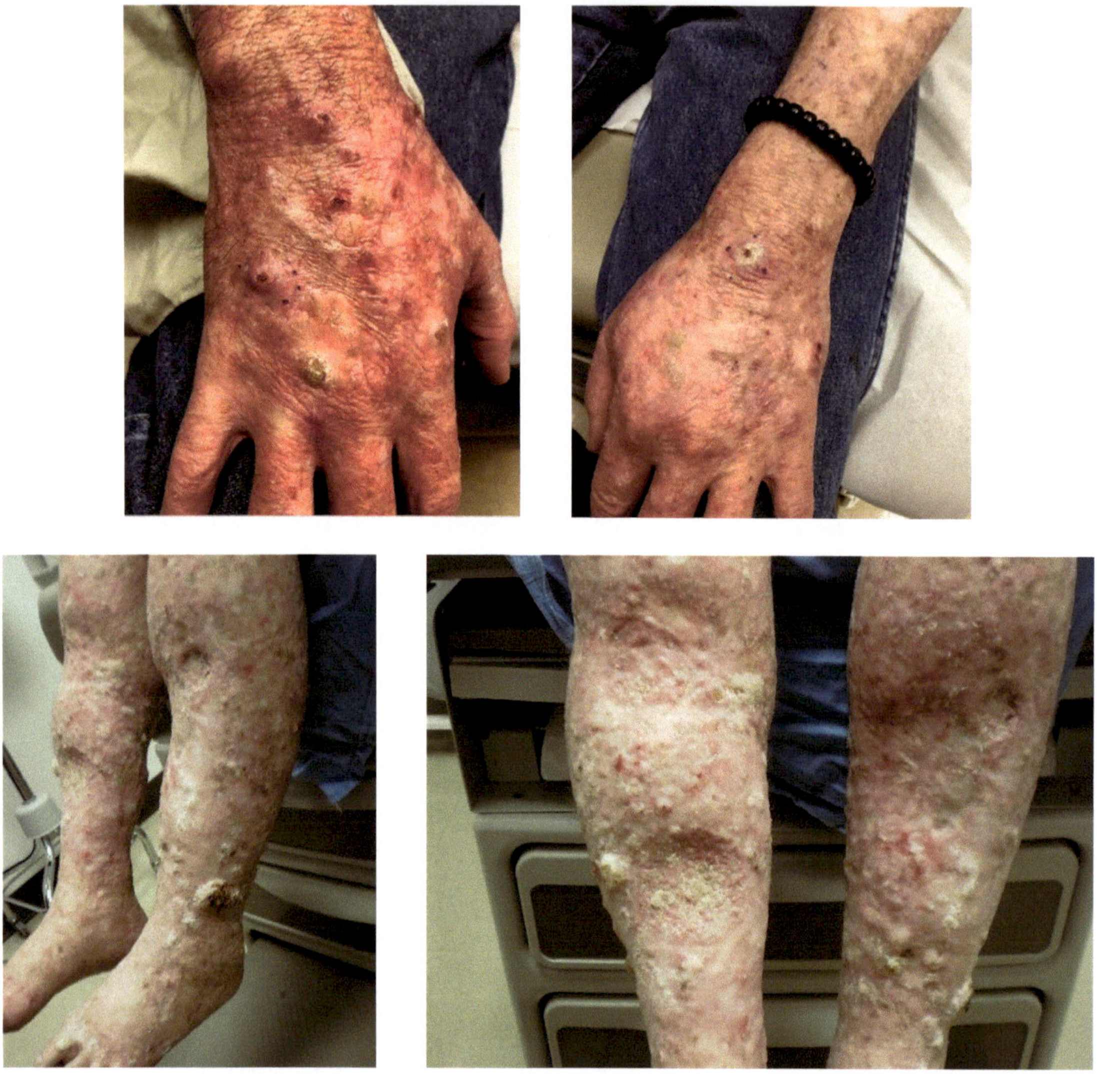

FIGURE 5.1 Field cancerization of the dorsal hands (top photos) and legs (bottom photos) showing multiple AK and NMSC in patients with a history of solid organ transplant.

hyperkeratotic actinic keratosis can be treated effectively with this destructive technique. A destructive technique may also be necessary when the effectiveness of topical treatments could be compromised by lack of drug penetration.

5- FLUOROURACIL

Topical 5-FU inhibits thymidylate synthetase, which inhibits DNA synthesis and leads to cell death. 5-FU cream has been used alone and in combination with topical tretinoin or alpha/beta hydroxy acids to reduce the number of NMSC and AK in SOTR.[14,16] The addition of topical tretinoin or alpha/beta hydroxy acids

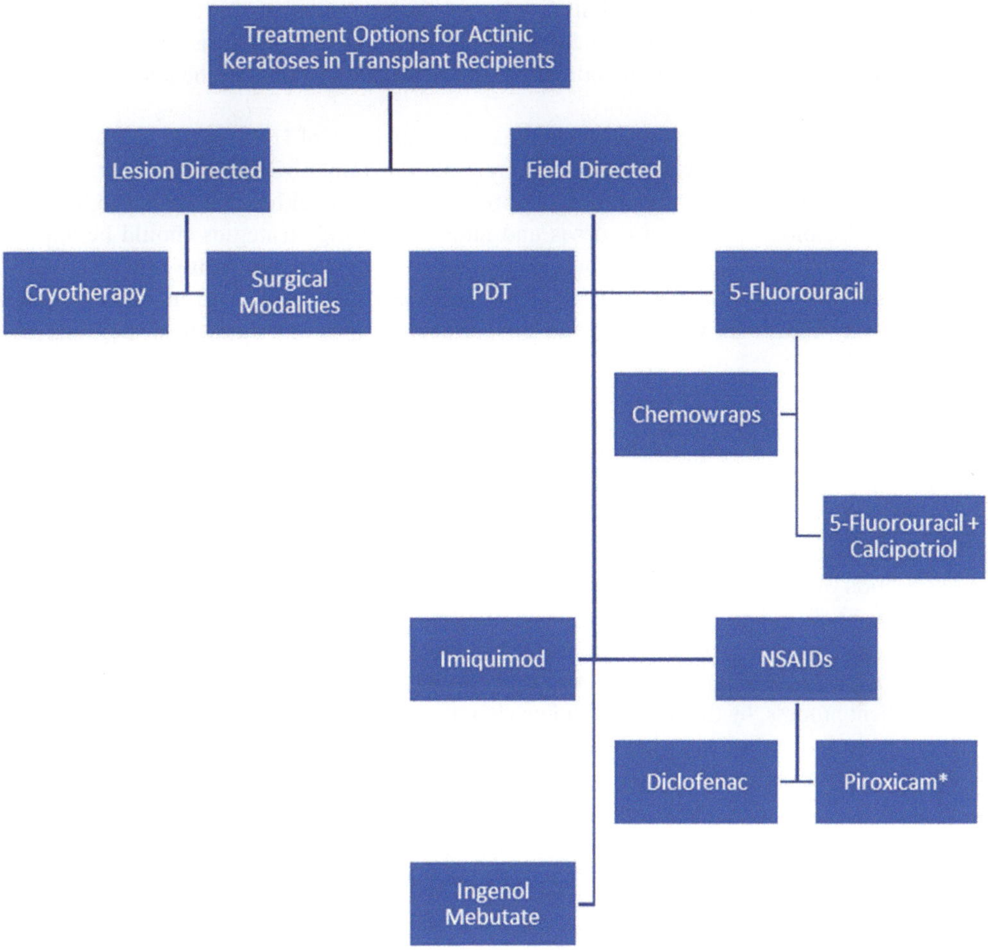

FIGURE 5.2 Topical treatment options for actinic keratoses in solid organ transplant recipients. *Evidence limited to a proprietary blend.

applied 1–2 times daily for 2 weeks prior to treatment with 5-FU is thought to assist in drug delivery by decreasing the thickness of the stratum corneum. In a study of renal transplant patients, 5-FU cream applied twice daily for 3 weeks resulted in 71% of patients with a 75% or greater clearance of AK sustained at 12 months.[17] Mean clearance rates were 98% at week 8 and 79% at 12 months.[17] Local skin reactions are common with 5-FU cream and include erythema, crusting, and erosions. Brisk responses may be treated with a low to mid potency topical corticosteroid to hasten healing and aid in patient comfort without compromising treatment results.[18]

Although there are few comparative studies, one study in SOTR showed the mean lesional area reduction for MAL-PDT to be 100% versus 79% for 5-FU.[16] However, complete clearance of lesional fields at 6 months was 89% in the MAL-PDT group and only 11% in the 5-FU group.[16] Treatment with PDT will be discussed further subsequently.

5-FU has demonstrated efficacy both as a monotherapy and in combination with calcipotriol (calcipotriene) for the treatment of AK. Calcipotriol induces production of thymic stromal lymphopoietin (TSLP), an epithelium-derived cytokine that induces tissue-resident T cells and generates robust antitumor immunity in barrier defective skin.[19] An RCT of 131 patients examined 5-FU (5%) combined 1:1

with calcipotriol (0.005%) applied twice daily for 4 days. Combination therapy showed an 87.8% mean reduction in the number of AK vs. 26.3% for 5-FU alone.[19] Although this study has not yet been replicated in the SOTR population, it shows the potential of the treatment as an effective therapeutic option with a shorter treatment course.

In practice, the authors use compounded 5-FU and calcipotriol (1:1) twice daily for 5 days for treatment of AK, and twice daily for 7 days for treatment of select SCCis. For patients with severe field cancerization, compounded 5FU and calcipotriol twice daily with occlusion at night for 7 days can be considered. Longer treatment courses and alternate dosing strategies should be approached with caution as this combination can produce an intense inflammatory response that peaks 4–5 days after cessation of treatment. Anecdotally, this treatment regimen is effective in immunocompetent patients and SOTR. Additional studies are needed to elucidate optimal treatment strategies and clearances rates in SOTR.

CHEMOWRAPS

Weekly application of 5-FU under occlusion, often referred to as chemowraps (Figure 5.3), provides an option for treatment of field cancerization of the extremities in SOTR.[20–24] A total of 20 grams of topical 5-FU is applied once weekly in the clinic and occluded with zinc oxide-impregnated gauze followed by a compression wrap that remains in place for 7 days. The wraps can be removed in the clinic at follow up or, for a more efficient process, by the patient at home prior to the next appointment. The wraps are replaced once weekly for a minimum of 4 weeks. The benefits of chemowraps include a high level of patient compliance as well as the combination of compression and zinc oxide to assist in wound healing, particularly in cases of venous insufficiency of the lower extremities.

Small case series using chemowraps in immunocompetent patients have shown a reduction in clinical lesions of hypertrophic AK (HAK) and SCC in patients treated with 4–20 weekly sessions with improvement lasting up to 3 years.[23,24] An open study of weekly chemowraps for AK showed a response rate of 60% and a complete response rate of 20% after an average of 9.6 sessions; the response rate for treatment of SCCis was 64% (22). Treatments were generally well-tolerated, and common side effects

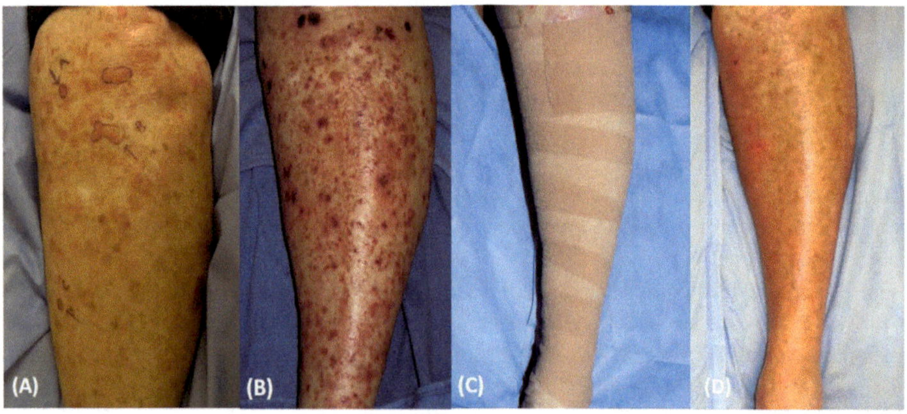

FIGURE 5.3 Chemowraps with 5% 5-fluorouracil cream in an immunocompetent patient. **(a)** Right leg before treatment; **(b)** right leg during treatment; **(c)** right leg with chemowrap in place; and **(d)** right leg following treatment. (Courtesy of Christopher J. Miller, MD).

included irritation and contact dermatitis.[22] Compressive chemowraps are contraindicated in patients with moderate-to-severe peripheral artery disease (PAD) and should be used with caution in patients with mild-to-moderate PAD.[25] Further studies are needed to determine the effectiveness of chemowraps in the transplant population.

IMIQUIMOD

Imiquimod is an immunomodulator of the imidazoquinolinone group that binds to toll-like receptor 7 (TLR-7), inducing a local and systemic innate immune response leading to antiviral and antitumor effects.[26,27] Imiquimod is approved for treatment of AK, external genital verruca, and sBCC. Although there is a theoretical concern that imiquimod could cause allograft rejection through increased levels of interferon (IFN), imiquimod has been used safely in limited areas in SOTR.[28,29] Rejection has not been reported when used in limited areas; the literature cites only a single report of reversible acute tubular necrosis in a patient with a third renal transplant after use of imiquimod 5% cream.[30]

Ulrich et al.[28] demonstrated the safety and efficacy of 5% imiquimod three times weekly for 16 weeks used to treat a 100 cm^2 field of AK in 43 SOTR (heart, liver, and kidney). The authors reported a 75% clearance of AK in the treated areas, and complete clearance was achieved in 62.1% of patients versus 0% in the vehicle group.[28] There was no indication of graft rejection in the treatment group. In a randomized study of immunocompetent patients, Krawtchenko et al.[12] found significantly higher rates of sustained histological clearance and improved cosmetic outcomes with the use of imiquimod to treat AK when compared with cryotherapy and 5-FU. Rates of sustained histological clearance and cosmetic outcomes with imiquimod have not been studied in the transplant population.

Although imiquimod has demonstrated safety for use in limited treatment areas in SOTR, alternative treatment modalities should be considered to cover large anatomical areas.

PHOTODYNAMIC THERAPY

Treatment of field disease with PDT has been relatively well-studied in the SOTR population when compared with other topical modalities.[13,31] A photosensitizing precursor of protoporphyrin IX (PpIX), such as aminolevulinic acid (ALA) or its methyl ester methyl aminolevulinate (MAL), is applied to the treatment area. Illumination with an appropriate wavelength of light (red or blue) results in generation of reactive oxygen species (ROS) that target rapidly dividing cells.[32] MAL-PDT has also been shown to correct abnormal proliferation-related gene profiles and aberrantly expressed cancer-associated genes while inducing expression of dermal extracellular matrix genes in photo-exposed skin.[33] ALA (10% gel or 20% solution) is the only Food and Drug Administration (FDA) approved photosensitizer in the United States, but MAL is available in Europe and several other countries. ALA and MAL are generally thought of as equivalent and produce comparable clearance rates.[34]

Clinical response to PDT varies with the anatomical site (i.e., lower clearance rates on hands than on the face and scalp) and treatment protocol. High initial complete clearance rates have been shown with serial sessions of PDT with an interval of 1–2 weeks between treatments.[35–37] In clinical practice, cyclic PDT is often performed every 3–6 months in high-risk patients. Debulking hyperkeratotic lesions with light curettage or use of topical keratolytics such as propylene glycol, carbamide, salicylic acid, paraffin, and urea may enhance efficacy via improved drug delivery.[35] Other modalities that may improve drug delivery include tape stripping, microdermabrasion, microneedling, and ablative fractional carbon dioxide laser (AFXL).[38]

A review of the evidence for local interventions in the treatment of AK in SOTR found the bulk of the available evidence was for the use of MAL-PDT.[39] MAL-PDT also produced the highest clearance rates of all interventions.[39] In one RCT, complete clearance was seen in 13 of 17 (76.4%) SOTR and a lesion reduction of 90% was seen after two consecutive treatments of MAL-PDT.[36] A randomized, intraindividual controlled trial in 28 SOTR found two treatments of PDT to be significantly more effective than imiquimod 5% cream with a lesion-specific clearance of 78% vs. 61% and a complete clearance of 40% vs. 28%, respectively.[29] Recent evidence suggests that PDT is effective both as a treatment *and* as a preventive measure for AK/SCC in SOTR.[40]

Combination treatments have also been studied. One study demonstrated 74% clearance of AK with AFXL used in conjunction with daylight PDT.[41] Another RCT with 10 patients compared AFXL-assisted MAL-PDT with AFXL alone.[42] Lesion clearance was significantly higher for AFXL-PDT (73%) compared with that of AFXL alone (31%) after 4 months.[42] Overall, 30% of patients in the AFXL-PDT group versus 10% in the monotherapy group experienced hypopigmentation. Side effects were more pronounced in the combination group. PDT should be considered as a first-line agent for field-directed therapy in SOTR given the current evidence. The benefits of PDT include its dual use for treatment of AK and NMSC, limited dependence on patient compliance, and ability to treat large anatomical areas. In addition, PDT may also play a preventive role in the development of AK/SCC, which makes it an ideal therapeutic option for SOTR.

INGENOL MEBUTATE

Evidence for use of Ingenol mebutate in SOTR is limited to two case reports and a small single-arm, open-label, investigator-initiated study. The case reports demonstrated clinical response to ingenol mebutate in renal transplant recipients without unexpected adverse events when applied once daily for 3 days.[43,44] The open-label study investigated the safety and tolerability of topical ingenol mebutate 0.015% gel in 20 SOTR (11 renal, 9 lung).[45] Patients with 4–20 AK in a 100-cm^2 area on the cheek or forehead were treated with four single-dose tubes of ingenol mebutate 0.015% gel per day for 3 consecutive days. Partial and complete clearance of AK occurred at rates of 60% and 40%, respectively, and no unexpected adverse events were noted.[45] More information is needed prior to recommendation of ingenol mebutate as a first-line agent for treatment of AK. Medication cost is also a consideration given the quantity of medication needed to cover larger anatomic areas, as ingenol mebutate is dispensed in limited quantities (0.47 g per tube).

NONSTEROIDAL ANTI-INFLAMMATORY DRUGS/DICLOFENAC

Chronically sun-damaged skin, AK, and NMSC have increased activity of inflammatory prostaglandins such as cyclooxygenase-2 (COX-2).[46] Nonsteroidal anti-inflammatory drugs (NSAIDs) including diclofenac (inhibits COX-2) and piroxicam (inhibits COX-1) have been used topically with variable results. A case series of 6 SOTR with multiple NMSC and AK treated with diclofenac 3% gel once daily for 16 weeks showed complete clearance in 50% (3/6) and partial clearance in 33% (1/6).[47] Ulrich et al.[48] investigated 32 SOTR in an RCT comparing diclofenac sodium 3% applied twice daily with vehicle. Complete clearance was achieved in 41% (9/22) of the active group vs. 0% (0/6) of the vehicle group, and lesion

TABLE 5.1 Topical Treatment Regimens for Actinic Keratoses and Field Cancerization in the Transplant Population.

TREATMENT AGENT	*DOSING*	*COMMENTS*
5-Fluorouracil 5% cream	Apply twice daily for 2–4 weeks	Pretreatment with a topical retinoid for 1–2 weeks may enhance drug delivery
5-Fluorouracil 5% cream + calcipotriol 0.005% cream	Mixed in a 1:1 ratio and applied twice daily for 4–7 days	Not studied in SOTR
Chemowraps (5-FU 5% cream)	Weekly applications of 20 g 5% 5-FU cream covered with zinc oxide-impregnated gauze and compression wraps in clinic for at least 4 weeks	Requires weekly visits Caution in patients with peripheral artery disease
Photodynamic therapy (PDT)	One treatment session with either red or blue light for mild disease (e.g., AK only). Repeat every 3–6 months.	For low-risk NMSC, two treatment cycles, preferably using a red light source. One cycle is the equivalent of two sessions of PDT 1–2 weeks apart with a period of 3–4 months between cycles.
Imiquimod 5% cream	Apply three times weekly for 16 weeks	Limit treatment areas to 100 cm^2 field in SOTR
Ingenol mebutate	Apply once daily for 3 days	Limited evidence in SOTR
NSAIDs		
Diclofenac 3% gel	Apply 1–2 times daily for 16 weeks	Long treatment regimen may limit adherence
Piroxicam + SPF 50 sunscreen filter		Evidence limited to proprietary medical device

Note: These are off label in the immunocompromised population.

clearance was 53% vs. 17% at week 16, respectively.[48] A case series of 10 SOTR showed reduction in AK and improvement in field cancerization with the use of a medical device containing piroxicam and SPF 50+ sunscreen filters.[49] Piroxicam also was shown to induce apoptosis and suppress the activity of metalloproteinase 2 and 9, both of which are associated with tumorigenesis.[49]

Although topical COX inhibitors have shown some efficacy in the treatment of AK, protracted treatment courses require a motivated and compliant patient. There are no comparative studies examining the use of diclofenac with other treatment modalities.

Table 5.1 summarizes the topical treatment regimens for AK and field cancerization in SOTR.

NONMELANOMA SKIN CANCER

Invasive Squamous Cell Carcinoma

Multiple population-based studies have demonstrated that invasive SCC in SOTR have an increased likelihood for aggressive disease and may be regarded as high-risk lesions.[50–54] The preferred treatments for invasive SCC are those that provide pathological confirmation of complete removal, such as Mohs micrographic surgery (MMS) or conventional surgical excision to prevent local recurrence and metastasis. When surgical treatment is not an option, alternative treatment methods such as topical or intralesional therapies may be considered. Carefully selected invasive SCC, such as small, well-differentiated lesions (e.g., keratoacanthomas, SCC/KA) on low-risk sites may be considered for destructive therapy (electrodessication and curettage, EDC) with the caveat that pathological confirmation of complete tumor extirpation is not achieved. Cryotherapy is rarely used for management of SCC because of the difficulty in achieving the uniform tissue destruction needed for tumor clearance and the potential for scarring associated with this treatment modality.

Squamous Cell Carcinoma In Situ

Surgical treatment options for SCCis in SOTR are similar to those of immunocompetent patients – MMS, conventional excision, and EDC. Topical treatment options include imiquimod, 5-FU, PDT, and combination therapies. Although topical therapy offers an element of convenience to patients, there are no large systematic studies that support the use of topical therapy for SCCis. The disadvantages of therapy include prolonged treatment periods requiring patient adherence to treatment. Clearance rates and application protocols vary widely. The clinician must keep in mind that treatment protocols for many topical therapies have not been fully elucidated, and more studies are needed to identify optimal treatment protocols for these agents in SOTR.

A review of topical treatments for SCCis in immunocompetent patients found that studies in the current literature report on <50 lesions with variable forms of medication and differing treatment protocols; the most efficacious regimens lasted more than 4 weeks.[55] Clearance rates for 5-FU in studies of 10 or more lesions ranged from 69.2% to 100% with a wide range of recurrence rates of 0% to 33.3%. Clearance rates of imiquimod were 73% to 93% with recurrence rate of 0% in the three largest studies.[55] Results of this review in non-SOTR demonstrated variable response rates for topical treatment of SCCis with overall clearance rates comparatively lower than that of surgical modalities.

Evidence for use of imiquimod and 5-FU in the treatment of SCCis in SOTR is limited to small studies. Imiquimod is safe for use in SOTR when applied to limited areas.[28,29,56,57] Off-label use of imiquimod to treat SCCis in immunocompetent patients has shown efficacy when applied once daily for 16 weeks.[58] Alternative dosing strategies have also been used in small studies of SOTR. One study demonstrated the clearance of 4 of 5 SCCis with the use of imiquimod applied under occlusion for 7 days in renal transplant recipients.[59]

Combinations therapies can be considered. Imiquimod and 5% 5-FU have been used in combination to treat SCCis.[60] A small study showed complete or near-complete clinical resolution of AK and SCCis in four SOTR treated sequentially with light curettage of hyperkeratotic lesions followed by application of 5-FU 5% cream twice daily for 5 days and PDT with a 1-hour incubation on day 6.[61]

Studies suggest that PDT (MAL-PDT and ALA-PDT) is equally or more efficacious in the treatment of SCCis when compared with topical therapy in immunocompetent patients.[62–64] However, there are no large RCTs evaluating the use of PDT to treat SCCis in SOTR. In an open-label, single-center, randomized, intrapatient comparative study, Perrett et al.[16] examined 5-FU versus MAL-PDT in eight SOTR with posttransplant epidermal dysplasia (SCCis, AK). Results showed that MAL-PDT was a more effective and cosmetically acceptable treatment for epidermal dysplasia when compared with 5-FU. Complete clearance rates were 89% for MAL-PDT versus 11% for 5-FU.[16] An open label, prospective trial in twenty SOTR found that PDT with 20% 5-ALA produced initial response rates for AK and SCCis comparable to those in immunocompetent patients.[65] Complete response rates at 4, 12, and 48 weeks were 86%, 68%, and 48%, respectively.[65]

Serial PDT with close monitoring is recommended in areas of field cancerization, particularly as an adjunctive therapy or in patients with contraindications to alternative options such as systemic chemoprophylaxis with acitretin. Additional, larger studies are needed to fully elucidate optimal treatment protocols and clearance rates for SCCis in SOTR.

Basal Cell Carcinoma

Nonsurgical treatment modalities for BCC in SOTR are similar to those for SCCis; however, there is relatively more data specific to treatment of BCC in SOTR.

Imiquimod

As previously discussed, the safety profile of imiquimod in SOTR has been demonstrated when used in limited areas. In immunocompetent patients, imiquimod is approved for treatment of sBCC with dosing 5 nights weekly for 6 weeks with clearance rates of up to 75%. However, multiple dosing strategies have been used, with more frequent dosing regimens yielding increased clearance rates. One study in immunocompetent patients showed 100% histological clearance of sBCC with twice daily dosing for 6 weeks when compared with once daily (87.9%) or three times weekly (69.7%) dosing.[66] For small, nodular BCC (nBCC), imiquimod was most effective when used daily for 12 weeks.[66]

A small, open-label study evaluated use of imiquimod 5% cream for treatment of BCC in transplant patients. Clearance rates were highest in sBCC > nBCC > infiltrative BCC (iBCC) when used 4 nights weekly for 6 weeks or 5 nights weekly for 5 weeks.[67] An Australian study of 10 renal transplant recipients showed complete clearance in 5 of 5 sBCC with imiquimod used under occlusion for 7 days.[59]

Imiquimod may be considered as a first-line therapy for small, low-risk subtypes of BCC in low-risk anatomical areas (e.g., trunk, extremities). Patient compliance with protracted treatment regimens may be problematic.

Photodynamic Therapy

PDT is an effective treatment for sBCC and thin (<2 mm) nBCC in both immunocompetent and immunosuppressed populations.[34,68–70] Clearance rates are highest for sBCC (87–97%); response rates for nBCC are lower but may increase up to 90% with prior tumor debulking.[70] Red light is the preferred illumination for PDT used to treat BCC given its greater depth of tissue penetration when compared to blue light. The largest study of PDT for treatment of BCC in SOTR showed no statistically significant difference in recurrence rates between SOTR and nontransplant patients (22.6% vs. 15.2%, respectively) with a 3-year follow up.[71]

One benefit of PDT is the ability to target a broad anatomical area with clinician-directed therapy that does not depend on patient adherence to a long-term daily treatment course. Additionally, PDT may provide improved post procedural cosmetic outcomes when compared with surgical intervention.[68]

The recommended treatment regimen for BCC based on European guidelines is two treatment cycles using a red-light source (one cycle is the equivalent of two sessions of PDT 1–2 weeks apart) with a period of 3–4 months between cycles.[72] Alternative light sources include blue light and daylight PDT.[72,73]

Limitations of PDT for treatment of BCC include procedural pain and variation of clinical response with anatomical site (i.e., lesions on the face and extremities are less responsive than those on the trunk) and subtype of BCC (i.e., sBCC and small nBCC are more responsive than iBCC).[74] Use of topical corticosteroids just prior to and following therapy was shown to reduce post-procedural erythema without compromising treatment efficacy.[18]

Kaposi Sarcoma

Kaposi sarcoma (KS) arises from lymphatic endothelial cells and is associated with human-herpesvirus 8 (HHV-8) infection. The incidence of KS is estimated to be increased between 84 and 500-fold in SOTR.[1,75,76] One study showed an increased risk of 23% in HHV-8 seropositive patients prior to transplantation versus 0.7% in seronegative patients, demonstrating that viral infection prior to transplantation is a key factor in development of KS in SOTR.[77] There are various modalities that have been used to successfully treat localized KS, including alitretinoin, imiquimod, intralesional (IL) antineoplastic drugs (vincristine, vinblastine, and bleomycin), IL sodium tetradecyl sulfate (STS), IL cidofovir, cryotherapy, and radiotherapy.[78–80] The bulk of the research for localized therapy has been performed in human immunodeficiency virus (HIV)-infected patients rather than SOTR. Although topical or IL modalities may be used as an adjunct for localized disease, the mainstay of treatment for KS in SOTR is alteration of the immunosuppressive regimen.[76]

INTRALESIONAL THERAPIES FOR NONMELANOMA SKIN CANCER

There are few studies describing the use of IL modalities for the treatment of NMSC, with the available studies primarily limited to immunocompetent populations. Well-differentiated SCC subtypes, such as SCC/KA, and less aggressive subtypes of BCC have shown the highest response rates to various IL modalities.[81,82] The cure rates with IL therapy for SCC/KA in immunocompetent patients approached 98% for 5-FU, 91% for methotrexate (MTX), 100% for bleomycin, 100% for interferon (IFN) alpha (α)-2, 83% for IFN α-2a, and 100% for IFN α-2b.[82] Table 5.2 outlines IL therapies for the treatment of NMSC in SOTR.

INTRALESIONAL 5-FLUOROURACIL

Injectable 5-FU is available in a 50 mg/mL solution and has been used with various dosing regimens and cumulative doses in the treatment of SCC with efficacies of 83%–100%.[81,82] A 1980 study showed clearance of 40 of 41 SCC/KA with an average of 3 weekly injections in aliquots of 0.5–1.0 mL of 50 mg/mL 5-FU.[83] A subsequent review showed that nearly all reported cases of SCC/KA treated with IL 5-FU

TABLE 5.2 Intralesional Therapies for Nonmelanoma Skin Cancer in Solid Organ Transplant Recipients

MALIGNANCY	*TREATMENT OPTIONS*	*COMMENTS*
Invasive SCC	5-Fluorouracil	Limited data on large SCC
	Methotrexate	Studied as a neoadjuvant treatment to decrease lesion size, particularly on the lip of immunocompetent patients. Caution in SOTR due to relatively higher risk of metastasis of SCC on the lip
	Cidofovir	Data limited to a single case report in an immunocompetent patient
SCC, KA type	5-Fluorouracil	Average of 3 weekly injections of 0.5–1.0 mL per injection (50 mg/mL)

(Continued)

TABLE 5.2 Intralesional Therapies for Nonmelanoma Skin Cancer in Solid Organ Transplant Recipients. (Continued)

MALIGNANCY	*TREATMENT OPTIONS*	*COMMENTS*
	Methotrexate	2–4 weekly injections of 0.5–1.0 mL per injection (25 mg/mL)
	Triamcinolone	Monthly injections
BCC	5-Fluorouracil	Limited data in immunocompetent patients only
Kaposi sarcoma		Mainstay of treatment is alteration of the immunosuppressive regimen
Other intralesional modalities		
	Bleomycin	Studied for SCC, SCC/KA, and BCC in immunocompetent patients. Most effective when combined with electroporation. Dosing varies with tumor volume and is repeated in 1–2 week intervals if clinically indicated.
	Interferon	Not recommended in transplant patients due to risk of allograft rejection

resolved (97%).[81] The data on large SCC are sparse and limited to a few case reports and a trial of 25 patients using a proprietary 5-FU/epinephrine gel.[84–86] Figure 5.4 shows a patient with biopsy-proven SCC of the ankles before and during therapy with IL 5-FU.

IL 5-FU has demonstrated success as a treatment for low risk BCC (sBCC and nBCC, <15 mm in diameter) as well as some large, recurrent, and multifocal tumors.[81,84,87] Although IL 5-FU may be considered as an alternative treatment option for NMSC, the authors recommend cautious use in carefully selected nonsurgical candidates based on a paucity of data. Additionally, the available data is limited to immunocompetent patients and may not be generalizable to treatment of the immunosuppressed population.

METHOTREXATE

MTX is a folic acid analog that blocks cellular proliferation via inhibition of dihydrofolate reductase and DNA synthesis. The use of IL MTX (25 mg/mL solution) has been primarily studied in the treatment of immunocompetent patients with low-risk, uncomplicated SCC/KA. A study of nine patients showed 8 of 9 SCC/KA with complete resolution after debulking and a range of 2–4 weekly injections ranging from 12.5 to 25 mg per injection.[88] Excision of the lesion with treatment failure showed moderately differentiated SCC.[88] A retrospective review of 38 cases found that IL MTX achieved resolution in 92% of cases with an average of 2.1 injections at average intervals of 18 days.[89] A study of 73 KAs in 54 patients found a cure rate of 88% compared with 100% with surgery.[90]

Use of IL MTX has also been studied as a neoadjuvant treatment for SCC (non-KA type) in an effort to decrease lesion size and reduce the need for complex reconstruction. The evidence is limited to case reports, a prospective observational study of 10 patients with SCC of the lip, and a retrospective cohort study of 43 patients.[91–94] The cohort study found that neoadjuvant IL MTX reduced the tumor size by a mean of 42.6%, and that tumors ≥2 cm in size required significantly fewer complex reconstructions.[94] The

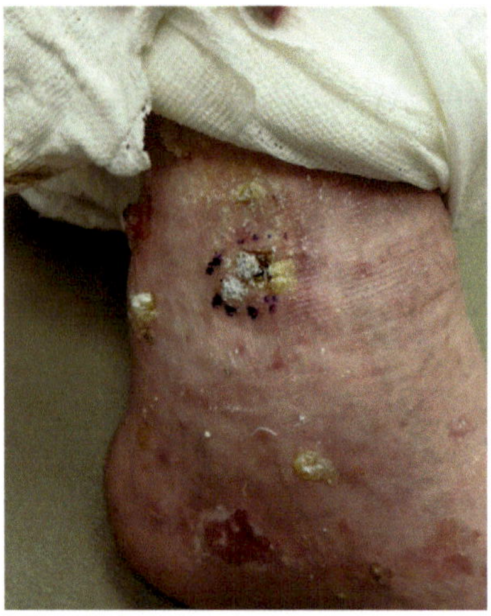

Initial biopsy.

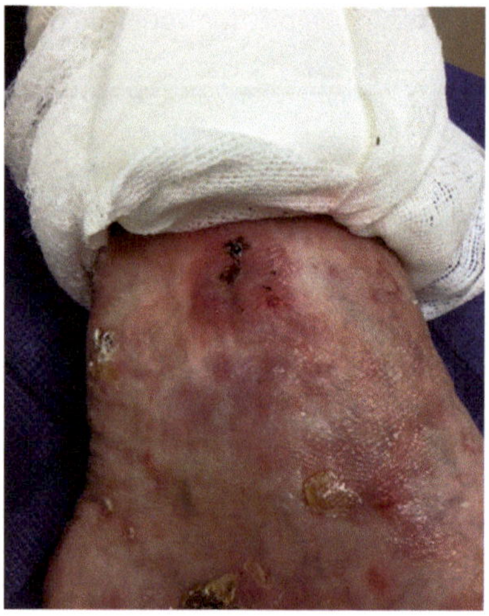

After three treatments with IL 5-FU.

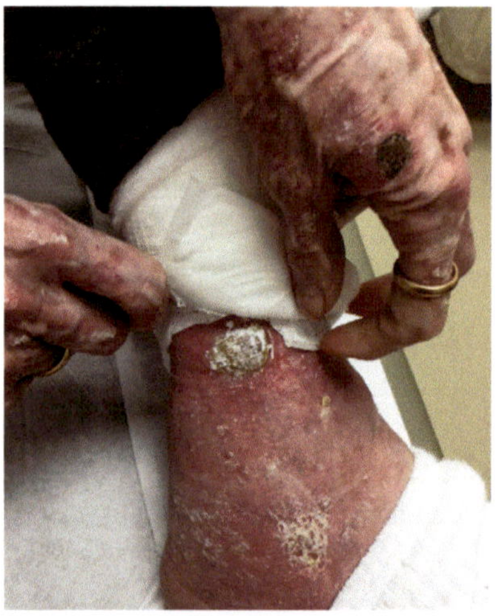

Initial biopsy.

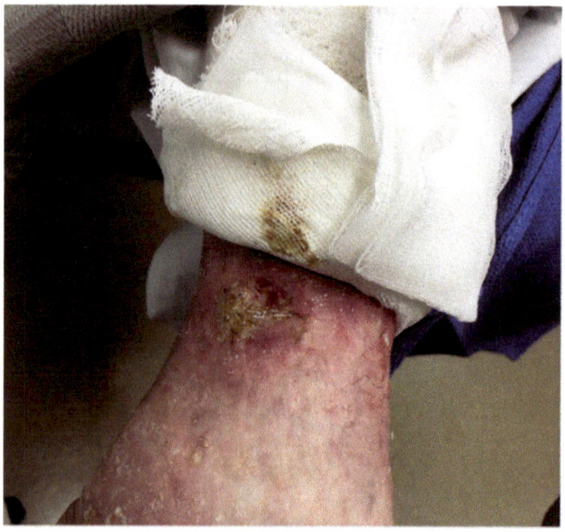

After two treatments with IL 5-FU.

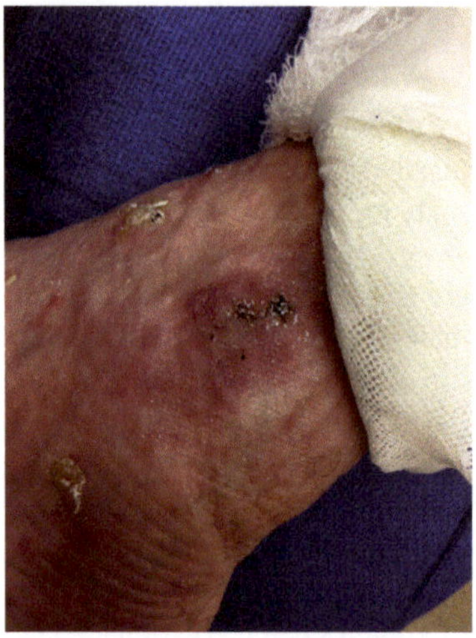

After four treatments of IL 5-FU.

FIGURE 5.4 A patient with SCC before and during therapy with IL 5-FU for SCC of the ankles. Although not a SOTR, the patient had a history significant for diffuse NMSC because of exposure to arsenic.

observational study found a response rate of 100% (i.e., size reduction) and a complete resolution rate of 30% when IL MTX was used for SCC of the lip.[89]

With the use of IL MTX, a screening complete blood count (CBC) is recommended at baseline and following treatment because of the risk of pancytopenia in patients with renal failure.[89,95] MTX should be avoided in patients with a glomerular filtration rate (GFR) <30 mL/min/1.73 m^2.[90]

As with systemic MTX, possible drug–drug interactions with the use of IL-MTX should be considered. Potential interactions with commonly used medications include but are not limited to nitrous oxide, NSAIDs, and sulfonamides (e.g., sulfamethoxazole).[96]

Evidence suggests that IL MTX may be considered either as solo therapy for low-risk SCC/KA or as a neoadjuvant therapy prior to surgical intervention, particularly for SCC of the lip. However, studies to date have been limited to the immunocompetent patient population. IL MTX should be used cautiously in the SOTR population given the relatively higher risk of metastasis of SCC (particularly of the lip) in immunocompromised patients.

BLEOMYCIN

Bleomycin, derived from the actinomycotic soil fungus *Streptomyces verticillus*, is classified as an antitumoral antibiotic that inhibits DNA synthesis. It has been used successfully to treat BCC, SCC, and SCC/KA in the immunocompetent patient population.[97–102] The highest clearance rates were achieved with IL bleomycin combined with electroporation, a technique that uses a configuration of electrode needles to deliver high-intensity currents directly into the tumor.[99] This method, referred to as bleomycin-mediated electrochemotherapy (ECT), demonstrated clearance rates of up to 94% for BCC after a single treatment.[100,101] IL bleomycin also was used alone and in combination with ECT to successfully treat KA.[98,102,103]

The dosing of bleomycin varies based on tumor volume. For KA, a common dosing regimen is bleomycin (1 mg/mL) solution diluted 1:1 with 0.5% lidocaine and injected into the lesion in 0.2–0.4 mg aliquots. The treatment can be repeated in 1–2 week intervals if clinically indicated. Overall, the evidence for use of IL bleomycin is sparse and limited to the immunocompetent population.

INTERFERON

IFN is an immunomodulatory cytokine. IFN-alpha increases the expression of the transcription factor IFN response factor 1 (IRF1), which is involved in cell cycle regulation and induction of apoptosis.[104–107] IRF1 induces lysyl oxidase (LOX) expression; loss of LOX expression and function is found in numerous cancers including SCC.[104–107] Multiple case series in immunocompetent patients show the efficacy of IL IFN-alpha 2b for the treatment of SCC with mild and dose-dependent side effects.[108–110] However, treatment with IFN is generally not recommended in the transplant population because of the risk of allograft rejection.

TRIAMCINOLONE

Intradermal triamcinolone has been used successfully as a treatment for solitary and multiple-reactive SCC/KA.[111–113] This once-popular treatment option has been eclipsed by the availability and growing data for the use of IL 5-FU. Nevertheless, it has shown efficacy in the treatment of SCC/KA and is worth consideration in the treatment armament.

CIDOFOVIR

Cidofovir acts via selective inhibition of DNA polymerase, blocking DNA synthesis and replication of human papilloma virus (HPV)-infected cells.[114,115] Although off label, IL and topical cidofovir have been used to treat HPV-associated disease in transplant recipients.[116] One case report showed clearance of an SCC of the lower eyelid with a single dose of IL cidofovir in in an immunocompetent patient.[117] Additional studies are needed to evaluate IL cidofovir as a treatment option for select SCC in SOTR.

CONCLUSION

The markedly increased risk of developing AK and NMSC in SOTR, with its associated morbidity and mortality, necessitates close follow up and an array of modalities aimed at prevention and treatment. Patients with diffuse disease may benefit from field-directed therapies such as 5-FU and PDT to reduce disease burden. There are many efficacious treatments to address field cancerization in SOTR, with the bulk of the current evidence on the use of PDT. However, treatment must be tailored to individual patients based on availability, patient preference, and comorbidities.

The treatment paradigm for NMSC in the SOTR remains largely surgical because of the high cure rates attained with pathological margin control. However, when surgical intervention is not an option, topical and IL agents may be considered, both as solo therapy and as neoadjuvant therapy prior to surgical intervention.

Despite the current paucity of high-quality RCTs specific to SOTR, there is a growing body of evidence delineating the efficacy and safety profiles of topical and IL therapies for AK and NMSC in the transplant population. Continued research and comparative studies are needed to identify optimal treatment regimens.

SUMMARY OF KEY POINTS

- SOTR have a markedly increased risk of developing AK and NMSC when compared with that of the general population because of long-term immunosuppression and impaired DNA-repair mechanisms.
- Precursor lesions like AK in SOTR are more resistant to conventional therapies with an increased risk of progression to malignancy and a lower likelihood of spontaneous regression.
- Surgical treatment is ideal for most NMSC given the high cure rates associated with pathological margin control.
- Photoprotection is an effective but underutilized preventive strategy.
- Field-directed therapy is indicated to treat large anatomical areas of field cancerization.
- The bulk of evidence for treatment of AK in SOTR is for PDT.
- Imiquimod is safe to use in SOTR in limited treatment areas.
- The mainstay of treatment for KS in SOTR is alteration of the immunosuppressive regimen.
- Topical or IL therapies may be considered for treatment of NMSC when surgical treatment is not an option.
- Some intralesional therapies may be used as neoadjuvant therapy to shrink large NMSC prior to surgical intervention.
- IFN is not recommended in the SOTR population because of the risk of allograft rejection.

REFERENCES

1. O'Reilly Zwald F, Brown M. Skin cancer in solid organ transplant recipients: advances in therapy and management: part I. Epidemiology of skin cancer in solid organ transplant recipients. J Am Acad Dermatol. 2011;65(2):253–61.
2. Ingvar A, Smedby KE, Lindelof B, Fernberg P, Bellocco R, Tufveson G et al. Immunosuppressive treatment after solid organ transplantation and risk of post-transplant cutaneous squamous cell carcinoma. Nephrol Dial Transplant. 2010;25(8):2764–71.
3. Wheless L, Jacks S, Mooneyham Potter KA, Leach BC, Cook J. Skin cancer in organ transplant recipients: more than the immune system. J Am Acad Dermatol. 2014;71(2):359–65.
4. Jiyad Z, Marquart L, O'Rourke P, Green AC. The natural history of actinic keratoses in organ transplant recipients. J Am Acad Dermatol. 2017;76(1):162–4.
5. Euvrard S, Kanitakis J, Pouteil-Noble C, Dureau G, Touraine JL, Faure M et al. Comparative epidemiologic study of premalignant and malignant epithelial cutaneous lesions developing after kidney and heart transplantation. J Am Acad Dermatol. 1995;33(2 Pt 1):222–9.
6. Ulrich C, Jurgensen JS, Degen A, Hackethal M, Ulrich M, Patel MJ et al. Prevention of non-melanoma skin cancer in organ transplant patients by regular use of a sunscreen: a 24 months, prospective, case-control study. Br J Dermatol. 2009;161(Suppl 3):78–84.
7. Donovan JC, Shaw JC. Compliance with sun protection following organ transplantation. Arch Dermatol. 2006;142(9):1232–3.
8. Seukeran DC, Newstead CG, Cunliffe WJ. The compliance of renal transplant recipients with advice about sun protection measures. Br J Dermatol. 1998;138(2):301–3.
9. Rose RF, Moniem K, Seukeran DC, Stables GI, Newstead CG. Compliance of renal transplant recipients with advice about sun protection measures. Transplant Proc. 2005;37(10):4320–2.
10. Hartman RI, Green AC, Gordon LG, Skin T, Allograft recipients S. Sun protection among OTR after participation in a skin cancer research study. JAMA Dermatol. 2018;154(7):842–4.
11. Torezan LA, Festa-Neto C. Cutaneous field cancerization: clinical, histopathological and therapeutic aspects. An Bras Dermatol. 2013;88(5):775–86.
12. Krawtchenko N, Roewert-Huber J, Ulrich M, Mann I, Sterry W, Stockfleth E. A randomised study of topical 5% imiquimod vs. topical 5-fluorouracil vs. cryosurgery in immunocompetent patients with actinic keratoses: a comparison of clinical and histological outcomes including 1-year follow-up. Br J Dermatol. 2007;157(Suppl 2):34–40.
13. Wennberg AM, Stenquist B, Stockfleth E, Keohane S, Lear JT, Jemec G et al. Photodynamic therapy with methyl aminolevulinate for prevention of new skin lesions in transplant recipients: a randomized study. Transplant. 2008;86(3):423–9.
14. O'Reilly Zwald F, Brown M. Skin cancer in solid organ transplant recipients: advances in therapy and management: part II. Management of skin cancer in solid organ transplant recipients. J Am Acad Dermatol. 2011;65(2):263–79.
15. Kokoszka A, Scheinfeld N. Evidence-based review of the use of cryosurgery in treatment of basal cell carcinoma. Dermatol Surg. 2003;29(6):566–71.
16. Perrett CM, McGregor JM, Warwick J, Karran P, Leigh IM, Proby CM et al. Treatment of post-transplant premalignant skin disease: a randomized intrapatient comparative study of 5-fluorouracil cream and topical photodynamic therapy. Br J Dermatol. 2007;156(2):320–8.
17. Ingham AI, Weightman W. The efficacy and safety of topical 5% 5-fluorouracil in renal transplant recipients for the treatment of actinic keratoses. Australas J Dermatol. 2014;55(3):204–8.
18. Wiegell SR, Petersen B, Wulf HC. Topical corticosteroid reduces inflammation without compromising the efficacy of photodynamic therapy for actinic keratoses: a randomized clinical trial. Br J Dermatol. 2014;171(6):1487–92.
19. Cunningham TJ, Tabacchi M, Eliane JP, Tuchayi SM, Manivasagam S, Mirzaalian H et al. Randomized trial of calcipotriol combined with 5-fluorouracil for skin cancer precursor immunotherapy. J Clin Invest. 2017;127(1):106–16.
20. Que SKT, Zwald FO, Schmults CD. Cutaneous squamous cell carcinoma: management of advanced and high-stage tumors. J Am Acad Dermatol. 2018;78(2):249–61.
21. Goon PK, Clegg R, Yong AS, Lee AS, Lee KY, Levell NJ et al. 5-Fluorouracil "chemowraps" in the treatment of multiple actinic keratoses: a Norwich experience. Dermatol Ther (Heidelb). 2015;5(3):201–5.

22. Peuvrel L, Saint-Jean M, Quereux G, Brocard A, Le Moigne M, Frenard C et al. 5-fluorouracil chemowraps for the treatment of multiple actinic keratoses. Eur J Dermatol. 2017;27(6):635–40.
23. Mann M, Berk DR, Petersen J. Chemowraps as an adjuvant to surgery for patients with diffuse squamous cell carcinoma of the extremities. J Drugs Dermatol. 2008;7(7):685–8.
24. Tallon B, Turnbull N. 5% fluorouracil chemowraps in the management of widespread lower leg solar keratoses and squamous cell carcinoma. Australas J Dermatol. 2013;54(4):313–16.
25. Lau JF, Weinberg MD, Olin JW. Peripheral artery disease. Part 1: clinical evaluation and noninvasive diagnosis. Nat Rev Cardiol. 2011;8(7):405–18.
26. Ulrich C. Topical treatment of field cancerization. Cancer Treat Res. 2009;146:439–46.
27. Firoz BF, Goldberg LH. When imiquimod fails. Dermatol Surg. 2010;36(5):717–20.
28. Ulrich C, Bichel J, Euvrard S, Guidi B, Proby CM, van de Kerkhof PC et al. Topical immunomodulation under systemic immunosuppression: results of a multicentre, randomized, placebo-controlled safety and efficacy study of imiquimod 5% cream for the treatment of actinic keratoses in kidney, heart, and liver transplant patients. Br J Dermatol. 2007;157(Suppl 2):25–31.
29. Togsverd-Bo K, Halldin C, Sandberg C, Gonzalez H, Wennberg AM, Sorensen SS et al. Photodynamic therapy is more effective than imiquimod for actinic keratosis in organ transplant recipients: a randomized intraindividual controlled trial. Br J Dermatol. 2018;178(4):903–9.
30. Santos-Juanes J, Esteve A, Mas-Vidal A, Coto-Segura P, Salgueiro E, Gomez E et al. Acute renal failure caused by imiquimod 5% cream in a renal transplant patient: review of the literature on side effects of imiquimod. Dermatology. 2011;222(2):109–12.
31. Wulf HC, Pavel S, Stender I, Bakker-Wensveen CA. Topical photodynamic therapy for prevention of new skin lesions in renal transplant recipients. Acta Derm Venereol. 2006;86(1):25–8.
32. Babilas P, Schreml S, Landthaler M, Szeimies RM. Photodynamic therapy in dermatology: state-of-the-art. Photodermatol Photoimmunol Photomed. 2010;26(3):118–32.
33. Joly F, Deret S, Gamboa B, Menigot C, Fogel P, Mounier C et al. Photodynamic therapy corrects abnormal cancer-associated gene expression observed in actinic keratosis lesions and induces a remodeling effect in photodamaged skin. J Dermatol Sci. 2018;91(2).
34. Savoia P, Deboli T, Previgliano A, Broganelli P. Usefulness of photodynamic therapy as a possible therapeutic alternative in the treatment of basal cell carcinoma. Int J Mol Sci. 2015;16(10):23300–17.
35. Basset-Seguin N, Baumann Conzett K, Gerritsen MJ, Gonzalez H, Haedersdal M, Hofbauer GF et al. Photodynamic therapy for actinic keratosis in organ transplant patients. J Eur Acad Dermatol Venereol. 2013;27(1):57–66.
36. Dragieva G, Prinz BM, Hafner J, Dummer R, Burg G, Binswanger U et al. A randomized controlled clinical trial of topical photodynamic therapy with methyl aminolaevulinate in the treatment of actinic keratoses in transplant recipients. Br J Dermatol. 2004;151(1):196–200.
37. Piaserico S, Belloni Fortina A, Rigotti P, Rossi B, Baldan N, Alaibac M et al. Topical photodynamic therapy of actinic keratosis in renal transplant recipients. Transplant Proc. 2007;39(6):1847–50.
38. Braun SA, Schrumpf H, Buhren BA, Homey B, Gerber PA. Laser-assisted drug delivery: mode of action and use in daily clinical practice. J Dtsch Dermatol Ges. 2016;14(5):480–8.
39. Heppt MV, Steeb T, Niesert AC, Zacher M, Leiter U, Garbe C et al. Local interventions for actinic keratosis in organ transplant recipients: a systematic review. Br J Dermatol. 2019;180(1):43–50.
40. Liew YCC, De Souza NNA, Sultana RG, Oh CC. Photodynamic therapy for the prevention and treatment of actinic keratosis/squamous cell carcinoma in solid organ transplant recipients: a systematic review and meta-analysis. J Eur Acad Dermatol Venereol. 2020;34(2):251–9.
41. Togsverd-Bo K, Lei U, Erlendsson AM, Taudorf EH, Philipsen PA, Wulf HC et al. Combination of ablative fractional laser and daylight-mediated photodynamic therapy for actinic keratosis in organ transplant recipients—a randomized controlled trial. Br J Dermatol. 2015;172(2):467–74.
42. Helsing P, Togsverd-Bo K, Veierod MB, Mork G, Haedersdal M. Intensified fractional CO2 laser-assisted photodynamic therapy vs. laser alone for organ transplant recipients with multiple actinic keratoses and wart-like lesions: a randomized half-side comparative trial on dorsal hands. Br J Dermatol. 2013;169(5):1087–92.
43. Muhlstadt M. Ingenol mebutate vs. daylight photodynamic therapy in a kidney transplant recipient. Dermatology. 2016;232(Suppl 1):20–3.
44. Mohanna M, Hofbauer G. Pronounced local skin reaction to ingenol mebutate against actinic keratosis in kidney transplant recipient without systemic adverse events. JAAD Case Rep. 2015;1(6):S19–22.
45. Crow LD, Yuan JT, Aroyan CS, Twigg AR, Singer JP, Roll GR et al. Ingenol mebutate .015% gel is safe for short-term tx of AK on the face of SOTC. Br J Dermatol. 2020;27.
46. Lonsdorf AS, Becker MR, Stockfleth E, Schakel K, Ulrich C. Primary and secondary prevention of skin cancer in organ transplant recipients. Hautarzt. 2010;61(3):195–206.

47. Ulrich C, Hackethal M, Ulrich M, Howorka A, Forschner T, Sterry W et al. Treatment of multiple actinic keratoses with topical diclofenac 3% gel in organ transplant recipients: a series of six cases. Br J Dermatol. 2007;156(Suppl 3):40–2.
48. Ulrich C, Johannsen A, Rowert-Huber J, Ulrich M, Sterry W, Stockfleth E. Results of a randomized, placebo-controlled safety and efficacy study of topical diclofenac 3% gel in organ transplant patients with multiple actinic keratoses. Eur J Dermatol. 2010;20(4):482–8.
49. Garofalo V, Ventura A, Mazzilli S, Diluvio L, Bianchi L, Toti L et al. Treatment of multiple actinic keratosis and field of cancerization with topical piroxicam 0.8% and sunscreen 50+ in organ transplant recipients: a series of 10 cases. Case Rep Dermatol. 2017;9(3):211–16.
50. Moloney FJ, Comber H, O'Lorcain P, O'Kelly P, Conlon PJ, Murphy GM. A population-based study of skin cancer incidence and prevalence in renal transplant recipients. Br J Dermatol. 2006;154(3):498–504.
51. Miller SJ, Alam M, Andersen J, Berg D, Bichakjian CK, Bowen G et al. Basal cell and squamous cell skin cancers. J Natl Compr Canc Netw. 2010;8(8):836–64.
52. Tessari G, Naldi L, Boschiero L, Nacchia F, Fior F, Forni A et al. Incidence and clinical predictors of a subsequent nonmelanoma skin cancer in solid organ transplant recipients with a first nonmelanoma skin cancer: a multicenter cohort study. Arch Dermatol. 2010;146(3):294–9.
53. Ramsay HM, Reece SM, Fryer AA, Smith AG, Harden PN. Seven-year prospective study of nonmelanoma skin cancer incidence in U.K. renal transplant recipients. Transplantation. 2007;84(3):437–9.
54. Fuente MJ, Sabat M, Roca J, Lauzurica R, Fernandez-Figueras MT, Ferrandiz C. A prospective study of the incidence of skin cancer and its risk factors in a Spanish mediterranean population of kidney transplant recipients. Br J Dermatol. 2003;149(6):1221–6.
55. Shimizu I, Cruz A, Chang KH, Dufresne RG. Treatment of squamous cell carcinoma in situ: a review. Dermatol Surg. 2011;37(10):1394–411.
56. Brown VL, Atkins CL, Ghali L, Cerio R, Harwood CA, Proby CM. Safety and efficacy of 5% imiquimod cream for the treatment of skin dysplasia in high-risk renal transplant recipients: randomized, double-blind, placebo-controlled trial. Arch Dermatol. 2005;141(8):985–93.
57. Ben M'barek L, Mebazaa A, Euvrard S, Frances C, Thervet E, Morel P et al. 5% topical imiquimod tolerance in transplant recipients. Dermatol. 2007;215(2):130–3.
58. Patel GK, Goodwin R, Chawla M, Laidler P, Price PE, Finlay AY et al. Imiquimod 5% cream monotherapy for cutaneous squamous cell carcinoma in situ (Bowen's disease): a randomized, double-blind, placebo-controlled trial. J Am Acad Dermatol. 2006;54(6):1025–32.
59. Das G, Tan B, Nicholls K. Safety and efficacy of a novel short occlusive regimen of imiquimod for selected non-melanotic skin lesions in renal transplant patients. Intern Med J. 2016;46(3):352–5.
60. Smith KJ, Germain M, Skelton H. Squamous cell carcinoma in situ (Bowen's disease) in renal transplant patients treated with 5% imiquimod and 5% 5-fluorouracil therapy. Dermatol Surg. 2001;27(6):561–4.
61. Jambusaria-Pahlajani A, Ortman S, Schmults CD, Liang C. Sequential Curettage, 5-fluorouracil, and photodynamic therapy for field cancerization of the scalp and face in solid organ transplant recipients. Dermatol Surg. 2016;42(Suppl 1):S66–72.
62. Morton C, Horn M, Leman J, Tack B, Bedane C, Tjioe M et al. Comparison of topical methyl aminolevulinate photodynamic therapy with cryotherapy or Fluorouracil for treatment of squamous cell carcinoma in situ: results of a multicenter randomized trial. Arch Dermatol. 2006;142(6):729–35.
63. Salim A, Leman JA, McColl JH, Chapman R, Morton CA. Randomized comparison of photodynamic therapy with topical 5-fluorouracil in Bowen's disease. Br J Dermatol. 2003;148(3):539–43.
64. Tarstedt M, Gillstedt M, Wennberg Larko AM, Paoli J. Aminolevulinic acid and methyl aminolevulinate equally effective in topical photodynamic therapy for non-melanoma skin cancers. J Eur Acad Dermatol Venereol. 2016;30(3):420–3.
65. Dragieva G, Hafner J, Dummer R, Schmid-Grendelmeier P, Roos M, Prinz BM et al. Topical photodynamic therapy in the treatment of actinic keratoses and Bowen's disease in transplant recipients. Transplant. 2004;77(1):115–21.
66. Marks R, Gebauer K, Shumack S, Amies M, Bryden J, Fox TL et al. Imiquimod 5% cream in the treatment of superficial basal cell carcinoma: results of a multicenter 6-week dose-response trial. J Am Acad Dermatol. 2001;44(5):807–13.
67. Vidal D, Alomar A. Efficacy of imiquimod 5% cream for basal cell carcinoma in transplant patients. Clin Exp Dermatol. 2004;29(3):237–9.
68. Wang H, Xu Y, Shi J, Gao X, Geng L. Photodynamic therapy in the treatment of basal cell carcinoma: a systematic review and meta-analysis. Photodermatol Photoimmunol Photomed. 2015;31(1):44–53.
69. Guleng GE, Helsing P. Photodynamic therapy for basal cell carcinomas in organ-transplant recipients. Clin Exp Dermatol. 2012;37(4):367–9.

70. Agostinis P, Berg K, Cengel KA, Foster TH, Girotti AW, Gollnick SO et al. Photodynamic therapy of cancer: an update. CA Cancer J Clin. 2011;61(4):250–81.
71. Collier NJ, Ali FR, Lear JT. Efficacy of photodynamic therapy for treatment of basal cell carcinoma in organ transplant recipients. Lasers Med Sci. 2015;30(4):1407–9.
72. Itkin A, Gilchrest BA. delta-Aminolevulinic acid and blue light photodynamic therapy for treatment of multiple basal cell carcinomas in two patients with nevoid basal cell carcinoma syndrome. Dermatol Surg. 2004;30(7):1054–61.
73. Wiegell SR, Skodt V, Wulf HC. Daylight-mediated photodynamic therapy of basal cell carcinomas—an explorative study. J Eur Acad Dermatol Venereol. 2014;28(2):169–75.
74. Fantini F, Greco A, Del Giovane C, Cesinaro AM, Venturini M, Zane C et al. Photodynamic therapy for basal cell carcinoma: clinical and pathological determinants of response. J Eur Acad Dermatol Venereol. 2011;25(8):896–901.
75. Berg D, Otley CC. Skin cancer in organ transplant recipients: epidemiology, pathogenesis, and management. J Am Acad Dermatol. 2002;47(1):1–17; quiz 8–20.
76. Cahoon EK, Linet MS, Clarke CA, Pawlish KS, Engels EA, Pfeiffer RM. Risk of Kaposi sarcoma after solid organ transplantation in the United States. Int J Cancer. 2018;143(11):2741–8.
77. Cattani P, Capuano M, Graffeo R, Ricci R, Cerimele F, Cerimele D et al. Kaposi's sarcoma associated with previous human herpesvirus 8 infection in kidney transplant recipients. J Clin Microbiol. 2001;39(2):506–8.
78. Facciola A, Venanzi Rullo E, Ceccarelli M, D'Aleo F, Di Rosa M, Pinzone MR et al. Kaposi's sarcoma in HIV-infected patients in the era of new antiretrovirals. Eur Rev Med Pharmacol Sci. 2017;21(24):5868–9.
79. Bodsworth NJ, Bloch M, Bower M, Donnell D, Yocum R, International panretin gel KSSG. Phase III vehicle-controlled, multi-centered study of topical alitretinoin gel 0.1% in cutaneous AIDS-related Kaposi's sarcoma. Am J Clin Dermatol. 2001;2(2):77–87.
80. Ramirez-Amador V, Esquivel-Pedraza L, Lozada-Nur F, De la Rosa-Garcia E, Volkow-Fernandez P, Suchil-Bernal L et al. Intralesional vinblastine vs. 3% sodium tetradecyl sulfate for the treatment of oral Kaposi's sarcoma: a double blind, randomized clinical trial. Oral Oncol. 2002;38(5):460–7.
81. Metterle L, Nelson C, Patel N. Intralesional 5-fluorouracil (FU) as a treatment for nonmelanoma skin cancer (NMSC): a review. J Am Acad Dermatol. 2016;74(3):552–7.
82. Chitwood K, Etzkorn J, Cohen G. Topical and intralesional treatment of nonmelanoma skin cancer: efficacy and cost comparisons. Dermatol Surg. 2013;39(9):1306–16.
83. Goette DK, Odom RB. Successful treatment of keratoacanthoma with intralesional fluorouracil. J Am Acad Dermatol. 1980;2(3):212–16.
84. Kraus S, Miller BH, Swinehart JM, Shavin JS, Georgouras KE, Jenner DA et al. Intratumoral chemotherapy with fluorouracil/epinephrine injectable gel: a nonsurgical treatment of cutaneous squamous cell carcinoma. J Am Acad Dermatol. 1998;38(3):438–42.
85. Morse LG, Kendrick C, Hooper D, Ward H, Parry E. Treatment of squamous cell carcinoma with intralesional 5-Fluorouracil. Dermatol Surg. 2003;29(11):1150–3; discussion 3.
86. Reisinger DM, Cognetta AB, Pynes LT, Paredes AA, Sweeney TJ, Dolson DJ. Treatment of a giant squamous cell carcinoma on the dominant thumb with intralesional 5-fluorouracil. J Am Acad Dermatol. 2011;65(1): 219–21.
87. Avant WH, Huff RC. Intradermal 5-fluorouracil in the treatment of basal cell carcinoma of the face. South Med J. 1976;69(5):561–3.
88. Patel NP, Cervino AL. Treatment of keratoacanthoma: is intralesional methotrexate an option? Can J Plast Surg. 2011;19(2):e15–8.
89. Annest NM, VanBeek MJ, Arpey CJ, Whitaker DC. Intralesional methotrexate treatment for keratoacanthoma tumors: a retrospective study and review of the literature. J Am Acad Dermatol. 2007;56(6):989–93.
90. Moss M, Weber E, Hoverson K, Montemarano AD. Management of keratoacanthoma: 157 tumors treated with surgery or intralesional methotrexate. Dermatol Surg. 2019;45(7):877–83.
91. Plascencia-Gomez A, Calderon-Rocher C, Proy-Trujillo H, Moreno-Coutino G. Neoadjuvant intralesional methotrexate before surgery in squamous cell carcinoma. Dermatol Surg. 2014;40(5):584–6.
92. Salido-Vallejo R, Cuevas-Asencio I, Garnacho-Sucedo G, Gonzalez-Menchen A, Alcantara-Reifs C, De la Corte-Sanchez S et al. Neoadjuvant intralesional methotrexate in cutaneous squamous cell carcinoma: a comparative cohort study. J Eur Acad Dermatol Venereol. 2016;30(7):1120–4.
93. Salido-Vallejo R, Garnacho-Saucedo G, Sanchez-Arca M, Moreno-Gimenez JC. Neoadjuvant intralesional methotrexate before surgical treatment of invasive squamous cell carcinoma of the lower lip. Dermatol Surg. 2012;38(11):1849–50.

94. Moye MS, Clark AH, Legler AA, Milhem MM, Van Beek MJ. Intralesional methotrexate for treatment of invasive squamous cell carcinomas in a patient taking vemurafenib for treatment of metastatic melanoma. J Clin Oncol. 2016;34(14):e134–6.
95. Flynn KN, Johnson MS, Brink WC, Smith DL. Pancytopenia, mucositis, and hepatotoxicity after intralesional methotrexate injection in a patient treated with peritoneal dialysis. Am J Health Syst Pharm. 2012;69(7):578–82.
96. Pfizer Canada ULC. Product monograph methotrexate injection USP. Kirkland Quebec; 2019. Submission Control No: 224776.
97. Mishima Y, Matunaka M. Effect of bleomycin on benign and malignant cutaneous tumours. Acta Derm Venereol. 1972;52(3):211–15.
98. Sayama S, Tagami H. Treatment of keratoacanthoma with intralesional bleomycin. Br J Dermatol. 1983;109(4):449–52.
99. Belehradek M, Domenge C, Luboinski B, Orlowski S, Belehradek J, Mir LM. Electrochemotherapy, a new antitumor treatment: first clinical phase I-II trial. Cancer. 1993;72(12):3694–700.
100. Glass LF, Jaroszeski M, Gilbert R, Reintgen DS, Heller R. Intralesional bleomycin-mediated electrochemotherapy in 20 patients with basal cell carcinoma. J Am Acad Dermatol. 1997;37(4):596–9.
101. Heller R, Jaroszeski MJ, Reintgen DS, Puleo CA, DeConti RC, Gilbert RA et al. Treatment of cutaneous and subcutaneous tumors with electrochemotherapy using intralesional bleomycin. Cancer. 1998;83(1):148–57.
102. de la Torre C, Losada A, Cruces MJ. Keratoacanthoma centrifugum marginatum: treatment with intralesional bleomycin. J Am Acad Dermatol. 1997;37(6):1010–11.
103. Pasquali P, Spugnini EP, Baldi A. Successful treatment of a keratoacanthoma with electrochemotherapy: a case report. Dermatol Ther (Heidelb). 2018;8(1):143–6.
104. Tanaka N, Ishihara M, Lamphier MS, Nozawa H, Matsuyama T, Mak TW et al. Cooperation of the tumour suppressors IRF-1 and p53 in response to DNA damage. Nature. 1996;382(6594):816–18.
105. Ogasawara S, Tamura G, Maesawa C, Suzuki Y, Ishida K, Satoh N et al. Common deleted region on the long arm of chromosome 5 in esophageal carcinoma. Gastroenterology. 1996;110(1):52–7.
106. Takaoka A, Tamura T, Taniguchi T. Interferon regulatory factor family of transcription factors and regulation of oncogenesis. Cancer Sci. 2008;99(3):467–78.
107. Payne SL, Hendrix MJ, Kirschmann DA. Paradoxical roles for lysyl oxidases in cancer-a prospect. J Cell Biochem. 2007;101(6):1338–54.
108. Kim KH, Yavel RM, Gross VL, Brody N. Intralesional interferon alpha-2b in the treatment of basal cell carcinoma and squamous cell carcinoma: revisited. Dermatol Surg. 2004;30(1):116–20.
109. Edwards L, Berman B, Rapini RP, Whiting DA, Tyring S, Greenway HT, Jr. et al. Treatment of cutaneous squamous cell carcinomas by intralesional interferon alfa-2b therapy. Arch Dermatol. 1992;128(11):1486–9.
110. Wickramasinghe L, Hindson TC, Wacks H. Treatment of neoplastic skin lesions with intralesional interferon. J Am Acad Dermatol. 1989;20(1):71–4.
111. McNairy DJ. Intradermal triamcinolone therapy of keratoacanthomas. Arch Dermatol. 1964;89:136–40.
112. Sanders S, Busam KJ, Halpern AC, Nehal KS. Intralesional corticosteroid treatment of multiple eruptive keratoacanthomas: case report and review of a controversial therapy. Dermatol Surg. 2002;28(10):954–8.
113. West L, Ayoade K, Vandergriff T, Nijhawan RI. Multiple reactive keratoacanthomas treated with zinc oxide wraps and intralesional corticosteroids. JAAD Case Rep. 2018;4(7):701–4.
114. Reusser NM, Downing C, Guidry J, Tyring SK. HPV Carcinomas in immunocompromised patients. J Clin Med. 2015;4(2):260–81.
115. Gormley RH, Kovarik CL. Human papillomavirus-related genital disease in the immunocompromised host: part II. J Am Acad Dermatol. 2012;66(6):883, e1–17; quiz 99–900.
116. Bonatti H, Aigner F, De Clercq E, Boesmueller C, Widschwendner A, Larcher C et al. Local administration of cidofovir for human papilloma virus associated skin lesions in transplant recipients. Transpl Int. 2007;20(3):238–46.
117. Calista D, Riccioni L, Coccia L. Successful treatment of squamous cell carcinoma of the lower eyelid with intralesional cidofovir. Br J Ophthalmol. 2002;86(8):932–3.

Advances in Photodynamic Therapy for the Treatment of Actinic Keratoses and Nonmelanoma Skin Cancer in Solid Organ Transplant Recipients

6

Jonathan Alvarez, Michael T. Olson, and Nathalie C. Zeitouni

INTRODUCTION

The long-term immunosuppressive regimens necessary for prolonged graft survival significantly increase the risk of malignancy in solid organ transplant recipients (SOTRs).[1] Skin cancer is the most common cancer in patients after transplantation, with cutaneous squamous cell carcinomas (cSCCs) and basal cell carcinomas (BCCs) being the most frequently detected.[2,3] Because of the early onset, high tumor burden, and unique tumor prognostic characteristics observed in transplant recipients, physicians face significant challenges in managing the treatment of cutaneous malignancies in these patients.

Photodynamic therapy (PDT) is a clinician-directed, field treatment modality that involves the combined action of a photosensitizing agent and light to destroy tumor cells. Although PDT has been used to treat internal malignancies, its most common application in dermatologic oncology clinical practice is for the treatment for actinic keratoses (AK), squamous cell carcinoma in situ (SCCIS), superficial BCCs (sBCC), and thin nodular BCCs (nBCC). Advantages of PDT include its ability to treat large and multiple

 DOI: 10.1201/9781003001461-6

lesions simultaneously, increased compliance and patient satisfaction, and favorable cosmesis.[4] In SOTRs, PDT has been used as both a primary treatment and as a preventive modality, as well as in combination with other therapies to improve overall patient outcomes. This chapter will focus its attention on the current status of PDT, including updated indications for treatment and evidence detailing its use in SOTRs.

PDT MECHANISM OF ACTION

PDT involves either the topical application or the systemic use of an exogenous photosensitizing agent, which is selectively taken up by cells in malignant or premalignant lesions. The target cells convert this agent, which is a prodrug, to protoporphyrin IX (PpIX) via the heme synthesis pathway.[5] Introduction of a light source causes activation of PpIX, formation of reactive oxygen species, and ultimately, cytotoxicity to malignant cells. PDT also induces an inflammatory response that promotes antitumor immunity through neutrophil migration to the treated tumor cells.[6] Localized damage to the tumor vasculature, with minimal normal tissue toxicity, can also occur during PDT.[7]

PHOTOSENSITIZERS AND LIGHT SOURCES

The most common topical photosensitizing agents used in PDT are 5-aminolevulinic acid (ALA) and methyl aminolevulinate (MAL). ALA formulations include an ALA 20% solution, a 10% nanoemulsion gel, and a self-adhesive ALA patch.[8] Systemic photosensitizers, such as porfimer sodium, offer deeper tumor penetration,[7] but their prolonged photosensitivity limits their use in dermatology.

A variety of light sources are available for PDT. A fluorescent tube blue light with a peak emission at 417 nm (BLU-U) is approved for use with the Levulan Kerastick (ALA 20% solution). Several narrow-band red-light lamps (BF RhodoLED, Aktilite, Omnilux) are also commercially available with activation peaks between 630 and 635 nm.[8] The depth of tissue penetration is related to the wavelength; red light, having a longer wavelength, will penetrate deeper than blue light and may be more suitable for deeper lesions. Other light sources such as coherent light sources (e.g., lasers), incoherent sources (e.g., broadband lamps, artificial white light), intense pulse lights, and natural sunlight can be used for PDT. Protocols using daylight PDT (dPDT) have license approval from the European Medicines Agency in select European countries and several other countries around the world.[8–10]

APPROVALS AND PROTOCOLS

Many PDT protocols have been approved for use across the world. The Levulan Kerastick is FDA approved with use of the BLU-U (10 J/cm^2, 1000 seconds) for the treatment of mild-to-moderate AKs of the face, scalp, or upper extremities. The approved incubation time is 14–18 hours without occlusion.[8] In clinical practice, however, the incubation time varies between 1 and 3 hours with or without occlusion with sessions appropriately repeated in 4–12 weeks for any remaining lesions (Figure 6.1).

The ALA 10% nanoemulsion gel (Ameluz), developed and approved in Europe, was also approved in the United States in combination with the BF-RhodoLED lamp (37 J/cm^2, 10 minutes) for lesion and field-directed treatment of mild-to-moderate AKs of the face and scalp. The recommended use is 3 hours

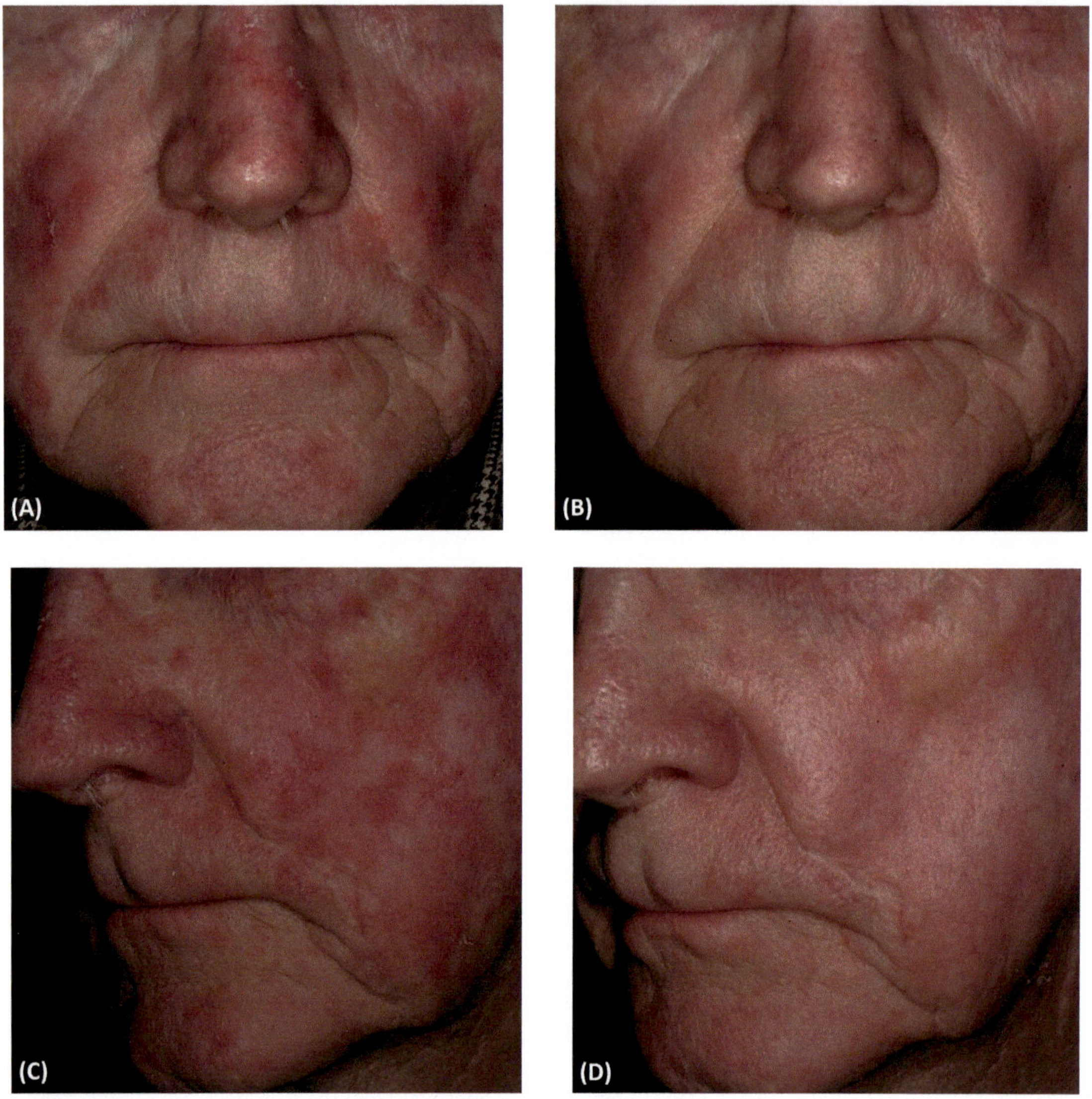

FIGURE 6.1 A 72-year-old non-transplant man with multiple areas of actinic keratosis on the face **(a)**, **(c)**. The redness and scaliness resolved following one PDT treatment with 5-aminolevulinic acid and a 417 nanometer blue light **(b)**, **(d)**. (Used with permission, C. William Hanke, MD.)

incubation under occlusion with treatment repeated at 3 months for persistent lesions. In Europe, ALA 10% gel was also approved for field cancerization, with dPDT (2-hour daylight exposure after 30 minutes incubation) and for nonaggressive BCC. The recommended treatment protocol for BCC is two PDT sessions 1 week apart and reassessment at 3 months.[8]

The use of MAL 16.8 % cream with red-light PDT has approved indications for the treatment of non-hyperkeratotic AKs of the face and scalp, as well as SCCIS, sBCC, and nBCC. MAL cream is available in Europe and in many countries worldwide with approved indications for PDT varying by country. MAL is also approved with dPDT for mild-to-moderate AKs in several countries around the world. In the United States, MAL red-light PDT was previously approved for use in June 2008 by the FDA, but it is no longer available on the market. One treatment of MAL-PDT is recommended for AK, repeated at 3 months if necessary. For superficial skin cancers deemed unsuitable for surgery, recommendations are for two treatment sessions, 1 week apart and reassessment at 3 months.[8]

EVIDENCE FOR PDT AS A PRIMARY MODALITY

Actinic Keratosis and Nonmelanoma Skin Cancer

Nonmelanoma skin cancer (NMSC) is the most common malignancy in SOTRs.[2,11] The risk of developing NMSC may be in part related to long-term immunosuppression after organ transplantation; lung transplant recipients, in particular, are commonly subjected to higher immunosuppressive dosages and experience higher rates of NMSC compared to other SOTRs.[12] Patients with a history of skin cancer prior to transplantation may be subject to a higher risk of NMSC after transplantation; additional risk factors may include certain medication use (e.g., voriconazole) and white race.[13] Higher mortality rates were documented in SOTRs, likely attributed to greater frequency and recurrence of aggressive lesions. Although surgery remains the gold-standard treatment modality for NMSC, PDT offers an alternative therapeutic modality as a field therapy for precancerous lesions and for select superficial cutaneous malignancies.[8,14,15]

Primary Treatment for AK and SCCIS

Initial studies conducted in SOTRs provided foundational evidence for PDT in managing precancerous skin lesions. In 2004, Dragieva and colleagues[16] performed one of the first studies investigating the efficacy of PDT in organ transplant recipients (OTRs) with AK or Bowen's disease. Twenty OTRs and 20 immunocompetent patients underwent 1–2 sessions of ALA with a 5-hour incubation period, followed by illumination with 75 J/cm^2 with an incoherent light source.[16] High initial complete response (CR) rates at 4 weeks were found in both the OTR (86%) and control (94%) groups. The long-term clearance decreased for both groups but was more significant in the OTR group than in the control group at 48 weeks (48% vs. 72%). Although PDT was deemed both safe and effective for OTRs, it appeared that they did not respond as well to PDT as did immunocompetent patients (Table 6.1).

Several other studies thereafter reported the use of MAL-PDT in OTRs. In one study, areas of mild-to-moderate AKs were randomized to two consecutive treatments of PDT at one week apart using either MAL or placebo cream. Sites were illuminated with 75 J/cm^2 of visible light delivered at 80 mW/cm^2. At 4 months, 13/17 patients enrolled in the study were clinically cleared of AK lesions, and a partial response was recorded in three others.[17] AKs unresponsive to conventional treatments in OTRs were treated with two sessions of MAL-PDT for 3 hours under occlusion and narrow-band red light. Overall response rate was 71% of AK lesions with a CR of 64% seen at 3 months.[18] Lower responses were observed on the dorsal hands (40%) versus the face and scalp (72%). In contrast, facial AKs showed a CR of 100% at 12 and 24 weeks using one to two sessions of MAL-PDT and red light, while photodamage also improved by 62.5%.[19]

Compared with topical 5-FU cream, MAL-PDT was found to be more effective for the treatment of epidermal dysplasia in OTRs. Cosmetic outcomes and patient preference were also superior in the PDT-treated group.[20] In a randomized trial comparing the efficacy and safety of field treatment with MAL-PDT versus imiquimod cream for AKs in OTRs, PDT achieved a higher rate of CR (78% versus 61%, $P < 0.001$) at 3 months with shorter lasting, but more intense, adverse skin reactions.[21] Interestingly, in a real-world analysis, CR rates with PDT in OTRs were both comparable to those of immunocompetent patients and durable at 12 months (80% vs. 73%). Overall, scalp lesions had the lowest responses.[22]

Several reviews have compiled evidence of sustained efficacy of PDT in OTRs.[23–26] In a qualitative synthesis of eight randomized trials with 242 OTRs, AK clearance rates were evaluated after MAL-PDT, ablative fractional laser (AFXL), diclofenac sodium 3%, imiquimod 5% cream, and topical 5-FU. MAL-PDT showed the highest rates of CR (40%–76.4%), followed by imiquimod (27.5%–62.1%), diclofenac (41%), and 5-FU (11%). Treatment with AFXL alone demonstrated particularly low lesion clearance (5%–31%). MAL-PDT is currently the best-studied intervention among the aforementioned treatment modalities.[26] Most recently in 2020, Liew and colleagues[24] published a systematic review and meta-analysis of 12 studies evaluating the

TABLE 6.1 Summary of PDT Studies in SOTRs for the Treatment of Actinic Keratoses and NMSC

STUDY	*DESIGN*	*REGIMEN*	*RESULTS*
ALA-cPDT Dragieva et al., 2004 [16]	Prospective case series 20 SOTRs with 44 lesions and 20 controls with 36 lesions AK and BD	ALA 20%-PDT[b] × 1–2 sessions, 5-hour incubation and incoherent visible light, 75 J/cm² light dose, at 80 mW/cm² one week apart	CR: immunosuppressed vs. control • at 4 weeks: 86% vs. 94% • at 12 weeks: 68% vs. 89% • at 48 weeks: 48% vs. 72%
MAL vs. placebo Dragieva et al., 2004 [17]	Double-blind intrapatient randomized prospective trial 17 SOTRs with 129 lesions Mild-to-moderate AK	MAL-PDT[a] × 2; 3-hour incubation and 630–730 nm incoherent visible light source, 75 J/cm² light dose, at 80 mW/cm² 1 week apart	CR: MAL vs. placebo • at 16 weeks: 76% vs. 0% Lesion complete response rate • 56/62 for PDT • 0/67 for placebo
ALA-PDT Schleier et al., 2004 [27]	Prospective case series 5 OTRs with 32 lesions AK, BCC, SCC, keratoacanthoma	ALA 40%-PDT × 1; 3–5-hour incubation and 635 nm diode laser with 120 J/cm² for 10 minutes	Complete remission in 24 tumors (75%)
MAL-PDT Perrett et al., 2006 [28]	Case Report 50-year-old patient with 1 lesion Small nBCC	MAL-PDT[a] ×2; 3-hour incubation and 633 nm red light, 75 J/cm² light dose, at 80 mW/cm² 1 week apart	CR of 100% at 4 weeks Durable response at 1 year
MAL-PDT vs. 5-FU Perrett et al., 2007 [20]	Randomized, intrapatient controlled comparative study 8 SOTRs with 18 lesional areas AK and BD	MAL-PDT[a] × 2; 3-hour incubation and 633 nm red light, 75 J/cm² light dose, at 80 mW/cm² one week apart or 5-FU BID for 3 weeks	CR: PDT vs. 5-FU • at 12 weeks: 89% vs. 11% • at 24 weeks: both groups unchanged
MAL-PDT Piaserico et al., 2007 [18]	Prospective case series 15 OTRs with 33 lesional areas including 245 AK lesions	MAL-PDT[a] 3-hour incubation and 633 nm red light, 37 J/cm² light dose × 2 sessions 2 weeks apart	Overall AK response rate: 71% Response rate was significantly higher on the scalp/face compared with the back of the hands (72% vs. 40%)
MAL-cPDT Hasson et al., 2012 [19]	Prospective case series 16 SOTRs with AK and photodamage of the face and scalp	MAL-PDT[a] × 1–2: 3-hour incubation and 635 nm red light, 37 J/cm² light dose; repeat at 12 weeks if AK present at >50% of baseline	CR 100% at 24 weeks Photodamage 62.5% improvement
MAL-cPDT Guleng et al., 2012 [29]	Prospective case series 18 SOTRs with BCCs (superficial and nodular)	MAL-PDT × 2: 3-hour incubation and 630 nm red light, 37 J/cm² light dose	CR of 94% Only 1 recurrence at 26 months

(Continued)

TABLE 6.1 Summary of PDT Studies in SOTRs for the Treatment of Actinic Keratoses and NMSC (Continued)

STUDY	*DESIGN*	*REGIMEN*	*RESULTS*
MAL-PDT Collier et al., 2015 [30]	Retrospective review 23 SOTRs with 53 lesions and 80 nontransplant patients with 269 lesions BCC	MAL-PDT × 2: 3-hour incubation and 630 nm red light one week apart	BCC Recurrence; average time • SOTR: 22.6%; 1.3 years • Nontransplant: 15.2%; 1.4 years No statistically significant difference between groups
MAL-PDT vs. IMIQ Togsverd-Bo et al., 2018 [21]	Randomized intraindividual controlled trial 35 SOTRs with 572 AK lesions	MAL-PDT[a] × 1; 3-hour incubation and 634 nm red light, 37 J/cm^2 light dose or IMIQ × 3 per week for 4 weeks. For incomplete clearance, MAL-PDT repeated after 3 months and IMIQ repeated after 2 months.	CR after one and two treatments • MAL-PDT: 66% and 78% • IMIQ: 49% and 61%
MAL-cPDT Lim et al., 2019 [22]	Retrospective chart review 25 SOTR, 33 lesions 167 nontransplant patients, 281 lesions AK, NMSC, lichen planus	MAL-PDT two sessions, 1–2 weeks apart	Clearance at 12 weeks and 12 months SOTR 74% and 80% Nontransplant 76 % and 73%

Abbreviations: AK, actinic keratoses; ALA, 5-aminolevulinic acid; BCC, basal cell carcinoma; BD, Bowen's disease; CR, complete response; cPDT, conventional PDT; IMIQ, imiquimod; MAL, methyl aminolevulinate; nBCC, nodular basal cell carcinoma; NMSC, nonmelanoma skin cancer; OTR, organ transplant recipient; SCC, squamous cell carcinoma; SOTR, solid organ transplant recipient. **Pretreatment**—[a]curettage, [b]curettage or salicylic acid.

use of PDT for the prevention (four randomized trials) and primary treatment (five randomized trials) of AKs and SCCs in OTRs. The remaining three studies reported treatment and prevention effects of PDT. The primary outcome for prevention was the 3-year incidence of AK/SCC, and the CR of lesions after PDT for the treatment group. The pooled risk-difference for preventive measure of NMSC was 0.14 (95% CI 0.08–0.19), showing significant association favoring the use of PDT in prevention. Furthermore, the CR rate was higher in those receiving PDT as a treatment, with a pooled risk difference of 0.77 (95% CI 0.6–0.94) and 0.50 (95% CI 0.22–0.79) in pre-divided lesional areas and number of lesions, respectively.[24] In summary, PDT remains a viable preventive and alternative treatment option for OTRs with AK or SCCIS, with superior cosmetic outcomes and good safety profile compared with those of other modalities. It remains important to continue investigating the use and optimization of PDT, particularly in light of the many combination therapies that may result in increased efficacy compared with monotherapy.

Primary Treatment for BCC

The feasibility and effectiveness of PDT for BCC has been evaluated in several reports. Schleier and colleagues[27] were the first to explore the use of PDT for BCC in five OTRs. Excellent response was noted in all tumors with a 75% CR rate at 12 weeks.[27] In 2006, Perrett and colleagues[28] published a case report of successful treatment of BCC on the nose in a liver transplant recipient. The patient was treated with two sessions of MAL-PDT for 3 hours under occlusion and a noncoherent red light source. After 1 month, there was a CR, which was durable up to 1 year, with excellent cosmetic outcome.[28] Subsequently, in a case series of 18 OTRs with BCC on the head and trunk, two sessions of MAL-PDT and red light delivered by an incoherent LED source obtained a CR rate of 94% at a mean follow-up of 22.6 months.[29] In a retrospective review involving 322 BCC lesions in 103 patients (23 OTRs and 80 immunocompetent hosts) treated with PDT, recurrence rates after treatment were similar between groups (22.6% vs. 15.2%, respectively) at a mean follow-up of 3.5 years.[30] Additionally, there was no evidence that PDT in OTRs produced inferior results compared with those in nontransplant patients.[30] Ultimately, fewer studies have characterized the treatment of BCC with topical PDT in OTRs; however, evidence based on existing experiences has shown similar clinical response rates compared with those of immunocompetent patients (Table 6.1).

COMBINATION METHODS TO ENHANCE PDT EFFICACY

Physical Pretreatment Modalities

Optimizing efficacy in OTRs has led to the use of various modalities to increase drug penetration and PpIX synthesis. In a randomized clinical trial comparing the relative potential of different physical pretreatments, curettage, microneedling, microdermabrasion, and the AFXL prior to PDT, all were found to increase intraepidermal PpIX compared with that in participants who did not undergo pretreatment.[31] The use of microneedling for resistant AKs was associated with an 83% CR rate at 9 months follow-up in one study of OTRs. Treatment was well tolerated, and pain was significantly reduced over further sessions.[32] Elevating temperature, or thermal PDT, also was shown to enhance PDT responses in both preclinical and clinical reports.[33]

Pretreatment with AFXL, used to create vertical channels and facilitate photosensitizer uptake, was shown in clinical practice to improve PDT efficacy.[34] A single session of AFXL-assisted PDT was more effective than AFXL alone in treating acral AKs (73% vs. 31%) and wart-like lesions (37% vs. 14%) in a series of ten OTRs.[35] No scarring was observed. Togsverd-Bo and colleagues[36] also assessed the use of AFXL-dPDT, dPDT, conventional PDT, and AFXL alone in 16 OTRs with 542 AKs. AFXL was delivered with a 2940 nm laser. In dPDT and AFXL-dPDT, MAL was applied for 30 minutes without occlusion, followed by 2-hour daylight exposure. For conventional PDT, MAL was occluded for 3 hours followed by red light (630 nm) irradiation at 37 J/cm^2. At 3 months, CRs were highest (74%) after AFXL-dPDT, followed by 50% after conventional PDT, 46% after dPDT, and 5% after AFXL alone. Although well tolerated, more intense adverse events were seen with AFXL-dPDT. Similar results were found for thick scalp and forehead AK treated with AFXL-dPDT.[37] A recent systematic review in all patients found that laser-assisted PDT for AKs offered higher clearance rates that PDT alone without a significant increase in pain[38] (Table 6.2).

Topical Neoadjuvant Therapy

To optimize response, the use of neoadjuvant agents, including 5-FU cream, retinoids, imiquimod, and most recently, vitamin D, were investigated in combination with PDT.[39] A mechanism-based combination approach using 5-FU as a neoadjuvant for ALA-PDT in mouse models of SCC found that pretreatment with 5-FU for 3 days followed by ALA for 4 hours led to large, tumor-selective increases in PpIX levels and enhanced cell death upon illumination.[40] Zhang and colleagues[41] validated these findings, demonstrating that the effects of apoptosis induced by ALA-PDT could be enhanced with 5-FU or 3-methyladenine treatment. This sequential approach was used to treat four OTRs with field cancerization of AKs and SCCIS involving either the scalp, face, or both. Light curettage of hyperkeratotic lesions, followed by 5-FU twice daily for 5 days and PDT with 1 hour incubation on day 6 showed good tolerance and excellent response.[42] Patients remained free of lesions at 1 and 6 months follow-up. In a group of immunocompetent

TABLE 6.2 Summary of PDT Studies with Combined Modalities for Actinic Keratoses and NMSC in SOTRs

STUDY	*DESIGN*	*REGIMEN*	*RESULTS*
MAL-PDT + microneedling Bencini et al., 2012 [32]	Prospective case series 12 OTRs 59 AK resistant to cPDT	Microneedling pretreatment MAL-PDT × 3 at 2-week intervals with 3-hour incubation followed by 10-minute irradiation at 90 J/cm² light dose	CR • at 4 months: 100% (12/12) • at 9 months: 83% (10/12) In 17% (2/12) of cases, there was a relapse of grade I and II in pts with multiple AKs
AFXL-PDT vs. AFXL Helsing, et al., 2013 [35]	Randomized half-side comparative trial 10 OTRs with 680 AK and 409 WLL	AFXL ± MAL-PDT × 1; 3-hour incubation and 632 nm red light, 37 J/cm² light dose	CR at 4 months: AFXL-PDT vs. AFXL • AK: 73% vs. 31% • WLL: 37% vs. 14% AFXL-PDT improved 82% of AKs to lower grade lesions vs. 52% with AFXL alone
AFXL-dPDT vs. dPDT vs. MAL-cPDT vs. AFXL Togsverd-Bo et al., 2015 [36]	Randomized controlled trial 16 OTRs. with 542 lesions AK	± AFXL pretreatment MAL-dPDT and 2.5 hours daylight exposure or MAL-cPDT for 3 hours under occlusion, with 630 nm red light, 37 J/cm² light dose or AFXL alone	CR at 3 months • AFXL-dPDT: 74% • dPDT: 46% • cPDT: 50% • AFXL: 5%
Sequential curettage, 5-FU, and PDT Jambusaria-Pahlajani et al., 2016 [42]	Prospective case series 4 SOTRs who previously failed monotherapy AK/SCCIS	Light curettage followed by 5-FU 5% cream BID × 5 days and PDT ×1 with 1-hour incubation on day 6 with either MAL followed by red light, 37 J/cm² light dose or ALA 20% and 400–450 nm blue light, 10 J/cm² light dose	All 4 patients had complete clearance or near-total clearance of their AKs Patients remained free of AK/SCCIS for 1 to 6 months after clearance
5-FU+PDT vs. PDT Maytin et al., 2018 [43]	Mechanism-based clinical pilot study 17 patients (4 OTRs and 13 nontransplant) with at least 4 AK lesions	± 6 days of 5-FU pretreatment MAL-PDT with 3-hour incubation and 635 nm red light, 37 J/cm² light dose	CR: 5-FU+PDT vs. PDT • at 3 months: 75% vs. 45% • at 6 months: 67% vs. 39%
AFXL-assisted dPDT vs. dPDT Rizvi et al., 2019 [37]	Prospective pilot study 12 OTRs with 209 AK on the scalp and forehead	MAL-dPDT ± AFXL for 30 minutes followed by 2 hours of sunlight	CR at 4 months • AFXL-dPDT: 75.5% • dPDT: 64%

Abbreviations: 5-FU, 5-fluorouracil; AFXL, ablative fractional laser; AK, actinic keratoses; ALA, 5-aminolevulinic acid; CR, complete response; cPDT, conventional PDT; dPDT, daylight PDT; MAL, methyl aminolevulinate; NMSC, nonmelanoma skin cancer; OTR, organ transplant recipient; SCCIS, squamous cell carcinoma in situ; SOTR, solid organ transplant recipient; WLL, wart like lesions.

and transplant patients, clearance rates of AK after 3 and 6 months were improved with serial 5-FU pretreatment and PDT (75 % and 67%) versus PDT alone (45% and 39%).[43] Improved AK clearance could be explained by enhanced photosensitizer accumulation as well as p53 induction.[43] Vitamin D as a neoadjuvant agent also was shown to promote preferential accumulation of PpIX and increase efficacy of PDT for AK and BCC.[44] Clinical trials are ongoing to further evaluate response, but its use in OTRs remains currently unexplored. Overall, in daily practice, the choice to employ combination therapy over monotherapy should be made on a case-by-case basis, considering resources and the patient's unique lesions and preference.[45]

EVIDENCE FOR PDT AS A PREVENTIVE MODALITY

In SOTRs, the risk of developing NMSC and its precursor lesions increases with organ graft survival time and duration of immunosuppression.[2,46] The need for early intervention to reduce the morbidity of widespread involvement has generated a great deal of interest in exploring the effectiveness of PDT as a preventive modality. Preclinical data have substantiated this interest by demonstrating that PDT could significantly delay UV-induced skin tumors in murine mouse models.[47] Early clinical studies also presented evidence for the concept of PDT use in cancer prevention, with significantly longer time to occurrence of new AK and other skin lesions in PDT-treated areas compared with control areas after 6–12 months[48,49] (Table 6.3).

Additional studies in case series confirmed PDT could reduce AK and SCC; however, mixed results were obtained at longer follow-up times. De Graff and colleagues[50] demonstrated a trend toward SCC prevention after one to two sessions of ALA violet light PDT at 12 months; however, no difference was observed after 2 years. Wennberg and colleagues[51] found a 46% reduction in new AKs at 3 months after two sessions of field MAL-PDT with red light. Single treatments were repeated at 3, 9, and 15 months, but the significance of that effect was lost at 27 months. Notably the patients that had undergone transplantation within 10 years tended to have a better response to PDT.

The observed diminishing efficacy of PDT as a preventive therapy underscores the fact that a single or even a limited series of treatments may not be sufficient to completely clear the signs of chronic actinic damage and thus the risk of NMSC,[52] and that long follow-up times are necessary. Additional studies found that frequent, ongoing, or cyclic treatments could have a preventive effect. In a small pilot study, Willey and colleagues[53] treated 12 high-risk OTRs with cyclic ALA-PDT blue light at 4- to 8-week intervals for 2 years. A median reduction in the development of new SCCs of 79% and 95% at 12 months and 24 months, respectively, was found compared to baseline.[53] Repeated PDT treatments served as an effective primary prevention for subclinical UV-induced skin dysplasia in renal transplant recipients. A randomized split-side study evaluated 25 patients with clinically normal skin who received MAL-PDT at 6-month intervals for 5 years. At 3 years, the authors observed AKs in 63% of the patients' untreated skin compared with 28% of the patients' PDT-treated skin.[54] More recently, consecutive treatments of dPDT showed potential effectiveness in preventing new AK and keratinocyte carcinoma in OTRs. Patients received two sessions of dPDT at baseline, at 3 months, and at 9 months. Field cancerization areas treated with dPDT showed significantly fewer new lesions with a higher patient preference compared with the results in the cryotherapy control group.[55] A primary prevention of AK and NMSC study is also currently investigating the long-term safety and efficacy of cyclic ALA-PDT in patients who have recently undergone organ transplantation (ClinicalTrials.gov: NCT03110159).

Due to the heterogeneity of the studied parameters, qualitative analysis of combined existing trial data may be challenging but has shown interesting trends. A recent systematic review of randomized controlled trials looking at interventions to prevent NMSC found that PDT was associated with lower risks of keratotic skin lesions (two trials, 53 participants, risk ratio [RR] 0.24 [95% CI, 0.12–0.48]), whereas the effect of PDT on NMSC was less certain (three trials, 93 participants, RR 1.42 [95% confidence interval [CI], 0.65–3.11]).[25] In contrast, a systematic review and meta-analysis of 12 treatment and/or prevention

TABLE 6.3 Summary of Studies of PDT as a Preventive Modality for Actinic Keratoses and NMSC in SOTRs

STUDY	*DESIGN*	*REGIMEN*	*RESULTS*
MAL-PDT vs. untreated control Wulf et al., 2006 [48]	Randomized, intrapatient controlled comparative trial 27 SOTRs Existing AKs and NMSCs	MAL-PDT[b] × 1: 3-hour incubation and 570–670 nm red light, 75 J/cm² light dose	Mean time to occurrence of new lesion • MAL-PDT: 9.6 months • Control: 6.8 months Lesion-free areas at 12 months • MAL-PDT: 62% (16/26) • Control: 35% (9/26)
ALA-PDT vs. untreated control de Graaf et al., 2006 [50]	Randomized, intrapatient controlled comparative trial 40 OTRs Existing NMSCs	ALA 20%-PDT × 1–2: 4-hour incubation and 400–450 nm violet light, 5.5–6 J/cm² light dose 2nd PDT treatment at 6 months	New SCC lesions at 2 years • ALA-PDT: 15 SCCs in 9/40 arms • Control: 10 SCCs in 9/40 arms No significant difference was seen in the occurrence of new SCCs. Number of keratotic lesions increased in both arms, but was less pronounced with PDT
MAL-PDT vs. cryotherapy control Wennberg et al., 2008 [51]	Randomized, intrapatient controlled comparative trial 81 OTRs with 889 lesions 90 % AK	MAL-PDT[b] × 2: 3-hour incubation and 630 nm red light, 37 J/cm² light dose 1 week apart Additional single treatments at 3, 9, and 15 months	New lesions: MAL-PDT vs. control • at 3 months: 65 vs. 103 • at 27 months: 253 vs. 312 46% new AK reduction at 3 months
Cyclic ALA-PDT Willey et al., 2010 [53]	Prospective case series 12 SOTRs SCCs	Cyclic ALA 20%-PDT[a] with 1- hour incubation and 417 nm blue light illumination at 4- to 8-week intervals for 2 years	Median SCC reduction • at 12 months: 79% • at 24 months: 95%
MAL-PDT vs. untreated control Togsverd-Bo et al., 2015 [54]	Randomized intrapatient controlled trial 25 OTRs No previous or current NMSCs	MAL-PDT with 3-hour incubation and 630 nm red light, 37 J/cm² light dose at 6-month intervals for 5 years	New AK lesions at 3 years • MAL-PDT: 28% of patients • Control: 63% of patient
MAL-dPDT vs. cryotherapy control Bernad et al., 2019 [55]	Randomized, intrasubject controlled, evaluator-blind, split-face and/or scalp trial 24 OTRs AK and KC	MAL[b] for 30 minutes then 2 hours of daylight: two sessions 15 days apart at baseline, 3 and 9 months Control received cryotherapy at baseline, 3, and 9 months	Total lesions at 21 months MAL-dPDT: 4.7 Control: 5.8 Mean of total new lesions: MAL-dPDT vs. Control. • 4.2 vs. 6.8 (3 mo), 3.0 vs. 4.3 (9 mo), 3.0 vs. 4.8 (15 mo), 3.7 vs. 5.0 (21 mo) *Nonsignificant at 21 months

Abbreviations: AK, actinic keratoses; ALA, 5-aminolevulinic acid; dPDT, daylight PDT; KC, keratinocyte carcinoma; MAL, methyl aminolevulinate; NMSC, nonmelanoma skin cancer; OTR, organ transplant recipient; SCC, squamous cell carcinoma; SOTR, solid organ transplant recipient. **Pretreatment**—[a]curettage, [b]debridement.

studies favored the use of PDT as a preventive measure for both AK and SCC, with PDT demonstrating a lower incidence of new lesions and pooled risk difference (RD) of 0.14 (95% CI 0.08–0.19).[24] Although findings have indicated that PDT may be effective in the reduction of new AKs, additional data may be needed to fully investigate SCC prevention.

Interest lies in understanding the mechanism of action of the PDT preventive effects. In one study, ALA-PDT displayed utility in inducing and eliminating apoptotic resistant senescent cells, which accumulate with age and following UV radiation, chemotherapy, and radiation therapy.[56] Investigations into the molecular and genetic changes with PDT showed that treatment can also correct abnormal cancer-associated gene expression in AKs of OTRs, while inducing the expression of dermal extracellular matrix genes in photo-exposed skin.[57] The latter study supports the use of PDT for field cancerization.

ADVERSE REACTIONS

PDT is generally a well-tolerated treatment modality without increased risk of major adverse reactions. A history of porphyria, preexisting photosensitivity, or allergy to any ingredient of the photosensitizer (including soybean, peanut, and almond oil) are contraindications to PDT. The main phototoxic effects seen are erythema and edema, which may be accompanied by desquamation, crusting, hypo- and hyperpigmentation, and a tingling and burning sensation posttreatment.[10,58] Pre- and posttreatment written instructions should be provided to patients and discussed with them, including posttreatment photoprotection, to better prepare them for the procedure. Transient amnesia during and post PDT therapy was reported in only one small series.[59] One of the main limitations of conventional PDT is treatment-related pain. Pain typically peaks at the onset of illumination and tends to improve over the duration of the treatment.[10,58] The perceived intensity of pain can vary greatly among patients and may be more pronounced in the SOTR population because of extensive lesion involvement.[58,60] Use of the 0–10 visual analog pain scale (VAS) can be useful during therapy to monitor the patient's discomfort level. A number of pain-relieving techniques have been described in the literature including supportive measures such as the use of cooling fans, nerve blocks, and topical anesthetics, as well as the use of fractionated irradiation and the use of modified delivery protocols.[61] Having the patient listen to music or talking to the patient during therapy may also alleviate some discomfort. Recent findings that showed a positive correlation between PDT-related pain and PpIX accumulation have led to the exploration of alternative strategies to limit PpIX buildup during treatment.[61–64]

One such strategy was the development of dPDT protocols, with a short incubation time and prolonged light exposure of low irradiance. The advent of dPDT has been a game changer with regards to treatment-related pain. In recent studies, dPDT was associated with no to minimal pain and was shown to have similar efficacy to conventional PDT.[8,10,61] The use of dPDT permits the treatment of large fields in routine practice, which would be especially beneficial to transplant recipients, while reducing office visit time and minimizing cost and equipment. Limitations of dPDT can include irradiance variability because of location and climate.[65] Some alternatives to dPDT include artificial white light (AWL), which could be used year round, and simulated indoor daylight.[66–68] In addition, a new illumination protocol with a fabric-based biophotonic device (the Phosistos protocol, reduced irradiance and light dose) has been found to be noninferior to conventional PDT for treating AKs, but with lower pain scores.[69] The advantage of textile PDT, or light-emitting fabrics, is that the device can adapt to the shape or convexity of the treated region. Additional protocols including the in-office "painless PDT" regimen also resulted in little to no pain, with an AK clearance rate of 52% (vs. 44% for conventional PDT) after a 15-minute ALA incubation followed by 60-minutes of blue light exposure.[63] Foregoing incubation altogether by initiating illumination for either 30, 45, or 60 minutes immediately after application of the photosensitizer (simultaneous or metronomic PDT) has resulted in a nearly identical efficacy compared with a conventional blue light regimen while significantly reducing pain.[62] Overall, reducing the drug-light interval with prolonged illumination can decrease pain while being therapeutically effective.[70] Zeitouni and colleagues[71,72] had previously introduced a two-step irradiance PDT protocol with red light, which demonstrated efficacy in preserving clinical outcomes while minimizing patient discomfort. Target lesions were irradiated at low levels until 90% of PpIX was photobleached before subsequently increasing the irradiance until the prescribed total light dose was delivered. Excellent pain control during AK treatment, including SOTR patients, was also seen with this protocol[73] (Table 6.4).

Progression to invasive SCC from either incompletely treated or nonresponding lesions is possible with PDT.[10] Any recurrent lesions, rapidly growing lesions, or nonresponding lesions should be promptly biopsied or excised to rule out an invasive or aggressive tumor. In addition, baseline and follow-up photographs of the treated areas could assist in evaluating new, recurrent, or progressive disease. Long-term and close follow ups are needed. The potential for paradoxical PDT-related induction of skin carcinogenesis was previously reported,[58] but there is currently no direct evidence that PDT causes skin cancer[10] (Table 6.4).

The risk of further immunosuppression in SOTRs is possible, but there is no clear data to support this risk. Following reports from murine studies suggesting that PDT may compromise immune clearance, healthy Mantoux-positive volunteers underwent narrow-band red light treatment, with and without prior application of MAL or ALA, and showed suppressed delayed-type hypersensitivity responses to tuberculin purified protein.[74] Harm to the allograft is another potential concern for transplant patients. However, an analysis of reported events involving >200 OTRs undergoing ALA/MAL-PDT and a recent systematic review involving 242 OTRs found no therapy-related transplant rejections or worsening graft function.[26,75]

CONCLUSION

PDT can be a highly effective strategy in the overall management of SOTRs and can offer numerous advantages in treating premalignant and select NMSCs. Notably, as a field therapy capable of treating large body surfaces, PDT may not only address precancerous lesions but may act as an effective long-term measure to possibly prevent field cancerization and the associated risk of malignant progression. In SOTRs, in whom surgery-fatigue can be seen, PDT may be integrated with other therapeutic options to potentially improve quality of life. Although pain continues to be the most notable limiting factor in clinical practice, the emergence of dPDT and alternative indoor PDT protocols and new illumination sources may minimize this adverse effect and facilitate adherence to treatment. Although PDT is one of the best-studied nonsurgical options in SOTRs, data analysis is frequently encumbered by several factors, including a relatively small study group or a lack of a control group, an overall high heterogeneity of treatment parameters, and to a certain extent, a variability in the subpopulation characteristics of the transplant patients. Future PDT research would benefit from larger, prospective randomized controlled studies and a more standardized approach. The emphasis of future studies should also be on translational research with a better understanding of the underlying molecular changes seen with PDT in transplant patients.

TABLE 6.4 Summary and Recommendations for the Treatment of Actinic Keratoses with PDT

PRETREATMENT		*TREATMENT OPTIONS*		*PAIN MANAGEMENT*		*FOLLOW UP*		
Patient selection Education Photographs **Skin Preparation** • Alcohol-soaked gauze scrub • Curettage or medical grade sandpaper **Physical Options** • Microneedling • Microdermabrasion • AFXL • Heat **Topical Neoadjuvant Options** • 5-FU • Retinoids • Imiquimod • Vitamin D	➔	ALA 20% for 1–3 hours with or without occlusion. Illuminate with blue light (10 J/cm^2, 1000 seconds) — OR — ALA 10% for 1–3 hours with/without occlusion Illuminate with red light (37 J/cm^2) or daylight (2-hour exposure after 30 minutes incubation) — OR — MAL 16.8% for 3 hours. Illuminate with red light (37 J/cm^2 or daylight (2-hour exposure after 30 minutes incubation)	➔	**Supportive Measures** • Fans • Short Breaks • Music/Talk • Monitor with VAS **Daylight PDT** (2-hour exposure after 30 minutes incubation) **Alternative indoor protocols** • "Painless" PDT 15 min ALA incubation followed by 60 min blue light activation • Simultaneous PS application and blue light activation for 30 minutes • Two-Step Irradiance 1–3 hours ALA incubation followed by initial irradiance of 35 mW/cm^2 then 70 mW/cm^2. Total light dose of 75 J/cm^2 • Textile PDT 30 minutes MAL incubation followed by 2.5 hours of red-light activation with fabric-based device. **Alternate light sources** • Artificial white light	➔	ALA 20%-PDT treatment may be repeated at 4–12 weeks — OR — ALA 10%-PDT treatment may be repeated at 3 months — OR — MAL 16.8%-PDT treatment may be repeated at 3 months	➔	**Biopsy** • Unresponsive lesions • Recurrent lesions **Prevention** • Sun protection • Regular follow-up visits • Cyclic PDT at 3–6-month intervals

Abbreviations: 5-FU, 5-fluorouracil; AFXL, ablative fractional laser; ALA, 5-aminolevulinic acid; MAL, methyl aminolevulinate; PDT, photodynamic therapy; PS, photosensitizer; VAS, visual analog scale

SUMMARY OF KEY POINTS

- PDT can be used safely and effectively to treat AK and select NMSCs in SOTRs, while offering favorable cosmetic results and high patient satisfaction.
- Use of physical pretreatments and neoadjuvant combination therapies may increase the efficacy of PDT treatment sessions.
- Early intervention and repeated/cyclic PDT treatments have the potential to be used as a long-term preventive strategy in high-risk patients.
- The advent of dPDT and alternative pain-relieving PDT protocols offer new options for PDT-associated treatment discomfort.
- Optimization of the PDT treatment parameters and better understanding of the molecular mechanisms are needed to improve outcomes.

REFERENCES

1. Engels EA, Pfeiffer RM, Fraumeni JF et al. Spectrum of cancer risk among US solid organ transplant recipients. JAMA. 2011;306(17):1891–901.
2. Mittal A, Colegio OR. Skin cancers in organ transplant recipients. Am J Transplant Off J Am Soc Transplant Am Soc Transpl Surg. 2017;17(10):2509–30.
3. Stockfleth E, Ulrich C, Meyer T, Christophers E. Epithelial malignancies in organ transplant patients: clinical presentation and new methods of treatment. Recent Results Cancer Res Fortschritte Krebsforsch Progres Dans Rech Sur Cancer. 2002;160:251–8.
4. Tierney EP, Eide MJ, Jacobsen G, Ozog D. Photodynamic therapy for actinic keratoses: survey of patient perceptions of treatment satisfaction and outcomes. J Cosmet Laser Ther Off Publ Eur Soc Laser Dermatol. 2008;10(2):81–6.
5. Kennedy JC, Pottier RH, Pross DC. Photodynamic therapy with endogenous protoporphyrin IX: basic principles and present clinical experience. J Photochem Photobiol B. 1990;6(1–2):143–8.
6. Gollnick SO, Evans SS, Baumann H et al. Role of cytokines in photodynamic therapy-induced local and systemic inflammation. Br J Cancer. 2003;88(11):1772–9.
7. Agostinis P, Berg K, Cengel KA et al. Photodynamic therapy of cancer: an update. CA Cancer J Clin. 2011;61(4):250–81.
8. Morton CA, Szeimies R-M, Basset-Seguin N et al. European dermatology forum guidelines on topical photodynamic therapy 2019 part 1: treatment delivery and established indications—actinic keratoses, Bowen's disease and basal cell carcinomas. J Eur Acad Dermatol Venereol JEADV. 2019;33(12):2225–38.
9. Morton CA, Szeimies R-M, Basset-Séguin N et al. European dermatology forum guidelines on topical photodynamic therapy 2019 part 2: emerging indications—field cancerization, photorejuvenation and inflammatory/infective dermatoses. J Eur Acad Dermatol Venereol JEADV. 2020;34(1):17–29.
10. Morton CA. A synthesis of the world's guidelines on photodynamic therapy for non-melanoma skin cancer. G Ital Dermatol E Venereol Organo Uff Soc Ital Dermatol E Sifilogr. 2018;153(6):783–92.
11. Garrett GL, Blanc PD, Boscardin J, Lloyd AA, Ahmed RL, Anthony T et al. Incidence of and risk factors for skin cancer in organ transplant recipients in the United States. JAMA Dermatol 2017;153(3):296–303.
12. Coghill AE, Johnson LG, Berg D, Resler AJ, Leca N, Madeleine MM. Immunosuppressive medications, and squamous cell skin carcinoma: nested case-control study within the skin cancer after organ transplant (SCOT) Cohort. Am J Transplant Off J Am Soc Transplant Surg. 2016;16(2):565–73.
13. Elnahas S, Olson MT, Kang P et al. Factors associated with skin cancer in lung transplant recipients: a single-center experience. Clin Transplant. 2019;33(12):e13718.
14. Fantini F, Greco A, Del Giovane C et al. Photodynamic therapy for basal cell carcinoma: clinical and pathological determinants of response. J Eur Acad Dermatol Venereol JEADV. 2011;25(8):896–901.

15. Collins A, Savas J, Doerfler L. Nonsurgical treatments for nonmelanoma skin cancer. Dermatol Clin. 2019;37(4):435–41.
16. Dragieva G, Hafner J, Dummer R et al. Topical photodynamic therapy in the treatment of actinic keratoses and Bowen's disease in transplant recipients. Transplantation. 2004;77(1):115–21.
17. Dragieva G, Prinz BM, Hafner J et al. A randomized controlled clinical trial of topical photodynamic therapy with methyl aminolaevulinate in the treatment of actinic keratoses in transplant recipients. Br J Dermatol. 2004;151(1):196–200.
18. Piaserico S, Belloni Fortina A, Rigotti P et al. Topical photodynamic therapy of actinic keratosis in renal transplant recipients. Transplant Proc. 2007;39(6):1847–50.
19. Hasson A, Navarrete-Dechent C, Nicklas C, de la Cruz C. Topical photodynamic therapy with methylaminolevulinate for the treatment of actinic keratosis and reduction of photodamage in organ transplant recipients: a case-series of 16 patients. Indian J Dermatol Venereol Leprol. 2012;78(4):448–53.
20. Perrett CM, McGregor JM, Warwick J et al. Treatment of post-transplant premalignant skin disease: a randomized intrapatient comparative study of 5-fluorouracil cream and topical photodynamic therapy. Br J Dermatol. 2007;156(2):320–8.
21. Togsverd-Bo K, Halldin C, Sandberg C et al. Photodynamic therapy is more effective than imiquimod for actinic keratosis in organ transplant recipients: a randomized intraindividual controlled trial. Br J Dermatol. 2018;178(4):903–9.
22. Lim CM, Grillo M, Harrison P, Nguyen A-M, Gordon L. Photodynamic therapy: a real-world analysis of outcomes of photodynamic therapy in an Australian tertiary dermatology clinic. Australas J Dermatol. 2019;60(4):339–40.
23. Lim CM, Gordon L. Photodynamic therapy: a targeted literature review focussing on outcomes and optimisation in solid organ transplant recipients. Australas J Dermatol. 2019;60(4):273–7.
24. Liew YCC, De Souza NNA, Sultana RG, Oh CC. Photodynamic therapy for the prevention and treatment of actinic keratosis/squamous cell carcinoma in solid organ transplant recipients: a systematic review and meta-analysis. J Eur Acad Dermatol Venereol JEADV. 2020;34(2):251–9.
25. Chung EYM, Palmer SC, Strippoli GFM. Interventions to prevent nonmelanoma skin cancers in recipients of a solid organ transplant: systematic review of randomized controlled trials. Transplantation. 2019;103(6):1206–15.
26. Heppt MV, Steeb T, Niesert AC et al. Local interventions for actinic keratosis in organ transplant recipients: a systematic review. Br J Dermatol. 2019;180(1):43–50.
27. Schleier P, Hyckel P, Berndt A et al. Photodynamic therapy of virus-associated epithelial tumours of the face in organ transplant recipients. J Cancer Res Clin Oncol. 2004;130(5):279–84.
28. Perrett CM, Tan SK, Cerio R et al. Treatment of basal cell carcinoma with topical methylaminolaevulinate photodynamic therapy in an organ-transplant recipient. Clin Exp Dermatol. 2006;31(1):146–7.
29. Guleng GE, Helsing P. Photodynamic therapy for basal cell carcinomas in organ-transplant recipients. Clin Exp Dermatol. 2012;37(4):367–9.
30. Collier NJ, Ali FR, Lear JT. Efficacy of photodynamic therapy for treatment of basal cell carcinoma in organ transplant recipients. Lasers Med Sci. 2015;30(4):1407–9.
31. Bay C, Lerche CM, Ferrick B, Philipsen PA, Togsverd-Bo K, Haedersdal M. Comparison of physical pretreatment regimens to enhance protoporphyrin IX uptake in photodynamic therapy: a randomized clinical trial. JAMA Dermatol. 2017;153(4):270–8.
32. Bencini PL, Galimberti MG, Pellacani G, Longo C. Application of photodynamic therapy combined with pre-illumination microneedling in the treatment of actinic keratosis in organ transplant recipients. Br J Dermatol. 2012;167(5):1193–4.
33. Champeau M, Vignoud S, Mortier L, Mordon S. Photodynamic therapy for skin cancer: how to enhance drug penetration? J Photochem Photobiol B. 2019;197:111544.
34. Togsverd-Bo K, Haak CS, Thaysen-Petersen D et al. Intensified photodynamic therapy of actinic keratoses with fractional CO2 laser: a randomized clinical trial. Br J Dermatol. 2012;166(6):1262–9.
35. Helsing P, Togsverd-Bo K, Veierød MB, Mørk G, Haedersdal M. Intensified fractional CO2 laser-assisted photodynamic therapy vs. laser alone for organ transplant recipients with multiple actinic keratoses and wart-like lesions: a randomized half-side comparative trial on dorsal hands. Br J Dermatol. 2013;169(5):1087–92.
36. Togsverd-Bo K, Lei U, Erlendsson AM et al. Combination of ablative fractional laser and daylight-mediated photodynamic therapy for actinic keratosis in organ transplant recipients—a randomized controlled trial. Br J Dermatol. 2015;172(2):467–74.
37. Rizvi SM, Veierød MB, Mørk G, Helsing P, Gjersvik P. Ablative fractional laser-assisted daylight photodynamic therapy for actinic keratoses of the scalp and forehead in organ transplant recipients: a pilot study. Acta Derm Venereol. 2019;99(11):1047–8.
38. Steeb T, Schlager JG, Kohl C, Ruzicka T, Heppt MV, Berking C. Laser-assisted photodynamic therapy for actinic keratosis: a systematic review and meta-analysis. J Am Acad Dermatol. 2019;80(4):947–56.

39. Lucena SR, Salazar N, Gracia-Cazaña T et al. Combined treatments with photodynamic therapy for non-melanoma skin cancer. Int J Mol Sci. 2015;16(10):25912–33.
40. Anand S, Rollakanti KR, Brankov N, Brash DE, Hasan T, Maytin EV. Fluorouracil enhances photodynamic therapy of squamous cell carcinoma via a p53-independent mechanism that increases protoporphyrin ix levels and tumor cell death. Mol Cancer Ther. 2017;16(6):1092–101.
41. Zhang L, Ji Z, Zhang J, Yang S. Photodynamic therapy enhances skin cancer chemotherapy effects through autophagy regulation. Photodiagnosis Photodyn Ther. 2019;28:159–65.
42. Jambusaria-Pahlajani A, Ortman S, Schmults CD, Liang C. Sequential curettage, 5-fluorouracil, and photodynamic therapy for field cancerization of the scalp and face in solid organ transplant recipients. Dermatol Surg Off Publ Am Soc Dermatol Surg Al. 2016;42(Suppl 1):S66–72.
43. Maytin EV, Anand S, Riha M et al. 5-fluorouracil enhances protoporphyrin IX accumulation and lesion clearance during photodynamic therapy of actinic keratoses: a mechanism-based clinical trial. Clin Cancer Res Off J Am Assoc Cancer Res. 2018;24(13):3026–35.
44. Maytin EV, Hasan T. Vitamin D and Other Differentiation-promoting agents as neoadjuvants for photodynamic therapy of cancer. Photochem Photobiol. 2020 Feb 19.
45. Steeb T, Wessely A, Leiter U, French LE, Berking C, Heppt MV. The more the better? An appraisal of combination therapies for actinic keratosis. J Eur Acad Dermatol Venereol JEADV. 2020;34(4):727–32.
46. Howard M, Su J, Chong A. Skin cancer following solid organ transplantation: a review of risk factors and models of care. Am J Clin Dermatol. 2018;19:585–97.
47. Sharfaei S, Juzenas P, Moan J, Bissonnette R. Weekly topical application of methyl aminolevulinate followed by light exposure delays the appearance of UV-induced skin tumours in mice. Arch Dermatol Res. 2002;294(5):237–42.
48. Wulf HC, Pavel S, Stender I, Bakker-Wensveen CA. Topical photodynamic therapy for prevention of new skin lesions in renal transplant recipients. Acta Derm Venereol.2006;86(1):25–8.
49. Apalla Z, Sotiriou E, Chovarda E, Lefaki I, Devliotou-Panagiotidou D, Ioannides D. Skin cancer: preventive photodynamic therapy in patients with face and scalp cancerization. A randomized placebo-controlled study. Br J Dermatol. 2010;162(1):171–5.
50. de Graaf YGL, Kennedy C, Wolterbeek R, Collen AFS, Willemze R, Bouwes Bavinck JN. Photodynamic therapy does not prevent cutaneous squamous-cell carcinoma in organ-transplant recipients: results of a randomized-controlled trial. J Invest Dermatol. 2006;126(3):569–74.
51. Wennberg A-M, Stenquist B, Stockfleth E et al. Photodynamic therapy with methyl aminolevulinate for prevention of new skin lesions in transplant recipients: a randomized study. Transplantation. 2008;86(3):423–9.
52. Bagazgoitia L, Cuevas Santos J, Juarranz A, Jaén P. Photodynamic therapy reduces the histological features of actinic damage and the expression of early oncogenic markers. Br J Dermatol. 2011;165(1):144–51.
53. Willey A, Mehta S, Lee PK. Reduction in the incidence of squamous cell carcinoma in solid organ transplant recipients treated with cyclic photodynamic therapy. Dermatol Surg Off Publ Am Soc Dermatol Surg Al. 2010;36(5):652–8.
54. Togsverd-Bo K, Omland SH, Wulf HC, Sørensen SS, Haedersdal M. Primary prevention of skin dysplasia in renal transplant recipients with photodynamic therapy: a randomized controlled trial. Am J Transplant Off J Am Soc Transplant Am Soc Transpl Surg. 2015;15(11):2986–90.
55. Bernad I, Aguado L, Núñez-Córdoba JM, Redondo P. Daylight photodynamic therapy for prevention of new actinic keratosis and keratinocyte carcinomas in organ transplants: a cryotherapy-controlled randomized clinical trial. J Eur Acad Dermatol Venereol JEADV. 2019 Nov 30.
56. Grigalavicius M, Juraleviciute M, Kwitniewski M, Juzeniene A. The influence of photodynamic therapy with 5-aminolevulinic acid on senescent skin cancer cells. Photodiagnosis Photodyn Ther. 2017;17:29–34.
57. Joly F, Deret S, Gamboa B et al. Photodynamic therapy corrects abnormal cancer-associated gene expression observed in actinic keratosis lesions and induces a remodeling effect in photodamaged skin. J Dermatol Sci. 2018 May 17.
58. Borgia F, Giuffrida R, Caradonna E, Vaccaro M, Guarneri F, Cannavò SP. Early and late onset side effects of photodynamic therapy. Biomedicines. 2018;6(1).
59. Reinholz M, Heppt MV, Hoffmann FS et al. Transient memory impairment and transient global amnesia induced by photodynamic therapy. Br J Dermatol. 2015;173(5):1258–62.
60. Arits AHMM, van de Weert MM, Nelemans PJ, Kelleners-Smeets NWJ. Pain during topical photodynamic therapy: uncomfortable and unpredictable. J Eur Acad Dermatol Venereol JEADV. 2010;24(12):1452–7.
61. Ang JM, Riaz IB, Kamal MU, Paragh G, Zeitouni NC. Photodynamic therapy and pain: a systematic review. Photodiagnosis Photodyn Ther. 2017 Sep;19:308–44.
62. Kaw U, Ilyas M, Bullock T et al. A regimen to minimize pain during blue light photodynamic therapy of actinic keratoses: bilaterally controlled, randomized trial of simultaneous versus conventional illumination. J Am Acad Dermatol. 2020;82(4):862–8.

63. Martin GM. In-office painless aminolevulinic acid photodynamic therapy: a proof of concept study and clinical experience in more than 100 patients. J Clin Aesthetic Dermatol. 2016;9(2):19–26.
64. Wiegell SR, Skiveren J, Philipsen PA, Wulf HC. Pain during photodynamic therapy is associated with protoporphyrin IX fluorescence and fluence rate. Br J Dermatol. 2008;158(4):727–33.
65. Wiegell SR, Fabricius S, Heydenreich J et al. Weather conditions and daylight-mediated photodynamic therapy: protoporphyrin IX-weighted daylight doses measured in six geographical locations. Br J Dermatol. 2013;168(1):186–91.
66. O'Gorman SM, Clowry J, Manley M et al. Artificial white light vs daylight photodynamic therapy for actinic keratoses: a randomized clinical trial. JAMA Dermatol. 2016;152(6):638–44.
67. Mordon S, Vignion-Dewalle AS, Thecua E et al. Can daylight-PDT be performed indoor? G Ital Dermatol E Venereol Organo Uff Soc Ital Dermatol E Sifilogr. 2018;153(6):811–16.
68. Marie C, Vignion-Dewalle AS, Cartier H et al. Artificial white light photodynamic therapy for actinic keratosis: a study of 38 patients in private practice. J Eur Acad Dermatol Venereol. 2020;34:e165–e167.
69. Mordon S, Vignion-Dewalle AS, Abi-Rached H et al. The conventional protocol vs. a protocol including illumination with a fabric-based biophotonic device (the Phosistos protocol) in photodynamic therapy for actinic keratosis: a randomized, controlled, noninferiority clinical study. Br J Dermatol. 2020;182(1):76–84.
70. Mordon S Painless and efficient ALA-PDT and MAL-PDT of actinic keratosis can be achieved by drastically reducing the drug-light interval. Dermatol Ther. 2020;33:e13423
71. Zeitouni NC, Paquette AD, Housel JP et al. A retrospective review of pain control by a two-step irradiance schedule during topical ALA-photodynamic therapy of non-melanoma skin cancer. Lasers Surg Med. 2013;45(2):89–94.
72. Zeitouni NC, Sunar U, Rohrbach DJ et al. A prospective study of pain control by a 2-step irradiance schedule during topical photodynamic therapy of nonmelanoma skin cancer. Dermatol Surg Off Publ Am Soc Dermatol Surg Al. 2014;40(12):1390–4.
73. Paragh G, Zeitouni NC. Two-step irradiance treatment can achieve excellent pain control during red light 5-aminolevulinic acid photodynamic therapy for actinic keratoses. Photomed Laser Surg. 2018;36(3):174–6.
74. Matthews YJ, Damian DL. Topical photodynamic therapy is immunosuppressive in humans. Br J Dermatol. 2010;162(3):637–41.
75. Basset-Seguin N, Baumann Conzett K, Gerritsen MJP et al. Photodynamic therapy for actinic keratosis in organ transplant patients. J Eur Acad Dermatol Venereol JEADV. 2013;27(1):57–66.

Pediatric Transplant Dermatology

7

Carrie C. Coughlin, James Lancaster, and Shivani Tripathi

INTRODUCTION

Many cutaneous sequelae of surgery and immunosuppression can follow pediatric organ transplantation. These occur as short-term reactions and long-term complications. As the life expectancy posttransplant and the number of pediatric organ transplant recipients (pOTRs) increases,[1,2] so too does the burden of disease from dermatologic side effects. Specifically, pOTRs have more time to develop more skin findings. Herein, common and rare cutaneous consequences of solid-organ transplantation are reviewed.

MAIN TOPICS

Skin Cancers and Tumors

Primary skin cancers (basal cell carcinoma: BCC, squamous cell carcinoma: SCC, and melanoma) and posttransplant lymphoproliferative disorders (PTLD) are the most common cancers in pOTRs.

BCC, SCC, and Melanoma

Time from transplant to development of skin cancer is longer in children than in many adults. Reported variably as median and mean years since transplant, time to skin cancer development in pOTRs ranges from 6 to 17 years (median)[3–6] and from 10 to 16 years (mean).[3,6–8] In adults, the time to onset decreases with increasing age at transplant, and high-risk patients should be screened within 2 years of transplant.[9] The broad range of time to first skin cancer for pOTRs means that studies without long-term follow-up and poor retention may be more likely to not identify skin cancers in their pOTR cohorts.[10,11] Of note, most of the skin cancers reported appear in adulthood, making continued follow-up and transition of care from pediatric to adult teams important.[4,6–8,12,13] Older age at transplant[4,13] and white race[4] may confer a higher risk of SCC and BCC. However, patients of all skin colors and skin types can develop these cancers (Figure 7.1), so careful examinations of all pOTRs with skin findings are warranted. Also of note, pOTRs develop keratinocyte carcinomas of the lip more frequently than adult OTRs.[6] Additionally, as in adults,

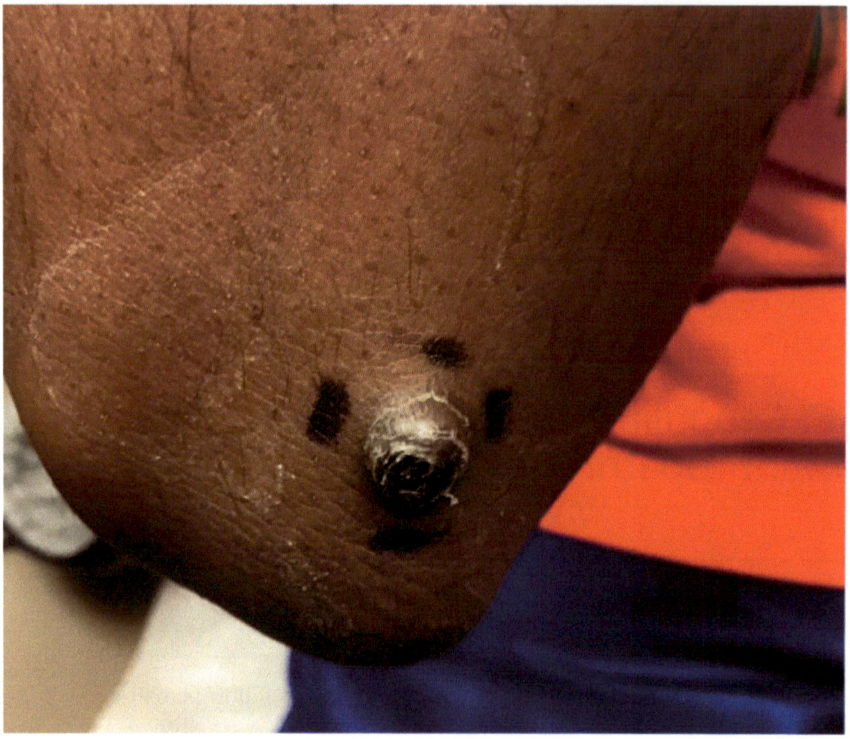

FIGURE 7.1 Squamous cell carcinoma at the elbow of a teenage lung transplant recipient.

voriconazole exposure has been associated with an increased risk of developing skin cancer in pOTRs.[14] The reported standardized incidence ratios (SIRs) of keratinocyte carcinomas vary widely from 65 to 222 for pOTRs[7,13]; one of these studies was limited to renal pOTRs.[7] Many smaller studies and some large studies do not report SIRs; more detailed analysis is needed to refine these estimates in children. Fogel et al.[15] showed the variability in some of these studies. As in adult OTRs, pOTRs develop SCC more frequently than they develop BCC.[3–7,15]

Melanoma risk in pOTRs appears to be similar to that of adult OTRs, with recent data in pediatric renal transplant recipients showing a SIR of 3.[4] However, some studies find higher risk in pOTRs compared with adult OTRs.[6,15] With a low absolute number of cases, it is difficult to know if the morphology of melanoma is the same in pOTRs and adult OTRs. Importantly, in the general pediatric population, melanoma can present differently than in adults. Children more commonly have amelanotic, raised lesions ("bumps"), of uniform color, of any diameter, that change. These characteristics make up the modified ABCDE criteria proposed for children, particularly younger children.[16] The lip has been reported as a common location of melanoma in pOTRs.[6] Thus, given the potential for atypical presentations in uncommon locations, a high index of suspicion is appropriate for solitary, persistent, changing lesions in pOTRs.

Treatment of BCC, SCC, and Melanoma

Treatment recommendations for skin cancers in pOTRs are the same as for adults.[15] With appropriate support in the office, some children can undergo excision or Mohs micrographic surgery (MMS) with local anesthesia for keratinocyte carcinomas (BCC or SCC). For children unable to tolerate surgery with local anesthesia, some practices have access to MMS with sedation. In groups without the option of MMS under sedation, excision with sedation can be substituted, with appropriate margin evaluation. Radiotherapy is rarely used in pOTRs.[15] The standard of care for melanoma is excision with appropriate margins, depending on the depth of invasion. This can be performed with or without sedation, depending on patient tolerance. As in adults, sentinel lymph node sampling should be considered in patients with thicker tumors.[17]

Studies of skin cancer in pOTRs often do not report outcomes, but there is a suggestion that pOTRs can have more aggressive and deadly tumors than adult OTRs.[6]

Prevention of BCC, SCC, and Melanoma

Photoprotection is the mainstay of BCC, SCC, and melanoma prevention in pOTRs. This involves using sunscreen, wearing photoprotective clothing, seeking shade, and avoiding peak sun hours, as well as avoiding tanning beds, which are known carcinogens.[18] Although skin cancer risk education is desired by patients and families,[19] multiple studies showed that even in "at-risk" populations, photoprotection was often not practiced effectively. Specifically, in a cohort of children who had undergone hematopoietic stem cell transplants (HSCTs), despite reporting the practice of photoprotective behaviors, the children had burns and tanning bed exposure at the same rate as that of their nonimmunosuppressed peers.[20] Similarly, children of parents with a history of melanoma applied sunscreen, but still burned as much as children in the general population.[21] In a cohort of 137 pOTRs, children who received in-person education with text message supplements or online education showed improved sun-protection knowledge at 6 weeks, but the online education group did not sustain the improved knowledge after a year, and neither group reported improved photoprotective behaviors after a year.[22] A multimodal (text, video, verbal) educational intervention for patients and guardians regarding sun protection knowledge and behaviors showed promise, with 6-month follow-up.[23] It is imperative to find ways to continue to modify ultraviolet (UV) light exposure-related behaviors in at-risk patients.

Of note, studies on skin cancer in pOTRs have not reported the incidence of skin cancer by race. Recommendations for photoprotection as the mainstay of prevention likely are most relevant to patients with lighter skin and greater tendency to burn. Whether the same recommendations apply across all skin types is unknown. Early detection of changing, growing, and/or symptomatic lesions, however, is important in all OTRs.

Chemoprevention, a mainstay of management in adult OTRs, is not well-described in pOTRs. Similar to adults, in pediatric patients with increasing numbers of skin cancer, consideration should be given to altering the immunosuppressive regimen.

The risk of vulvar SCC is important in this population.[5] Vaccination for human papilloma virus (HPV) is relevant for anogenital cancers. A nonavalent HPV vaccine is now available and approved for patients 9 years of age and older. Vaccination is recommended before transplantation.[24] Best-practices for vaccine schedules (number of vaccines, intervals, timing) posttransplant are not well defined, but vaccination post-transplant is still encouraged for unvaccinated children.[24,25] Particularly as pOTRs age, total body skin exam, with appropriate timing, consent, and counseling, is important to detect cancers at the groin.[26]

Resources for photoprotection education and skin cancer detection include handouts from the Society for Pediatric Dermatology,[27] information from the International immunosuppression and Transplant Skin Cancer Collaborative (itscc.org), and local multimodal educational programs, several of which were reviewed by the Community Guide.[28]

Other Tumors

PTLD rarely presents in the skin. However, it is important to recognize, as it can be mistaken for benign conditions like eczema. Biopsy is needed for diagnosis of new disease. Cutaneous PTLD can appear before systemic involvement or symptoms of systemic involvement, indicating the need for close monitoring of patients without known internal disease.[29,30] Both B-cell and T-cell disease can present in the skin. The morphology varies from typical scaly patches of mycosis fungoides to folliculotropic variants,[31,32] ulcerations,[29] and nodules.[30] Cutaneous PTLD was reported in cardiac, renal, liver, and multivisceral pOTRs.[29] Epstein-Barr virus (EBV)-naïve status is often a risk factor for B-cell PTLD, but its role is not as clear-cut in T-cell disease. Treatment depends on the extent of the disease and can involve topical corticosteroids, phototherapy, and changes to immunosuppression.[29] For refractory disease, surgical and/or medical therapies can be employed. PTLD can be one of the most serious complications of transplantation.[29]

The risk of Kaposi's sarcoma (caused by human herpes virus 8 infection) may be increased in pOTRs (about 3%–4% of all posttransplant cancers).[3,6,15] Large series and reviews report few cases,[3,6,33] and even fewer that are limited to cutaneous involvement.[6,34] Case reports of posttransplant Kaposi's sarcoma detaile systemic involvement along with cutaneous findings; treatment included reduction or revision of immunosuppression and medical therapy.[35,36]

Increased risk of Merkel cell carcinoma has not been reported in pOTRs.

Summary

Skin cancers can cause significant morbidity and mortality in pOTRs. Patient and family education is a first step in prevention. Families want to learn about their risks before or immediately after transplant.[19] However, photoprotection education, although associated with reporting some behavioral change,[23] is not enough to ultimately decrease risk. Early detection is important to decrease the negative effects of these tumors.

Infections

Pediatric OTRs are at risk for common and rare skin infections. Importantly, bacterial infections frequently seen in children, such as staphylococcal and streptococcal infections, are also seen in pOTRs (Figure 7.2).

Viral Infections

Common viral infections, such as herpes simplex virus and varicella zoster virus (VZV), should be considered in patients presenting with vesicles, pustules, erosions or ulcers, as immunosuppression could make these eruptions more severe. Vaccination for VZV is important, including attempting to vaccinate children before transplantation and considering updating the vaccines of family members and close contacts to decrease the risk of infection posttransplant.[24] When possible, administration of live vaccines should occur before transplantation, as there are safety questions posttransplantation. Additionally, immune response to vaccines is typically more robust without immunosuppression.[24] See "Skin Cancers and Tumors" earlier in this chapter for specifics about HPV vaccination.

Cutaneous verrucae are common in children, although the prevalence varies in different populations. In a US cohort of children (n = 9417, 0–17 years of age), the prevalence of verrucae was 3.3%, whereas in a Dutch cohort of school-age children (n = 1001, 4–12 years of age), the prevalence was 33%.[37,38] In pOTRs, verrucae were even more common (Figure 7.3). For example, prevalences of 53.8% (French renal, liver, and heart transplant cohort; 78/145; <18 years of age), 45% (Norwegian renal transplant cohort; 17/38; </=18 years of age), and 28.3% (United Kingdom renal transplant cohort; 17/60, <20 years of age) were reported.[39–41] Additionally, in an Italian cohort of children and adults who received renal, liver, cardiac, and lung transplants before age 18, the prevalence of verrucae was 24.4% (53/217).[42] Verrucae in these patients were difficult to treat,[39,40,42] and the authors reported more verrucae with increasing levels of immunosuppression.[39,40] When considering less common treatment options for recalcitrant verrucae, there are case reports of success using topical cidofovir 1%–3% (recommendations for frequency and duration of application vary)[43,44] and squaric acid (strength varies depending on frequency of application and home versus in-office application).[45] At times, verrucae can be extensive enough to merit changes in immunosuppression regimens.[46] It will be interesting to see if routine HPV vaccination has collateral effects on the development of verrucae at nongenital sites in OTRs.

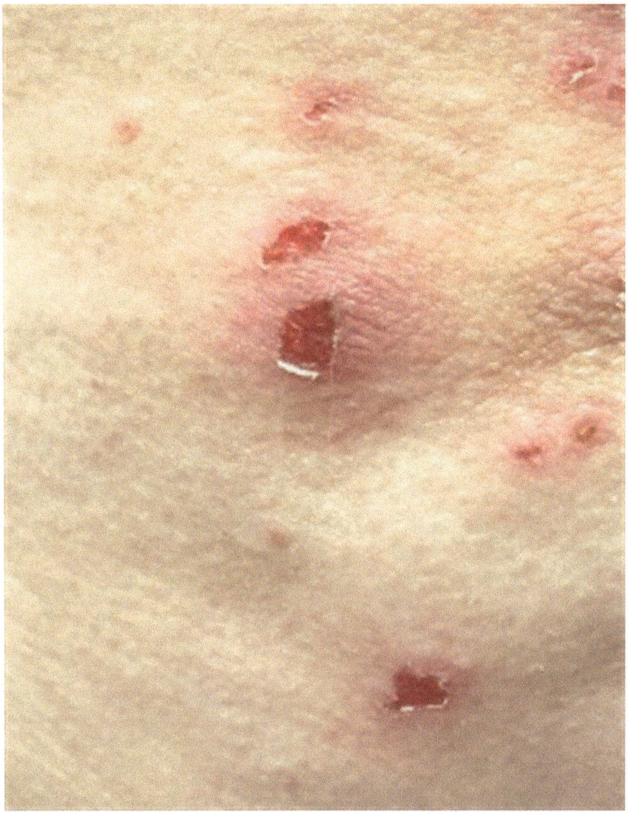

FIGURE 7.2 Recurrent staphylococcal infection in a teenage cardiac transplant recipient.

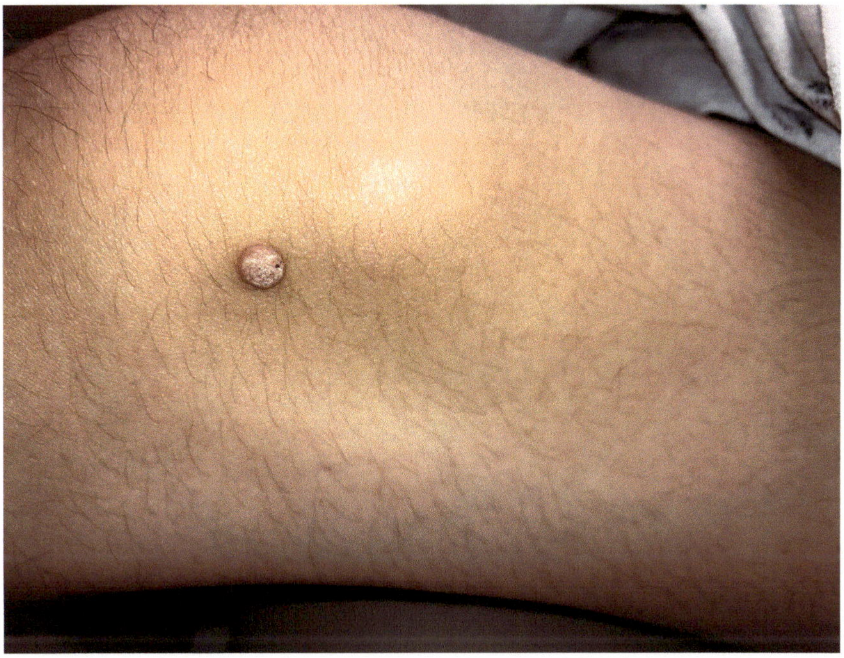

FIGURE 7.3 One of four verrucae vulgaris scattered on a liver transplant recipient. Note that although some pOTRs can have many recalcitrant viral lesions, others have small, focal lesions.

Unusual HPV infections were also reported in pOTRs, including HPV-7 causing anal condyloma[47] and acquired epidermodysplasia verruciformis.[48]

Molluscum contagiosum also occurs in pOTRs, but with reported prevalences much lower than those seen for verrucae (7% in the French cohort and 1% in the Italian cohort detailed previously).[39,42] However, in rare patients, molluscum infections can be bothersome enough for changes in immunosuppressive medications to be considered.[46,49]

Trichodysplasia spinulosa (TS), on the other hand, is specific to immunosuppressed patients and was first described in OTRs.[50] Patients infected with TS polyomavirus present with follicular, hyperkeratotic papules located predominantly on the face, but also on the body, as well as varying degrees of alopecia. See Chapter 15 for more detailed information about TS. Table 7.1 shows pediatric renal, cardiac, pulmonary, bowel, and multivisceral transplant recipients have developed TS months to years after transplantation.[51–65] The current literature points to the association of TS with immunosuppression, rather than a specific underlying disease or medication. Diagnosis is only achieved with a high index of suspicion for this eruption. Importantly for children, noninvasive techniques (such as skin scraping) can avoid the need for skin biopsy.[66] Successful treatments in pOTRs include topical cidofovir, systemic valganciclovir, and reduction of immunosuppression. Looking to treatment results in other pediatric populations, manual spicule extraction was helpful in a child with acute lymphoblastic leukemia.[66]

TABLE 7.1 Pediatric OTRs with Trichodysplasia Spinulosa Reported in the Literature

FIRST AUTHOR (DATE)	*AGE AT ONSET (Y)*	*TIME FROM TRANSPLANT TO ONSET*	*SEX*	*TRANSPLANT*	*IMMUNOSUPPRESSION AT PRESENTATION*
Satesteban (2015)	1	6 months	F	Multivisceral	Tacrolimus, prednisone
Schwieger-Briel (2010)	5	9 months	F	Cardiac	Tacrolimus, MMF, AZA, sirolimus
Benoit (2010)	5	1 year	M	Cardiac	Tacrolimus, prednisone, cyclophosphamide, rituximab, intravenous immunoglobulin
Kazem (2012)	5	NR	M	Renal	NR
Stephan (2020)	6	15 months	M	Cardiac	Tacrolimus, prednisone, MMF
Chamseddin (2019)	6	NR	F	Bowel	Tacrolimus, prednisone, sirolimus
Borgogna (2019)	7	2 years*	M	Renal	Tacrolimus, prednisone, mycophenolic acid
Wyatt (2005)	8	8 months	M	Renal	Tacrolimus, prednisone, MMF
Barone (2019)	9	5 years	F	Renal	Tacrolimus, MMF
Rouanet (2016)	12	6 months	M	Renal	Tacrolimus, MMF
Coogle (2016)	12	15 months	M	Renal	Tacrolimus, MMF
Sperling (2004)	13	9 months	F	Renal	Tacrolimus, prednisone, MMF
Chastain (2000)	13	3 years	F	Cardiac	Cyclosporine, prednisone, MMF, MTX
Van der Meijden (2010)	14**	2.5 years	M	Cardiac	Tacrolimus, methylprednisolone, MMF
Berk (2013)	14	3 years	F	Lung	Cyclosporine, prednisone, MMF, MTX, muromonab-CD3

Abbreviations: AZA, azathioprine; MMF, mycophenolate mofetil; MTX, methotrexate; NR, not reported.

**2 years since second transplant; first transplant 4 years before eruption with early loss of graft.*
***Presented at age 15 with a 1.5-year history of the eruption.*

Fungal Infections

The superficial fungal infection tinea (pityriasis) versicolor was variably present, with prevalences of 0%–20% in the cohorts discussed previously.[39,40,42]

Cutaneous deep fungal infections have been reported rarely in pediatric OTRs.[67–69] However, infections with endemic mycoses (such as histoplasmosis, blastomycosis, and coccidiomycosis) present a high risk of morbidity and mortality.[68] Morphologies were not well described in the literature. Extrapolating data from deep fungal infections in other immunosuppressed patients, lesions that are erythematous, violaceous, ulcerated, necrotic, or pustular papules, plaques, or nodules should raise suspicion for these infections.[69,70] Receiving an infected organ and residence in an area with endemic mycoses were primary risk factors.[68] Biopsy for microscopic evaluation and culture was encouraged.[66] Additionally, touch preparation (smearing or touching a biopsy to a glass slide, letting this dry, and then applying a fungal stain) can help with diagnosis.[71,72] This technique can demonstrate fungal forms within minutes, helping with empiric therapy while awaiting confirmatory pathology and culture results.

Summary

Thus, common and rare cutaneous infections present in pOTRs. They provide a window into the shifting balance of needs for immune suppression and regulation. Interestingly, some infections can indicate the need to decrease immunosuppressive medications.

Surgical Sequelae

Surgical scars are long-lasting, visual reminders of transplantation (Figure 7.4). Showing their importance, the American Society for Transplantation's patient and family guide for pediatric renal transplantation recommends discussing scars and diagramming for children what they will look like as part of their preparation for surgery.[73]

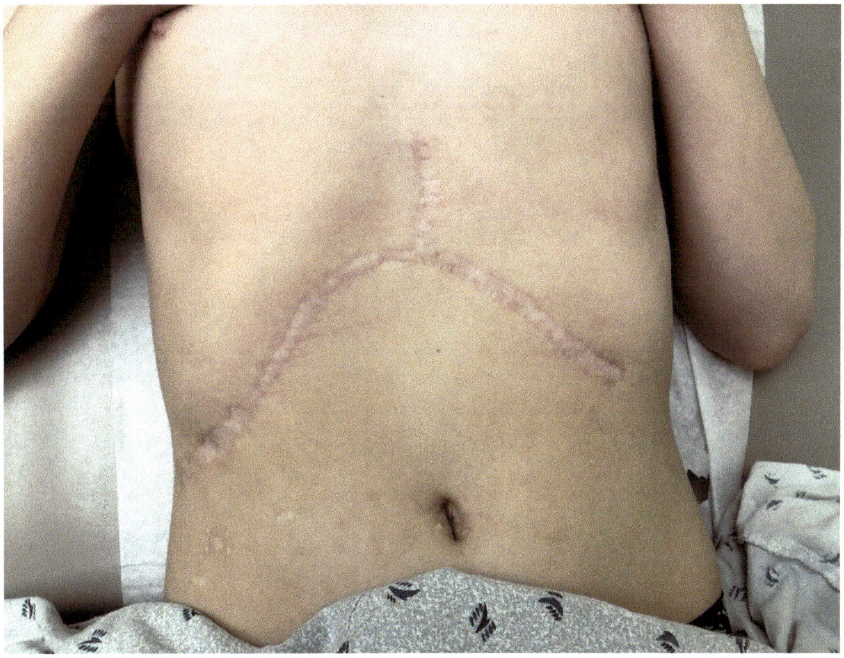

FIGURE 7.4 Surgical scars of a liver transplant recipient.

When visible outside of clothing, scars can trigger others to ask pOTRs questions.[74] Thus, not only do scars remind the children of their transplants, they reveal to others that a child has gone through a surgery, exposing them to potentially unwanted scrutiny. Further, some report more concerns about scars as pOTRs age.[75] On the other hand, some patients report being proud of what their scars represent (personal communication and anecdotal reports).

Fortunately, therapies for problematic scars have advanced markedly in recent years. For symptomatic or distressing scars, consultation with a procedural dermatologist or plastic surgeon is indicated. Surgical, medical, and laser treatments (and at times combinations of these modalities) provide many options for scar management.[76]

Multiple types of alopecia can be associated with transplant surgery. First, telogen effluvium, which can be triggered by physiological and/or psychological stress, is possible. The shift from anagen to telogen hairs with subsequent shedding can occur before or after surgery. Importantly, it can also occur because of nutritional deficiency, which should be considered in a chronically ill patient. Acute telogen effluvium can occur more quickly than the often reported 3-month interval after an inciting event.[77] Diffuse alopecia areata is the primary clinical differential diagnosis.[77] A chronic form of telogen effluvium is possible as well.

Second, postsurgical pressure-related alopecia can occur. It presents as localized alopecia at a place under pressure for a long period of time. It often occurs at the occipital or vertex scalp.[78,79] It is sometimes associated with crusting and ulceration because of tissue necrosis. Hair loss is often temporary, but can be permanent.[78,79] Onset soon after a period of prolonged immobilization (transplant surgery) and location can be clues to this diagnosis. Pressure-related injuries after surgery also can occur at sites other than the scalp. Morphology, location, and appearance proximate to surgery are clues to the diagnosis.

Medication-Related Skin Findings

As in adults, steroid-induced cutaneous side effects (acne, striae, body composition changes) were also seen in pOTRs.[39,40,42,80] Similarly, cyclosporine-induced changes (gingival hyperplasia, hypertrichosis) were common in children.[39,40,42,80] Though we may see these commonly as providers, it is important to remember that patients may find these cutaneous side effects very distressing. In one series, a patient reported suicidal ideation linked to her hypertrichosis.[80] Examples like this serve as a reminder to continue involving patients in their care and elicit values and preferences during encounters, following the tenets of shared decision-making.[81] Tacrolimus has been associated with alopecia, although the type and mechanism were not explained in the literature.[82] This alopecia was reversible with the reduction of the tacrolimus dosage.

Atopic Dermatitis

Atopic dermatitis (AD), variably related to other manifestations of atopy (asthma, allergies, allergic rhinitis), is increasingly reported in pOTRs. Prevalence varies widely and is incompletely captured in the literature. Further, when compared with the general pediatric population, prevalence of atopy in pOTRs might not differ.[83]

Mechanism

The pathophysiology of AD after transplantation is likely multifactorial and is not fully understood. Multiple investigators suggested that an altered T-cell repertoire may account for this heightened risk.[84–86] Lopez-Abente et al.[85] observed low regulatory T-cell levels among a group of 11 pediatric cardiac transplant recipients who developed atopic dermatitis, in the setting of reduced Th1/Th2 ratios, eosinophilia, and elevated IgE levels.

Risk Factors and Associations

Table 7.2 provides a review of potential risk factors for posttransplant AD, including age,[83,84,86–89] organ type,[84,86,87] immunosuppressive medication,[90] and thymectomy.[84,85] Some have investigated EBV status as a risk factor,[87] but it is variably reported in studies.

AD is often associated with food allergies in pOTRs.[83,91] The prevalence of food allergies may decrease over time in patients who were transplanted at a young age[92]; the natural history of AD post-transplant is not well-described. Tacrolimus, which can increase intestinal permeability,[93] may be a common risk factor for the development of AD and food allergies. However, kidney transplant recipients, who often receive tacrolimus immunosuppression, do not seem to have the same risk of these manifestations of atopy as other pOTRs,[87,94] and exposure to tacrolimus in a cohort of cardiac transplant recipients was the same in those with and without AD.[85] Thus, an interplay of risk factors likely leads to development of AD after transplantation.

Interestingly, eosinophilia, elevated IgE (total and food-specific), and/or positive skin-prick tests are reported in pOTRs on tacrolimus with and without symptoms of food allergy or asthma.[95,96] Further, there are conflicting reports on whether the level of eosinophilia correlates or does not correlate with allergic symptoms.[97] These findings remind providers of the importance of clinical context when interpreting laboratory findings. More work is needed to sort out the contributions of medications to risk.

Investigators have looked at associations of posttransplant AD and rejection episodes, seeing if alterations in immune response leading to AD were related to risk of rejection. Researchers suggested that the Th2 skewing present in the transplant recipients with AD could have prevented the rejection episodes normally facilitated by Th1 cells. Data were mixed, with some reports supporting an association[85] and others finding no association.[87]

Interestingly, other manifestations of atopy and eosinophilic disease were even more commonly reported after transplantation. Food allergy and eosinophilic esophagitis were both seen. Although outside the scope of this chapter, their potential associations with the type of transplant, medications, and age at transplant are useful to consider when thinking about the development and treatment of AD in this population.[85,98,99]

Treatment

Atopic dermatitis treatment involves elimination of exacerbating factors (such as irritants and contact allergens), application of emollients, and use of pharmacologic treatment. Concerns particularly relevant to treating AD in pediatric transplant recipients are discussed here.

TABLE 7.2 Risk Factors for Atopic Dermatitis Posttransplantation

RISK FACTOR	*DETAILS*	*REFERENCE(S)*
Age	Younger age conferring higher risk	Avdimiretz (2018), Ozdemir (2013), Marcus (2018), Niemeier (2005), Shroff (2012), Topal (2014)
Organ type	Liver recipients at higher risk because of the portal circulation's role in antigen presentation; cardiac transplant recipients may be at higher risk.	Avdimiretz (2018), Ozdemir (2013), Marcus (2018)
Immunosuppression	Tacrolimus potentially implicated because of its effects suppressing interleukin 2, shifting towards a Th2 response, and inhibition of Treg function	Kehar (2020)
Thymectomy	Altered T-cell response	Avdimiretz (2018), Lopez-Abente (2019)

Topical treatment is first-line. The general principles of using topical corticosteroids of low, intermediate, and high potency based on the severity and location of AD still apply to pOTRs. Steroid-sparing topical agents, such as topical calcineurin inhibitors (pimecrolimus cream or tacrolimus ointment), may also be used for face involvement or for areas (such as flexures and the groin) where it is desirable to avoid topical steroids when possible. However, transplant recipients have special circumstances to consider with these agents. First, many transplant recipients take systemic calcineurin inhibitors. Transplant teams may want to follow tacrolimus levels, for example, more closely for patients starting topical tacrolimus therapy. Although rare, and not reported to date in pOTRs, systemic absorption can lead to elevated, even toxic, tacrolimus levels. Patients with markedly impaired barriers (Netherton's syndrome, graft versus host disease) have had elevated levels reported.[100–102] Occlusion, strength, surface area, concomitant systemic therapy, and impaired skin barrier can be indications for following systemic levels. Given these concerns, discussing treatment plans (even topical-only plans) with a patient's transplant team is advised.

Second, although topical tacrolimus is a US Food and Drug Administration (FDA)-approved treatment for AD, systemic therapy with this agent has been implicated as a trigger for posttransplantation AD. It was implicated in the development of AD after islet-cell,[103] cardiac,[104] and liver transplantation.[90] Thus, for patients with recalcitrant and severe AD on tacrolimus, considerations of dose changes or changing immunosuppression are warranted.[87,100,101] However, most patients on tacrolimus do not develop AD or other forms of atopy. Moreover, given the risks of rejection with changes in regimens otherwise working well and the lack of guaranteed improvement of AD, these discussions are complicated.[90]

Third, pimecrolimus cream and tacrolimus ointment both have "black box" warnings from the US FDA, added in 2006, cautioning about the risk of lymphoma with the use of these agents. The warnings were not supported in the literature,[106–109] but remain on the labels. Explanation of these warnings is important for families before they pick up their medications at the pharmacy. Some families might not be comfortable with using these medications despite reassurances. In these cases, alternative therapies should be used.

Fourth, for severe disease, systemic treatment may be considered. Phototherapy with narrow-band UVB (nbUVB) can be considered. Review of any medications that predispose to UVB sensitivity is required. Compared with psoralen-UVA phototherapy, which increases the risk of skin cancer, nbUVB is less likely to have this side effect.[110] However, when combined with immunosuppression, this risk may be increased and patients should still be monitored for new or changing growths on the skin. Many systemic agents used to treat AD off-label in children, such as cyclosporine and methotrexate, are challenging to consider in the transplant population. Any use of prednisone, methotrexate, or cyclosporine should be reviewed with a patient's transplant team; dosing and laboratory monitoring should be decided only in conjunction with the team. As of May 2020, dupilumab (a monoclonal antibody that inhibits IL4 and IL13 signaling) is FDA-approved for use in pediatric patients aged 6 years and over with AD.[111] Early reports of adult OTRs (including a patient in her 20s)[105] treated with the dupilumab showed that this might be an alternative when there is more data on its use in combination with immunosuppressive agents. However, there were few reports of its use in OTRs of any age.[112,113] Further, dupilumab therapy has been associated with progression of cutaneous T-cell lymphoma, making it even more important to differentiate AD from scaly patches of PTLD. Thus, studies are needed to evaluate its safety and efficacy in pOTRs.

Fifth, treatment for many patients involves consideration and modification of the cutaneous microbiome. Patients with AD have increased colonization with *Staphylococcus aureus* and can have overt staphylococcal infections, as well.[114–116] Attempts to decrease *S. aureus* colonization, such as intermittent application of topical antimicrobials (particularly to the nares) and incorporation of biweekly dilute bleach (0.005% sodium hypochlorite) was shown to improve AD severity.[114] However, improvement of AD with dilute bleach baths was not consistently reported[117]; the utility of dilute bleach baths and targeting of *S. aureus* are under study.[115] Moreover, the cutaneous microbiome in pOTRs is not currently described; this is an area needing more investigation. Understanding the "typical" cutaneous bacterial microbiome in pOTRs (if this exists) can give insight into potential specific therapeutic interventions for this population.

Summary

Thus, management of AD, which is already complex in many patients, presents more challenges in the pOTR population. Emerging therapies may provide much needed treatment options for these patients.

Graft-versus-Host Disease

Graft-versus-host disease (GVHD) is rare following solid organ transplantation. It is most commonly thought of in patients receiving visceral transplants. Intestinal transplant recipients are most at risk, but liver and kidney recipients also develop GVHD.[118–120] Cutaneous involvement can point to the diagnosis, and the skin is the most commonly affected organ.[118,119] The morphology varies from unspecified "rash" to maculopapular eruptions, desquamation, and bullae.[119,121,122] Presentations can be severe, and a differential of epidermal necrolysis and severe drug eruption must be considered.[121] Recalcitrant or severe GVHD can lead to death.[118,119] Although blood chimerism is often thought to be a risk factor for GVHD, others have demonstrated macrochimerism without GVHD and with donor tolerance.[123]

Corticosteroids remain the mainstay of GVHD treatment. Topical corticosteroid therapy was useful for localized cutaneous involvement, whereas systemic therapy was required for diffuse or multisystem disease.[118,119,124] Alteration of the immunosuppression regimen (withdrawal or addition of medications) was also used, with variable success.[118,119] Discussed more in the post-HSCT GVHD literature, nbUVB therapy is a GVHD treatment option.[124] Additionally, Janus kinase inhibitors are under study in HSCT recipients.[125] Also reported in pOTRs with GVHD, extracorporeal photopheresis can be considered as a treatment in refractory cases.[118,119] Mesenchymal stem cells[118,119] and donor-specific antibodies[120] are newer therapies under investigation.

Alternatively, instead of complicating organ transplantation, acute and chronic GVHD after HSCT can be an indication for transplantation, particularly as therapy for liver and lung GVHD.[126,127]

Special Considerations in Pediatric OTRs

Pediatric OTRs may face challenges different than their peers dealing with dermatologic issues. Executive function has been reported to be lower in pOTRs than that children without transplants. Specifically, a meta-analysis showed deficits with small-to-medium effect sizes for working memory, processing speed, and metacognitive skills.[128] Attentional control was also lower, with a medium effect size.[128] Thus, pOTRs likely need more support in receiving instructions for care and planning to perform their care. The need for support extends to the discussion of transitioning care from pediatric to adult clinics. Many centers are looking at and implementing transition models and care teams, and key aspects of successful plans are under investigation.[129,130] Additionally, work in health-related quality of life (QOL) in pOTRs is still in its early stages. A pOTR-specific QOL measure was developed to aid in research and clinical care.[131,132] Importantly, one of the eight domains included is "perceived physical appearance," showing the importance of cutaneous findings in health-related QOL for pOTR.

SUMMARY OF KEY POINTS

- Onset of skin cancer in pOTRs is typically more delayed from transplant than in adults.
- Cutaneous infections, particularly verrucae, are common after transplant.
- Cutaneous sequelae can prompt a change in the immunosuppression regimen.
- GVHD is rare after organ transplantation, but the skin is the most commonly involved site.
- Children aging out of pediatric care require coordinated efforts to support transitions in care.

REFERENCES

1. Van Arendonk KJ, Boyarsky BJ, Orandi BJ, James NT, Smith JM, Colombani PM, Segev DL. National trends over 25 years in pediatric kidney transplant outcomes. Pediatrics. 2014 Mar 13;133(4):594–601. PubMed PMID:24616363; PMCID:PMC4530294.
2. Mogul DB, Luo X, Bowring MG, Chow EK, Massie AB, Schwarz KB, Cameron AM, Bridges JFP, Segev DL. Fifteen-year trends in pediatric liver transplants: split, whole deceased, and living donor grafts. J Pediatr. 2018 Jan 9;196:148–53, e2. PubMed PMID:29307689; PMCID:PMC5924625.
3. Euvrard S, Kanitakis J, Cochat P, Claudy A. Skin cancers following pediatric organ transplantation. Dermatol Surg. 2004 Apr 6;30(4 Pt 2):616–21. PubMed PMID:15061845.
4. Francis A, Johnson DW, Craig JC, Wong G. Incidence and predictors of cancer following kidney transplantation in childhood. Am J Transplant. 2017 Apr 4;17(10):2650–8. PubMed PMID:28371054.
5. Huang JT, Coughlin CC, Hawryluk EB, Hook K, Humphrey SR, Kruse L, Lawley L, Al-Sayegh H, London WB, Marghoob A, Phung TL, Pope E, Gerami P, Schmidt B, Robinson S, Bartenstein D, Bahrani E, Brahmbhatt M, Chen L, Haddock E, Mansour D, Nguyen J, Raisanen T, Tran G, Travis K, Wolner Z, Eichenfield LF. Risk factors and outcomes of nonmelanoma skin cancer in children and young adults. J Pediatr. 2019 May 20;211:152–8. PubMed PMID:31103258.
6. Penn I. De novo malignances in pediatric organ transplant recipients. Pediatr Transplant. 1998;2(1):56–63. Epub 1999/03/20. PubMed PMID:10084762.
7. Coutinho HM, Groothoff JW, Offringa M, Gruppen MP, Heymans HS. De novo malignancy after paediatric renal replacement therapy. Arch Dis Child. 2001 Nov 24;85(6):478–83. PubMed PMID:11719332; PMCID:PMC1719000.
8. Koukourgianni F, Harambat J, Ranchin B, Euvrard S, Bouvier R, Liutkus A, Cochat P. Malignancy incidence after renal transplantation in children: a 20-year single-centre experience. Nephrol Dial Transplant. 2010;25(2):611–16. PubMed PMID:19820249.
9. Crow LD, Jambusaria-Pahlajani A, Chung CL, Baran DA, Lowenstein SE, Abdelmalek M et al. Initial skin cancer screening for solid organ transplant recipients in the United States: Delphi method development of expert consensus guidelines. Transpl Int. 2019;32(12):1268–76. PubMed PMID:31502728.
10. Debray D, Baudouin V, Lacaille F, Charbit M, Rivet C, Harambat J, Iserin F, Di Filippo S, Guyot C. Pediatric transplantation working group of the french speaking society of T. De novo malignancy after solid organ transplantation in children. Transplant Proc. 2009;41(2):674–5. PubMed PMID:19328954.
11. Foo SH, Nightingale PG, Gazzani P, Bader E, Ogboli M, Martin-Clavijo A, Milford DV, Kelly DA, Moss C, Thomson MA. A 10-year longitudinal follow-up study of a U.K. paediatric transplant population to assess for skin cancer. Br J Dermatol. 2018 Apr 28;179(6):1368–75. PubMed PMID:29701240.
12. Penn I. De novo malignancy in pediatric organ transplant recipients. J Pediatr Surg. 1994 Feb 1;29(2):221–6; discussion 7–8. PubMed PMID:8176596.
13. Simard JF, Baecklund E, Kinch A, Brattstrom C, Ingvar A, Molin D, Adami J, Fernberg P, Wilczek H, Ekbom A, Smedby KE. Pediatric organ transplantation and risk of premalignant and malignant tumors in Sweden. Am J Transplant. 2011 Jan 5;11(1):146–51. PubMed PMID:21199354.
14. Wong JY, Kuzel P, Mullen J, Lien D, Mahmood M, Conrad C, Fiorillo L. Cutaneous squamous cell carcinoma in two pediatric lung transplant patients on prolonged voriconazole treatment. Pediatr Transplant. 2014 Jul 22;18(6):E200–7. PubMed PMID:25039541.
15. Fogel AL, Miyar M, Teng JM. Cutaneous malignancies in pediatric solid organ transplant recipients. Pediatr Dermatol. 2016 Jul 30;33(6):585–93. PubMed PMID:27470071.
16. Cordoro KM, Gupta D, Frieden IJ, McCalmont T, Kashani-Sabet M. Pediatric melanoma: results of a large cohort study and proposal for modified ABCD detection criteria for children. J Am Acad Dermatol. 2013 Feb 12;68(6):913–25. PubMed PMID:23395590.
17. Swetter SM, Tsao H, Bichakjian CK, Curiel-Lewandrowski C, Elder DE, Gershenwald JE, Guild V, Grant-Kels JM, Halpern AC, Johnson TM, Sober AJ, Thompson JA, Wisco OJ, Wyatt S, Hu S, Lamina T. Guidelines of care for the management of primary cutaneous melanoma. J Am Acad Dermatol. 2019;80(1):208–50. Epub 2018/11/06. PubMed PMID:30392755.
18. El Ghissassi F, Baan R, Straif K, Grosse Y, Secretan B, Bouvard V, Benbrahim-Tallaa L et al. A review of human carcinogens-part D: radiation. Lancet Oncol. 2009;10(8):751–2. Epub 2009/08/06. PubMed PMID:19655431.

19. Chen L, Gao F, Coughlin CC. Optimal time to provide skin cancer and photoprotection education to pediatric solid organ transplant recipients. J Am Acad Dermatol. 2017;77(1):166–7. Epub 2017/06/18. PubMed PMID:28619555.
20. Li EB, Song JS, Huang JT, Hawryluk EB, London WB, Guo D, Sridharan M, Fisher DE, Rea CJ, Lehmann LE, Duncan CN. Sun exposure and protection practices in children after allogeneic hematopoietic stem cell transplantation: a survey-based cross-sectional cohort study. Pediatr Dermatol. 2019;36(6):882–6. Epub 2019/08/15. PubMed PMID:31410910; PMCID:PMC6883116.
21. Glenn BA, Lin T, Chang LC, Okada A, Wong WK, Glanz K, Bastani R. Sun protection practices and sun exposure among children with a parental history of melanoma. Cancer Epidemiol Biomarkers Prev. 2015;24(1):169–77. Epub 2015/01/15. PubMed PMID:25587110; PMCID:PMC4295624.
22. Bottcher S, Buck C, Zeeb H, Laschewski G, Hauer C, Wagner G, Sachse MM. Randomised controlled trial to evaluate the influence of mHealth and eHealth skin cancer prevention education among young organ transplant recipients: the HIPPOlino intervention study. BMJ Open. 2019;9(12):e028842. Epub 2019/12/19. PubMed PMID:31848158; PMCID:PMC6937057.
23. Coughlin CC, Perez M, Kumar MG, Jeffe DB, Bayliss SJ, Sternhell-Blackwell K. Skin cancer risk education in pediatric solid organ transplant patients: an evaluation of knowledge, behavior, and perceptions over time. Pediatr Transplant. 2017;21(2). Epub 2016/11/03. PubMed PMID:27804197; PMCID:PMC5591957.
24. Danziger-Isakov L, Kumar D, Practice AICo. Vaccination of solid organ transplant candidates and recipients: guidelines from the American society of transplantation infectious diseases community of practice. Clin Transplant. 2019;33(9):e13563. Epub 2019/04/20. PubMed PMID:31002409.
25. Fox TG, Nailescu C. Vaccinations in pediatric kidney transplant recipients. Pediatr Nephrol. 2019;34(4):579–91. Epub 2018/04/20. PubMed PMID:29671067.
26. Nadhan KS, Larijani M, Abbott J, Doyle AM, Linfante AW, Chung CL. Prevalence and Types of Genital Lesions in Organ Transplant Recipients. JAMA Dermatol. 2018;154(3):323–9. Epub 2018/02/02. PubMed PMID:29387873; PMCID:PMC5885815.
27. Patient perspectives: pediatric skin cancer. Pediatr Dermatol. 2017;34(2):187–8. Epub 2017/03/16. PubMed PMID:28297146.
28. Community Preventive Services Task Force. Preventing skin cancer: primary and middle school interventions; 2014. p. 1–4. Available from: https://www.thecommunityguide.org/findings/skin-cancer-primary-and-middle-school-based-interventions.
29. Rogers TS, McGevna L, Cook DL. Pediatric cutaneous T-cell post-transplant lymphoproliferative disorder: case report and review of the literature. J Cutan Pathol. 2018;45(11):858–63. Epub 2018/07/29. PubMed PMID:30054921.
30. Chen KY, Lin CY, Kuo TT, Shih LY, Chang CH, Chen WT, Yang CY. Cutaneous involvement of polymorphic post-transplant lymphoproliferative disorder in a child after liver transplantation. Pediatr Dermatol. 2019;36(5):681–5. Epub 2019/06/20. PubMed PMID:31215060.
31. Spence-Shishido A, Streicher JL, George RP, Parker SR, Lawley LP. Folliculotropic Mycosis Fungoides as a Posttransplant Lymphoproliferative Disorder. Pediatrics. 2015;136(3):e701–5. Epub 2015/08/19. PubMed PMID:26283779.
32. Wang RF, Sokumbi O, Chiu YE. Folliculotropic mycosis fungoides in a pediatric patient mimicking black dot tinea capitis. Pediatr Dermatol. 2019;36(3):386–7. Epub 2019/02/23. PubMed PMID:30791127.
33. Dow DE, Cunningham CK, Buchanan AM. A Review of Human Herpesvirus 8, the Kaposi's Sarcoma-Associated Herpesvirus, in the Pediatric Population. J Pediatric Infect Dis Soc. 2014;3(1):66–76. Epub 2014/02/26. PubMed PMID:24567845; PMCID:PMC3933043.
34. Ozen S, Saatci U, Karaduman A, Buyukpamukcu M, Gokoz A, Besbas N, Bakkaloglu A. Kaposi sarcoma in a paediatric renal transplant recipient. Nephrol Dial Transplant. 1996;11(6):1162–3. Epub 1996/06/01. PubMed PMID:8671991.
35. Celtik C, Unuvar A, Aydogan A, Gokce S, Ozturk G, Gulluoglu M, Yilmaz G, Turkoglu S, Anak S, Sokucu S, Durmaz O. Human herpes virus type 8-associated Kaposi sarcoma in a pediatric liver transplant recipient. Pediatr Transplant. 2011;15(5):E100–4. Epub 2010/03/11. PubMed PMID:20214749.
36. Yuksekkaya HA, Arikan C, Yazici A, Baran M, Aydogdu S, Kilic M. Successful treatment of a child having generalized Kaposi's sarcoma after living donor liver transplantation with conversion to sirolimus. Pediatr Transplant. 2009;13(3):375–8. Epub 2008/05/03. PubMed PMID:18452496.
37. Bruggink SC, Eekhof JA, Egberts PF, van Blijswijk SC, Assendelft WJ, Gussekloo J. Warts transmitted in families and schools: a prospective cohort. Pediatrics. 2013;131(5):928–34. Epub 2013/04/24. PubMed PMID:23610204.
38. Silverberg JI, Silverberg NB. The U.S. prevalence of common warts in childhood: a population-based study. J Invest Dermatol. 2013;133(12):2788–90. Epub 2013/05/10. PubMed PMID:23657500.

39. Euvrard S, Kanitakis J, Cochat P, Cambazard F, Claudy A. Skin diseases in children with organ transplants. J Am Acad Dermatol. 2001;44(6):932–9. Epub 2001/05/23. PubMed PMID:11369903.
40. Sitek JC, Tangeraas T, Bjerre A, Helsing P. The prevalence of skin disorders in Norwegian paediatric renal transplant recipients. Acta Derm Venereol. 2014;94(4):421–4. Epub 2013/11/30. PubMed PMID:24287733.
41. Lunn A, Ravenscroft J, Watson AR. Cutaneous warts in children before and after renal transplantation. Pediatr Nephrol. 2010;25(5):941–6. Epub 2009/12/22. PubMed PMID:20024587.
42. Fortina AB, Piaserico S, Alaibac M, Caforio AL, Brandolisio L, Zacchello G, Zanon GF, Zancan L, Peserico A. Skin disorders in patients transplanted in childhood. Transpl Int. 2005;18(3):360–5. Epub 2005/02/26. PubMed PMID:15730499.
43. Cleary A, Watson R, McMahon CJ. Successful treatment of refractory cutaneous warts using topical 3% cidofovir in a child after heart transplant. J Heart Lung Transplant. 2014;33(9):971–2. Epub 2014/04/15. PubMed PMID:24726426.
44. Das BB, Anton K, Knox L, Jarin J, Sue PK. Successful treatment of giant condyloma in a pediatric heart transplant recipient with topical cidofovir. Transpl Infect Dis. 2018;20(6):e12989. Epub 2018/09/06. PubMed PMID:30184307.
45. Huang W, Morrell D. Successful treatment of recalcitrant warts with topical squaric acid in immunosuppressed child. Pediatr Dermatol. 2008;25(2):275–6. Epub 2008/04/24. PubMed PMID:18429804.
46. Nguyen L, McClellan RB, Chaudhuri A, Alexander SR, Chen SF, Concepcion W, Grimm P. Conversion from tacrolimus/mycophenolic acid to tacrolimus/leflunomide to treat cutaneous warts in a series of four pediatric renal allograft recipients. Transplantation. 2012;94(5):450–5. Epub 2012/09/11. PubMed PMID:22960763.
47. Garaix F, Hery G, Tsimaratos M, Colson P, Tamalet C. Human papillomavirus type 7-associated anal condyloma after renal transplantation in a child. Pediatr Transplant. 2019;23(5):e13470. Epub 2019/05/14. PubMed PMID:31081227.
48. Hirschman D, Tacastacas J, Rady PL, Tyring SK, Cooper K, Honda K. Acquired epidermodysplasia verruciformis associated with human papilloma virus type 14 in a small bowel transplanted child: a case report. Pediatr Dermatol. 2016;33(1):e1–5. Epub 2015/12/10. PubMed PMID:26646304.
49. Kemper MJ, Laube G, Blasius M, Neuhaus TJ. The child with initially refractory skin infection after renal transplantation. Nephrol Dial Transplant. 2002;17(5):927–8. Epub 2002/05/01. PubMed PMID:11981086.
50. Haycox CL, Kim S, Fleckman P, Smith LT, Piepkorn M, Sundberg JP, Howell DN, Miller SE. Trichodysplasia spinulosa-a newly described folliculocentric viral infection in an immunocompromised host. J Investig Dermatol Symp Proc. 1999;4(3):268–71. Epub 2000/02/16. PubMed PMID:10674379.
51. Barone H, Brockman R, Johnson L, Al-Uzri A, Wright M, Mengden-Koon S, Funk T. Trichodysplasia spinulosa mimicking lichen nitidus in a renal transplant patient. Pediatr Transplant. 2019;23(4):e13394. Epub 2019/03/28. PubMed PMID:30916861.
52. Benoit T, Bacelieri R, Morrell DS, Metcalf J. Viral-associated trichodysplasia of immunosuppression: report of a pediatric patient with response to oral valganciclovir. Arch Dermatol. 2010;146(8):871–4. Epub 2010/08/18. PubMed PMID:20713819.
53. Berk DR, Lu D, Bayliss SJ. Trichodysplasia spinulosa in an adolescent with cystic fibrosis and lung transplantation. Int J Dermatol. 2013;52(12):1586–8. Epub 2013/11/23. PubMed PMID:24261736.
54. Borgogna C, Albertini S, Zavattaro E, Veronese F, Peruzzi L, van der Meijden E, Feltkamp MCW, Tosoni A, Volpe A, Boldorini R, Gariglio M. Primary trichodysplasia spinulosa polyomavirus infection in a kidney transplant child displaying virus-infected decoy cells in the urine. J Med Virol. 2019;91(10):1896–900. Epub 2019/06/19. PubMed PMID:31209897.
55. Chamseddin BH, Tran B, Lee EE, Pastrana DV, Buck CB, Wang RC, Kirkorian AY. Trichodysplasia spinulosa in a child: identification of trichodysplasia spinulosa-associated polyomavirus in skin, serum, and urine. Pediatr Dermatol. 2019;36(5):723–4. Epub 2019/06/14. PubMed PMID:31190328.
56. Chastain MA, Millikan LE. Pilomatrix dysplasia in an immunosuppressed patient. J Am Acad Dermatol. 2000;43(1 Pt 1):118–22. Epub 2000/06/23. PubMed PMID:10863236.
57. Coogle LP, Holland KE, Pan C, Van Why SK. Complete resolution of trichodysplasia spinulosa in a pediatric renal transplant patient: case report and literature review. Pediatr Transplant. 2017;21(2). Epub 2016/12/27. PubMed PMID:28019062.

58. Kazem S, van der Meijden E, Kooijman S, Rosenberg AS, Hughey LC, Browning JC, Sadler G, Busam K, Pope E, Benoit T, Fleckman P, de Vries E, Eekhof JA, Feltkamp MC. Trichodysplasia spinulosa is characterized by active polyomavirus infection. J Clin Virol. 2012;53(3):225–30. Epub 2011/12/27. PubMed PMID:22196870.
59. Rouanet J, Aubin F, Gaboriaud P, Berthon P, Feltkamp MC, Bessenay L, Touze A, Nicol JT, Franck F, D'Incan M. Trichodysplasia spinulosa: a polyomavirus infection specifically targeting follicular keratinocytes in immunocompromised patients. Br J Dermatol. 2016;174(3):629–32. Epub 2015/12/15. PubMed PMID:26663358.
60. Santesteban R, Feito M, Mayor A, Beato M, Ramos E, de Lucas R. Trichodysplasia spinulosa in a 20-month-old girl with a good response to topical cidofovir 1%. Pediatrics. 2015;136(6):e1646–9. Epub 2015/12/02. PubMed PMID:26620059.
61. Schwieger-Briel A, Balma-Mena A, Ngan B, Dipchand A, Pope E. Trichodysplasia spinulosa: a rare complication in immunosuppressed patients. Pediatr Dermatol. 2010;27(5):509–13. Epub 2010/08/28. PubMed PMID:0796236.
62. Sperling LC, Tomaszewski MM, Thomas DA. Viral-associated trichodysplasia in patients who are immunocompromised. J Am Acad Dermatol. 2004;50(2):318–22. Epub 2004/01/17. PubMed PMID:14726896.
63. Stephan C, Kurban M, Khalil S, Bitar F, El-Rassi I, Assy J. Viral-associated trichodysplasia spinulosa in a paediatric cardiac transplant recipient. Clin Exp Dermatol. 2020;45(2):244–6. Epub 2019/06/21. PubMed PMID:31219640.
64. van der Meijden E, Janssens RW, Lauber C, Bouwes Bavinck JN, Gorbalenya AE, Feltkamp MC. Discovery of a new human polyomavirus associated with trichodysplasia spinulosa in an immunocompromized patient. PLoS Pathog. 2010;6(7):e1001024. Epub 2010/08/06. PubMed PMID:20686659; PMCID:PMC2912394.
65. Wyatt AJ, Sachs DL, Shia J, Delgado R, Busam KJ. Virus-associated trichodysplasia spinulosa. Am J Surg Pathol. 2005;29(2):241–6. Epub 2005/01/13. PubMed PMID:15644782.
66. Barton M, Lockhart S, Sidbury R, Wang R, Brandling-Bennett H. Trichodysplasia spinulosa in a 7-year-old boy managed using physical extraction of keratin spicules. Pediatr Dermatol. 2017;34(2):e74–6. Epub 2016/12/19. PubMed PMID:27990673; PMCID:PMC5788291.
67. Ferguson-Paul K, Park C, Childress S, Arnold S, Ault B, Bagga B. Disseminated histoplasmosis in pediatric kidney transplant recipients-A report of six cases and review of the literature. Pediatr Transplant. 2018;22(7):e13274. Epub 2018/08/05. PubMed PMID:30076688.
68. Kauffman CA, Freifeld AG, Andes DR, Baddley JW, Herwaldt L, Walker RC, Alexander BD, Anaissie EJ, Benedict K, Ito JI, Knapp KM, Lyon GM, Marr KA, Morrison VA, Park BJ, Patterson TF, Schuster MG, Chiller TM, Pappas PG. Endemic fungal infections in solid organ and hematopoietic cell transplant recipients enrolled in the transplant-associated infection surveillance network (TRANSNET). Transpl Infect Dis. 2014;16(2):213–24. Epub 2014/03/05. PubMed PMID:24589027; PMCID:PMC5664161.
69. Smith RJ, Klieger SB, Sulieman SE, Berger E, Treat JR, Fisher BT. Retrospective review of immunocompromised children undergoing skin biopsy for suspected invasive infection: analysis of factors predictive of invasive mold. Pediatr Dermatol. 2018;35(1):104–11. Epub 2017/12/13. PubMed PMID:29231258.
70. Zampogna JC, Hoy MJ, Ramos-Caro FA. Primary cutaneous north american blastomycosis in an immunosuppressed child. Pediatr Dermatol. 2003;20(2):128–30. Epub 2003/03/27. PubMed PMID:12657008.
71. Kingsley J, Clarey D, Lauer SR, Trowbridge RM. Disseminated histoplasmosis diagnosed by "touch prep". Am J Dermatopathol. 2020. Epub 2020/05/31. PubMed PMID:32472769.
72. Singer HM, Reddy BY, Grossman ME. Touch preparation for the rapid diagnosis of disseminated aspergillosis. JAAD Case Rep. 2017;3(3):202–4. Epub 2017/04/27. PubMed PMID:28443309; PMCID:PMC5394196.
73. BSDACB. Pediatric kidney transplantation: a guide for patients and families. Transplantation ASo; 2015. Available from: https://www.myast.org/sites/default/files/Pediatric%20Kidney%20Transplantation%20BrochureAST%20%20-%20final%20copy%202015-06-27_0.pdf.
74. Green A, McSweeney J, Ainley K, Bryant J. In my shoes: children's quality of life after heart transplantation. Prog Transplant. 2007;17(3):199–207; quiz 8. Epub 2007/10/20. PubMed PMID:17944159; PMCID:PMC2241742.

75. Nicholas DB, Otley AR, Taylor R, Dhawan A, Gilmour S, Ng VL. Experiences and barriers to health-related quality of life following liver transplantation: a qualitative analysis of the perspectives of pediatric patients and their parents. Health Qual Life Outcomes. 2010;8:150. Epub 2010/12/24. PubMed PMID:21176211; PMCID:PMC3024277.
76. Krakowski AC, Totri CR, Donelan MB, Shumaker PR. Scar management in the pediatric and adolescent populations. Pediatrics. 2016;137(2):e20142065. Epub 2016/01/09. PubMed PMID:26743819.
77. Castelo-Soccio L. Diagnosis and management of alopecia in children. Pediatr Clin North Am. 2014;61(2):427–42. Epub 2014/03/19. PubMed PMID:24636654.
78. Ben-Amitai D, Garty BZ. Alopecia in children after cardiac surgery. Pediatr Dermatol. 1993;10(1):32–3. Epub 1993/03/01. PubMed PMID:8493163.
79. Ravaioli GM, Starace M, Alessandrini AM, Guicciardi F, Piraccini BM. Pressure alopecia in pediatric and adult patients: clinical and trichoscopic findings in 12 cases. J Am Acad Dermatol. 2019;81(4):1021–3. Epub 2019/08/25. PubMed PMID:31443909.
80. Silverberg NB, Singh A, Laude TA. Cutaneous manifestations of chronic renal failure in children of color. Pediatr Dermatol. 2001;18(3):199–204. Epub 2001/07/05. PubMed PMID:11437998.
81. Hoffmann TC, Montori VM, Del Mar C. The connection between evidence-based medicine and shared decision making. JAMA. 2014;312(13):1295–6. Epub 2014/10/01. PubMed PMID:25268434.
82. Pirsch JD, Miller J, Deierhoi MH, Vincenti F, Filo RS. A comparison of tacrolimus (FK506) and cyclosporine for immunosuppression after cadaveric renal transplantation. FK506 Kidney Transplant Study Group. Transplantation. 1997;63(7):977–83. Epub 1997/04/15. PubMed PMID:9112351.
83. Shroff P, Mehta RS, Chinen J, Karpen SJ, Davis CM. Presentation of atopic disease in a large cohort of pediatric liver transplant recipients. Pediatr Transplant. 2012;16(4):379–84. Epub 2012/04/12. PubMed PMID:22489822.
84. Avdimiretz N, Seitz S, Kim T, Murdoch F, Urschel S. Allergies and autoimmune disorders in children after heart transplantation. Clin Transplant. 2018;32(10):e13400. Epub 2018/09/04. PubMed PMID:30176068.
85. Lopez-Abente J, Bernaldo-de-Quiros E, Camino M, Gil N, Panadero E, Campos-Dominguez M, Seoane-Reula E, Gil-Jaurena JM, Pion M, Correa-Rocha R. Immune dysregulation and Th2 polarization are associated with atopic dermatitis in heart-transplant children: a delicate balance between risk of rejection or atopic symptoms. Am J Transplant. 2019;19(5):1536–44. Epub 2019/01/08. PubMed PMID:30614192.
86. Ozdemir O. New developments in transplant-acquired allergies. World J Transplant. 2013;3(3):30–5. Epub 2013/11/21. PubMed PMID:24255880; PMCID:PMC3832858.
87. Marcus N, Amir AZ, Grunebaum E, Dipchand A, Hebert D, Ng VL, Walters T, Avitzur Y. De novo allergy and immune-mediated disorders following solid-organ transplantation-prevalence, natural history, and risk factors. J Pediatr. 2018;196:154–60 e2. Epub 2018/02/06. PubMed PMID:29395171.
88. Niemeier V, Passoth PR, Kramer U, Bauer J, Oschmann P, Kupfer J, Gieler U. Manifestation of atopic eczema in children after heart transplantation in the first year of life. Pediatr Dermatol. 2005;22(2):102–8. Epub 2005/04/05. PubMed PMID:15804295.
89. Topal E, Catal F, Selimoglu MA, Karabiber H, Klc T, Baskran A, Senbaba E, Ylmaz S. Acquired atopic disease after liver transplantation in children; similarities to and differences from adults: a preliminary study. Eur J Gastroenterol Hepatol. 2014;26(9):1055–9. Epub 2014/06/21. PubMed PMID:24949707.
90. Kehar M, Grunebaum E, Jimenez-Rivera C, Mozer-Glassberg Y, Jamal A, Ng VL, Avitzur Y. Conversion from tacrolimus to sirolimus as a treatment modality in de novo allergies and immune-mediated disorders in pediatric liver transplant recipients. Pediatr Transplant. 2020:e13737. Epub 2020/05/20. PubMed PMID:32428390.
91. Almaas R, Haflidadottir S, Kaldestad RH, Matthews IL. Asthma, eczema, and food allergy in children following liver transplantation. J Pediatr. 2019;204:263–9. Epub 2018/10/03. PubMed PMID:30270158.
92. Lee Y, Lee YM, Kim MJ, Lee SK, Choe YH. Long-term follow-up of de novo allergy in pediatric liver transplantation-10 yr experience of a single center. Pediatr Transplant. 2013;17(3):251–5. Epub 2013/02/15. PubMed PMID:23405954.
93. Gabe SM, Bjarnason I, Tolou-Ghamari Z, Tredger JM, Johnson PG, Barclay GR, Williams R, Silk DB. The effect of tacrolimus (FK506) on intestinal barrier function and cellular energy production in humans. Gastroenterology. 1998;115(1):67–74. Epub 1998/07/03. PubMed PMID:9649460.

94. Levy Y, Davidovits M, Cleper R, Shapiro R. New-onset post-transplantation food allergy in children-is it attributable only to the immunosuppressive protocol? Pediatr Transplant. 2009;13(1):63–9. Epub 2008/01/09. PubMed PMID:18179638.
95. Granot E, Yakobovich E, Bardenstein R. Tacrolimus immunosuppression—an association with asymptomatic eosinophilia and elevated total and specific IgE levels. Pediatr Transplant. 2006;10(6):690–3. Epub 2006/08/17. PubMed PMID:16911492.
96. Dehlink E, Gruber S, Eiwegger T, Gruber D, Mueller T, Huber WD, Klepetko W, Rumpold H, Urbanek R, Szepfalusi Z. Immunosuppressive therapy does not prevent the occurrence of immunoglobulin E-mediated allergies in children and adolescents with organ transplants. Pediatrics. 2006;118(3):e764–70. Epub 2006/09/05. PubMed PMID:16950967.
97. Asante-Korang A, Boyle GJ, Webber SA, Miller SA, Fricker FJ. Experience of FK506 immune suppression in pediatric heart transplantation: a study of long-term adverse effects. J Heart Lung Transplant. 1996;15(4):415–22. Epub 1996/04/01. PubMed PMID:8732602.
98. Obayashi N, Suzuki M, Yokokura T, Naritaka N, Nakano S, Ohtsuka Y, Sugo H, Kawasaki S, Shimizu T. Management of tacrolimus-associated food allergy after liver transplantation. Pediatr Int. 2015;57(6):1205–7. Epub 2015/11/07. PubMed PMID:26541649.
99. Wisniewski J, Lieberman J, Nowak-Wegrzyn A, Kerkar N, Arnon R, Iyer K, Miloh T. De novo food sensitization and eosinophilic gastrointestinal disease in children post-liver transplantation. Clin Transplant. 2012;26(4):e365–71. Epub 2012/06/15. PubMed PMID:22694084.
100. Allen A, Siegfried E, Silverman R, Williams ML, Elias PM, Szabo SK, Korman NJ. Significant absorption of topical tacrolimus in 3 patients with Netherton syndrome. Arch Dermatol. 2001;137(6):747–50. Epub 2001/06/19. PubMed PMID:11405764.
101. Olson KA, West K, McCarthy PL. Toxic tacrolimus levels after application of topical tacrolimus and use of occlusive dressings in two bone marrow transplant recipients with cutaneous graft-versus-host disease. Pharmacotherapy. 2014;34(6):e60–4. Epub 2014/04/05. PubMed PMID:24700567.
102. Prot-Labarthe S, Therrien R, Champagne MA, Duval M, Joubert C. Toxic serum levels of tacrolimus after topical administration in an infant with severe cutaneous graft-versus-host disease. Bone Marrow Transplant. 2007;40(3):295–6. Epub 2007/06/06. PubMed PMID:17549052.
103. Ponte GM, Baidal DA, Romanelli P, Faradji RN, Poggioli R, Cure P, Froud T, Selvaggi G, Pileggi A, Ricordi C, Alejandro R. Resolution of severe atopic dermatitis after tacrolimus withdrawal. Cell Transplant. 2007;16(1):23–30. Epub 2007/04/18. PubMed PMID:17436852.
104. Jackson Cullison SR, Siegfried EC. Paradoxic eczema in infants after heart transplantation. Pediatr Dermatol. 2018;35(1):e29-e34. Epub 2017/12/02. PubMed PMID:29194735.
105. Hamid RN, Bomar L, Strowd L. Dupilumab for treatment of severe atopic dermatitis in a heart transplant recipient. Cutis. 2019;103(6):E1-E2. Epub 2019/07/28. PubMed PMID:31348459.
106. Arellano FM, Wentworth CE, Arana A, Fernandez C, Paul CF. Risk of lymphoma following exposure to calcineurin inhibitors and topical steroids in patients with atopic dermatitis. J Invest Dermatol. 2007;127(4):808–16. Epub 2006/11/11. PubMed PMID:17096020.
107. Luger T, Boguniewicz M, Carr W, Cork M, Deleuran M, Eichenfield L, Eigenmann P, Folster-Holst R, Gelmetti C, Gollnick H, Hamelmann E, Hebert AA, Muraro A, Oranje AP, Paller AS, Paul C, Puig L, Ring J, Siegfried E, Spergel JM, Stingl G, Taieb A, Torrelo A, Werfel T, Wahn U. Pimecrolimus in atopic dermatitis: consensus on safety and the need to allow use in infants. Pediatr Allergy Immunol. 2015;26(4):306–15. Epub 2015/01/06. PubMed PMID:25557211; PMCID:PMC4657476.
108. Margolis DJ, Abuabara K, Hoffstad OJ, Wan J, Raimondo D, Bilker WB. Association between malignancy and topical use of pimecrolimus. JAMA Dermatol. 2015;151(6):594–9. Epub 2015/02/19. PubMed PMID:25692459; PMCID:PMC4465068.
109. Remitz A, Reitamo S. Long-term safety of tacrolimus ointment in atopic dermatitis. Expert Opin Drug Saf. 2009;8(4):501–6. Epub 2009/05/14. PubMed PMID:19435404.
110. Crall CS, Rork JF, Delano S, Huang JT. Phototherapy in children: considerations and indications. Clin Dermatol. 2016;34(5):633–9. Epub 2016/09/18. PubMed PMID:27638444.
111. Drugs@FDA: FDA-Approved Drugs, BLA: 761055 2020 [cited 2020 August 2]. Available from: www.accessdata.fda.gov/scripts/cder/daf/index.cfm?event=overview.process&ApplNo=761055.
112. Ludriksone L, Elsner P, Malessa C, Settmacher U, Schliemann S. Effectiveness and safety of dupilumab for atopic dermatitis in a liver transplant recipient: a case report. J Dtsch Dermatol Ges. 2020. Epub 2020/03/27. PubMed PMID:32212242.

113. Sklover L, Nielson C, De Benedetto A. The use of selective Th2 blocker dupilumab for the treatment of atopic dermatitis in a heart transplant patient: case report. Dermatol Ther. 2019;32(6):e13144. Epub 2019/10/31. PubMed PMID:31664753.
114. Huang JT, Abrams M, Tlougan B, Rademaker A, Paller AS. Treatment of Staphylococcus aureus colonization in atopic dermatitis decreases disease severity. Pediatrics. 2009;123(5):e808–14. Epub 2009/05/01. PubMed PMID:19403473.
115. Paller AS, Kong HH, Seed P, Naik S, Scharschmidt TC, Gallo RL, Luger T, Irvine AD. The microbiome in patients with atopic dermatitis. J Allergy Clin Immunol. 2019;143(1):26–35. Epub 2018/11/27. PubMed PMID:30476499; PMCID:PMC7163929.
116. Totte JE, van der Feltz WT, Hennekam M, van Belkum A, van Zuuren EJ, Pasmans SG. Prevalence and odds of Staphylococcus aureus carriage in atopic dermatitis: a systematic review and meta-analysis. Br J Dermatol. 2016;175(4):687–95. Epub 2016/03/20. PubMed PMID:26994362.
117. Chopra R, Vakharia PP, Sacotte R, Silverberg JI. Efficacy of bleach baths in reducing severity of atopic dermatitis: a systematic review and meta-analysis. Ann Allergy Asthma Immunol. 2017;119(5):435–40. Epub 2017/11/19. PubMed PMID:29150071; PMCID:PMC5726436.
118. Clouse JW, Kubal CA, Fridell JA, Pearsall EJ, Mangus RS. Post-intestine transplant graft-vs-host disease associated with inclusion of a liver graft and with a high mortality risk. Clin Transplant. 2019;33(1):e13409. Epub 2018/09/18. PubMed PMID:30222903.
119. Green T, Hind J. Graft-versus-host disease in paediatric solid organ transplantation: a review of the literature. Pediatr Transplant. 2016;20(5):607–18. Epub 2016/05/21. PubMed PMID:27198497.
120. Zuber J, Boyer O, Neven B, Jollet I, Renac V, Berthaud R et al. Donor-targeted serotherapy as a rescue therapy for steroid-resistant acute GVHD after HLA-mismatched kidney transplantation. Am J Transplant. 2020. Epub 2020/02/18. PubMed PMID:32065452.
121. Cruysmans C, Ferneiny MG, Fraitag S, Frange P, Chardot C, Bodemer C, Goulet O, Lacaille F. Severe skin complications after small bowel transplantation: graft-versus-host disease, DRESS, virus, or drug toxicity? Transplantation. 2016;100(10):2222–5. Epub 2016/03/08. PubMed PMID:26950725.
122. Yashar S, Wu SS, Binder SW, Cotliar J. Acute graft-versus-host disease after pediatric solid organ transplant. J Drugs Dermatol. 2008;7(5):467–9. Epub 2008/05/29. PubMed PMID:18505140.
123. Zuber J, Rosen S, Shonts B, Sprangers B, Savage TM, Richman S, Yang S, Lau SP, DeWolf S, Farber D, Vlad G, Zorn E, Wong W, Emond J, Levin B, Martinez M, Kato T, Sykes M. Macrochimerism in intestinal transplantation: association with lower rejection rates and multivisceral transplants, without GVHD. Am J Transplant. 2015;15(10):2691–703. Epub 2015/05/20. PubMed PMID:25988811; PMCID:PMC4575629.
124. Hymes SR, Alousi AM, Cowen EW. Graft-versus-host disease: part II. Management of cutaneous graft-versus-host disease. J Am Acad Dermatol. 2012;66(4):535 e1–16; quiz 51–2. Epub 2012/03/17. PubMed PMID:22421124; PMCID:PMC7357210.
125. Schroeder MA, Choi J, Staser K, DiPersio JF. The role of Janus Kinase signaling in graft-versus-host disease and graft versus leukemia. Biol Blood Marrow Transplant. 2018;24(6):1125–34. Epub 2018/01/01. PubMed PMID:29289756; PMCID:PMC5993569.
126. Bunin N, Guzikowski V, Rand ER, Goldfarb S, Baluarte J, Meyers K, Olthoff KM. Solid organ transplants following hematopoietic stem cell transplant in children. Pediatr Transplant. 2010;14(8):1030–5. Epub 2010/09/18. PubMed PMID:20846242.
127. Faraci M, Bertaina A, Dalissier A, Ifversen M, Schulz A, Gennery A, Burkhardt B, Badell Serra I, Diaz-de-Heredia C, Lanino E, Lankester AC, Gruhn B, Matthes-Martin S, Kuhl JS, Varotto S, Paillard C, Guilmatre A, Sastre A, Abecasis M, Garwer B, Sedlacek P, Boelens JJ, Beohou E, Bader P, Party EPDW. Solid organ transplantation after hematopoietic stem cell transplantation in childhood: a multicentric retrospective survey. Am J Transplant. 2019;19(6):1798–805. Epub 2018/12/27. PubMed PMID:30586230.
128. Cushman GK, Stolz MG, Blount RL, Reed B. Executive functioning in pediatric solid organ transplant recipients: a meta-analytic review. Transplantation. 2020;104(2):357–66. Epub 2019/09/14. PubMed PMID:31517786; PMCID:PMC7201367.
129. Kosola S, Ylinen E, Finne P, Ronnholm K, Ortiz F. Implementation of a transition model to adult care may not be enough to improve results: national study of kidney transplant recipients. Clin Transplant. 2019;33(1):e13449. Epub 2018/11/16. PubMed PMID:30431669.
130. Michaud V, Achille M, Chainey F, Phan V, Girardin C, Clermont MJ. Mixed-methods evaluation of a transition and young adult clinic for kidney transplant recipients. Pediatr Transplant. 2019;23(4):e13450. Epub 2019/05/08. PubMed PMID:31062926.

131. Weissberg-Benchell J, Zielinski TE, Rodgers S, Greenley RN, Askenazi D, Goldstein SL, Fredericks EM, McDiarmid S, Williams L, Limbers CA, Tuzinkiewicz K, Lerret S, Alonso EM, Varni JW. Pediatric health-related quality of life: feasibility, reliability and validity of the PedsQL transplant module. Am J Transplant. 2010;10(7):1677–85. Epub 2010/07/21. PubMed PMID:20642689.
132. Killian MO, Triplett KN, Masood SS, Boehler J, Mayersohn GS. Measurement of health-related quality of life in pediatric organ transplantation recipients: a systematic review of the PedsQL transplant module. Qual Life Res. 2020 Jan 3;29(5):1137–46. PubMed PMID:31894507.

Melanoma in Solid Organ Transplant Recipients

8

Alexandra Gosh, Mohammed Almashali, Susan Pei, and Gyorgy Paragh

INTRODUCTION

Solid organ transplantations offer hope for a longer and higher quality life for over 139,000 people annually in the world.[1] However, this opportunity comes at a high price. Immunosuppression not only helps allograft organs survive but also enables more efficient immune evasion by malignancies.[2] Among the cutaneous malignancies seen in solid organ transplant recipients (OTRs), melanomas are one of the less frequently seen malignancies, but their impact in OTRs is nonetheless important given the high metastatic potential and the increasing incidence of melanomas.

MELANOMA EPIDEMIOLOGY

Melanoma has shown the greatest rise in incidence of all major malignancies with an over three-fold rise in incidence since the mid-1970s. Fortunately, mortality rates have remained consistently low during the decades of the rapid incidence increase, and in the past 5 years, there has been a slow decline in melanoma mortality because of the wider use of molecular targeted therapy and immunotherapy. In 2020, we expected just over 100,000 people to be diagnosed with invasive melanoma in the United States, and we are projecting to see 6850 patients succumb to the disease.[3] Excluding in-situ carcinomas and nonmelanoma skin cancers, invasive melanoma is currently the fifth leading cause of cancer diagnosis.[4] Most melanomas affect non-Hispanic whites, with an incidence rate of 28/100,000. Hispanics and African Americans show markedly lower incidence rates; 5 and 1 per 100,000, respectively. Men are 1.49 times more likely to be diagnosed and 1.9 times more likely to die of melanoma compared with women.[4] Besides invasive melanomas, we expect to diagnose 95,710 in-situ melanomas in the United States in 2020.[4] Although the median age at melanoma diagnosis is 65 years, melanoma is a common invasive cancer in young adults. It is the most common malignancy

 DOI: 10.1201/9781003001461-8

in men and the third most common cancer in women below 50 years of age.[4] Over 1.2 million people in the United States have a history of invasive melanoma.[3]

RISK FACTORS FOR MELANOMA

Melanoma is a multifactorial malignant neoplasm arising from both genetic susceptibility and environmental exposure. Solar ultraviolet (UV) radiation is the most important environmental risk factor for developing malignant melanoma, and intermittent UV exposure appears to be a major contributor to melanoma risk.[5] Acute sun exposure, childhood sun exposure, and early life sunburns are associated with the highest melanoma risk.[6] This is in stark contrast to how chronic continuous UV exposure is associated with cutaneous squamous cell carcinoma risk.[7] Tanning bed use and other artificial UV exposures are also increasingly recognized contributors to melanoma risk.[8] Moreover, psoralen plus ultraviolet A (PUVA) therapy has also been linked with an increased risk of developing melanoma.[9] Other important risk factors include the number of melanocytic nevi and genetic susceptibility. About 25% of melanoma cases arise in preexisting nevi.[10] Melanomas arising in preexisting nevi mostly present on the trunk with superficial spreading histological features.[11] Melanoma risk varies based on the size, type, and number of nevi.[12–14] Larger nevi show a significantly higher risk of melanoma.[15] Atypical nevi are not only directly associated with an increased risk of developing melanoma, but their presence also increases de novo melanoma risk. The existence of five atypical nevi increases the risk of developing melanoma by sixfold.[16,17] Patients with over 100 nevi have a sevenfold increased risk for melanoma.[16]

A family history of melanoma is also an important risk factor. In families with inherited melanoma, the most common genetic abnormalities are cyclin-dependent kinase inhibitor 2A (*CDKN2A* or p16) mutations, whereas mutations in cyclin-dependent kinase 4 (*CDK4*) are less common.[18] Dysfunctional nuclear excision repair in patients with xeroderma pigmentosum subtypes also greatly increases melanoma risk.[19] Patients with other inherited cancer syndromes (Li-Fraumeni, Lynch syndrome, retinoblastoma) may also have an elevated melanoma risk.[20] Other genetic factors responsible for phenotypic characteristics of light complexion (light colored hair and eyes, easy freckling) also raise the risk of developing melanoma.[21] These latter features are in part because of melanocortin 1 receptor gene polymorphisms, which are known risk factors for melanoma.[22]

CLINICAL FEATURES OF MELANOMAS

Melanomas are best viewed as a group of closely related melanocytic neoplasms with marked similarities but some distinct clinical and histological features (Figure 8.1). The most common clinical variants of melanoma include superficial spreading melanoma (SSM), nodular melanoma (NM), lentigo maligna melanoma (LMM), and acral lentiginous melanoma (ALM). Other less common and thus less well-characterized subtypes include desmoplastic melanoma, mucosal melanoma, malignant blue nevus, spitzoid melanoma, and deep dermal melanoma.[20]

SSM is the most common melanoma variant, representing up to 70% of the cases. It is closely associated with intermittent sun-exposure and thus is often localized to the posterior lower leg in women and the back in men. SSM may arise de novo or in association with a nevus. The clinical features usually fit the classic "ABCDE" criteria with asymmetry, irregular border, color variation, diameter of >6 mm, and evolution.[17,20]

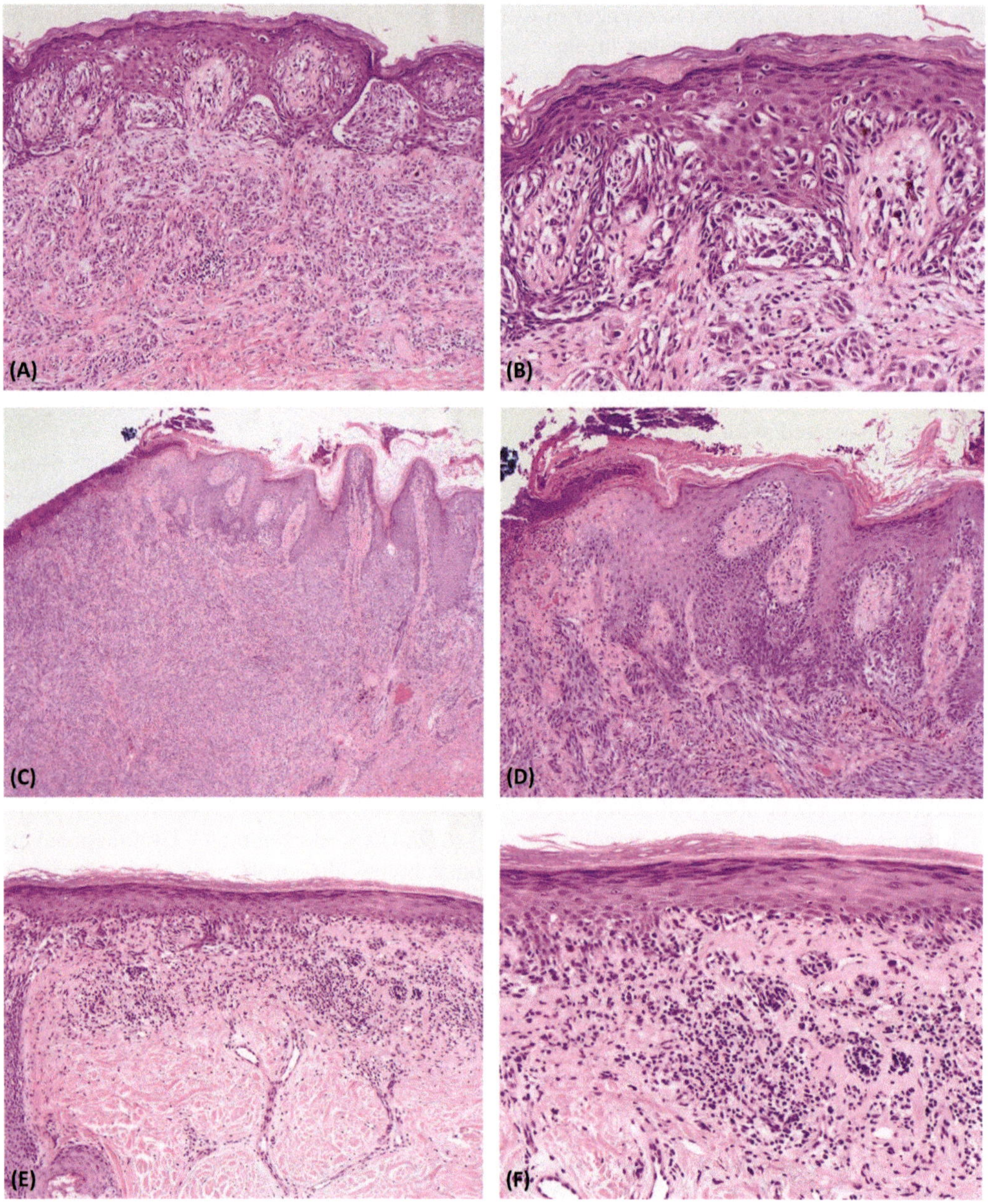

FIGURE 8.1 Common histological features of melanoma. (**a**), (**b**) Superficial spreading melanoma. Confluent proliferation of single and nested atypical melanocytes in the epidermis with extensive pagetoid spread. An invasive component is present in the dermis (hematoxylin and eosin, 100×, **a**). Atypical melanocytes are pleomorphic and hyperchromatic. Nests are elongated and bizarre in shape. (hematoxylin and eosin, 200×, **b**). (**c**), (**d**) Superficial spreading melanoma with ulceration and predominantly nodular component (vertical growth phase). An ulceration is present with full-thickness loss of the epidermis. Atypical melanocytes invade the dermis in irregular nests with lack of maturation (hematoxylin and eosin, 40×, **c**). A radial growth phase component, comprised of single and poorly nested melanocytes with pagetoid spread, is present in the epidermis adjacent to the ulcer (hematoxylin and eosin, 100×, **d**). (**e**), (**f**) Lentigo maligna melanoma. Confluent junctional proliferation of single and poorly nested atypical melanocytes with adnexal extension and effacement of the rete ridges on skin with solar damage (hematoxylin and eosin, 100×, **e**). Small nests of atypical melanocytes invade the superficial dermis (hematoxylin and eosin, 200×, **f**)

NM represents 15%–30% of melanomas and most commonly involves the trunk and limbs of patients in the fifth or sixth decade of life with a male predominance. NM is thought to begin almost immediately in the vertical growth phase, which correlates with its more rapid growth and higher rate of metastasis.[23] Clinically, NM typically appears as an ulcerated and deeply pigmented, smooth-surfaced papule, nodule, or tumor. It can also appear as an ulcerated polyp or as an elevated plaque with irregular outlines. NM may also appear amelanotic and harder to clinically differentiate from other skin malignancies.[17,20]

LMM accounts for 4% to 15% of cutaneous melanomas and occurs mainly in the head and neck area of older individuals with chronic sun-damaged skin. Clinically, the lesion appears as a slowly growing macule with irregular borders and a variety of colors, including black, brown, or brown on a tan background. The tumor is often relatively large and flat and develops slowly over years to decades. The focus of invasion may be detected as a papule and the invasive component may progress more rapidly.[17,20]

ALM is the most common melanoma subtype in patients with more pigmented skin types; however, it only represents 5% of melanomas in white people. There is a female predilection and the affected persons are usually elderly patients. ALM is mainly located in glabrous skin and the adjacent skin of digits, palms, and soles; it usually involves the nail bed of the great toe or thumb.[17,20]

MELANOMA PATHOGENESIS

The distinct clinical variants of melanoma arise under slightly different environmental conditions and have different genetic features.[24] There is epidemiological and genetic evidence that UV exposure contributes to melanoma initiation by both direct and indirect mutagenesis.[25,26] Furthermore, based on indirect evidence, trauma and trauma-induced reparative changes may drive mutagenesis in ALM.[27] The importance of activating mutations in oncogenes (*BRAF*, *NRAS*, *KIT*, Rac1) and inactivating mutations in tumor suppressors (*TP53*, *PTEN*, *NF1*, *CDKN2A*) in melanoma is clear, but the complex mechanism of melanoma initiation and progression orchestrated by these genetic changes are to date not well understood.[25,28] Although *BRAF* V600E mutations are present in half of melanomas, leading to melanoma growth and driving metastatic disease, the same mutations are more frequent in benign nevi and contribute to oncogenic senescence.[29]

MELANOMA AND IMMUNITY

Melanomas are human malignancies with one of the highest mutations and neoantigen burden.[30–32] Melanomas are amongst the first malignancies in which the importance of immunotherapy has been shown; first when bacillus Calmette-Guérin (BCG) administration demonstrated survival benefits and later when high dose interleukin 2 (IL2) offered long-term cure for a small subset of melanoma patients.[33,34] However, melanomas actively evade the immune response by creating an immune exhausted niche in and around the tumor cells by releasing paracrine mediators and modifying cell surface markers.[35] Early immunotherapies mostly failed to overcome this local immunosuppression and thus could not markedly modify melanoma prognosis. Recently, the excellent therapeutic response to immune checkpoint inhibitors in metastatic melanoma redirected the attention to the role of the immune response in melanoma and highlighted the risks of melanoma in immunosuppressed populations, specifically OTRs. After providing a brief introduction to melanoma, in the remainder of chapter, we will focus on melanoma in OTRs.

MELANOMA IN SOLID ORGAN TRANSPLANT RECIPIENTS

We have come a long way since the first successful kidney transplantation in 1954.[36] Today, over 350,000 people live with allograft solid organ transplants.[37] The long-term success of grafts relies on the adequate suppression of the recipients' immune response to prohibit graft rejection. Although transplanted organs provide a new chance for life, the burden of immunosuppression carries new dangers—increased risk of infectious diseases, and relevant to this topic, increased risk for numerous malignancies, including melanoma (Figure 8.2).

The incidence of melanoma was previously reported to be anywhere from 0 to 8-fold higher in OTRs compared with that in the general papulation.[38–41] More contemporary data from Europe suggested that there was a 2.4-fold increase (95% CI, 1.9–3.0) in the standardized incidence ratio of melanoma in OTRs compared with that in the general population.[42] A systematic review of 12 cohort studies from around the world also found a 2.4-fold (95% CI, 2.0–2.9) overall increase in melanoma incidence in OTRs.[43] However, the observed increase in incidence in the different studies varied based on the characteristics of the assessed OTR populations. In a cohort of 105,174 renal transplant recipients of whom 488 had a record of melanoma in the US Renal Data System, the age-standardized relative rate of melanoma was 4.9 compared with the Surveillance, Epidemiology, and End Results.[44] In a meta-analysis of cohort studies published in 2014, melanoma risk was reported to be 2.7-fold increased among OTRs in general, but the risk of melanoma was 2.54-fold increased in kidney transplant patients and over 2-fold increased in liver and heart transplant patients, with a 5.27-fold increased risk of melanoma compared with that in the general population.[45] Not all studies found similar incidence increase based on the grafted organ. In a retrospective cohort study of 1164 patients who underwent cardiothoracic transplant in a single center, the incidence of melanoma post cardiothoracic transplant was similar to that of renal transplant, but a markedly shorter period of latency to melanoma post transplantation was seen, with a median of 2.5 years in cardiothoracic transplantation compared with a median of 6.1 years in renal transplantation.[46]

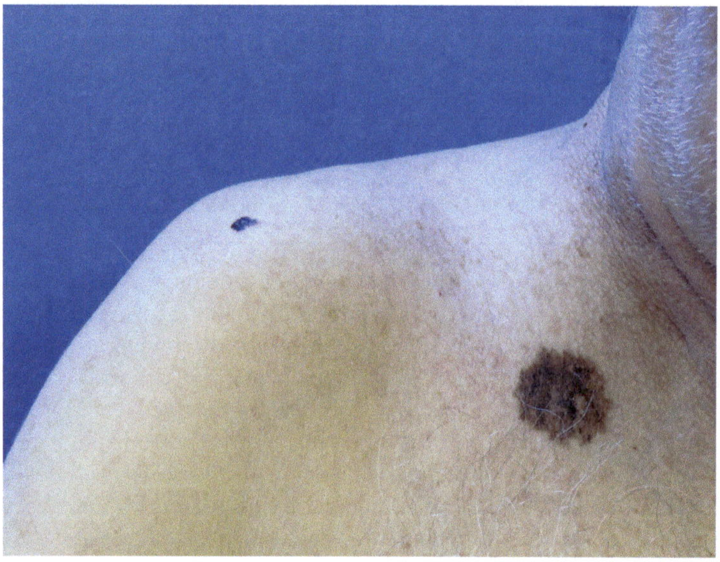

FIGURE 8.2 Double lung transplant patient with two primary invasive melanomas of the right shoulder and right clavicle. (Nathalie C. Zeitouni, MDCM)

There are numerous factors influencing melanoma risk in OTRs. In the US Renal Data System, the significant risk factors for developing melanoma were older age and white race of both recipients and donors, male sex of recipient, less than 4 HLA mismatches, living donor transplant, and history of immunosuppressive sirolimus and cyclosporine therapy.[44]

Other reported risk factors include azathioprine maintenance therapy, polyclonal antibody induction therapy, and lower latitude.[47]

Unfortunately, this increase in melanoma incidence in OTRs is unlikely to be only because of overdiagnosis and better surveillance; worse outcomes for melanoma were observed in OTRs compared with those of non-immunosuppressed controls.[48] There was contemporary evidence that melanoma-specific mortality was almost threefold greater among solid organ transplant patients than in controls.[47] Although OTRs with more advanced melanomas were previously found to do disproportionally worse, recent data indicated that the overall increase in melanoma-specific mortality was mostly because of a mortality increase resulting from thin invasive melanomas, not locoregionally advanced tumors or distant metastatic tumors.[47,48] Given the limitations of melanoma therapy in OTRs, both the difference in outcomes in OTRs and the general population is expected to further worsen in the coming years, thus highlighting the importance of better melanoma prevention and treatment in OTRs.

SOURCE OF MELANOMA

Solid organ transplantation creates unique scenarios for the emergence of melanoma. After transplantation, melanoma may emerge as a primary melanoma or may also recur from preexisting melanoma in the recipient or from the donor. Primary melanoma developing *de novo* after transplantation represents the most common presentation of melanoma. The mean time to primary melanoma ranges from 17.4 to 61 months post transplantation.[44,49] The primary melanomas after transplantation may arise in normal skin or can also arise from preexisting nevi.[49]

Unfortunately, melanoma may also recur after solid organ transplantation.[50] To date, we have limited data about the risk for recurrence of a preexisting melanoma in OTRs. An initial report on the subject in 1996 showed that 6 out of 31 patients (19.4%) with preexisting melanoma developed recurrences after transplantation, and all patients succumbed to melanoma within 6 to 30 months after recurrence.[50] According to more recent data, no increased risk of recurrence of melanoma was identified in 59 patients with preexisting melanomas after transplantation during the follow-up period up to 10.5 years.[51] This lack of increased recurrence risk was also found by others.[48,52] Although lately no elevated risk of melanoma recurrence in OTRs has been seen, the true recurrence risk may be difficult to measure and to accurately compare with that of controls as there is a selection bias in transplant candidate identification. Patients with higher risk melanomas are less likely to undergo transplantation, and even patients with lower risk melanomas will only be chosen for transplantation after a safety period, as will be discussed later in this chapter.

Solid organ transplantation creates an environment in which melanoma may not only recur from the recipient's preexisting melanoma but can also arise from the donor organ.[50] The risk of a donor transmitting cancer was reported to be 0.2% as there was 1.3% risk of having a donor with an undetected malignancy.[53] Melanomas are responsible for 17% of transmitted malignancy leading to distant metastasis and are one of the most likely malignancies transmitted during organ transplantation.[54] In several reports, organ donors whose initial cause of death was thought to be cerebral hemorrhage were sources of organ-derived melanoma.[50] Donors with unidentified metastatic melanoma are highly likely to transmit melanoma to OTRs. A summary of a few reports and case series showed a total of 17 donors who provided organs to 44 recipients—35 of whom developed melanoma between 3–24 months and a subsequent 23 of those 35 recipients (65%) died as result of malignant melanoma.[49,55,56]

MANAGEMENT OF MELANOMA IN SOLID ORGAN TRANSPLANT RECIPIENTS MELANOMA PREVENTION

Donor Selection

The potential for metastasis even a decade after surgical removal of a primary melanoma suggests that "dormant" clinically unnoticeable melanoma cells may be present in tissues of melanoma patients.[57,58] Donor-derived melanomas indicate that these cells can become reactivated in the recipients and may lead to devastating metastatic melanoma—occasionally 16 and 32 years after the diagnosis and presumed successful treatment of the primary melanoma.[56–59] Therefore, a personal history of melanoma is an absolute contraindication to solid organ donation.[60,61] Despite our best efforts, organ donation with unidentified melanoma history is still a possibility and melanomas are one of the most common malignancies transmitted via organ donation.[61] Given the metastatic risk of small primary tumors and the high incidence of melanoma, all potential donors must receive a careful skin examination to exclude the presence of previously unrecognized melanoma.[61,62] Special care is needed in donors with a history of sudden cerebrovascular hemorrhage.[62] Furthermore, autopsies should be performed on all cadaver donors to look for unexpected malignancies.[63] If a suspicious pigmented lesion is found during a living donor exam, a biopsy is the recommended standard of care. Donors with atypical nevi may pose diagnostic difficulty, and therefore collaboration between donor organizations and hospitals, dermatologists, and dermatopathologists can provide prompt diagnosis of a suspicious lesion.[61]

If donor-derived melanoma is identified in OTRs, the diagnosis has therapeutic implications for both the patient with the donor-derived melanoma and other recipients of organs from the same donor. The identification of melanoma in one recipient should prompt investigation of the remaining recipients of multiorgan donations.[60] If donor-derived melanoma is diagnosed in a renal transplant recipient, immediate cessation of immunosuppression and removal of the graft may need to be considered. In transplantation of organs essential to life, a decrease in the depth of immunosuppression followed by retransplantation, if possible, is advised. Transplant teams of other recipients need to be notified to be able to consider options on the case-by-case basis.[50,56,61,63]

Transplant Candidate Identification

As melanoma cells can spread and lay dormant for decades after the surgical removal of the primary tumor, there is a potential risk of melanoma recurrence after transplantation.[57,58] Review of recent literature as summarized previously suggests that the risk of posttransplant melanoma recurrence varies between 0% and 11%, although limitations including the sparsity of staging data and Breslow depth as well as bias in transplant candidate selection make interpretation of the data difficult.[43,48,64] In 2015, the International immunosuppression and Transplant Skin Cancer Collaborative (ITSCC) created an American Joint Committee on Cancer (AJCC) cancer stage-based model resulting in a newer approach for determining pretransplantation wait times[64] (Table 8.1). It must be recognized, though, that these recommendations were derived from analysis of 5-year and 10-year melanoma survival rates in the nonimmunosuppressed population from the AJCC 7th edition Cancer Staging Manual. The AJCC 7th edition data indicated greater than twofold higher melanoma-specific mortality for all Stage I–II subgroups than the more contemporary AJCC 8th edition staging dataset (see Table 8.2).[65–67] Since these recommendations were adapted, it is also clear that novel immunotherapy and molecular therapy offer potential long-term cure for some nonimmunosuppressed patients with Stage III and IV melanoma. Therefore, all the

TABLE 8.1 ITSCC Recommended Wait Times Between Melanoma Diagnosis and Transplantation in a Transplant Candidate Based on AJCC 7th Edition Melanoma Mortality Risk Data.

PRETRANSPLANT MELANOMA STAGE	*CANCER STAGE-BASED MODEL RECOMMENDED WAIT TIME*
0 *(In situ)*	No waiting period
IA	2 years
IB	5 years
IIA, IIB, IIIA	5–10 years
IIC, IIIB	10–15 years

Source: Adapted based on: Zwald et al.[64]

TABLE 8.2 10-Year Melanoma-Specific Survival in the AJCC 7th and the AJCC 8th Edition Datasets.

STAGE	*10-YEAR MELANOMA-SPECIFIC SURVIVAL IN MELANOMA*	
	AJCC 7TH EDITION	*AJCC 8TH EDITION*
IA	95%	98%
IB	88%	94%
IIA	67%	88%
IIB	57%	82%
IIC	40%	75%

Abbreviation: AJCC, American Joint Committee on Cancer.

Source: The AJCC 7th Edition Dataset Showed 2-Fold Increased Mortality for All Stage I–II Subgroups Compared with that of the More Contemporary AJCC 8th Dataset.[65,66]

preceding considerations must be considered when determining individual candidate pretransplantation wait times, and close adherence to the previously published recommendations is expected to overexaggerate the risk of melanoma recurrence and will likely prove overly restrictive.

Appropriate Selection of Immunosuppression

The most important difference between control populations and OTRs is the need for ongoing deep immunosuppression. Appropriate selection of immunosuppressive agents has long been postulated to influence the risk of posttransplant cancer and to also contribute to melanoma risk. Common posttransplant immunosuppressant therapies include calcineurin inhibitors (tacrolimus and cyclosporine), antiproliferative agents (azathioprine and mycophenolate mofetil), mammalian target of rapamycin (mTOR) inhibitors (sirolimus and everolimus), and steroids such as prednisone.[68] Table 8.3 compiles findings from the most recent literature on the risk of developing malignancy with different immunosuppressive therapies.

There was limited data specifically addressing melanoma risk after immunosuppression with different immunosuppressive medications.[44] Cyclosporine, tacrolimus, azathioprine, and steroids have been associated with an increased risk of posttransplant malignancies.[69–71] Cyclosporine is known to have direct cellular effects that cause an increased production of growth factors. Azathioprine's photosensitizing properties may accelerate ultraviolet radiation (UVR)-induced DNA damage, contributing to its increased posttransplant malignancy rates. Although conclusive data on mycophenolate mofetil remains unclear, it does appear to be associated with lower rates of cutaneous malignancies compared with those of azathioprine.[68,69] Recent studies suggested mTOR inhibitors were associated with a reduced risk of any posttransplant malignancy. Particularly, sirolimus use in renal transplant patients was associated with a reduced risk of malignancy; the most pronounced benefit was found in patients who switched to sirolimus from established immunosuppressive regimens.[72] However, its use was not recommended for most renal transplant patients as it was also associated with an increased risk of all-cause mortality.[72] In heart transplant patients, mTOR inhibitors and mycophenolate mofetil were associated with a lower risk of developing any malignancy, and mTOR inhibitors showed a lower recurrence rate of cutaneous malignancy at the 5-year follow-up of diagnosis of initial malignancy.[69] It was postulated that mTOR inhibitors reduced tumor growth through antiangiogenic activities.[73] It is also recognized that the associated reduction in posttransplant malignancy risk with mTOR inhibitor use may be attributed to the removal of oncogenic immunosuppressive agents such as cyclosporine.[72,74] However, contradicting the expected reduced melanoma risk with mTOR inhibitors, sirolimus and cyclosporine were both associated with higher risk of melanoma in renal OTRs and also higher melanoma mortality.[44]

TABLE 8.3 Immunosuppressive Medications and Risk of Malignancy: A Summary of the Most Recent Literature.

IMMUNOSUPPRESSIVE AGENT	*REFERENCE*	*ALLOGRAFT*	*INFLUENCE ON CANCER RISK*	*OTHER CONSIDERATIONS*	*POSTULATED MECHANISM AFFECTING MALIGNANCY RISK*
Calcineurin inhibitors					
Cyclosporine	[69] [71]	Heart Liver	Increased Increased		Direct cellular effect to increase production of growth factors.
Tacrolimus	[70] [71] [69]	Renal Liver Heart	Increased Increased Decreased	Findings might be explained by shorter follow-up period compared with that of cyclosporine.	Induces VEGF expression. Inhibits cancer cell apoptosis.
Antiproliferative agents					
Azathioprine	[69]	Heart	Increased		Photosensitization accelerating UVR-induced DNA damage.
Mycophenolate mofetil	[69]	Heart	Decreased	Lower incidence of skin cancer compared with azathioprine in this study. Influence on risk of malignancy is unclear in other studies.	

(*Continued*)

TABLE 8.3 Immunosuppressive Medications and Risk of Malignancy: A Summary of the Most Recent Literature (Continued)

IMMUNOSUPPRESSIVE AGENT	*REFERENCE*	*ALLOGRAFT*	*INFLUENCE ON CANCER RISK*	*OTHER CONSIDERATIONS*	*POSTULATED MECHANISM AFFECTING MALIGNANCY RISK*
Steroids					
Prednisolone	[69]	Heart	Increased		
mTOR inhibitors					
Sirolimus	[72]	Renal	Decreased	Increased all-cause mortality. Research needed to determine if populations at high risk of cancer may benefit.	
	[69] *	Heart	Decreased	Cutaneous malignancy recurrence at 2 and 5 years of follow-up after initial diagnosis of tumor was lower. Lower mortality was observed with noncutaneous malignancies after initial diagnosis of malignancy.	Inhibits angiogenesis.

Abbreviations: DNA, deoxyribonucleic acid; mTOR, mammalian target of rapamycin; UVR, ultraviolet radiation; VEGF, vascular endothelial growth factor.

*Everolimus was found to have similar impact as sirolimus.

MELANOMA TREATMENT

Workup, Staging, and Surgical Treatment

Workup and treatment of local melanoma in the immunosuppressed population parallels that in the immunocompetent population. No data is available based on which modified guidelines for OTRs could be recommended. If available, dermoscopy should be performed prior to biopsy as it improves both the sensitivity and specificity of the clinical diagnosis of melanoma, and perhaps more importantly, improves the confidence in the diagnosis of benign pigmented lesions, thereby reducing the number of unnecessary biopsies.[75] If a suspicious pigmented lesion is found on examination, a complete full-thickness excisional biopsy with 1–3 mm margins is advised.[76]

Once a biopsy is performed, diagnosis is usually based on histological features on H&E (hematoxylin and eosin) staining, although in some cases, immunohistochemical stains such as S-100, MART-1, HMB-45, and SOX10 can aid in the diagnosis.[77] If a diagnosis of melanoma is made, the National Comprehensive Cancer Network (NCCN) guidelines recommend wide local excision with clinical margins based on Breslow depth.[76] This excision depth should be down to, but not including, the muscle fascia.[78] In recent years, the use of Mohs surgery has been described in the literature for the treatment of select melanomas, but currently there is no data regarding its use in OTRs.[79]

Concerning indications for sentinel lymph node biopsy (SLNB), the NCCN 2019 guidelines recommended discussion and consideration of SLNB in patients with stage IB, T1b melanoma (Breslow depth <0.8 mm with ulceration or 0.8–1 mm with or without ulceration), or T1a melanoma with Breslow depth <0.8 mm and with other adverse features. For patients with stage IB (T2a) or stage II (>1 mm thick), the recommendation was to offer SLNB.[76] If performed, the results of SLNB may aid in melanoma staging using the 8th edition AJCC TMN system, and thereby may help stratify risk and establish whether or not a patient may benefit from adjuvant treatment and more aggressive reduction in immunosuppression.[56,68] For patients with positive lymph nodes or other concerning features of locoregional or distant disease, imaging studies should be performed to aid staging.[63,76] There are no specific guidelines on the use of radiation therapy for melanoma in transplant patients. Recommendations on radiation use are based on the general NCCN melanoma guidelines. There is evidence that primary melanoma gene expression profiles (GEPs) may also aid melanoma risk assessment but the use of GEPs is still controversial and there is no data on the utility of GEPs in OTRs.[80]

Modification of Immunosuppression

Melanomas exert local immunosuppression on their tumor microenvironment.[81,82] This local immunosuppression is thought to play a crucial role in melanoma progression.[81,82] In a limited immunohistochemistry-based study, markers of the localized immunosuppression indicated more prominent local immunosuppression in melanomas of OTRs than that in melanomas from controls.[83] Indoleamine-2, 3-dioxygenase 1 (IDO), an enzyme that catabolizes tryptophan and suppresses T-cell function, on immunohistochemistry was shown to be highly expressed in the tumors of OTRs.[83,84] CD8, FoxP3, PD1, and PD-L1 are poorly expressed in the melanoma microenvironment of OTRs, further contributing to local immunosuppression.[83] These findings, together with reports of regression of melanoma metastases following the withdrawal of immunosuppressive therapy,[85] and the effect of immunosuppressive treatment choice on melanoma risk,[44] point to the importance of systemic immunosuppression in shifting the immune balance towards melanoma survival and progression. Thus, current evidence suggests that modification of immunosuppression may have a therapeutic role in OTRs with melanoma.

There are three major approaches to modifying immunosuppression regimens for prevention and management of melanoma. We can reduce the overall level of immunosuppression, reduce or remove pro-oncogenic immunosuppressive agents (i.e., cyclosporine, tacrolimus), and add or increase the agents that may reduce malignancy risk (i.e., mTOR inhibitors).[68]

The ITSCC and its European counterpart, the Skin Care in Organ Transplant Patients-Europe (SCOPE) Reduction of Immunosuppression Task Force, established expert consensus guidelines for indications that warrant discussion of the of mild, moderate, and severe reduction of immunosuppression in solid organ transplant recipients (SOTRs) with high-risk skin cancer, including melanoma.[86] Table 8.4 shows recommendations provided for melanoma. These guidelines were formulated

TABLE 8.4 Recommended Immunosuppression Reduction Based on AJCC 6th Edition Staging and Melanoma Mortality Risk Data.

MELANOMA STAGE	*RECOMMENDED LEVEL OF REDUCTION OF IMMUNOSUPPRESSION*		
	ALLOGRAFT		
	KIDNEY	*LIVER*	*HEART*
0	None	None	None
IA	Moderate	Mild	Moderate
IB	Moderate	Moderate	Moderate
IIA	Severe	Moderate	Moderate
IIB	Severe	Moderate	Moderate to severe
IIC-III	Severe	Severe	Severe
IV	Severe	Severe	Severe

Abbreviations: AJCC, American Joint Committee on Cancer; ITSCC, International immunosuppression and Transplant Skin Cancer Collaborative; SCOPE, Skin Care in Organ Transplant Patients-Europe.

Source: Table based on data presented by Otley et al.[86]

Note: Guidelines per ITSCC and SCOPE Expert Panel Consensus. Reduction Level Based on the Risk to the Allograft. Examples of Risks to the Allograft Include: None—No Risk of Dysfunction; Mild—Risk of Reversible Dysfunction Needing Medical Treatment; Moderate—Risk of Partial Permanent Dysfunction to the Allograft from Rejection; and Severe—Risk of Failure with Potential for Death.

by assessing the risk of mortality from the tumors and judging the immunosuppression risk to the allografts.[86] Melanoma mortality risk was based on AJCC 6th edition of melanoma staging data. As the mortality risks in melanoma stage groups in the more contemporary datasets are lower and novel treatments are available for melanoma, adaptation of the original recommendations to the more contemporary mortality risk and treatment repertoire is important. When deciding on reduction in immunosuppression, it is also important to take into consideration how organs tolerate reduction in immunosuppressive therapy. Renal transplant patients can return to dialysis if reduction in the regimen leads to graft rejection. Liver transplant patients tend to tolerate reductions in immunosuppressive therapy well, and liver tissue was shown to have a greater ability to recover from rejection, should it occur, compared with other organs.[68,86]

As we discussed previously in our chapter, the use of calcineurin inhibitors has been associated with increased posttransplant risk of malignancy. Therefore, reduction or removal of these oncogenic agents and/or conversion to or addition of proposed anti-oncogenic agents, such as mTOR inhibitors, is another option to consider. Although long-term data on the efficacy of this approach to reduce melanoma mortality are lacking, and mTOR inhibitors may paradoxically even increase melanoma risk.[44] Azathioprine may also be switched to mycophenolate mofetil in the proper patients to reduce the accumulation of mutations and possibly inhibit the growth of cutaneous malignancies.[87–89] Ultimately, modifying therapy requires a multidisciplinary approach in which factors including patient age, medication levels, risk of graft rejection, allograft source, and use of melanoma-directed therapy must be considered by the health care team.[63]

Targeted Therapy

The mutation profile of melanoma in the immunosuppressed population correlates with that of the immunocompetent population, including mutations of *BRAF* and *NRAS* oncogenes.[83] Therefore, many melanomas in OTRs are amenable to treatment targeting activating mutations of these oncogenes (Figure 8.3). BRAF is a serine-threonine kinase associated with the activation of the mitogen-activated protein kinase

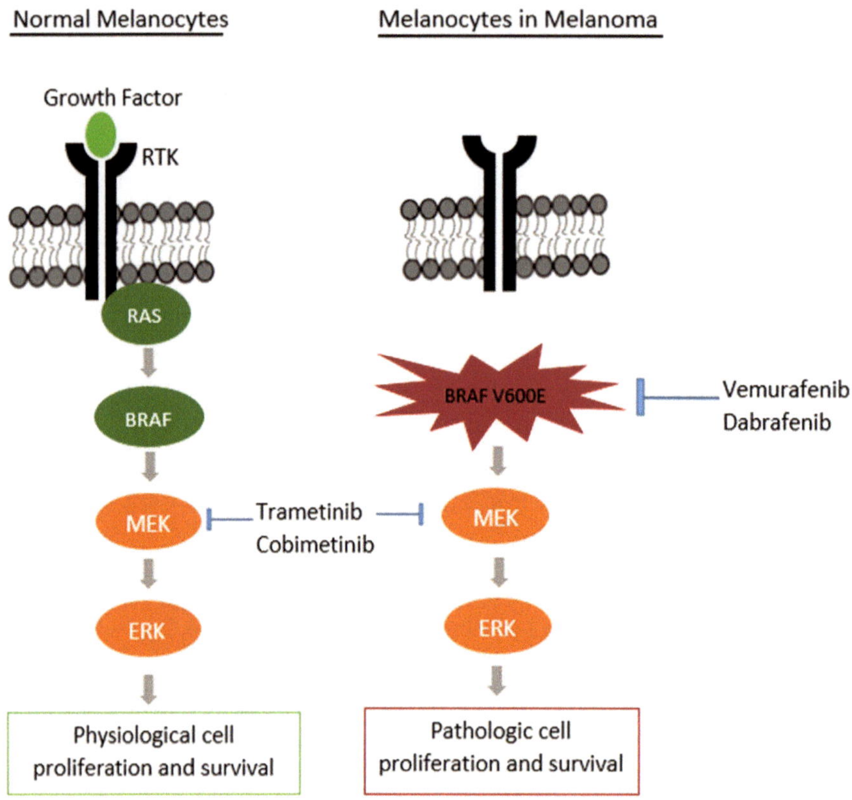

FIGURE 8.3 Targeted therapy of advanced melanoma. In the physiological pathway, growth factor activation of receptor tyrosine kinase (RTK) activates the MEK pathway leading to signaling for normal cell survival. Vemurafenib and dabrafenib inhibit V600E mutated *BRAF* found in some melanomas, thus they counter constitutive activation of the MEK pathway and inhibit tumorigenic growth signals. Trametinib and cobimetinib are MEK inhibitors, which block downstream signaling, thus decreasing the emergence of resistance and improving efficacy of BRAF inhibitors.

(MAPK) pathway and cancer cell proliferation. Vemurafenib and dabrafenib are small molecule inhibitors that selectively inhibit *BRAF* V600E mutants[90] and are approved by the FDA for use in unresectable or metastatic melanomas with these mutations.[90] Prior to initiating treatment, mutational tissue analysis should be performed.[76] Patients with tumors harboring *BRAF* mutations could undergo treatment with a BRAF inhibitor, but not patients with known *RAS* mutations.[90] Although trials in the general population have shown better survival compared with that of dacarbazine, a conventional chemotherapy agent approved for melanoma treatment in the 1970s, the extent of overall benefit in monotherapy and in early combination treatments was limited.[91] There are a limited number of case reports of single agent targeted therapy in OTRs. Vemurafenib use in a lung transplant recipient with metastatic melanoma was associated with a partial extracerebral response and manageable adverse effects.[92] Dabrafenib use in a heart transplant recipient with metastatic melanoma was associated with a partial response and the emergence of resistance.[93]

In an attempt to decrease the emergence of resistance, BRAF inhibitors have been lately used almost exclusively in combination with inhibitors of an important resistance pathway, MEK.[94] MEK inhibitors also have activity in *NRAS* mutant melanomas.[90] Such therapies include dabrafenib + trametinib, vemurafenib + cobimetinib, and encorafenib + binimetinib. In a heart transplant recipient with metastatic melanoma, dabrafenib with trametinib (MEK1/2 inhibitor) was well tolerated and the combination treatment resulted in a better than anticipated (15 months) progression-free survival.[95]

Molecular inhibitors are widely used in the treatment of advanced melanoma in OTRs, but few reports are available and reports often lack details.[96] Hopefully, systematically collected data will soon become available to compare the efficacy of these molecular inhibitors in OTRs with that in the nonimmunosuppressed patients.

Important drug interactions and toxicities have been reported with the use of small molecular inhibitors. In the previously mentioned heart transplant patient on BRAF inhibitor monotherapy, interactions between dabrafenib and everolimus and tacrolimus metabolism (drugs metabolized by CYP3A4) were observed, necessitating increased immunosuppression levels to avoid graft rejection.[93] Both vemurafenib and dabrafenib have nephrotoxic effects; vemurafenib appears to be more nephrotoxic, and this toxicity is potentiated when it is used in combination with MEK inhibitors.[97] In contrast, dabrafenib appears to be less nephrotoxic, even when used in combination with trametinib.[98] Vemurafenib can also induce a phototoxic reaction.[99] BRAF inhibitor monotherapy leads to a marked increase in cutaneous squamous cell carcinoma (cSCC) incidence (12.5%–18%).[98,100] According to a recent meta-analysis, although BRAF and MEK inhibitor combination therapy also showed higher than expected cSCC incidence (3.0%), MEK inhibitor use reduced cSCC incidence by almost fivefold compared with unopposed BRAF inhibitor use.[100] Thus the risk of BRAF inhibitor-induced cSCC incidence increase needs to also be taken into consideration, although no data exists on the risk of cSCC in OTRs after melanoma small molecular inhibitor treatment.[100]

Immunotherapy

Melanoma therapy has been revolutionized in the past decade by immunotherapy.[101,102] There is ample evidence for the efficacy of immune check point inhibitors in metastatic melanoma in immunocompetent patients.[101] However, in the immunosuppressed population, administration of immunotherapy is complex because of two central issues surrounding immunotherapy: 1) immunotherapy requires a functioning immune system in order to elicit a tumor response, and 2) the immunotherapy effect is not tumor specific and thus can also enhance immune response against the graft, increasing the risk of organ rejection. Consequently, the issue of immunosuppression modification becomes a complex balancing act for OTRs on immunotherapy.

Previously used agents, such as IL2, peginterferon alfa-2b, and high-dose interferon alfa-2b, because of their low efficacy, were replaced by newer agents. Given the low efficacy but increased allograft rejection risk in OTRs, these first-generation immunotherapy agents had little utility.[63] The advent of checkpoint inhibitors brought promising survival results for patients with metastatic melanoma in the general population.[102] Programmed cell death protein (PD-1) inhibitors, such as pembrolizumab and nivolumab, and monoclonal antibodies against cytotoxic T-lymphocyte-associated antigen-4 (CTLA-4), such as ipilimumab, are the most commonly used checkpoint inhibitors in current use for melanoma therapy.[101,102] Immunotherapy can induce profound autoimmune side effects including hepatitis, interstitial nephritis, myocarditis, and a whole range of cutaneous eruptions resembling autoimmune dermatitides from atopic dermatitis to lichen planus to bullous pemphigoid.[103,104]

There are a limited number of case reports and case series for the use of checkpoint inhibitor therapy in OTRs with advanced cutaneous malignancy.[105]

Highlights of the current literature on the tumor response and signs of organ rejection of people undergoing immunotherapy are summarized in Table 8.5. Organ rejection is more frequent with PD-1 inhibitors vs. CTLA-4 blockade.[106] In the prior systematic review, graft rejection was not the most common cause of death, rather it was disease progression. Some OTRs require organ transplantation because of autoimmune disease. Immune checkpoint inhibition raises the theoretical possibility of a repeated flare of a prior autoimmune disease, destroying the graft or other organs. Other autoimmune adverse events may also be initiated by immunotherapy. Given the limited number of studies performed in OTRs and the resulting lack of available recommendations for their use in transplant patients, currently fine-tuning

TABLE 8.5 Summary of Case Reports on the Use of Checkpoint Inhibitor Therapy in SOTRs with Advanced Cutaneous Malignancies

ALLOGRAFT AND SAMPLE SIZE	*MALIGNANCY*	*CHECKPOINT INHIBITOR*	*ALLOGRAFT RESPONSE*	*TUMOR RESPONSE*	*REFERENCE*
Liver n = 1	Metastatic melanoma	Ipilimumab	None	None	[115]
Liver n = 1	Metastatic melanoma	Ipilimumab	Transaminitis but no graft loss	Partial	[116]
Liver n = 1	Metastatic melanoma	Not specified	None	Unclear	[96]
Liver n = 2	Metastatic melanoma	Pembrolizumab	1 patient with acute rejection	1 patient with complete response	[117]
Liver n = 1	Metastatic melanoma	Ipilimumab followed by pembrolizumab	None	Partial response	[118]
Cardiac n = 1	Metastatic melanoma	Ipilimumab followed by pembrolizumab	None	None	[119]
Cardiac n = 1	Metastatic squamous cell carcinoma	Nivolumab (1 dose)	Acute rejection	None	[120]
Combined cardiac and renal n = 1	Metastatic melanoma	Ipilimumab followed by an unspecified PD-1 inhibitor	Acute kidney graft rejection following ipilimumab and again following PD-1 inhibitor	None	[121]
Renal n = 6	Metastatic melanoma	Ipilimumab	1 acute rejection	1 partial response, 1 stable disease, 4 disease progression	[122]
Renal n = 2	Metastatic melanoma	Ipilimumab	None	Partial response	[123]
Renal n = 1	Metastatic melanoma	Ipilimumab followed by Nivolumab	None	None	[124]
Renal n = 1	Metastatic melanoma	Ipilimumab followed by Nivolumab	Acute rejection (after starting nivolumab)	Partial response	[125]
Renal n = 1	Metastatic melanoma	Nivolumab	Acute rejection	Ongoing clinical and radiologic response	[126]
Renal n = 1	Metastatic melanoma	Ipilimumab followed by pembrolizumab	Acute rejection (after starting pembrolizumab)	Not discussed	[127]
Renal n = 3	Metastatic melanoma	Not specified per patient	1 Acute rejection on pembrolizumab	2 partial responses	[96]

Abbreviation: PD-1, programmed cell death protein 1

immunosuppression levels in OTRs on immune checkpoint inhibitors requires a careful interdisciplinary approach and should always take patient expectations and wishes into account. Given the potential for autoimmune adverse events and organ rejection, systemic immunotherapy is currently reserved for OTRs with advanced melanoma in which melanoma-specific mortality greatly outweighs the risk of organ dysfunction,[107] or in clinical trials.

Besides systemic immunotherapy, recently the first localized immunotherapy treatment, an oncolytic virus, also became available for melanoma treatment when the FDA approved Talimogene laherparepvec (T-VEC) in 2015 for the treatment of advanced melanoma.[108] It is a genetically modified attenuated type 1 herpes simplex virus. T-VEC is injected into accessible cutaneous metastasis or nodal lesions and selectively replicates in tumor cells and lyses them. The modified oncolytic virus also expresses granulocyte-macrophage colony-stimulating factor (GM-CSF) to induce a local immune response. Its effects are mostly local and locoregional but it may also trigger a systemic anticancer immune response, potential abscopal effect.[109] To date, T-VEC use in OTRs has only been documented in a few case reports. A 2019 study in a combined heart and kidney transplant recipient with melanoma showed complete tumor response without any graft loss after 11 cycles of T-VEC.[109] A 2017 study in a heart transplant patient with metastatic melanoma showed complete tumor response without any signs of graft loss after 5 cycles.[106] A recent case report documented the combination use of T-VEC and imiquimod for in transit melanoma in a renal transplant patient.[110]

Intralesional melanoma therapy with T-VEC holds the promise of offering antitumor effects at limited systemic toxicity risk in OTRs and may become a mainstream treatment in high-risk, surgically unresectable, locoregional disease. However, given the limited safety and efficacy data, the use of T-VEC in OTRs should be considered on a case-by-case basis after multidisciplinary discussion or in a clinical trial.

Other currently developed intralesional immunotherapies for advanced melanoma may also hold promise in OTRs, although most of these treatments are currently tested in combination with PD-1 inhibitors and thus they do not eliminate the risks posed by systemic immunotherapy. Intertumoral injection of plasmid interleukin-12 (pIL-12) followed by electroporation in combination therapy with systemic PD-1 inhibitors were tested for enhancing response to immunotherapy.[111] Additionally, intralesional toll-like receptor 9 (TLR9) agonists are currently also being studied for their synergistic effects with systemic PD-1 inhibitors.[112] Lastly, PV-10 (10% solution of rose bengal), a fluorescein derivative that accumulates in the lysosomes of tumor cells and causes necrosis, has also been proposed as an intralesional treatment enhancing melanoma systemic immunotherapy.[113] The future of intralesional therapies in combination with systemic therapies holds promise for individuals with advanced disease and may later also help better target immunotherapy in OTRs.

Follow Up Considerations

The management of melanoma in OTRs is challenging. It is often further complicated by the patients' other skin cancers, medication sides effects, and iatrogenic complications of immunosuppression. Unfortunately, contemporary data indicates that OTRs with even thin melanomas tend to do markedly worse than nonimmunosuppressed patients. Melanoma also signals risk for novel other melanomas.[114] Therefore, even if a melanoma has been successfully treated, patients should continue regular full-body skin exams with examination of lymph node basins. Although definitive guidelines have not yet been established for OTRs, recommendations for the frequency of skin checks should be based on factors affecting skin cancer risk, including amongst other factors the type of transplant, age at transplant, other skin cancer history, and immunosuppression regimens. In general, all post-transplant melanoma patients should be screened every 3 months for at least 2 years, then total-body skin exams at least every 6 months lifelong are reasonable. Those with metastatic melanoma should be screened every 4–6 weeks. Patient education about sun-protective behavior and monthly self-skin exams are also key.[63,68]

SUMMARY OF KEY POINTS

- Melanoma incidence has risen 3-fold over the last decades.
- The incidence of melanoma in OTRs is overall 2–3-fold higher than that in the public.
- Invasive melanoma shows higher mortality risk in OTRs than that in nonimmunosuppressed patients.
- Donor-derived melanomas are a potentially devastating complication of organ transplantation.
- Treatment of early primary melanoma in OTRs is similar to that of nonimmunosuppressed patients.
- Locoregional and distant melanoma therapy in OTRs is complicated by immunosuppression and the risk of organ rejection.
- Management of advanced melanoma in OTRs is an evolving field, requires a multidisciplinary approach, and needs to be streamlined to patient wishes and priorities.

REFERENCES

1. Global Observatory on Donation & Transplantation. Global database on donation and transplantation; 2017. Available from: www.transplant-observatory.org/.
2. Martinez OM, de Gruijl FR. Molecular and immunologic mechanisms of cancer pathogenesis in solid organ transplant recipients. Am J Transplant. 2008;8(11):2205–11.
3. Surveillance E, End results (SEER) program. Cancer stat facts: melanoma of the skin. surveillance, epidemiology, and end results (SEER) program. 2019. Available from: https://seer.cancer.gov/statfacts/
4. American Cancer Society. Cancer facts & figures 2020. Atlanta: American Cancer Society; 2020. Available from: www.cancer.org/content/dam/cancer-org/research/cancer-facts-and-statistics/annual-cancer-facts-and-figures/2020/cancer-facts-and-figures-2020.pdf.
5. Gandini S et al. Meta-analysis of risk factors for cutaneous melanoma: II. Sun exposure. Eur J Cancer. 2005;41(1):45–60.
6. Tannous ZS et al. Progression to invasive melanoma from malignant melanoma in situ, lentigo maligna type. Hum Pathol. 2000;31(6):705–8.
7. Lacour JP et al. Daylight photodynamic therapy with methyl aminolevulinate cream is effective and nearly painless in treating actinic keratoses: a randomised, investigator-blinded, controlled, phase III study throughout Europe. J Eur Acad Dermatol Venereol. 2015;29(12):2342–8.
8. International Agency for Research on Cancer Working Group on artificial ultraviolet, l. and c. skin, The association of use of sunbeds with cutaneous malignant melanoma and other skin cancers: a systematic review. Int J Cancer. 2007;120(5):1116–22.
9. Stern RS, up study. The risk of melanoma in association with long-term exposure to PUVA. J Am Acad Dermatol. 2001;44(5):755–61.
10. Survellance End Results Program. SEER stat fact sheets: melanoma of the skin. 2016. Available from: https://seer.cancer.gov/statfacts/html/melan.html
11. Purdue MP et al. Etiologic and other factors predicting nevus-associated cutaneous malignant melanoma. Cancer Epidemiol Biomarkers Prev. 2005;14(8):2015–22.
12. Walling HW et al. Staged excision versus Mohs micrographic surgery for lentigo maligna and lentigo maligna melanoma. J Am Acad Dermatol. 2007;57(4):659–64.
13. Kasprzak JM, Xu YG, Diagnosis and management of lentigo maligna: a review. Drugs Context. 2015;4:212281.
14. NAACC Registries. NAACCR fast stats: an interactive quick tool for quick access to key NAACCR cancer statistics. Available from: https://www.naaccr.org/interactive-data-on-line/
15. Watt AJ, Kotsis SV, Chung KC. Risk of melanoma arising in large congenital melanocytic nevi: a systematic review. Plast Reconstr Surg. 2004;113(7):1968–74.
16. Gandini S et al. Meta-analysis of risk factors for cutaneous melanoma: I. common and atypical naevi. Eur J Cancer. 2005;41(1):28–44.

17. Gautschi M et al. Prognostic markers in lentigo maligna patients treated with imiquimod cream: a long-term follow-up study. J Am Acad Dermatol. 2016;74(1):81–7, e1.
18. Tsao H, Niendorf K. Genetic testing in hereditary melanoma. J Am Acad Dermatol. 2004;51(5):803–8.
19. English JS, Swerdlow AJ. The risk of malignant melanoma, internal malignancy and mortality in xeroderma pigmentosum patients. Br J Dermatol. 1987;117(4):457–61.
20. Markovic SN et al. Malignant melanoma in the 21st century, part 1: epidemiology, risk factors, screening, prevention, and diagnosis. Mayo Clin Proc. 2007;82(3):364–80.
21. Titus-Ernstoff L et al. Pigmentary characteristics and moles in relation to melanoma risk. Int J Cancer. 2005;116(1):144–9.
22. Beaumont KA, Liu YY, Sturm RA. The melanocortin-1 receptor gene polymorphism and association with human skin cancer. Prog Mol Biol Transl Sci. 2009;88:85–153.
23. Kalkhoran S et al. Historical, clinical, and dermoscopic characteristics of thin nodular melanoma. Arch Dermatol. 2010;146(3):311–18.
24. Greenwald HS, Friedman EB, Osman I. Superficial spreading and nodular melanoma are distinct biological entities: a challenge to the linear progression model. Melanoma Res. 2012;22(1):1–8.
25. Hocker T, Tsao H. Ultraviolet radiation and melanoma: a systematic review and analysis of reported sequence variants. Hum Mut. 2007;28(6):578–88.
26. Emri G et al. Ultraviolet radiation-mediated development of cutaneous melanoma: an update. J Photochem Photobiol B. 2018;185:169–75.
27. Jung HJ et al. A clinicopathologic analysis of 177 acral melanomas in koreans: relevance of spreading pattern and physical stress. JAMA Dermatol. 2013;149(11):1281–8.
28. Hodis E et al. A landscape of driver mutations in melanoma. Cell. 2012;150(2):251–63.
29. Wajapeyee N et al. Oncogenic BRAF induces senescence and apoptosis through pathways mediated by the secreted protein IGFBP7. Cell. 2008;132(3):363–74.
30. Alexandrov LB et al. Signatures of mutational processes in human cancer. Nature. 2013;500(7463):415–21.
31. Brown SD et al. Neo-antigens predicted by tumor genome meta-analysis correlate with increased patient survival. Genome Res. 2014;24(5):743–50.
32. Cancer Genome Atlas. Genomic classification of cutaneous melanoma. Cell. 2015;161(7):1681–96.
33. Morton DL et al. BCG immunotherapy of malignant melanoma: summary of a seven-year experience. Ann Surg. 1974;180(4):635–43.
34. Rosenberg SA. Treatment of 283 consecutive patients with metastatic melanoma or renal cell cancer using high-dose bolus interleukin 2. JAMA. 1994;271(12):907–13.
35. Tucci M et al. Immune system evasion as hallmark of melanoma progression: the role of dendritic cells. Front. Oncol. 2019;9(1148).
36. Barker CF, Markmann JF. Historical overview of transplantation. Cold Spring Harb Perspect Med. 2013;3(4):a014977.
37. Murray JE, Merrill JP, Harrison JH. Kidney transplantation between seven pairs of identical twins. Ann Surg. 1958;148(3):343–59.
38. Le Mire L et al. Melanomas in renal transplant recipients. Br J Dermatol. 2006;154(3):472–7.
39. Engels EA et al. Spectrum of cancer risk among US solid organ transplant recipients. JAMA. 2011;306(17):1891–901.
40. Ali FR, Lear JT, Melanoma in organ transplant recipients: incidence, outcomes and management considerations. J Skin Cancer. 2012:404615.
41. Lindelöf B et al. Incidence of skin cancer in 5356 patients following organ transplantation. Br J Dermatol. 2000;143(3):513–19.
42. Rizvi SMH et al. Long-term change in the risk of skin cancer after organ transplantation: a population-based nationwide cohort study. JAMA Dermatol. 2017;153(12):1270–7.
43. Dahlke E et al. Systematic review of melanoma incidence and prognosis in solid organ transplant recipients. Transplant Res. 2014;3:10.
44. Ascha M et al. Risk factors for melanoma in renal transplant recipients. JAMA Dermatol. 2017;153(11):1130–6.
45. Green AC, Olsen CM. Increased risk of melanoma in organ transplant recipients: systematic review and meta-analysis of cohort studies. Acta Derm Venereol. 2015;95(8):923–7.
46. Puza CJ, Cardones AR, Mosca PJ. Examining the incidence and presentation of melanoma in the cardiothoracic transplant population. JAMA Dermatol. 2018;154(5):589–91.
47. Robbins HA et al. Melanoma risk and survival among organ transplant recipients. J Invest Dermatol. 2015;135(11):2657–65.
48. Matin RN et al. Melanoma in organ transplant recipients: clinicopathological features and outcome in 100 cases. Am J Transplant. 2008;8(9):1891–900.

49. Dzambova M et al. Malignant melanoma in organ transplant recipients: incidence, outcomes, and management strategies: a review of literature. Dermatol Ther. 2016;29(1):64–8.
50. Penn I. Malignant melanoma in organ allograft recipients. Transplant. 1996;61(2):274–8.
51. Brewer JD et al. Malignant melanoma in solid transplant recipients: collection of database cases and comparison with surveillance, epidemiology, and end results data for outcome analysis. Arch Dermatol. 2011;147(7):790–6.
52. Dapprich DC et al. Outcomes of melanoma in recipients of solid organ transplant. J Am Acad Dermatol. 2008;59(3):405–17.
53. Birkeland SA, Storm HH. Risk for tumor and other disease transmission by transplantation: a population-based study of unrecognized malignancies and other diseases in organ donors. Transplant. 2002;74(10):1409–13.
54. Xiao D et al. Donor cancer transmission in kidney transplantation: a systematic review. Am J Transplant. 2013;13(10):2645–52.
55. Penn I. Transmission of cancer from organ donors. Ann Transplant. 1997;2(4):7–12.
56. Zwald FO et al. Melanoma in solid organ transplant recipients. Am J Transplant. 2010;10(5):1297–304.
57. Kauffman HM et al. Deceased donors with a past history of malignancy: an organ procurement and transplantation network/united network for organ sharing update. Transplant. 2007;84(2):272–4.
58. Strauss DC, Thomas JM. Transmission of donor melanoma by organ transplantation. Lancet Oncol. 2010;11(8):790–6.
59. MacKie RM, Reid R, Junor B. Fatal melanoma transferred in a donated kidney 16 years after melanoma surgery. N Engl J Med. 2003;348(6):567–8.
60. Morris-Stiff G et al. Transmission of donor melanoma to multiple organ transplant recipients. Am J Transplant. 2004;4(3):444–6.
61. Juszczak H et al. Potential for overlooked melanoma in solid organ donors with a severely dysplastic nevus. JAAD Case Rep. 2018;4(7):682–3.
62. National Kidney Foundation. Living donor evaluation. 2019. Available from: www.kidney.org/transplantation/livingdonors/evaluation.
63. O'Reilly Zwald F, Brown M. Skin cancer in solid organ transplant recipients: advances in therapy and management: part II. Management of skin cancer in solid organ transplant recipients. J Am Acad Dermatol. 2011;65(2):263–79.
64. Zwald F et al. Recommendations for solid organ transplantation for transplant candidates with a pretransplant diagnosis of cutaneous squamous cell carcinoma, merkel cell carcinoma and melanoma: a consensus opinion from the international transplant skin cancer collaborative (ITSCC). Am J Transplant. 2016;16(2):407–13.
65. Balch CM et al. Final version of 2009 AJCC melanoma staging and classification. J Clin Oncol. 2009;27(36):6199–206.
66. Gershenwald JE, Scolyer RA. Melanoma staging: American joint committee on cancer (AJCC) 8th edition and beyond. Ann Surg Oncol. 2018;25(8):2105–10.
67. Almashali MER, Paragh G. Melanoma epidemiology, staging and prognostic factors. In: Faries MB, Lee DJ editors, Practical manual for dermatologic and surgical melanoma management. Cham: Springer; 2021.
68. Collins L, Quinn A, Stasko T. Skin cancer and immunosuppression. Dermatol Clin. 2019;37(1):83–94.
69. Rivinius R et al. Analysis of malignancies in patients after heart transplantation with subsequent immunosuppressive therapy. Drug Des Devel Ther. 2015;9:93–102.
70. Stallone G, Infante B, Grandaliano G. Management and prevention of post-transplant malignancies in kidney transplant recipients. Clin Kidney J. 2015;8(5):637–44.
71. Tjon AS et al. Increased incidence of early de novo cancer in liver graft recipients treated with cyclosporine: an association with C2 monitoring and recipient age. Liver Transpl. 2010;16(7):837–46.
72. Knoll GA et al. Effect of sirolimus on malignancy and survival after kidney transplantation: systematic review and meta-analysis of individual patient data. BMJ. 2014;349:g6679.
73. Guba M et al. Rapamycin inhibits primary and metastatic tumor growth by antiangiogenesis: involvement of vascular endothelial growth factor. Nat Med. 2002;8(2):128–35.
74. Lim WH et al. The risk of cancer in kidney transplant recipients may be reduced in those maintained on everolimus and reduced cyclosporine. Kidney Int. 2017;91(4):954–63.
75. Vestergaard ME et al. Dermoscopy compared with naked eye examination for the diagnosis of primary melanoma: a meta-analysis of studies performed in a clinical setting. Br J Dermatol. 2008;159(3):669–76.
76. Coit DG et al. Cutaneous melanoma (Version 1.2020). NCCN Clini Prac Guidelines in Oncol; 2019 Feb 12. Available from: www.nccn.org/professionals/physician_gls/pdf/cutaneous_melanoma.pdf.
77. Filosa A Filosa G. Melanoma diagnosis: the importance of histopathological report. Dermatopathology (Basel). 2018;5(1):41–3.
78. Grotz TE et al. Preservation of the deep muscular fascia and locoregional control in melanoma. Surg. 2013;153(4):535–41.

79. Ellison PM, Brodland DG. Mohs micrographic surgery for melanoma: a prospective multicenter study. J Am Acad Dermatol. 2019 Sep;81(3):767–74.
80. Ferris LK, Middlebrook B et al. Identification of high-risk cutaneous melanoma tumors is improved when combining the online American joint committee on cancer individualized melanoma patient outcome prediction tool with a 31-gene expression profile-based classification. J Am Acad Dermatol. 2017;76(5): 818–25, e3.
81. Polak ME et al. Mechanisms of local immunosuppression in cutaneous melanoma. Br J Cancer. 2007;96(12): 1879–87.
82. Brochez L, Chevolet I, Kruse V. The rationale of indoleamine 2,3-dioxygenase inhibition for cancer therapy. Eur J Cancer. 2017;76:167–82.
83. Brocard A et al. Clinical, genetic and innate immunity characteristics of melanoma in organ transplant recipients. Acta Derm Venereol. 2017;97(4):483–8.
84. Krahenbuhl L et al. A longitudinal analysis of IDO and PDL1 expression during immune- or targeted therapy in advanced melanoma. Neoplasia. 2018;20(2):218–25.
85. Dillon P et al. Regression of advanced melanoma upon withdrawal of immunosuppression: case series and literature review. Med Oncol. 2010;27(4):1127–32.
86. Otley CC et al. Reduction of immunosuppression for transplant-associated skin cancer: expert consensus survey. Br J Dermatol. 2006;154(3):395–400.
87. Ritchie SA, Patel MJ, Miller SJ. Therapeutic options to decrease actinic keratosis and squamous cell carcinoma incidence and progression in solid organ transplant recipients: a practical approach. Dermatol Surg. 2012;38(10):1604–21.
88. Coghill AE et al. Immunosuppressive medications and squamous cell skin carcinoma: nested case-control study within the skin cancer after organ transplant (SCOT) Cohort. Am J Transplant. 2016;16(2):565–73.
89. Einollahi B et al. Skin cancer after renal transplantation: results of a multicenter study in Iran Ann Transplant. 2010;15(3):44–50.
90. Domingues B et al. Melanoma treatment in review. Immunotargets Ther. 2018;7:35–49.
91. Eggermont AM, Kirkwood JM. Re-evaluating the role of dacarbazine in metastatic melanoma: what have we learned in 30 years? Eur J Cancer. 2004;40(12):1825–36.
92. Afshar K et al. BRAF inhibition in a lung transplant recipient with metastatic melanoma. JAMA Dermatol. 2016;152(2):228–30.
93. Levavasseur M et al. Drug interaction between dabrafenib and immunosuppressive drugs: about one case. Melanoma Res. 2016;26(5):532–4.
94. Sullivan RJ, Flaherty KT. Resistance to BRAF-targeted therapy in melanoma. Eur J Cancer. 2013;49(6):1297–304.
95. Garrett GL et al. Combined dabrafenib and trametinib therapy in metastatic melanoma and organ transplantation: case report and review of the literature. JAAD Case Rep. 2015;1(6):S23–5.
96. Tripathi SV et al. Metastatic melanoma after solid organ transplantation: an interdisciplinary, institution-based review of management with systemic and targeted therapies. J Am Acad Dermatol. 2018;78(1):184–5.
97. Larkin J et al. Combined vemurafenib and cobimetinib in BRAF-mutated melanoma. N Engl J Med. 2014;371(20):1867–76.
98. Robert C et al. Improved overall survival in melanoma with combined dabrafenib and trametinib. N Engl J Med. 2015;372(1):30–9.
99. Peacock M et al. DNA repair inhibition by UVA photoactivated fluoroquinolones and vemurafenib. Nucleic Acids Res. 2014;42(22):13714–22.
100. Peng L et al. Incidence and relative risk of cutaneous squamous cell carcinoma with single-agent BRAF inhibitor and dual BRAF/MEK inhibitors in cancer patients: a meta-analysis. Oncotarget. 2017;8(47):83280–91.
101. da Silveira Nogueira Lima JP et al. A systematic review and network meta-analysis of immunotherapy and targeted therapy for advanced melanoma. Cancer Med. 2017;6(6):1143–1153.
102. Rothermel LD et al. Current immunotherapy practices in melanoma. Surg Oncol Clin N Am. 2019;28(3):403–18.
103. Murakami N et al. Severe acute interstitial nephritis after combination immune-checkpoint inhibitor therapy for metastatic melanoma. Clin Kidney J. 2016;9(3):411–17.
104. Mahmood SS et al. Myocarditis in patients treated with immune checkpoint inhibitors. J Am Coll Cardiol. 2018;71(16):1755–64.
105. Fisher J, Fan W, Samie FH. Immune checkpoint inhibitor therapy in solid organ transplant recipients: a patient-centered systematic review (includes cases in your table). J Am Acad Dermatol. 2020 Jun;82(6):1490–500.
106. Schvartsman G et al. Safe and effective administration of T-VEC in a patient with heart transplantation and recurrent locally advanced melanoma. J Immunother Cancer. 2017;5:45.
107. Lai HC et al. Programmed cell death 1 (PD-1) inhibitors in renal transplant patients with advanced cancer: a double-edged sword? Int J Mol Sci. 2019;20(9).

108. Lisa A. Raedler, imlygic (talimogene laherparepvec): first oncolytic viral therapy for the treatment of patients with recurrent melanoma. J Hematol Oncol Phar. 2016 Mar;6.
109. Ressler J et al. Talimogene laherparepvec (T-VEC) in advanced melanoma: complete response in a heart and kidney transplant patient. A case report. Br J Dermatol. 2019;181(1):186–9.
110. Sunshine JC, Shetty A, Choi JN. Successful treatment of in-transit metastatic melanoma in a renal transplant patient with combination T-VEC/imiquimod immunotherapy. J Immunother. 2020 May;43(4):149–52.
111. Canton DA et al. Melanoma treatment with intratumoral electroporation of tavokinogene telseplasmid (pIL-12, tavokinogene telseplasmid). Immunother. 2017;9(16):1309–21.
112. Wang S et al. Intratumoral injection of a CpG oligonucleotide reverts resistance to PD-1 blockade by expanding multifunctional CD8+ T cells. Proc Natl Acad Sci USA. 2016;113(46):e7240–9.
113. Agarwala SS, Ross MI, Zager JS, Shirai K, Essner R, Smithers BM, Atkinson V, Wachter EA. Phase 1B study of PV-10 and anti-PD-1 in advanced cutaneous melanoma. J Clin Oncol. 2019 May 20;37.
114. Yang GB et al. Risk and survival of cutaneous melanoma diagnosed subsequent to a previous cancer. Arch Dermatol. 2011;147(12):1395–402.
115. Ranganath HA, Panella TJ. Administration of ipilimumab to a liver transplant recipient with unresectable metastatic melanoma. J Immunother. 2015;38(5):211.
116. Morales RE et al. Safety and efficacy of ipilimumab to treat advanced melanoma in the setting of liver transplantation. J Immunother Cancer. 2015;3:22.
117. DeLeon TT et al. Pilot evaluation of PD-1 inhibition in metastatic cancer patients with a history of liver transplantation: the Mayo clinic experience. J Gastrointest Oncol. 2018;9(6):1054–62.
118. Kuo JC, Lilly LB, Hogg D. Immune checkpoint inhibitor therapy in a liver transplant recipient with a rare subtype of melanoma: a case report and literature review. Melanoma Res. 2018;28(1):61–4.
119. Qin R, Salama AK. Report of ipilimumab in a heart transplant patient with metastatic melanoma on tacrolimus. Melanoma Manag. 2015;2(4):311–14.
120. Owonikoko TK et al. Cardiac allograft rejection as a complication of PD-1 checkpoint blockade for cancer immunotherapy: a case report. Cancer Immunol Immunother. 2017;66(1):45–50.
121. Soellradl I, Kehrer H, Cejka D. Use of ipilimumab and pembrolizumab in metastatic melanoma in a combined heart and kidney transplant recipient: a case report. Transplant Proc. 2020;52(2).
122. Zehou O et al. Ipilimumab for the treatment of advanced melanoma in six kidney transplant patients. Am J Transplant. 2018;18(12):3065–71.
123. Lipson EJ et al. Successful administration of ipilimumab to two kidney transplantation patients with metastatic melanoma. J Clin Oncol. 2014;32(19):e69–71.
124. Herz S et al. Checkpoint inhibitors in chronic kidney failure and an organ transplant recipient. Eur J Cancer. 2016;67:66–72.
125. Spain L et al. Acute renal allograft rejection after immune checkpoint inhibitor therapy for metastatic melanoma. Ann Oncol. 2016;27(6):1135–7.
126. Ong M et al. Antitumor activity of nivolumab on hemodialysis after renal allograft rejection. J Immunother Cancer. 2016;4:64.
127. Alhamad T et al. Checkpoint inhibitors in kidney transplant recipients and the potential risk of rejection. Am J Transplant. 2016;16(4):1332–3.

Cutaneous Squamous Cell Carcinoma in Solid Organ Transplant Recipients

9

Ali Rajabi-Estarabadi, Caiwei Zheng, Courtney J. Ensslin, and Ally-Khan Somani

INTRODUCTION

Skin cancers are the most frequent malignant neoplasm found in solid organ transplant recipients (OTRs), 95% of which are nonmelanoma skin cancers (NMSCs).[1] Cutaneous squamous cell carcinoma (cSCC), in particular, is the most common, with a 65-fold to 250-fold higher incidence in patients subject to immunomodulatory therapy (Figure 9.1a).[2] Other cutaneous malignancies such as basal cell carcinoma (BCC), Merkel cell carcinoma, and Kaposi's sarcoma are also seen in OTRs, although less commonly.[3,4] Figure 9.2 shows a graph of time to first malignancy after childhood organ transplant for different cancer types.[5]

cSCC in OTRs expresses a different molecular phenotype compared with those seen in the immunocompetent,[6] and it is well-documented in the literature to be associated with a more aggressive disease course (Figure 9.1 b, c), higher risk of metastasis, and higher mortality compared with those of primary occurrence in the general population.[7] Risk factors for developing NMSCs in OTRs are similar to those seen in the general population, which include older age, smoking, presence of premalignant skin lesions, a past medical history of skin cancer, history of significant sun exposure, and a Fitzpatrick skin type I–II.[3,4,8] In addition, the incidence of skin cancer in OTRs is directly proportional to the level[8] and duration of immunosuppression. However, the strongest predictor of posttransplantation cSCC risk is a history of pretransplantation cSCC.[9]

EPIDEMIOLOGY

The incidence of cSCC in solid organ transplantations is well documented. In general, as many as 40%–70% of transplant patients may eventually develop skin cancer, and the risk increases over time.[10] For instance, the risk of cSCC as reported in the United States. and western Europe ranges from 10% to 27%

DOI: 10.1201/9781003001461-9

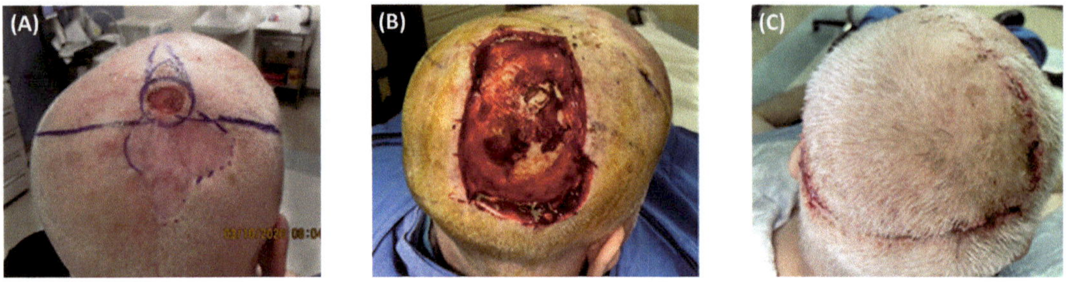

FIGURE 9.1 (**a**) Recurrent squamous cell carcinoma on the scalp in a cardiac transplant patient with extensive periosteal and perineural invasion. (**b**) Mohs micrographic surgical defect. (**c**) Two weeks follow-up after large bilateral-rotation flaps.

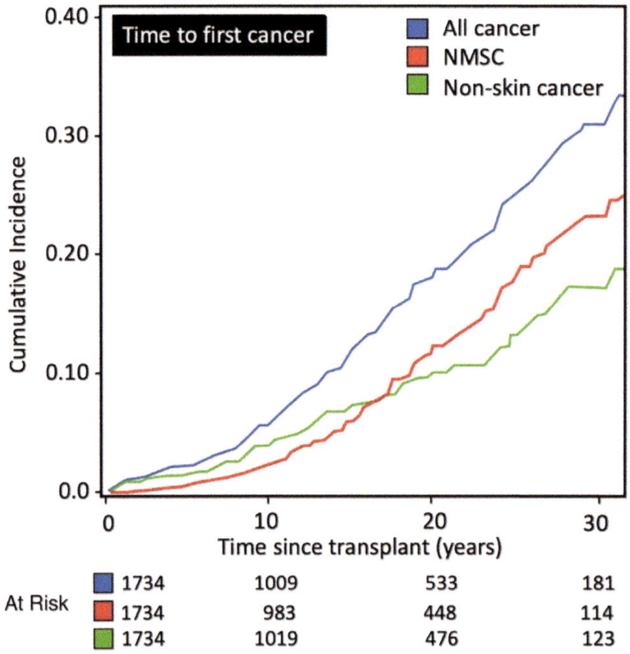

FIGURE 9.2 Time to first cancer, stratified by type (adjusted for competing risk of death). (From Francis et al.[5] with permission.)

at 10 years after transplantation but increases to 40%–60% at 20 years posttransplant.[3] Patients with heart and lung transplants, in particular, are found to have a higher incidence of cSCC than that in those with kidney and liver transplants, although the kidney is the most common organ transplanted.[3,4] This is presumed to be because of the relatively more intensive immunosuppressive regimens required after heart and lung transplants and the fact that the heart and lung transplant recipients are often of an older age.[11] In kidney transplant patients, the pooled incidence of NMSC was 12.6% (95% CI: 12%–14%) with a majority being cSCC 55% (95% CI: 47%–63%).[12] A recent study reported that the hazard ratios for cSCC in 8026 patients who underwent heart, lung, and liver transplantation from 1968 through 2012 was 1.59 (1.29–1.96), 1.53 (0.99–2.36), and 0.37 (0.21–0.64) in reference to kidney transplant patients.[13] Also, treatment with more than two immunosuppressive agents was significantly associated with the development of new skin cancers in OTRs.[14] The class of immunosuppressant also played an important role in the incidence of skin cancer in OTRS, as the study by Murray et al.[15] showed that in kidney and liver transplant recipients there was a lower incidence of NMSC in recipients treated with mammalian target of rapamycin inhibitors (mTORi) compared with that in those treated with calcineurin inhibitors.

In general, patients on medications with photosensitizing properties were found to face a higher risk of NMSC. A 2013 case-control study investigating NMSC's association with the use of photosensitizing medication reported a modest increase in the risk of SCC (odds ratio (OR) = 1.2, 95% confidence interval (CI) = 1.0–1.4) and BCC (OR = 1.2, 95% CI = 0.9–1.5).[16] Although its association with specific OTRs is unknown, it is important to note its potential contribution to the risk of NMSC in OTRs.

PATHOGENESIS

As in the general population, the cause of cSCC in OTRs is multifactorial, including both intrinsic and extrinsic factors, of which ultraviolet (UV) radiation is arguably the most important causative factor.[8,17] UVB radiation, especially, is a potent carcinogen that directly induces covalent bond formation between adjacent pyrimidines, creating pyrimidine dimers that damage deoxyribonucleic acid (DNA) structurally.[18] Although UVA has a less mutagenic role, it contributes to carcinogenesis indirectly via creation of reactive oxygen species.[19] UV radiation also was reported to cause mutations in the p53 tumor-suppressor gene, leading to local immunodeficiency. When combined with the chronic systemic immunosuppressive therapy used for OTRs, mechanisms of immune-mediated tumor suppression are severely impaired, leading to a significantly increased risk of carcinogenesis.[17,20] Because of the known effects of the mTORi on the PI3K/Akt/mTOR signaling pathway, a switch to mTORi has been proposed to provide both immunosuppressive effects for organ viability as well as antitumoral effects against cutaneous malignancy.[21] However, a recent study by Koletsa et al.[21] reported that use of mTORi did not significantly change the immunohistochemical expression of upstream molecules in the pathway (mTOR, PI3K, pAkt) in cSCC, suggesting the need for combination treatment that targets multiple pathways for more efficient tumor prevention.

Role of Human Papillomavirus

The role of oncogenic viruses in cSCC development in OTRs is actively being studied because of the known susceptibility of transplant patients to oncogenic viral infections.[22] In particular, human papillomavirus (HPV), a small, circular, double-stranded DNA virus with a genome of about 8kb, is frequently associated with cSCC. In fact, HPV DNA was identified in 65%–90% of cSCC from transplant recipients.[22,23] A case-control study done by Proby et al.[24] reported that people who had both beta HPV DNA and antibodies for the same HPV type were at significantly increased risk for cSCC. Most studies suggested that β-HPV strains were more commonly associated with cutaneous malignancy compared with the α-HPV strains, which were more commonly found in genital and oropharyngeal mucosal lesions.[23] β-HPV's greater contribution to carcinogenesis was attributed to its inhibition of notch-dependent tumor suppression in immunosuppressed patients.[23] This mechanism works in conjunction with the HPV-related E6 protein that causes degradation of the Bak protein, blocking the p53 apoptotic response.[25] β-HPV E7 is also known to promote keratinocyte invasion, a finding supported by a study reporting spontaneous carcinogenesis in HPV8 transgenic mice.[24,26] Unlike its alpha counterpart, β-HPV rarely integrates into the human cell genome, which explains its limited carcinogenic capability in immunocompetent hosts.[24] It is important to note that despite these findings, studies have found no HPV ribonucleic acid (RNA) in cSCC lesions of OTRs, suggesting that active viral replication is not a requirement for cSCC progression.[24,27] In addition, HPV is thought to play a much smaller role in tumor maintenance compared with initial oncogenesis, as HPV prevalence and viral load are actually higher in premalignant lesions.[3]

Role of Immunosuppression

Immune cells are thought to be crucial in the antitumoral response on a broad level. Specific cell types such as CD4+ cells, CD8+ cells, tumor-associated macrophages, and dermal dendritic cells were found to be the main participants in the large inflammatory response infiltrating cSCC.[28] Selection of the immunosuppressive regimen contributes to the increased risk of carcinogenesis by altering the antitumoral immune response. Older immunosuppressive agents such as calcineurin inhibitors and azathioprine are generally believed to contribute more to increased cancer risks compared with newer agents like sirolimus.[18] The mechanism is because of azathioprine's photosensitizing effects on the skin, making it more sensitive to UVA radiation and leading to accumulation of 6-thioguanine in DNA.[29,30] It was later found that 6-thioguanine and UVA work synergistically to generate high levels of mutagenic reactive oxygen species, which further contributed to SCC formation.[30]

Cyclosporin A, commonly used in OTRs, is another drug that is often implicated in the formation of SCC in the posttransplant population. Normally, keratinocytes respond to excessive UV radiation-induced oxidative stress by undergoing a process called the mitochondrial permeability transition (MPT), which consists of a sequence of events that eventually lead to necrosis or apoptosis.[31] The opening of mitochondrial permeability transition pores (MPTPs) is a key step to start the MPT. When opened, solutes with molecular mass of up to 1500 Da can diffuse across the mitochondrial inner membrane nonselectively, causing subsequent mitochondrial depolarization, uncoupling of oxidative phosphorylation, mitochondrial swelling, and ultimately cell death because of adenosine triphosphate (ATP) depletion.[31] Cyclosporin inhibits MPTP opening, which causes resistance to stress-induced apoptosis, allowing genotoxic insults to propagate.[17] Cyclosporin also acts by inhibiting interleukin 2 (IL-2) transcription, which leads to inhibition of T-cell function. A recent study by Santana et al.[28] examined the cSCC microenvironment using gene expression profiling and compared it with that of cSCC in transplant patients. It was reported that cSCC in OTRs experienced a shift in immune infiltrate that favored malignancy with an increased ratio of Treg to CD8+ T cells and a lower percentage of CD4+ T cells.[28] It also was noted that cyclosporine increased the proportion of T cells capable of producing IL-22, a cytokine known to increase the tumorigenic potential of cells via enhancement of inducible nitric oxide synthase (iNOS) expression.[28] However, calcineurin inhibitors have remained the mainstay of posttransplant regimens, despite their potential contribution to accelerating the development of skin cancer (see Chapter 2).

Role of Antifungal Agents

Voriconazole is an antifungal agent that is widely used as prophylaxis for and treatment of fungal infections in lung transplant patients. The drug is generally well-tolerated but its side effects of photosensitivity and phototoxicity are well documented.[32] In a large multicenter, retrospective cohort study, it was found that of 900 lung transplant patients, the crude incidence rate per 1000 person-years was 33.4 for patients exposed to voriconazole alone, compared with 21.7 in patients exposed to both voriconazole and another azoles, and 10.4 in patients only exposed to other azoles.[33] After controlling for confounders such as immunosuppression and time, it was reported that the adjusted hazard ratio for developing cSCC was 2.39 (95% CI, 1.31–4.37) after voriconazole exposure alone and 3.45 for those exposed to both voriconazole and other azoles.[33] The association was further supported by a new study by Tang et al.,[34] which reported a risk ratio of 1.86 (95% CI, 1.36–2.55), demonstrating an increased risk of SCC with voriconazole use in both lung and hematopoietic cell transplant patients. Numerous recent studies also have reported similar increases in cSCC risk in hematopoietic cell transplant recipients exposed to voriconazole. One such study by Wojenski et al.[35] reported a cumulative SCC incidence of 19% at 5 years post-allotransplant and a hazard ratio of 1.86 for each 180 days of use ($P < 0.001$).

In a cohort study by D'Arcy et al.,[36] the associations of voriconazole with the risk of SCC were evaluated in lung recipients; 9793 lung transplants among 9599 non-Hispanic white patients were included in this study. During a median follow-up of 3.0 (interquartile range [IQR], 1.4–5.0) years after transplant, 1031 SCCs were reported. Compared with lung recipients with no observed voriconazole use, those with 1–3 months of voriconazole use had an increased adjusted hazard ratio (AHR) for SCC of 1.09 (95% CI, 0.90–1.31); 4–7 months use, 1.42 (95% CI, 1.16–1.73); 8–15 months use, 2.04 (95% CI, 1.67–2.50); and >15 months use, 3.05 (95% CI, 2.37–3.91).[36]

The exact mechanism of voriconazole-induced cutaneous malignancy in not well understood. Current popular hypotheses implicate both the drug itself and its metabolite, voriconazole N-oxide (VNO)—which is arguably more carcinogenic than the drug itself. It is thought that the two act as UVA sensitizers that generate reactive oxygen species, leading to the production of oxidative DNA damage and inhibition of gene repair mechanisms.[32,37] Voriconazole is also known to inhibit the enzymes CYP3A4 and CYP2C9, both of which are crucial to retinol metabolism. Such inhibition leads to increased accumulation of the phototoxic compound tretinoin, which contributes to the development of premalignant lesions.[38] Recent studies investigating voriconazole's regulation of cell cycle and terminal differentiation pathways in keratinocytes reported no similar effect from fluconazole, suggesting voriconazole's carcinogenic effects is unique rather than a class effect.[39] Itraconazole and posaconazole are effective alternative triazole prophylactic agents that are thought to have better side-effect profiles.

PREVENTION OF SCC IN OTRS

In light of the evidence of increased SCC development associated with OTRs, active efforts are in place to prophylactically reduce the posttransplantation skin cancer incidence. Prior to transplantation, a dermatologic consultation is recommended to screen for and treat skin cancer and its associated precursor lesions. Skin lesions that are suspicious for malignancy should be biopsied and further evaluated pathologically. If present, actinic keratoses, porokeratoses, and viral warts should be treated before transplantation.[40,41] A thorough past medical history of skin cancer also should be obtained to determine the follow-up frequency and the wait time before transplantation.[40,41] In addition, because cSCC in OTRs share some of the same risk factors as cSCC in the general population, patient education regarding the importance of sun protection and the recognition of the early signs of cutaneous malignancies are imperative in the peritransplant period.

Disease prevention efforts aimed at identifying those at risk for poor outcomes are also available. The Skin and Ultraviolet Neoplasia Transplant Risk Assessment Calculator (SUNTRAC) was developed based on 6340 patients and utilizes multivariate analysis to generate a risk score for solid OTRs that informs transplant care providers of a patient's risk of skin cancer.[42] SUNTRAC uses data collected through the Transplant Skin Cancer Network Database, which incorporates data from 26 transplant centers across the United States between the years 2003 and 2008. Risk factors used to formulate the point system include white race (9 points), pretransplant history of skin cancer (6 points), age ≥50 years (4 points), male sex (2 points), and thoracic transplant (1 point). The output is classification into 4 risk categories, 0–6 points indicating low risk, 7–13 points indicating medium risk, 14–17 points indicating high risk, and 18–22 points indicating very high risk. The 5-year cumulative incidence of development of skin cancer was 1.01%, 6.15%, 15.14%, and 44.75%, for the Low, Medium, High, and Very High SUNTRAC categories, respectively.[42]

In conjunction with the recommendations from a recent Delphi study citing 2% as the screening threshold, an algorithm was created to determine the time to first skin cancer screening (Figure 9.3).[43] In 2019, Crow and et al.[44] conducted three rounds of Delphi method surveys with a panel of 84 U.S. dermatologists and transplant physicians to establish skin cancer screening recommendations for

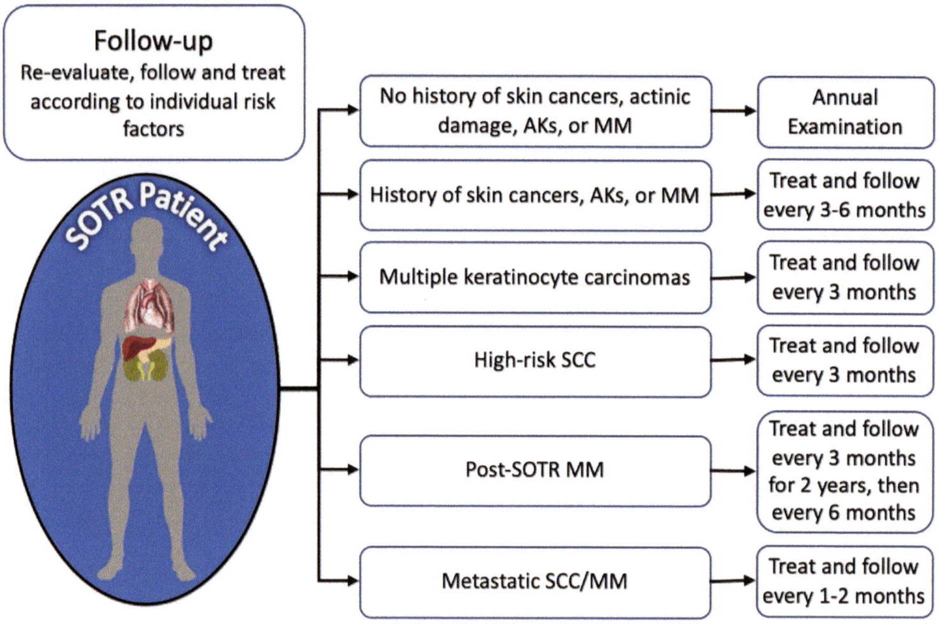

FIGURE 9.3 Skin cancer screening algorithm in OTRs. (Incorporating material from Stevenson et al.[43] with permission.)

SOTR. The panelists recommended that the transplant team should conduct skin cancer risk assessment, either at the time of listing or at the time of transplant. Patients with a history of skin cancer should follow-up regularly with a dermatologist in order to determine the appropriate intervals for continued skin cancer surveillance. Patients were defined "high risk" according to any of the following: thoracic organ transplant, age over 50 at the time of transplant, or male gender. The absence of all of these features was defined as low risk. A consensus of panelists also agreed that there was a need for an evidence-based risk assessment or risk stratification tool. The risk stratification tool should be time-efficient and could be completed by office staff using basic patient health information. The summary of the panelist's screening recommendations for each SOTR patient demographic is shown in Table 9.1.[44]

Chemoprevention

Low-dose systemic retinoids (isotretinoin and acitretin), capecitabine, and nicotinamide have been actively studied as a means of chemoprevention of SCC in transplant patients. Studies supporting the use of systemic retinoids in chemoprevention date back to 1995, although recent, large scale randomized trials are limited. One of the most recent studies reported that solid OTRs who received prophylactic systemic retinoids at dosages of 0.2–0.4 mg/kg/day developed significantly less SCCs in the first 3 years of treatment compared with rates in those who did not.[45] In addition, the study found that in patients who had been on retinoids therapy for more than 12 months, interruption of therapy led to a significant increase in SCC numbers in the 12-month interval after interruption, with a mean increase of 4.67 SCCs (95% CI, 1.3–8.03; $P = .02$).[45] This "rebound" phenomenon was supported by observations made by several previous studies. It was then postulated that low-dose retinoids can reduce SCC development in high-risk OTRs for at least 3 years and probably as long as 9 years.[45]

TABLE 9.1 Screening Recommendations for Each SOTR Patient Demographic

SOTR PATIENT CHARACTERISTICS	*SCREENING RECOMMENDATION*
Caucasian: high risk*	Within 2 years
Caucasian: low risk**	Within 5 years
Hispanic	Within 5 years
Asian	Within years
African American: high risk	Within years
African American: low risk	No consensus

Abbreviation: SOTR, solid organ transplant recipient.

* *Any individuals with one of the following risk factors:* thoracic organ, age >50 years at the time of transplant, male sex.
** *Any individuals without the following additional risk factors:* thoracic organ, age >50 years at the time of transplant, male sex.

Source: Crow et al.44 with permission.

Use of capecitabine as a chemopreventive agent is relatively more robustly supported. One report found that treatment with capecitabine thwarted the development of new cutaneous carcinomas and improved existing lesions in three transplant patients with an extensive history of SCCs.[46] Subsequent studies have provided further support of benefit, including a case series reporting reductions in the incidence of SCCs in 9 of 10 solid OTRs following a 21-day cycle of capecitabine treatment (0.5–1.5 g/m^2 per day on days 1–14 for 5–24 months).[47] In contrast, nicotinamide's chemopreventive effects are not yet consistently supported. A phase 2 randomized trial including 22 renal transplant recipients compared the effects of nicotinamide at 500 mg twice daily with that of a placebo and found a nonsignificant 35% reduction rate in the incidence of new skin cancers at 6 months.[48]

A switch to sirolimus has also been proposed for its lower risk of carcinogenesis compared with that of older immunosuppressive agents. Studies have consistently reported a lower incidence of SCC in patients on sirolimus therapy compared with that in those on calcineurin therapy. Euvrard et al.[49] conducted a randomized, controlled trial comparing the two in kidney transplant recipients who had had at least one SCC. It was reported that only 22% of the patients in the sirolimus group developed at least one additional SCC compared with a much higher 39% in the calcineurin group.[18,49] In a retrospective study, Murray et al.[15] showed that transitioning from calcineurin- to sirolimus-based immunosuppression reduced the occurrence of NMSCs without a consequent deterioration in renal function. However, the benefit was not without cost, as sirolimus was associated with a much higher occurrence of adverse events (0.938 vs. 0.250), including edema (37%), acneiform eruption (28%), aphthous ulcers (24%), and proteinuria (20%) as well as increased mortality driven by cardiovascular and infection-related deaths.[18,50]

WAIT TIME TO TRANSPLANT

Solid organ transplantation successfully extends the lives of thousands of patients. In order to prevent the futile transplantation of scarce donor organs into patients with a high risk of mortality, there are recommendations and guidelines regarding an appropriate wait period pretransplantation for candidates with a history of preexisting conditions. One of the greatest risk factors for cSCC is a personal prior history; one meta-analysis found the 3-year cumulative risk of subsequent cSCC was 18%, at least a 10-fold increase compared with that of the general population.[51]

For solid organ transplant candidates with a pretransplant diagnosis of cSCC, the consensus opinion from the International immunosuppression and Transplant Skin Cancer Collaborative (ITSCC) regarding the wait time to transplantation was based upon high-risk features, nodal status, and appropriate treatment. For patients with a history of low-risk cSCC, no delay to transplant is needed after appropriate surgical treatment (either wide local excision [WLE] or Mohs micrographic surgery [MMS]) with negative margins. For patients with a history of high-risk cSCC, a wait time of 2 years before transplantation is recommended if there is no evidence of metastasis on computed tomography (CT) or positron emission tomography-CT (PET-CT) imaging and the tumor has been cleared with negative surgical margins.[40] High-risk features are defined by ITSCC as tumor size >2 cm, high-risk location, recurrent lesion, and poorly differentiated on histology. In patients with tumors that have evidence of perineural invasion (PNI) or ≥2 high-risk features, the ITSCC recommends that the wait time to transplantation should be extended to 2– 3 years, and that the addition of adjuvant radiation therapy (ART) is considered after negative surgical margins have been achieved. For high-risk cSCC with positive local nodal disease, the group recommends combination therapy of surgical excision with appropriate lymph node dissection plus ART and a wait time of 5 years, beginning once appropriate treatment has been completed with no radiological evidence of residual disease. Patients with a history of cSCC with distant metastasis should be referred to oncology but are not eligible for transplantation[40] (Figure 9.4).

PATIENT EDUCATION

The National Comprehensive Cancer Network (NCCN) recommends that patient education regarding sun avoidance and protection methods, as well as an assessment of individual risk factors for the development of SCC, begin at the time of transplantation. Transplant patients should be educated on how to recognize suspicious lesions and taught how to perform monthly self-examinations of all skin surfaces. Randomized trials have shown that educational interventions can be effective in changing sun protective

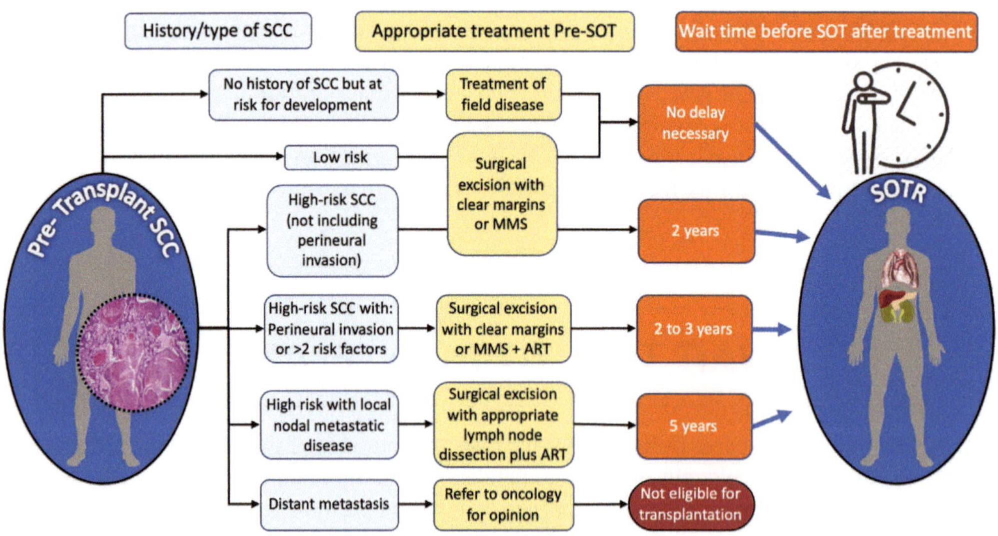

FIGURE 9.4 Recommended wait times before transplant for patients with a history of squamous cell carcinoma (SCC). ART, adjuvant radiation therapy; MMS, Mohs micrographic surgery; SOT, solid organ transplant; SOTR, solid organ transplant recipient. (Incorporating material from Zwald et al.[40] with permission.)

behaviors in transplant patients.[52,53] However, extensive and repeated education is needed in this patient population as other medical concerns may make them initially unreceptive, especially during the first year of transplantation.[54]

SUMMARY OF KEY POINTS

- NMSCs are the most frequent malignant neoplasm found in OTRs, with cSCC being the most common.
- The incidence of skin cancer in OTRs is directly proportional to the level of immunosuppressive therapy utilized.
- Patients with thoracic transplants (heart and lung) have a higher incidence of SCC than that of those with abdominal transplants (kidney, liver, and pancreas).
- Pretransplantation SCC is the strongest predictor of posttransplantation SCC risk.
- The immunosuppressive regimen contributes to an increased risk of carcinogenesis by altering the antitumoral immune response.
- Low-dose systemic retinoids (isotretinoin and acitretin), capecitabine, and nicotinamide are current options for chemoprevention of SCC in transplant patients, although high-quality evidence in the literature are limited.
- Appropriate wait time to transplantation for patients with a history of cSCC is based on tumor high-risk features, nodal status, and appropriate treatment.

REFERENCES

1. Ulrich C et al. Skin cancer in organ transplant recipients-where do we stand today? Am J Transplant. 2008;8(11):2192–8.
2. Cheng JY et al. Cutaneous squamous cell carcinomas in solid organ transplant recipients compared with immunocompetent patients. JAMA Dermatol. 2018;154(1):60–6.
3. Chockalingam R, Downing C, Tyring SK. Cutaneous squamous cell carcinomas in organ transplant recipients. J Clin Med. 2015;4(6):1229–39.
4. Oliveira WRP et al. Skin lesions in organ transplant recipients: a study of 177 consecutive Brazilian patients. Int J Dermatol. 2019;58(4):440–8.
5. Francis A et al. Incidence and predictors of cancer following kidney transplantation in childhood. Am J Transplant. 2017;17(10):2650–8.
6. Geissler EK, Skin cancer in solid organ transplant recipients: are mTOR inhibitors a game changer? Transplant Res. 2015;4(1).
7. Lanz J et al. Aggressive squamous cell carcinoma in organ transplant recipients. JAMA Dermatol. 2019;155(1):66–71.
8. Euvrard S, Kanitakis A, Fau Claudy J, Claudy A. Skin cancers after organ transplantation. N Engl J Med. 2003;348(17):1681–91.
9. Ramsay HM et al. Factors associated with nonmelanoma skin cancer following renal transplantation in Queensland, Australia. J Am Acad Dermatol. 2003;49(3):397–406.
10. Berg D, Otley CC. Skin cancer in organ transplant recipients: epidemiology, pathogenesis, and management. J Am Acad Dermatol. 2002;47(1):1–17; quiz 18–20.
11. Zwald FO, Brown M. Skin cancer in solid organ transplant recipients: advances in therapy and management. part I: epidemiology of skin cancer in solid organ transplant recipients. J Am Acad Dermatol. 2011;65(2):253–61.
12. Matinfar M, Shahidi S, Feizi A. Incidence of nonmelanoma skin cancer in renal transplant recipients: a systematic review and meta-analysis. J Res Med Sci. 2018;1735–995.

13. Rizvi SMH et al. Long-term change in the risk of skin cancer after organ transplantation: a population-based nationwide cohort study. JAMA Dermatol. 2017;153(12):1270–7.
14. Kim YJ et al. Twenty-eight-year incidence and characteristics of post-transplant skin cancers: comparative analysis of past and recent 10-year experience. J Dermatol. 2020;47(10):1131–40.
15. Murray SL et al. The impact of switching to mTOR inhibitor-based immunosuppression on long-term non-melanoma skin cancer incidence and renal function in kidney and liver transplant recipients. Ren Fail. 2020;42(1):607–12.
16. Robinson SN et al. Photosensitizing agents and the risk of non-melanoma skin cancer: a population-based case-control study. J Invest Dermatol. 2013;133(8):1950–5.
17. Mittal A, Colegio OR. Skin cancers in organ transplant recipients. Am J Transplant. 2017;17(10):2509–30.
18. Kim C, Cheng J, Colegio OR. Cutaneous squamous cell carcinomas in solid organ transplant recipients: emerging strategies for surveillance, staging, and treatment. Semin Oncol. 2016;43(1532–8708 [Electronic]):390–4.
19. Madan V, Lear J, Szeimies RM. Non-melanoma skin cancer. Lancet. 2010;375:673–85.
20. Yu SH, Bordeaux J, Baron ED. The immune system and skin cancer. Adv Exp Med Biol. 2014;810:182–91.
21. Koletsa T et al. mTOR signalling pathway-protein expression in post-transplant cutaneous squamous-cell carcinomas before and after conversion to mTOR-inhibitors. Anticancer Res. 2018.;38(6):3319–22.
22. Harwood CA et al. Human papillomavirus infection and non-melanoma skin cancer in immunosuppressed and immunocompetent individuals. J Med Virol. 2000;61(3):289–97.
23. Connolly K et al. Papillomavirus-associated squamous skin cancers following transplant immunosuppression: one notch closer to control. Cancer Treat Rev. 2014;40(2):205–14.
24. Proby CM et al. A case-control study of betapapillomavirus infection and cutaneous squamous cell carcinoma in organ transplant recipients. Am J Transplant. 2011;11(7).
25. Athar M, Walsh S., Kopelovich L, Elmets CA. Pathogenesis of nonmelanoma skin cancers in organ transplant recipients. Arch Biochem Biophys. 2011;508:159–63.
26. Schaper ID et al. Development of skin tumors in mice transgenic for early genes of human papillomavirus type 8. Cancer Res. 2005;65(4):1394–400.
27. Arron ST, Ruby J, Dybbro E, Ganem D, Derisi JL. Transcriptome sequencing demonstrates that human papillomavirus is not active in cutaneous squamous cell carcinoma. J Invest Dermatol. 2011;131:1745–53.
28. Santana AL, Felsen D, Carucci JA. Interleukin-22 and cyclosporine in aggressive cutaneous squamous cell carcinoma. Dermatol Clin. 2017;35(1):73–84.
29. Perrett CM, O'Donovan P et al. Azathioprine treatment photosensitizes human skin to ultraviolet A radiation. Br J Dermatol. 2008;159:198–204.
30. O'Donovan P, Perrett CM, Zhang X, Montaner B, Xu YZ, Harwood CA et al., Azathioprine and UVA light generate mutagenic oxidative DNA damage. Science. 2005;309:1871–4.
31. Kim JS, He L, Lemasters JJ. Mitochondrial permeability transition: a common pathway to necrosis and apoptosis. Biochem Biophys Res Comm. 2003;304(3):463–70.
32. Ona K, Oh DH. Voriconazole N-oxide and its ultraviolet B photoproduct sensitize keratinocytes to ultraviolet A. Br J Dermatol. 2016;173(3):751–9.
33. Hamandi B et al. Voriconazole and squamous cell carcinoma after lung transplantation: a multicenter study. Am J Transplant. 2018;18(1):113–24.
34. Tang H et al. Voriconazole exposure and risk of cutaneous squamous cell carcinoma among lung or hematopoietic cell transplant patients: a systematic review and meta-analysis. J Am Acad Dermatol. 2019;80(2):500–7.
35. Wojenski DJ et al. Voriconazole exposure and the risk of cutaneous squamous cell carcinoma in allogeneic hematopoietic stem cell transplant patients. Transpl Infect Dis. 2015;17(2):250–8.
36. D'Arcy ME et al. Voriconazole and the risk of keratinocyte carcinomas among lung transplant recipients in the United States. JAMA Dermatol. 2020;156(7):1–9.
37. Kuklinski LF et al. Effect of voriconazole on risk of nonmelanoma skin cancer after hematopoietic cell transplantation. J Am Acad Dermatol. 2017;77(4):706–12.
38. Levine MT, Chandrasekar PH. Adverse effects of voriconazole: over a decade of use. Clin Transplant. 2016;30(11):1377–86.
39. Mansh M et al. Voriconazole exposure regulates distinct cell-cycle and terminal differentiation pathways in primary human keratinocytes. Br J Dermatol. 2017;176(3):816–20.
40. Zwald F et al. Recommendations for solid organ transplantation for transplant candidates with a pretransplant diagnosis of cutaneous squamous cell carcinoma, Merkel cell carcinoma and melanoma: a consensus opinion from the international transplant skin cancer collaborative (ITSCC). Am J Transplant. 2016;16(2):407–13.
41. Kang W, Sampiao M, Huang E, Bunnapradist S. Association of pretransplant skin cancer with posttransplant malignancy, graft failure and death in kidney transplant recipients. Transplant. 2017;101(6):1303–9.

42. Jambusaria-Pahlajani A et al. Predicting skin cancer in organ transplant recipients: development of the SUNTRAC screening tool using data from a multicenter cohort study. Transplant Int 2019;32(12):1259–67.
43. Stevenson ML, Carucci J, Colegio OR. Skin cancer in transplant recipients: scientific retreat of the international immunosuppression and transplant skin cancer collaborative and skin care in organ transplant patients—Europe. Cli Transplant. 2019;33(12):e13736.
44. Crow LD et al. Initial skin cancer screening for solid organ transplant recipients in the United States: Delphi method development of expert consensus guidelines. Transplant Int. 2019;32(12):1268–76.
45. Harwood CA, Leedham-Green M, Leigh IM, Proby CM. Low-dose retinoids in the prevention of cutaneous squamous cell carcinomas in organ transplant recipients: a 16-year retrospective study. Arch Dermatol. 2005;141:456–64.
46. Endrizzi BT, Lee P, Management of carcinoma of the skin in solid organ transplant recipients with oral capecitabine. Dermatol Surg. 2009;35(10):1567.
47. Endrizzi B, Ahmed R, Ray T, Dudek A, Lee P. Capecitabine to reduce nonmelanoma skin carcinoma burden in solid organ transplant recipients. Dermatol Surg. 2013;39(4):634–45.
48. Chen AC, Martin A, Dalziell RA, McKenzie CA, Lowe PM, Eris JM, Scolyer RA, Dhillon HM, Vardy JL, Bielski VA, Halliday GM, Damian DL. A phase II randomized controlled trial of nicotinamide for skin cancer chemoprevention in renal transplant recipients. Br J Dermatol. 2016;175(5):1073.
49. Euvrard S, Morelon E, Rostaing L, Goffin E, Brocard A, Tromme I et al. Sirolimus and secondary skin-cancer prevention in kidney transplantation. N Engl J Med. 2012;367(4):329–39.
50. Badve SV, Pascoe E., Burke M, Clayton PA, Campbell SB, Hawley CM, Lim WH, McDonald SP, Wong G, Johnson DW. Mammalian target of rapamycin inhibitors and clinical outcomes in adult kidney transplant recipients. Clin J Am Soc Nephrol. 2016;11(10):1845.
51. Marcil I, Stern RS. Risk of developing a subsequent nonmelanoma skin cancer in patients with a history of nonmelanoma skin cancer: a critical review of the literature and meta-analysis. Arch Dermatol. 2000;136(12):1524–30.
52. Clowers-Webb HE et al. Educational outcomes regarding skin cancer in organ transplant recipients: randomized intervention of intensive vs standard education. Arch Dermatol. 2006;142(6):712–18.
53. Robinson JK et al. Response across the health-literacy spectrum of kidney transplant recipients to a sun-protection education program delivered on tablet computers: randomized controlled trial. JMIR Cancer. 2015;1(2):e8.
54. Kim NN et al. Squamous cell carcinoma in solid organ transplant recipients: influences on perception of risk and optimal time to provide education. Arch Dermatol. 2009;145(10):1196–7.

Management of Squamous Cell Carcinoma in Solid Organ Transplant Recipients

10

Courtney J. Ensslin and Faramarz H. Samie

INTRODUCTION

Most cases of cutaneous squamous cell carcinoma (cSCC, Figure 10.1) have excellent outcomes with single-modality surgical clearance; however, there exists a small but important subset of tumors that display more aggressive behavior. Because of the lack of data collection regarding these tumors by population-based registries in the United States, the specific numbers regarding this cohort, locoregional recurrences, nodal metastasis, and disease-specific death are poorly understood. Consequently, these high-risk cases are often not identified until they develop recurrence or more advanced disease.

Conversely, solid organ transplant recipients (SOTRs) are a demographic group that is known to have a 65-fold to 100-fold increased risk of developing cSCC compared with that of the general population. Although the majority of these cases are also cured by surgical monotherapy, there is a growing body of data that suggests that high-risk features and aggressive tumor types are more likely to occur in the immunosuppressed population.[1–3] In the immunocompetent population, rates of locoregional recurrence and distant metastasis are rare. However, in the immunosuppressed population, reported locoregional recurrence rates range between 13% and 48%, and rates of distant metastasis range between 7% and 19%, especially after treatment with surgery alone.[4–6]

Because SOTRs on chronic immunosuppression are more likely to develop high-risk tumors and present with more aggressive disease, they are at a higher likelihood of requiring multimodality treatment. Management of these patients requires a multidisciplinary team-based approach, with collaboration and communication among the transplant team, dermatology, dermatologic surgery, medical oncology, radiation oncology, and otolaryngology/surgical oncology. Although there have been many advances in the treatment of cSCC in this high-risk cohort, there is a paucity of evidence-based therapeutic strategies to guide management in this specific patient population.

 DOI: 10.1201/9781003001461-10

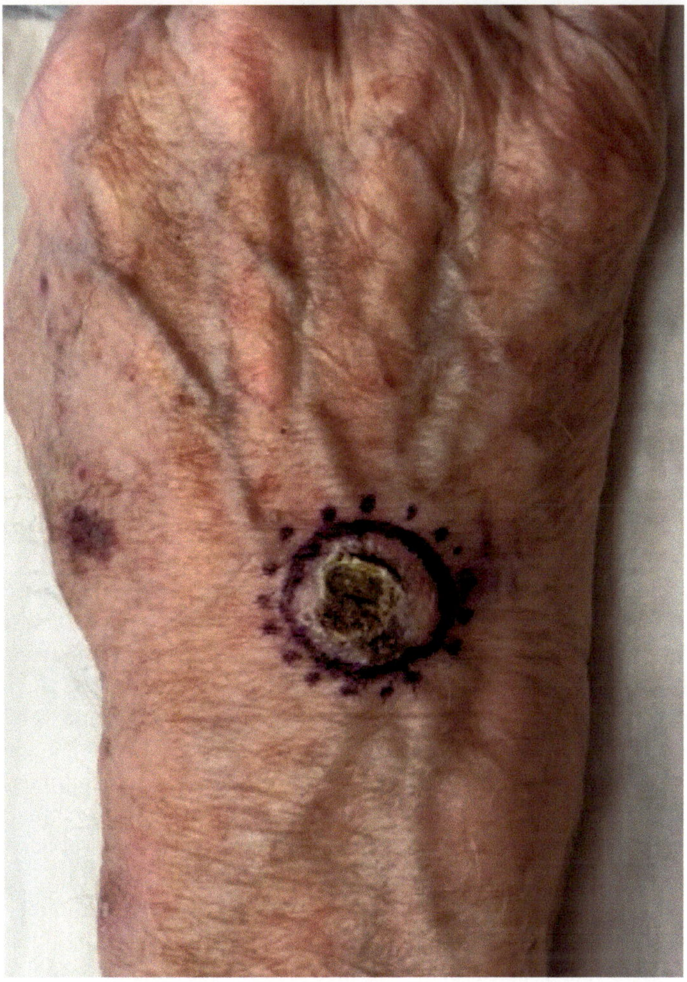

FIGURE 10.1 Cutaneous SCC (cSCC).

In this chapter, the authors hope to guide the appropriate management of SOTRs with cSCC by summarizing the evidence behind patient selection, the role of imaging, and treatment with surgical monotherapy, adjuvant radiation therapy, and sentinel lymph node biopsy.

EVALUATION AND RISK ASSESSMENT

A rational therapeutic plan should be designed for each SOTR with a diagnosis of cSCC based upon an assessment of the patient's preferences, comorbidities, tumor histopathology, and immunosuppression. Providers should take into consideration the duration, growth rate, symptoms related to the lesion, history of prior therapy, pathologic findings, and clinical presentation. A history of localized neurologic symptoms such as anesthesia, paresthesia, and pain should raise suspicion of possible perineural involvement. Any of the classic high-risk factors for recurrence or metastasis, such as size >2 cm, poorly differentiated on histology, lymphovascular or perineural invasion, or depth of invasion beyond the dermis should be identified (Table 10.1), along with any history of prior treatment or radiation therapy to the site.[7] Ideally, the biopsy report should include a histopathologic subtype, degree of differentiation, presence of ulceration, perineural or vascular involvement, and an estimate or actual measurement of depth. In addition, it is not uncommon during treatment of cSCC with Mohs micrographic surgery (MMS) to find discrepancies between the initial preoperative biopsy results and the frozen sections from MMS. A study of 1000 cases of MMS reviewed pathology margins and found a positive margin on the first stage of MMS was seen in 30% of cases that had showed clear margins on biopsy.[8] Another study of 513 cases of biopsy-proven basal cell carcinoma (BCC) or cSCC treated with MMS found that in 21.1% of the cases, intraoperative examination revealed an aggressive subtype that was not diagnosed on biopsy, including 10 SCC in situ that were found to be invasive cSCC, and 1 superficial BCC that was found to be invasive cSCC.[9] Thus, when the tumor staging is potentially incomplete, it is recommended that intraoperatively the entirety of the remaining tumor be submitted for pathologic evaluation with paraffin-embedded sections in order to provide all possible information for staging.[10]

The provider should perform a comprehensive physical examination including careful observation of the tumor and its surrounding skin to determine tumor borders, assess for evidence of previous treatment, and exclude the presence of satellite lesions (Figure 10.2). The tumor should be palpated to determine whether there is any induration suggestive of underlying connections to muscle or bone. The draining lymph node basin should also be palpated to assess for lymphadenopathy as high-risk tumors are more common and more aggressive in SOTRs.[1] The presence of clinically palpable or suspicious nodes should prompt a fine-needle aspiration (FNA) or core biopsy. Per the National Comprehensive Cancer Network (NCCN) guidelines for cSCC, if the initial pathology results are negative, reevaluation is recommended by clinical examination, computed tomography (CT) with contrast imaging, and/or biopsy of an additional lymph node specimen. For patients with an initial positive pathology report showing evidence of nodal disease, preoperative imaging of the nodal basin by CT with contrast is recommended to further evaluate the size, number, and location of pathologic nodes. In addition, positron emission tomography/CT (PET/CT) or chest/abdominal/pelvic CT with contrast are recommended to evaluate for distant metastatic disease.[10]

The NCCN guidelines for cSCC (version 1.2020, published October 2019) recognizes immunosuppressed patients, and specifically SOTRs, as a certain patient group at high risk for developing multiple and potentially aggressive tumors. In order to further identify individual high-risk patients within this group, they note important individual risk factors as the total number of tumors, frequency of tumor development, and occurrence of aggressive tumors (Table 10.1). The NCCN recommends a low threshold for performing a skin biopsy of suspicious lesions in this population and places an emphasis on urgent diagnosis and treatment. In regards to treatment of life-threatening or rapidly developing tumors in SOTRs, the NCCN recommends considering decreasing the level of immunosuppressive therapy and/or incorporating mammalian target of rapamycin (mTOR) inhibitors[10] in addition to treating the tumor. Large multivariate analyses of SOTRs have determined that the duration and dose of immunosuppression

TABLE 10.1 Classically Defined Risk Factors for Recurrent or Metastatic Squamous Cell Carcinoma

Diameter ≥2 cm
Recurrent tumor
Depth of invasion beyond the dermis
Poorly differentiated on histology
Perineural invasion
Lymphovascular invasion
Immunosuppressed patient

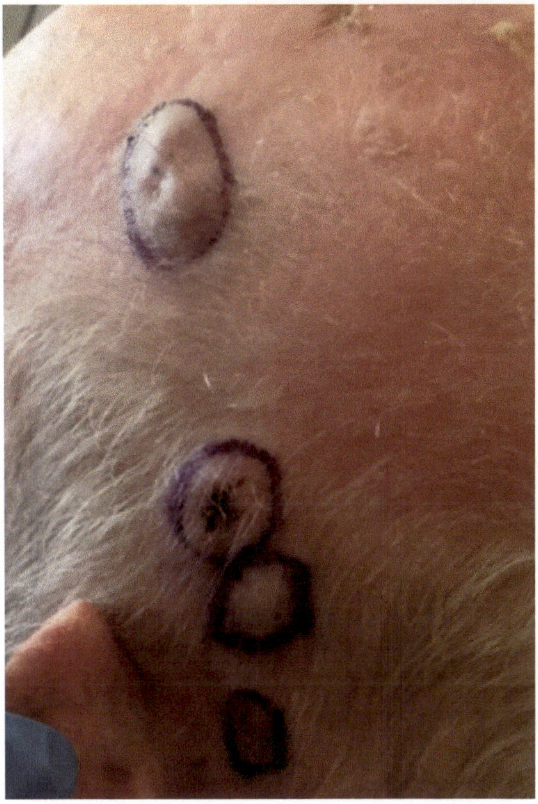

FIGURE 10.2 Multiple firm subcutaneous nodules in a patient with high-risk cSCC of the scalp, consistent with in-transit metastases.

is linked to the incidence of new skin cancers.[11–13] Prospective randomized trials have found that switching from other immunosuppressants to mTOR inhibitors decreases the risk of developing new cSCC lesions, especially in those who have a prior history of cSCC.[14–21]

TUMOR STAGING

With these data, an individual tumor may be stratified into a low- or high-risk category. Although there is no single universally accepted definition of high-risk cSCC,[22] the NCCN guidelines, American Joint Committee on Cancer (AJCC)[23] and Brigham and Women's Hospital (BWH) cSCC staging systems[24–25] can be used as guides to identifying high-risk patients and stratify disease-related outcomes (Table 10.2). In 2010, the AJCC published the first staging system for cSCC, the AJCC 7th edition (AJCC-7).[26] Unfortunately, this system was found to poorly prognosticate which patients were at risk for local recurrence and nodal metastasis and lacked distinctiveness (outcomes differ between categories), homogeneity (outcomes are similar within categories), and monotonicity (outcomes worsen with increasing categories).[27] The AJCC recently published a revised staging system, the 8th edition (AJCC-8), for cSCC located on the head and neck, but there is currently little data to validate this system. However, an alternative staging system developed by BWH in 2013 has been validated in a larger study.[24,25] The BWH staging system

TABLE 10.2 Comparison of Squamous Cell Carcinoma Tumor Staging Systems

	AJCC-7[26]	*AJCC-8*[23]	*BWH*[25]
T STAGE	*RISK FACTORS*	*RISK FACTORS*	*RISK FACTORS*
T1	Tumor ≤2 cm with <2 high-risk features	Tumor <2 cm	No high-risk features
T2	Tumor >2 cm or any size tumor with ≥2 high-risk features	Tumor ≥2 cm but <4 cm in greatest dimension	T2a: 1 high-risk feature T2b: 2–3 high-risk features
T3	Tumor with invasion of the orbit, maxilla, mandible, or temporal bones	Tumor ≥4 cm, or perineural invasion ≥0.1 mm, or deep invasion beyond the subcutaneous fat, or minor bone erosion	≥4 high-risk features or bone invasion
T4	Tumor with invasion into other bone or direct perineural invasion of the skull base	Tumor with gross invasion into cortical bone or marrow	Not applicable
High risk features	>2 mm thickness, Clark level ≥IV, perineural invasion, primary site of ear or non-hair-bearing lip, poorly differentiated histology		Tumor diameter ≥2 cm, depth of invasion beyond subcutaneous fat (excluding bone), poorly differentiated histology, perineural invasion ≥0.1 mm

Abbreviations: AJCC-7, American Joint Committee on Cancer, 7th edition; AJCC-8, American Joint Committee on Cancer, 8th edition; BWH, Brigham and Women's Hospital

stratifies tumors of all locations with a division between favorable stages (T1 and T2a) and higher-risk stages (T2b and T3), making it a valuable prognostic tool for the clinician. For example, although BWH stage T2b tumors only represented 5% of the cohort in their validation study, they accounted for 70% of nodal metastases and 83% of deaths related to cSCC.[28] The BWH staging system also may prove useful as a guide for patient selection in future prospective clinical trials. However, one limitation of the BWH staging system when compared with the AJCC-8 is that it does not incorporate nodal status or distant metastasis. Of note, neither staging system includes in-transit metastases.

For SOTRs, a comparison of the AJCC-7 and the BWH staging systems found the BWH staging criteria to better risk-stratify cSCC in immunosuppressed patients in regards to nodal metastasis and local recurrence.[29] The recently released AJCC-8 incorporates many of the high-risk factors of cSCC into staging and has demonstrated improved homogeneity compared with the previous edition of staging guidelines.[27,30] They both overlap in terms of predicting poor prognosis. However, additional studies of the AJCC-8 are needed to determine its prognostic accuracy, especially in the immunosuppressed population.[25,31] The current NCCN guidelines only list the AJCC-8 staging system, but note the development of alternative staging systems that more accurately define high-risk groups. The NCCN notes that such emerging data has led to significant revisions for determination of T-stage in the recently published AJCC-8.[10] Blechman and colleagues[32] compared the new AJCC-8 staging system with the BWH staging system in 58 immunosuppressed patients with 63 cSCCs and concluded that the AJCC-8 and BWH staging systems stratify cSCC in immunosuppressed patients with similar distinctiveness, homogeneity, and monotonicity. However, additional studies are needed to further refine staging criteria in this patient population.

Although immune status is not currently accounted for in either staging system, it should be considered in future staging systems given the higher risk of poor outcomes in immunosuppressed patients. Many poor outcomes related to cSCC in immunosuppressed patients have been described with low T stages,[29] suggesting that early detection of even low-stage cSCC and definitive treatment is crucial. In clinical practice, the consensus amongst transplant physicians is to manage all cSCC in SOTRs as higher risk for recurrence and metastasis.[33] Close follow-up is recommended for SOTRs diagnosed with high-risk cSCC, as the majority of recurrences occur within 2 years of the initial diagnosis.[5,25] In general, it is recommended that transplant patients with a history of skin cancer be seen every 3–6 months for a full body skin evaluation and lymph node examination; however, follow-up should be titrated to the frequency of tumor development. For patients who are felt to be at very high risk for recurrence or metastasis, such as those with multiple high-risk features or extensive perineural invasion (PNI), repeat imaging (CT of the nodal basis when concerned for metastasis, magnetic resonance imaging [MRI] for cases with named nerve invasion) may be considered every 6 months for 2 years following treatment.[34]

ROLE OF RADIOLOGIC IMAGING

As the overall risk of metastasis from cSCC is low, radiologic imaging is not routinely recommended. However, in tumors with high-risk features, imaging should be considered to evaluate for locoregional or metastatic disease. The NCCN guidelines recommend imaging studies for cases of cSCC with suspected bone or deep soft tissue involvement, and perineural, lymphatic, or vascular invasion, as the results of these studies may alter management.[10,35,36] CT, MRI, ultrasonography, and PET/CT have all been used for the evaluation and workup of cSCC, with retrospective analyses identifying CT as the most common radiologic modality used[36,37] (Figure 10.3).

The imaging modality of choice is dependent on the clinical question. For evaluation of perineural disease or deep soft tissue involvement, MRI with contrast is preferred over CT with contrast, as MRI has a higher sensitivity (65% versus 52%, respectively) for head and neck nodal disease.[38–40] If suspicion is high for bony involvement (including the orbit), CT with contrast is preferred to evaluate the depth of extension.[10] The use of PET/CT has been shown to increase the sensitivity of nodal detection and has a potential role in initial staging and management.[41] However, it is an expensive tool and has not been

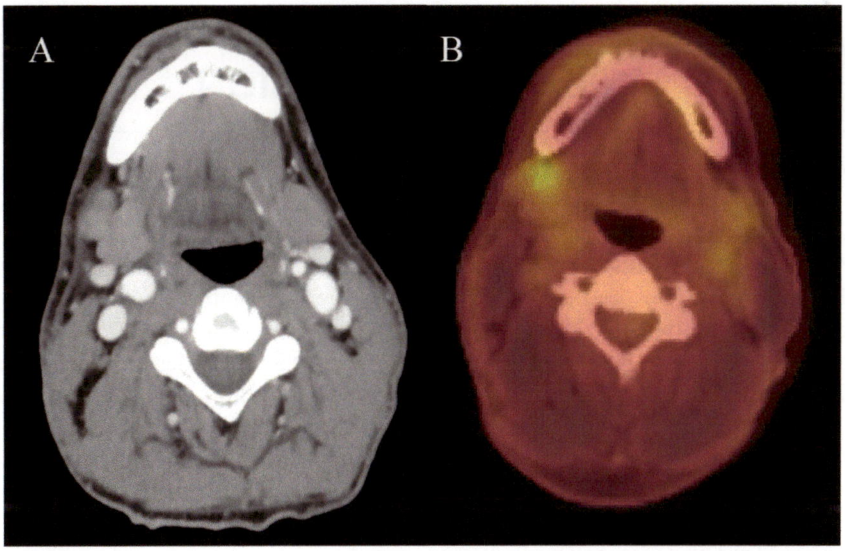

FIGURE 10.3 (**a**) Computed tomography (CT) with contrast and (**b**) Positron emission tomography (PET)/CT both demonstrate an enlarged right level 1B lymph node, denoted by the red arrow, in a patient with metastatic cSCC.

proven to alter management in the majority of patients with cSCC of the head and neck with regional nodal metastases.[42] The NCCN has no guidelines on the use of imaging for the management of high-risk or high-stage cSCCs.[10] One retrospective review found that only 46% of patients with high-risk cSCC (BWH stage T2b or T3) had imaging performed, and that the results of these imaging studies resulted in a change in treatment in 33%. In this cohort, the 5-year disease-free survival rate was higher in patients who were imaged (78%) when compared with that of those who were not (51%), suggesting that imaging allowed for earlier detection of nodal disease and may improve outcomes.[36] Maher and colleagues[43] evaluated the impact of baseline and surveillance imaging on management of high-risk cSCC and found that management was altered in 24% of the patients by the results of the imaging studies, and subclinical disease was detected in 21% of cases. Furthermore, the majority (56%) of subclinical disease was detected during surveillance imaging within 2 years of treatment. These findings support the role of imaging for detection of subclinical disease and management, but prospective studies are needed to determine the best practice for screening and surveillance.

In addition to the NCCN, other groups have proposed criteria for the role of radiologic imaging in cSCC.[44] Que et al.[34] recommended CT imaging of draining nodal basins in patients with BWH T2b/T3 stage cSCC, given that the risk of nodal metastases in these advanced tumors is in excess of 20%.[25] Breuninger et al.[45] recommended ultrasonography to evaluate for lymph node involvement in tumors that were >2 mm in thickness and CT or MRI for destructive or infiltrative tumors. In Europe, ultrasonography is the most commonly used initial imaging modality for evaluation of regional nodal basins in high-risk cSCC.[46–48] Ultrasonography was shown to diagnose extranodal spread of head and neck cSCC with a higher specificity and similar accuracy when compared with MRI but at a lower cost.[49] However, the accuracy of nodal detection with ultrasonography is operator and technique dependent.

As there are no universal guidelines for imaging in cSCC, specific guidelines for the transplant population do not currently exist. Additional studies are needed to further evaluate the role of radiologic imaging in cSCC to establish which patients will benefit most, especially in immunosuppressed patients who are at higher risk of aggressive disease. While awaiting more robust data, clinicians should strongly consider imaging in SOTRs according to the aforementioned recommendations including NCCN guidelines, as current evidence supports that radiologic imaging may influence management and positively impact outcomes.[36]

WIDE LOCAL EXCISION

The aim in excision of any cSCC is complete removal of the tumor with negative surgical margins, taking into consideration anatomic location and maximal preservation of function and cosmesis. The NCCN panel recommends that any peripheral rim of erythema around a cSCC be assumed to be part of the tumor.[10] There is no consensus with regards to the most appropriate surgical margin, with published recommendations ranging between 3 and 10 mm,[50] most often depending on tumor size. It is generally accepted that for low-risk tumors <2 cm in diameter, wide local excision (WLE) with 4 mm margins to the subcutaneous fat is adequate for removal of 95% of tumors.[51] A wider surgical margin of at least 6 mm is recommended for WLE of tumors with any high-risk feature, including size >2 cm in diameter (Table 10.1). The NCCN panel does not recommend a standard margin for WLE of high-risk cSCC because of the wide variability of clinical characteristics. Instead, the panel recommends modification of margins based upon tumor and/or patient-specific factors, including awareness of the subclinical extension of the tumor.[10]

Studies have shown that larger excision margins are required as the diameter of the tumor increases and when additional risk factors are present (i.e., high-risk location, PNI, poorly differentiated).[52–54] Recurrent tumors have also been found to require larger margins for removal, with studies finding extensive subclinical spread when compared with that of primary tumors.[54,55] Retrospective and observational analyses of cSCC removed by WLE have found a significant association between incomplete excision and the following factors: lesion thickness, location, PNI, degree of differentiation, invasion beyond the subcutaneous fat, and recurrent tumors.[56–62] For patients with positive margins after WLE, reexcision with postoperative margin assessment is the recommended treatment, as studies support that reexcision often yields clean margins.[56,63–67] It is considered highly inappropriate to merely observe an cSCC that is incompletely excised with positive surgical margins, as recurrent cSCC is associated with a significantly higher incidence of regional metastases.[68]

Although WLE with clear surgical margins is curative in most patients, 3% develop local recurrence, 2%–5% develop lymph node metastasis, and 1.5% ultimately succumb from their disease.[69] As SOTRs have a higher incidence of cSCC and often present with more aggressive disease when compared with immunocompetent hosts,[70–72] the basic tenets of obtaining negative surgical margins and examining for high-risk features such as PNI are of utmost importance. SOTRs have also been reported to develop cSCCs that are thicker and more infiltrative.[73–74] No studies have been performed to determine the minimum margin needed in WLE for complete tumor extirpation in immunosuppressed patients such as SOTRs. Although there is no data evaluating persistent or recurrent cSCC after WLE in SOTRs,[50] Ilyas and colleagues[75] evaluated residual cSCC after shave biopsy in SOTRs compared to immunocompetent controls and found a significantly higher prevalence of residual tumor (49% vs. 26.5%, odds ratio: 2.59). The authors hypothesized that SOTRs have a higher prevalence of residual cSCC after biopsy because tumor clearance is diminished by immunosuppression. Previous studies found that spontaneous resolution of BCC and cSCC was associated with infiltrating CD4+ T cells.[76–77] As the majority of immunosuppressive medications impair CD4+ regulatory T-cell functions,[78] it follows that in SOTRs, there is less clearance of residual tumor after biopsy. In addition, immunosuppression is associated with impaired wound healing, and wound healing after shave biopsy has been implicated as a contributing factor for spontaneous regression of cSCC.[79]

Based on these data, although clear histologic margins after WLE can be expected to provide a high cure rate for primary cSCC in immunocompetent patients, the same high cure rate cannot be assumed for transplant recipients. Both patient and tumor characteristics must be carefully weighed when determining whether surgical removal should be performed by WLE or intraoperative margin-controlled surgery. SOTRs with cSCC, especially with the presence of any additional high-risk features beyond immunosuppression, should at least have treatment with MMS or excision with intraoperative margin assessment considered rather than WLE with postoperative margin assessment. In any patient, regardless of immune status, if the surgical defect cannot be closed linearly, with a skin graft, or by secondary intention and necessitates tissue rearrangement, the NCCN panel recommends intraoperative margin assessment prior to closure.[10]

MOHS MICROGRAPHIC SURGERY

MMS was initially developed in the 1930s by Dr. Frederic Mohs as a method of margin control when surgically excising skin cancer. MMS employs a fresh frozen-section technique that allows for evaluation of 100% of the surgical margin. To allow for evaluation of the entire margin, MMS uses horizontal sections (versus vertical, which are used in standard sectioning such as in postoperative margin assessment after WLE). The use of horizontal sections alongside the precise mapping of specimens with ink allows for the highest cure rate for cutaneous neoplasms such as BCC and cSCC.[80] In addition, MMS allows for tissue conservation in sensitive anatomic areas, which can improve both cosmesis and functional outcomes.

MMS has been demonstrated to be highly effective as monotherapy for the treatment of high-risk cSCC with one or more high risk features, including PNI, and superior to WLE with postoperative margin assessment. Based on retrospective review of MMS versus non-MMS modalities for treatment of primary cSCC, local recurrence rates in immunocompetent patients were: 3.1% vs. 10.9% on the skin and lip, 5.3%

vs. 18.7% on the ear, 10% vs. 23.3% for locally recurrent cSCC, and 0% vs. 47% for cSCC with perineural involvement.[68] For cSCC of the head and neck, MMS has been shown to be superior to WLE with a lower rate of recurrence (3% after MMS vs. 8% after WLE).[81] A recent retrospective analysis of 260 tumors described extremely low overall rates of local recurrence (1.2%) and nodal metastasis (2.3%), but was published prior to the creation of the BWH staging system and did not stratify patient outcomes related to the AJCC-7 or AJCC-8 tumor staging systems.[53] A larger 2019 retrospective analysis of 647 high-risk cSCC tumors found an overall rate of local recurrence of 2.9%, rate of nodal metastasis of 4.8%, and rate of distant metastasis and disease-specific death of 1.1%.[35] The authors stratified their patient outcomes by BWH stage and observed that the BWH stage T2b patients in their cohort had a local recurrence rate of 7.8% compared with a local recurrence rate of 17.2% in T2b patients treated with WLE, with or without radiation. In addition, their BWH stage T3 patients treated with MMS had a lower rate of disease-specific death than that of T3 patients treated with WLE, with or without radiation. The authors found poor histologic differentiation and invasion beyond the subcutaneous fat to be the only two factors significantly associated with poor outcomes, suggesting that MMS may mitigate the risk conferred by other high-risk factors such as size >2 cm or PNI. Overall, there is a large body of evidence to support the use of MMS as the gold standard for the management of high-risk primary or recurrent cSCC over the use of WLE.[35,53,55,82,83]

Consideration of tumor treatment by MMS is based upon both tumor and patient characteristics. In order to help physicians identify which patients and tumors are high-risk and warrant treatment with MMS, a 2012 joint task force amongst the American Academy of Dermatology, the American College of Mohs Surgery, the American Society for Dermatologic Surgery Association, and the American Society for Mohs Surgery established guidelines for appropriate-use criteria.[84] The consensus amongst the task force regarding indications for MMS included: recurrent or incompletely excised nonmelanoma skin cancer; tumors with aggressive histologic subtypes; tumors with poorly defined clinical margins; high-risk location >0.4 cm (H-zone of the face, eyes, ears, nose); large tumors (>1.0 cm on the face, >2.0 cm on the trunk or extremities); cosmetically and functionally important areas, including genital, anal, perianal, hand, foot, and nail units; tumors arising in immunosuppressed patients; tumors arising in previously irradiated skin or scar; and genetic conditions with increased risk of neoplasms (such as basal cell nevus syndrome or xeroderma pigmentosa). The appropriate use criteria are available as a phone app and aim to optimize the use of MMS for clinical scenarios with the greatest benefit.

For cSCC, most physicians consider MMS appropriate if there is one or more high-risk factor present (Table 10.1). Because immune status is considered to be a risk factor for recurrence and metastasis, the appropriate use criteria support the use of MMS for treatment of most cSCC lesions in immunocompromised patients such as SOTRs, even without the presence of additional high-risk features. However, it should be noted that these criteria are suggested guidelines. The ultimate decision regarding the use of MMS should be determined by the clinician as a summation of individual patient and tumor factors, clinical expertise, and experience. Although MMS is the preferred treatment option for cSCC in immunocompromised patients, other treatment modalities may be considered in patients with a high volume of tumors or if patients are unable to tolerate the procedure.

MMS is reported to be very safe, with a low incidence of intra- and postoperative complications.[85] The most commonly reported adverse events after MMS were wound infection, dehiscence, partial or full necrosis, bleeding, and hematoma formation.[86–87] Although overall complication rates from MMS were very low, newer data have shown that solid organ transplantation and immunosuppressive medications are associated with an 8.8-times higher risk of complications.[88] The most common complications seen in immunocompromised patients were surgical site infection and wound dehiscence. Factors that may contribute to this increased risk include more aggressive tumors with subclinical extension, multiple lesions, prolonged duration of the procedure, and impaired healing. Specifically, heart transplant recipients on immunosuppressive therapy were found to primarily account for the increased complication risk amongst SOTRs and were 7.89 times more likely to have a postoperative complication compared with immunocompetent patients.[88] This may be attributed to additional factors that increase the risk of skin cancer in heart transplant recipients, including intensive immunosuppression, older age at the time of transplantation, and predominance of white race and male sex.[89,90] Patients taking immunosuppressive medications, such as tacrolimus, prednisone, or sirolimus, were found to have a 5.78-times higher odds for complications, with the greatest complication risk associated with sirolimus. This finding is of interest as prior studies have associated this drug with a reduced risk of skin cancer, thus rendering sirolimus a favorable option for patients at risk of developing skin cancer posttransplant.[14–16,91] Overall, clinicians should consider that SOTRs, especially heart transplant recipients and/or those taking sirolimus, may benefit from close monitoring during the postoperative period and careful counseling regarding wound care.

ADJUVANT RADIATION THERAPY

Although the primary treatment modality for cSCC is surgical removal, there are clinical settings in which primary radiotherapy is considered favorable, including treatment of inoperable carcinoma or for those patients who cannot tolerate surgery. In tumors with a high risk of recurrence, such as those with extensive perineural involvement, incomplete resection, and when reexcision is not possible, adjuvant radiation therapy (ART) is sometimes used to reduce the risk of recurrence. The goal of ART is to eradicate residual microscopic disease and prevent recurrence. However, radiation therapy is associated with morbidity, mortality, high cost, and can confound future efforts at resection if recurrence occurs. It is therefore necessary to clearly define which patients may benefit from ART.

The most important factors in deciding a patient's need for ART are postoperative margin status and presence of PNI. An incompletely excised cSCC has a 30%–50% recurrence rate[92] and higher incidence of nodal metastases.[68] In addition, recurrent cSCC has been shown to be larger, more likely to have PNI, and to invade deeper with greater subclinical extension.[93] In patients with close or positive surgical margins, when reexcision is not possible, ART may be considered to reduce the risk of local relapse. In one patient series of cSCC on the lip, those who underwent excision alone (27% with close or positive margins) had a 37% local recurrence rate, in comparison with a 6% local recurrence rate in those treated with surgery plus ART (94% with close or positive margins).[94]

PNI in cSCC is an uncommon but serious finding that has been associated with an increased risk of poor outcomes (Figure 10.4). Between 2.5% and 14% of cSCC are noted to have PNI,[95–97] and local recurrence rates range between 16% and 45% with nodal metastasis rates of 10% to 50%.[5,70,98,99] Risk factors for PNI include male gender, recurrent tumors, location on the midface (H zone), poorly differentiated on histology, and deep subclinical extension.[68] Suggestive symptoms that may herald diagnosis include

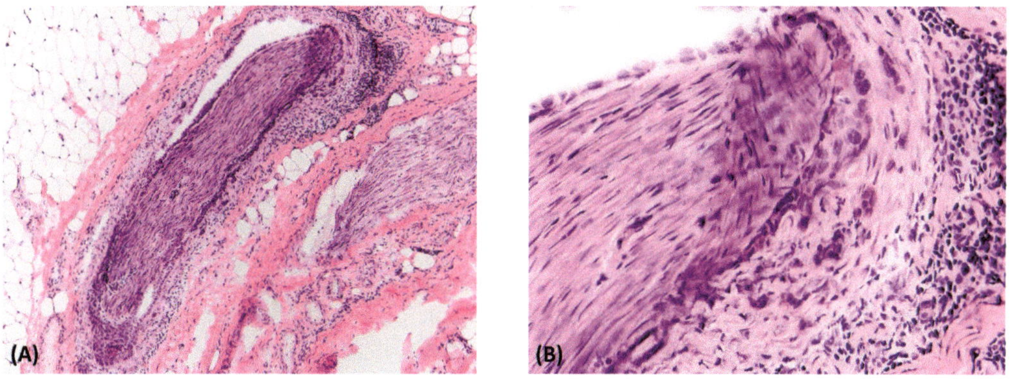

FIGURE 10.4 (**a**) A large peripheral nerve (diameter >0.1 mm) with enlarged, atypical keratinocytes surrounding and within the perineurium, consistent with perineural invasion of cSCC (H&E, original magnification ×10). (**b**) Higher magnification (original magnification ×40) reveals an intraneural island of carcinoma.

formication, anesthesia, paresthesias, dysesthesias, and pain; however, PNI is more often found incidentally on histologic examination. A high degree of nerve involvement carries a poorer prognosis, with invasion of named nerves associated with a worse prognosis than involvement of smaller, uninvolved nerves. Similarly, invasion of nerves <0.1 mm in diameter has not been associated with a poorer prognosis unless additional risk factors are present.[98,99] The NCCN guidelines recommend ART for cSCC with extensive, large caliber (> 0.1 mm) PNI or named-nerve involvement, regardless of surgical margins.[10]

There is conflicting evidence regarding the indications for and benefits of ART for aggressive cSCC after negative surgical margins.[69,100–102] Although there are multiple high-risk features for cSCC, only PNI and regional metastatic disease are currently recognized indications for adjuvant therapy.[103–105] Although PNI is considered an indication for ART, there is limited evidence for this recommendation. A large systemic review by Jambusaria-Pahlajani et al.[101] in 2009 found no benefit to postoperative ART for cSCC with PNI. Warren et al.[106] found improved survival from the addition of ART in advanced cSCC of the head and neck, but did not directly compare results with those of patients who received surgery alone. However, recently published data in head and neck surgery suggest that patients with advanced cSCC of the head and neck with PNI who are treated with ART after primary surgery have improved survival.[107] The extent of PNI appears to be helpful in defining the potential benefit of ART; "clinical PNI" is used to describe patients with clinical symptoms (i.e., paresthesias, pain) and radiographic disease, whereas patients with PNI on histology but without clinical symptoms or radiologic evidence are described as "incidental PNI". Clinical PNI has been determined to be a poor prognostic indicator for local control, and Balamucki et al.[108] found that patients with clinical PNI who were treated with ART had a higher disease-free survival rate. After surgery and pre- or post-radiotherapy, the local control rate for those with incidental PNI was 80%–90%, compared with 50%–55% for those with clinical PNI.[109] These findings underscore the importance of thoroughly examining and questioning for symptoms of PNI during clinical examination and thorough histologic evaluation for pathologic evidence of PNI, especially in immunosuppressed patients such as SOTRs. Ideally, ART should be initiated within 6–7 weeks of excision.

In patients with high-risk cSCC without extensive PNI, the role of ART is even more unclear. Treatment of high-risk cSCC with MMS alone has a low rate of local recurrence (2.9%) and nodal metastasis (4.8%),[35] and there is limited data to determine which high-risk tumor features or combination of features may benefit from the addition of ART to surgery.[101] In one of the largest studies to date on patients who received ART after resection (either MMS or WLE) with negative margins, Miller and colleagues[69] performed a retrospective analysis of 32 tumors and stratified outcomes by primary tumor stage, both AJCC-8 and BWH. Their cohort was dominated by high-stage tumors; 72% of the tumors had PNI, of which 61% were >0.1 mm in diameter. However, the two staging systems appeared to stratify patients similarly; 88% of tumors were BWH staging system T2b/T3 and 78% were AJCC-8 staging system stage T3. Within their cohort, the three patients who developed recurrent disease had poorly differentiated tumors, >2 cm in size, with PNI, supporting that there is still a small subset of these patients who may succumb to disease-related death. Despite the predominance of advanced stage tumors within the cohort, 91% showed no evidence of disease at the last follow-up, suggesting that surgery plus ART can achieve high rates of efficacy in patients with high BWH stage tumors (T2b/T3), and that these patients are reasonable candidates for aggressive bimodal treatment.[69] After treatment with MMS alone, tumors defined as BWH T2b/T3 were shown to have a risk of locoregional recurrence (LR) of 10%.[35] A 10% risk of LR for higher stage cSCC may not be high enough for ART to significantly impact the risk of recurrence,[110] and therefore may explain why improved outcomes have not been seen in previous studies comparing surgery plus ART with surgical monotherapy alone.[100–111]

As previously discussed, there is a growing body of data to support that immunosuppressed patients with cSCC have more aggressive phenotypes and poorer outcomes compared with those of their immunocompetent peers, with one study finding PNI in 7.8% of cSCC in SOTRs compared with 0.6% of immunocompetent controls.[112] Although current data is limited and further studies are needed to fully elucidate how much higher the risk of PNI is in SOTRs compared with their immunocompetent counterparts, these findings suggest that radiation therapy may be better able to influence outcomes in SOTR.[48,73,112–114]

Transplant patients have been shown to tolerate radiotherapy well, without an increased degree of acute toxicity.[93] The largest comparative study to date analyzed 206 patients over multiple institutions who received surgery plus ART and compared outcomes between immunocompetent patients and a heterogeneous group of immunosuppressed patients (including SOTRs, patients with hematologic malignancies, and patients with HIV).[113] Consistent with other studies, the authors found immunosuppression to be independently associated with inferior outcomes.[115,116] Within their cohort, those who were immunosuppressed had worse outcomes despite similar, aggressive bimodal therapy, with higher rates of LR (48% vs. 24%) and lower disease-free survival at 2 years (45% vs. 62%). In the immunosuppressed cohort, one-half of patients had LR despite receiving ART, suggesting that intensification of treatment or addition of systemic therapy in this cohort may be warranted. These results suggested that immune status should be considered a strong prognostic factor, and inclusion of immune status in AJCC and BWH staging systems may enhance their prognostic capabilities.[113]

In general, immunosuppression is strongly associated with inferior outcomes in patients with high-risk cSCC. These patients should be treated with MMS with negative surgical margins and close follow-up for at least 5 years. Although there are no definitive guidelines available as to which high-risk patients should be offered elective ART, most recommendations support bimodal therapy for the management of tumors with incomplete resection, extensive PNI, or BWH stage T2b/T3. The diagnosis and management of high-risk cSCC, regardless of immune status, should involve palpation of the regional lymph nodes. Patients with palpable lymphadenopathy should be referred to a head and neck surgeon and proceed to ultrasound-guided fine-needle aspiration or biopsy to confirm the involved lymph nodes. A positive specimen will usually result in lymphadenectomy of the associated nodal basin, often with ART.[34] The risk of relapse is high with nodal metastases even after surgery, and ART is almost always recommended to improve locoregional control. With the combination of surgery and ART in this patient population, expected 5-year disease-free survival is 70%–75%.[117] ART is particularly helpful in patients who have multiple nodes involved or extracapsular involvement, or those with parotid metastases.[118,119]

SENTINEL LYMPH NODE BIOPSY

The potential role for sentinel lymph node biopsy (SLNB) in patients with cSCC is for early detection of microscopic nodal metastases that will benefit outcomes and/or provide a survival benefit. The overall risk of nodal metastasis for cSCC is estimated to be 4%–6% in immunocompetent patients,[5,70,120,121] with an elevated risk of up to 37% for high-risk tumors of the head and neck.[122] Mortality in advanced stage cSCC is secondary to uncontrolled regional and nodal metastases, rather than distant metastasis, in 85% of cases.[5] Even with radiologic imaging, sensitivity is not high enough to detect smaller disease foci; to be considered positive for nodal disease on imaging, there must be evidence of >1 lymph node that is >1 cm in size.[34] SLNB has been shown to have a high sensitivity (79%) and negative predictive value for cSCC (96%) and to be more sensitive than MRI or CT at detecting occult metastases.[34,99,123]

The use of SLNB in the staging of high-risk cSCC is just starting to be investigated. The majority of data pertaining to this topic are limited by small cohort numbers, limited follow-up, low rates of sentinel lymph node (SLN) positivity and are largely retrospective in nature. Furthermore, most studies evaluating SLNB for cSCC only included patients who underwent SLNB and do not compare treatment and outcomes between patients who have had SLNB versus those who have not; thus, the impact of SLNB on outcomes currently cannot be assessed. For most studies that compared outcomes for cSCC patients with a negative versus a positive SLN, the results showed that even after receiving completion lymph node dissection, patients with a positive SLN had higher rates (33% to 45%) of postoperative recurrence/metastases.[124–127] In addition, patients with a positive SLN were more likely to die from cSCC.[99,125,127] These findings support that SLNB may have prognostic value, but it is unclear whether current interventions for

SLN-positive patients (such as completion lymph node dissection or ART) improve patient outcomes. It is also important to recognize that the production of higher-level evidence from large retrospective multi-institutional analysis is hindered by the lack of a cSCC National Tumor Registry.[124]

Although conclusions cannot be drawn regarding whether SLNB for cSCC provides a survival benefit, there is growing evidence that it may serve as a promising option for the detection of sub-radiologic disease. A systematic review of the current evidence for SLNB in patients with cSCC found a wide range of reported SLN positivity,[7,28,99,125–146] with an overall rate of 14%.[138] Current studies suggested that risk factors for SLN positivity included tumor diameter and thickness, angiolymphatic invasion, PNI, and the presence of multiple high-risk features.[124,125,127] The majority of these studies excluded anogenital cSCC, but one study of 585 patients with anogenital SCC who received SLNB reported subclinical nodal metastases in 24% of patients.[99] Among patients with cSCC and negative SLNB, some studies reported nodal metastases subsequently developing in 2%–7% of patients.[28,99,123–126,136–137,143,147] Overall, a recent meta-analysis reported the false-negative risk of SLNB in cSCC to be 5%.[138]

The criteria for selecting patients with cSCC for SLNB are unclear. In melanoma, SLNB is recommended for patients with at least a 10% risk of nodal metastasis, which corresponds to at least Stage T1b and a SLN positivity rate of 8%–10%.[148,149] Only BWH staging was used to evaluate the risk of nodal metastasis in cSCC relative to stage and risk factors. In the BWH cohort study from 2000 to 2009, the risk of nodal metastasis was 21% for BWH stage T2b tumors and 67% for BWH stage T3 tumors.[24,25] The rate of SLN positivity in BWH stage T2b tumors was 29.4% and, when combined with T3 tumors, increased to 34.7%[28] (Table 10.3). These rates are in line with the 10% risk threshold generally thought to warrant SLNB for melanoma,[30,140–150] suggesting that it may be reasonable to recommend SLNB in cSCC classified as BWH stage T2b and higher without palpable lymphadenopathy for staging, prognostication, and therapeutic planning.[7,28,138] Surgeons should also consider the cost-benefit when deciding whether to perform SLNB, as one study investigating cost-effectiveness of SLNB for cSCC of the head and neck found that only when nodal metastasis rates approached 20% did SLNB become cost-effective.[151]

The accuracy of SLNB may be affected by several factors including the experience of the provider performing the procedure, the technique used, prior surgery or scar in the areas where the tracer is injected, accuracy of tracer injection sites, and specimen processing.[124] Technique and tissue processing protocols are well-described and fairly standardized, but there is a learning curve for the surgeon to perform SLNB for cSCC. The sensitivity of SLNB can be enhanced through the use of combined radioisotope and blue dye for nodal identification, followed by comprehensive serial sectioning and immunohistochemistry to ensure identification of microscopic foci of disease.[124] For example, after performing more thorough tissue processing and immunohistochemistry, one study identified metastatic cSCC in 2 of 5 cases previously deemed negative.[124]

Another challenge in the application of SLNB to cSCC is that most tumors are staged either intra- or postoperatively. In these situations, SLNB is performed by injecting dye and radioactive tracer into the dermis around the area of cSCC tumor resection, rather than into the perimeter of a small intact tumor, such as in melanoma. Although literature regarding SLNB in melanoma suggests that previous WLE does not negatively impact detection of nodal metastasis,[152] the impact has not been studied for cSCC and cannot be assumed to be the same because of previously described differences in SLNB technique.[7]

TABLE 10.3 Incidence Rates of Local Recurrence, Nodal Metastasis, and Sentinel Lymph Node (SLN) Positivity Occurring in High and Low T Stages in the BWH Staging System

T STAGE	*LOCAL RECURRENCE (%)*[25]	*NODAL METASTASIS (%)*[25]	*SLN POSITIVITY (%)*[28]
T1	**0.6**	**0.1**	**0.0**
T2a	5.0	3.0	7.1
T2b	21.0	21.0	29.4
T3	82.0	67.0	50.0

Abbreviations: BWH, Brigham and Women's Hospital; SLN, sentinel lymph node.

The accuracy of SLNB likely decreases after complex reconstruction has been performed because of disruption of the draining lymphatic beds. Similarly, reconstruction on the head and neck may decrease the yield and efficacy of SLNB because of the involvement of multiple potential lymph node basins. In high-risk cases, delayed repair may be considered to prevent potential lymphatic disruption. Future studies should prospectively investigate the optimal SLNB technique and sectioning to increase accuracy and utility.

Despite the lack of consensus on when to perform SLNB in cSCC, current recommendations from the High-Risk Cutaneous cSCC Workgroup of the Association of Professors of Dermatology include consideration of SLNB or ultrasonography in patients with advanced stage cSCC (BWH stage T2b and T3 tumors) because of the high risk of nodal metastasis and low morbidity of nodal staging.[7] Adverse events associated with SLNB are low and include lymphedema, infection, hematoma, seroma, wound dehiscence, and allergic reaction to dye. Some authors also suggested consideration of SLNB in BWH stage T2a patients with tumors >2 cm in diameter.[22] As immunosuppression is considered a high-risk feature in cSCC, it may be reasonable to consider SLNB at a lower threshold for SOTRs with cSCC, especially for those with tumors that have additional high-risk features. At a minimum, future trials are needed to evaluate outcomes for SLNB in cSCC and should include immunosuppressed patients to determine its utility in this high-risk patient population.

GENE EXPRESSION PROFILE

More recently, there has been investigation into the development of a prognostic gene expression profile to identify risk for metastasis in localized, high-risk cSCC. A 40-gene expression profile (40-GEP) was developed and validated using a cohort of 586 patients from 23 independent centers.[153] The 40-GEP test stratified patients into three classes based on metastasis risk: Class 1 (low-risk), Class 2A (high-risk), and Class 2B (highest-risk). The validation cohort had 3-year metastasis free survival rates of 91.4%, 80.6%, and 44.0%, respectively, with a positive predictive value of 60% for Class 2B (the highest-risk group). These findings suggested that the 40-GEP test may prove valuable in identifying high-risk cSCC alongside current staging systems,[153] although it is unclear how the results would impact clinician management decisions. A clinical impact study was undertaken by Litchman and colleagues[154] to better assess the potential utility of the 40-GEP test. The authors found that 40-GEP test results indicating a reduced risk of metastasis (Class 1) or an increased risk of metastasis (Class 2B) may impact management decisions in a significant and risk-appropriate manner, such as more frequent recommendations of adjuvant therapies, nodal imaging, and follow-ups.[154] At this time, there is no data to support that a more aggressive management regimen would change outcomes. Further studies are needed to determine how test results would affect clinical decision-making and align with a risk-directed management plan.

SUMMARY OF KEY POINTS

- All cSCC in SOTRs should be managed as high risk for recurrence and metastasis. These patients require close follow-up, as the majority of recurrences occur within 2 years of initial diagnosis.
- High-risk factors for cSCC include size >2 cm, poorly differentiated on histology, lymphovascular or perineural invasion, depth of invasion beyond the dermis, immunosuppression, and history of prior treatment or radiation therapy to the site.

- Treatment of cSCC in SOTR should be individualized and based upon the patient's preferences, comorbidities, tumor histopathology, and immunosuppression. A comprehensive history and physical exam should be performed in all patients, including evaluation for clinical symptoms of PNI and palpation of draining lymph node basins, to determine the need for radiologic imaging, nodal pathology, and/or referral to head and neck surgery.
- Imaging studies are recommended for tumors with perineural, lymphatic, or vascular invasion or suspected bone or deep soft tissue involvement, as the results of these studies may alter management.
- The AJCC-8 and BWH cSCC staging systems should be used as a guide to identify patients at high risk of recurrence and local or distant spread and to stratify disease-related outcomes. Although immune status is not included in either staging system, both appear to stratify immunosuppressed patients similarly.
- Surgical treatment may be performed by WLE or MMS and the treatment method should be determined by the patient and tumor characteristics. MMS has been demonstrated to be highly effective and superior to WLE for the treatment of high-risk cSCC with one or more high-risk features, including PNI.
- There is variability in the literature in regards to the efficacy of ART after negative surgical margins. Nonetheless, most recommendations support bimodal therapy for tumors with incomplete resection, extensive PNI, regional metastatic disease, or BWH stage T2b/T3 tumors.
- Investigations are underway to define the role of SLNB in patients with high-risk cSCC. Current data suggests that SLNB may allow for early detection of microscopic nodal metastases. Whether earlier detection impacts outcomes and/or provides a survival benefit is uncertain.
- A recently validated prognostic 40-GEP test may aid in early identification of high-risk cSCC at risk for metastasis. Further studies are needed to determine how test results would affect clinical decision-making and align with a risk-directed management plan.

REFERENCES

1. Berg D, Otley CC. Skin cancer in organ transplant recipients: epidemiology, pathogenesis, and management. J Am Acad Dermatol. 2002;47(1):1–17.
2. Karia PS, Han J, Schmults CD. Cutaneous squamous cell carcinoma: estimated incidence of disease, nodal metastasis, and deaths from disease in the United States, 2012. J Am Acad Dermatol. 2013;68(6):957–66.
3. Silberstein E, Sofrin E, Bogdanov-Berezovsky A, Nash M, Segal N. Lymph node metastasis in cutaneous head and neck squamous cell carcinoma. Dermatol Surg. 2015;41(10):1126–9.
4. Zavos G, Karidis NP, Tsourouflis G et al. Nonmelanoma skin cancer after renal transplantation: a single-center experience in 1736 transplantations. Int J Dermatol. 2011;50(12):1496–500.
5. Schmults CD, Karia PS, Carter JB, Han J, Qureshi AA. Factors predictive of recurrence and death from cutaneous squamous cell carcinoma: a 10-year, single-institution cohort study. JAMA Dermatol. 2013;149(5):541–7.
6. Velez NF, Karia PS, Vartanov AR, Davids MS, Brown JR, Schmults CD. Association of advanced leukemic stage and skin cancer tumor stage with poor skin cancer outcomes in patients with chronic lymphocytic leukemia. JAMA Dermatol. 2014;150(3):280–7.
7. Fox M, Brown M, Golda N et al. Nodal staging of high-risk cutaneous squamous cell carcinoma. J Am Acad Dermatol. 2019;81(2):548–57.
8. Koslosky CL, El Tal AK, Workman B, Tamim H, Durance MC, Mehregan DA. Reliability of skin biopsies in determining accurate tumor margins: a retrospective study after Mohs micrographic surgery. Dermatol Surg. 2014;40(9):964–70.
9. Izikson L, Seyler M, Zeitouni NC. Prevalence of underdiagnosed aggressive non-melanoma skin cancers treated with Mohs micrographic surgery: analysis of 513 cases. Dermatologic Surg. 2010;36(11):1769–72.
10. National Comprehensive Cancer Network. NCCN guidelines; 2019 [cited 2019 Dec 15]. Available from: www.nccn.org/store/login/login.aspx?ReturnURL=www.nccn.org/professionals/physician_gls/pdf/squamous.pdf.

11. Bordea C, Wojnarowska F, Millard PR, Doll H, Welsh K, Morris PJ. Skin cancers in renal-transplant recipients occur more frequently than previously recognized in a temperate climate. Transplant. 2004;77(4):574–9.
12. Fortina AB, Piaserico S, Caforio ALP et al. Immunosuppressive level and other risk factors for basal cell carcinoma and squamous cell carcinoma in heart transplant recipients. Arch Dermatol. 2004;140(9):1079–85.
13. McGeown MG, Douglas JF, Middleton D. One thousand renal transplants at Belfast city hospital: post-graft neoplasia 1968–1999, comparing azathioprine only with cyclosporin-based regimes in a single centre. Clin Transpl. 2000:193–202 [cited 2019 Dec 29]. Available from: www.ncbi.nlm.nih.gov/pubmed/11512313
14. Euvrard S, Morelon E, Rostaing L et al. Sirolimus and secondary skin-cancer prevention in kidney transplantation. N Engl J Med. 2012;367(4):329–39.
15. Campbell SB, Walker R, Tai SS, Jiang Q, Russ GR. Randomized controlled trial of sirolimus for renal transplant recipients at high risk for nonmelanoma skin cancer. Am J Transplant. 2012;12(5):1146–56.
16. Salgo R, Gossmann J, Schöfer H et al. Switch to a sirolimus-based immunosuppression in long-term renal transplant recipients: reduced rate of (pre-)malignancies and nonmelanoma skin cancer in a prospective, randomized, assessor-blinded, controlled clinical trial. Am J Transplant. 2010;10(6):1385–93.
17. Alberú J, Pascoe MD, Campistol JM et al. Lower malignancy rates in renal allograft recipients converted to sirolimus-based, calcineurin inhibitor-free immunotherapy: 24-month results from the CONVERT trial. Transplant. 2011;92(3):303–10.
18. Hoogendijk-van Den Akker JM, Harden PN, Hoitsma AJ et al. Two-year randomized controlled prospective trial converting treatment of stable renal transplant recipients with cutaneous invasive squamous cell carcinomas to sirolimus. J Clin Oncol. 2013;31(10):1317–23.
19. Tedesco-Silva H, Peddi VR, Sánchez-Fructuoso A et al. Open-label, randomized study of transition from tacrolimus to sirolimus immunosuppression in renal allograft recipients. Transplant Direct. 2016;2(4):e69.
20. Gu YH, Du JX, Ma ML. Sirolimus and non-melanoma skin cancer prevention after kidney transplantation: a meta-analysis. Asian Pac J Cancer Prev. 2012;13(9):4335–9.
21. Lim WH, Russ GR, Wong G, Pilmore H, Kanellis J, Chadban SJ. The risk of cancer in kidney transplant recipients may be reduced in those maintained on everolimus and reduced cyclosporine. Kidney Int. 2017;91(4):954–63.
22. Baum CL, Wright AC, Martinez J-C et al. A new evidence-based risk stratification system for cutaneous squamous cell carcinoma into low, intermediate, and high risk groups with implications for management. J Am Acad Dermatol. 2018;78(1):141–7.
23. Amin MB, Greene FL, Edge SB et al. AJCC cancer staging manual. 8th ed. New York, NY: Springer; 2017.
24. Jambusaria-Pahlajani A, Kanetsky PA, Karia PS et al. Evaluation of AJCC tumor staging for cutaneous squamous cell carcinoma and a proposed alternative tumor staging system. JAMA Dermatol. 2013;149(4):402–10.
25. Karia PS, Jambusaria-Pahlajani A, Harrington DP, Murphy GF, Qureshi AA, Schmults CD. Evaluation of American joint committee on cancer, international union against cancer, and Brigham and women's hospital tumor staging for cutaneous squamous cell carcinoma. J Clin Oncol. 2014;32(4):327–34.
26. Edge S, Byrd D, Compton C, Fritz A, Greene F, Trotti A. AJCC cancer staging manual. 7th ed. New York, NY: Springer; 2010.
27. Karia PS, Morgan FC, Califano JA, Schmults CD. Comparison of tumor classifications for cutaneous squamous cell carcinoma of the head and neck in the 7th vs 8th edition of the AJCC cancer staging manual. JAMA Dermatol. 2018;154(2):175–81.
28. Schmitt AR, Brewer JD, Bordeaux JS, Baum CL. Staging for cutaneous squamous cell carcinoma as a predictor of sentinel lymph node biopsy results: meta-analysis of american joint committee on cancer criteria and a proposed alternative system. JAMA Dermatol. 2014;150(1):19–24.
29. Gonzalez JL, Cunningham K, Silverman R, Madan E, Nguyen BM. Comparison of the American joint committee on cancer seventh edition and Brigham and women's hospital cutaneous squamous cell carcinoma tumor staging in immunosuppressed patients. Dermatologic Surg. 2017;43(6):784–91.
30. Cañueto J, Burguillo J, Moyano-Bueno D et al. Comparing the eighth and the seventh editions of the American joint committee on cancer staging system and the Brigham and women's hospital alternative staging system for cutaneous squamous cell carcinoma: implications for clinical practice. J Am Acad Dermatol. 2019;80(1):106–13, e2.
31. Collins L, Quinn A, Stasko T. Skin cancer and immunosuppression. Dermatol Clin. 2019;37(1):83–94.
32. Blechman AB, Carucci JA, Stevenson ML. Stratification of poor outcomes for cutaneous squamous cell carcinoma in immunosuppressed patients using the American joint committee on cancer eighth edition and Brigham and women's hospital staging systems. Dermatol Surg. 2019;45(9):1117–24.

33. Cheng JY, Li FY, Ko CJ, Colegio OR. Cutaneous squamous cell carcinomas in solid organ transplant recipients compared with immunocompetent patients. JAMA Dermatol. 2018;154(1):60–6.
34. Que SKT, Zwald FO, Schmults CD. Cutaneous squamous cell carcinoma: management of advanced and high-stage tumors. J Am Acad Dermatol. 2018;78(2):249–61.
35. Marrazzo G, Zitelli JA, Brodland D. Clinical outcomes in high-risk squamous cell carcinoma patients treated with Mohs micrographic surgery alone. J Am Acad Dermatol. 2019;80(3):633–8.
36. Ruiz ES, Karia PS, Morgan FC, Schmults CD. The positive impact of radiologic imaging on high-stage cutaneous squamous cell carcinoma management. J Am Acad Dermatol. 2017;76(2):217–25.
37. Marrazzo G, Thorpe R, Condie D, Pinho MC, Srivastava D. Clinical and pathologic factors predictive of positive radiologic findings in high-risk cutaneous squamous cell carcinoma. Dermatologic Surg. 2015;41(12):1405–10.
38. Gandhi MR, Panizza B, Kennedy D. Detecting and defining the anatomic extent of large nerve perineural spread of malignancy: comparing "targeted" MRI with the histologic findings following surgery. Head Neck. 2011;33(4):469–75.
39. Williams LS, Mancuso AA, Mendenhall WM. Perineural spread of cutaneous squamous and basal cell carcinoma: CT and MR detection and its impact on patient management and prognosis. Int J Radiat Oncol Biol Phys. 2001;49(4):1061–9.
40. Nemzek WR, Hecht S, Gandour-Edwards R, Donald P, McKennan K. Perineural spread of head and neck tumors: how accurate is MR imaging? Am J Neuroradiol. 1998;19:701–6.
41. Mahajan S, Barker CA, Singh B, Pandit-Taskar N. Clinical value of 18F-FDG-PET/CT in staging cutaneous squamous cell carcinoma. Nucl Med Commun. 2019;40(7):744–51.
42. Supriya M, Suat-Chin N, Sizeland A. Use of positron emission tomography scanning in metastatic head and neck cutaneous squamous cell cancer: does it add to patient management? Am J Otolaryngol—Head Neck Med Surg. 2014;35(3):347–52.
43. Maher JM, Schmults CD, Murad F, Karia PS, Benson CB, Ruiz ES. Detection of subclinical disease with baseline and surveillance imaging in high-risk cutaneous squamous cell carcinomas. J Am Dermatology. 2020;82:920–6.
44. Bander TS, Nehal KS, Lee EH. Cutaneous squamous cell carcinoma: updates in staging and management. Dermatol Clin. 2019;37(3):241–51.
45. Breuninger H, Bootz F, Hauschild A et al. Short German guidelines: squamous cell carcinoma. J der Dtsch Dermatologischen Gesellschaft. 2008;6:S5–8.
46. Bonerandi JJ, Beauvillain C, Caquant L et al. Guidelines for the diagnosis and treatment of cutaneous squamous cell carcinoma and precursor lesions. J Eur Acad Dermatol Venereol. 2011;25:1–51.
47. Breuninger H, Brantsch K, Eigentler T, Häfner HM. Comparison and evaluation of the current staging of cutaneous carcinomas. JDDG—J Ger Soc Dermatol. 2012;10(8):579–86.
48. Manyam BV, Gastman B, Zhang AY et al. Inferior outcomes in immunosuppressed patients with high-risk cutaneous squamous cell carcinoma of the head and neck treated with surgery and radiation therapy. J Am Acad Dermatol. 2015;73(2):221–7.
49. de Bondt RBJ, Nelemans PJ, Hofman PAM et al. Detection of lymph node metastases in head and neck cancer: a meta-analysis comparing US, USgFNAC, CT and MR imaging. Eur J Radiol. 2007;64(2):266–72.
50. Stasko T, Brown MD, Carucci JA et al. Guidelines for the management of squamous cell carcinoma in organ transplant recipients. Dermatol Surg. 2004;30(4 Pt 2):642–50.
51. Kunishige JH, Brodland DG, Zitelli JA. Surgical margins for melanoma in situ. J Am Acad Dermatol. 2012;66(3):438–44.
52. Schell AE, Russell MA, Park SS. Suggested excisional margins for cutaneous malignant lesions based on Mohs micrographic surgery. JAMA Facial Plast Surg. 2013;15(5):337–43.
53. Pugliano-Mauro M, Goldman G. Mohs surgery is effective for high-risk cutaneous squamous cell carcinoma. Dermatologic Surg. 2010;36(10):1544–53.
54. Sonia Batra R, Kelley LC. Predictors of extensive subclinical spread in nonmelanoma skin cancer treated with Mohs micrographic surgery. Arch Dermatol. 2002;138(8):1043–51.
55. Leibovitch I, Huilgol SC, Selva D, Hill D, Richards S, Paver R. Cutaneous squamous cell carcinoma treated with Mohs micrographic surgery in Australia I. Experience over 10 years. J Am Acad Dermatol. 2005;53(2):253–60.
56. Baker NJ, Webb AAC, Macpherson D. Surgical management of cutaneous squamous cell carcinoma of the head and neck. Br J Oral Maxillofac Surg. 2001;39(2):87–90.

57. Mourouzis C, Boynton A, Grant J et al. Cutaneous head and neck SCCs and risk of nodal metastasis—UK experience. J Cranio-Maxillofacial Surg. 2009;37(8):443–7.
58. Bogdanov-Berezovsky A, Cohen AD, Glesinger R, Cagnano E, Rosenberg L. Risk factors for incomplete excision of squamous cell carcinomas. J Dermatolog Treat. 2005;16(5–6):341–4.
59. Tan PY, Ek E, Su S, Giorlando F, Dieu T. Incomplete excision of squamous cell carcinoma of the skin: a prospective observational study. Plast Reconstr Surg. 2007;120(4):910–16.
60. Khan AA, Potter M, Cubitt JJ et al. Guidelines for the excision of cutaneous squamous cell cancers in the United Kingdom: the best cut is the deepest. J Plast Reconstr Aesthetic Surg. 2013;66(4):467–71.
61. Carducci M, Bozzetti M, De Marco G, Foscolo AM, Betti R. Preoperative margin detection by digital dermoscopy in the traditional surgical excision of cutaneous squamous cell carcinomas. J Dermatolog Treat. 2013;24(3):221–6.
62. Ribero S, Osella Abate S, Di Capua C et al. Squamocellular carcinoma of the skin: clinicopathological features predicting the involvement of the surgical margins and review of the literature. Dermatol. 2016;232(3):279–84.
63. Bovill ES, Cullen KW, Barrett W, Banwell PE. Clinical and histological findings in re-excision of incompletely excised cutaneous squamous cell carcinoma. J Plast Reconstr Aesthetic Surg. 2009;62(4):457–61.
64. Stewart CMM, Garlick J, Mcmullin J et al. Surgical excision of non—melanoma skin cancer in an elderly veteran's affairs population. Plast Reconstr Surg—Glob Open. 2014;2(12).
65. Yuan Y, Duff ML, Sammons DL, Wu S. Retrospective chart review of skin cancer presence in the wide excisions. World J Clin Cases. 2014;2(3):52.
66. Brinkman JN, Hajder E, Van Der Holt B, Den Bakker MA, Hovius SER, Mureau MAM. The effect of differentiation grade of cutaneous squamous cell carcinoma on excision margins, local recurrence, metastasis, and patient survival: a retrospective follow-up study. Ann Plast Surg. 2015;75(3):323–6.
67. Griffiths RW, Suvarna SK, Feeley K. Audit of clinical and histological prognostic factors in primary invasive squamous cell carcinoma of the skin: assessment in a minimum 5 year follow-up study after conventional excisional surgery. Br J Plast Surg. 2002;55(4):287–92.
68. Rowe DE, Carroll RJ, Day CL. Prognostic factors for local recurrence, metastasis, and survival rates in squamous cell carcinoma of the skin, ear, and lip: implications for treatment modality selection. J Am Acad Dermatol. 1992;26(6):976–90.
69. Miller J, Chang T, Schwartz D, Peters M, Baum C. Outcomes of adjuvant radiotherapy following negative surgical margins for cutaneous squamous cell carcinoma. Dermatol Surg. 2019;45(9):1111–16.
70. Brantsch KD, Meisner C, Schönfisch B et al. Analysis of risk factors determining prognosis of cutaneous squamous-cell carcinoma: a prospective study. Lancet Oncol. 2008;9(8):713–20.
71. Song SS, Goldenberg A, Ortiz A, Eimpunth S, Oganesyan G, Jiang SIB. Nonmelanoma skin cancer with aggressive subclinical extension in immunosuppressed patients. JAMA Dermatol. 2016;152(6):683–90.
72. Brunner M, Veness MJ, Ch'Ng S, Elliott M, Clark JR. Distant metastases from cutaneous squamous cell carcinoma-analysis of AJCC stage IV. Head Neck. 2013;35(1):72–5.
73. Smith KJ, Hamza S, Skelton H. Histologic features in primary cutaneous squamous cell carcinomas in immunocompromised patients focusing on organ transplant patients. Dermatol Surg. 2004;30(4 Pt 2):634–41.
74. Schmults CD. High-risk cutaneous squamous cell carcinoma: identification and management. Adv Dermatol. 2005;21:133–52.
75. Ilyas M, Zhang N, Sharma A. Residual squamous cell carcinoma after shave biopsy in solid organ transplant recipients. Dermatol Surg. 2018;44(3):370–4.
76. Hunt MJ, Halliday GM, Weedon D, Cooke BE, Barnetson RSC. Regression in basal cell carcinoma: an immunohistochemical analysis. Br J Dermatol. 1994;130(1):1–8.
77. Halliday GM, Patel A, Hunt MJ, Tefany FJ, Barnetson RS. Spontaneous regression of human melanoma/nonmelanoma skin cancer: association with infiltrating CD4+ T cells. World J Surg. 19(3):352–8.
78. Zhang C, Shan J, Feng L et al. The effects of immunosuppressive drugs on CD4(+) CD25(+) regulatory T cells: a systematic review of clinical and basic research. J Evid Based Med. 2010;3(2):117–29.
79. Swetter SM, Boldrick JC, Pierre P, Wong P, Egbert BM. Effects of biopsy-induced wound healing on residual basal cell and squamous cell carcinomas: rate of tumor regression in excisional specimens. J Cutan Pathol. 2003;30(2):139–46.
80. Bolognia JL, Jorizzo JL, Schaffer JV. Dermatology; 2012 [cited 2019 Dec 15]. Available from: www.elsevier.com/books/dermatology-2-volume-set/bolognia/978-0-7234-3571-6.

81. van Lee CB, Roorda BM, Wakkee M et al. Recurrence rates of cutaneous squamous cell carcinoma of the head and neck after Mohs micrographic surgery vs. standard excision: a retrospective cohort study. Br J Dermatol. 2019;181(2):338–43.
82. Blomberg M, He SY, Harwood C et al. Research gaps in the management and prevention of cutaneous squamous cell carcinoma in organ transplant recipients. Br J Dermatol. 2017;177(5):1225–33.
83. Khan K, Mykula R, Kerstein R et al. A 5-year follow-up study of 633 cutaneous SCC excisions: rates of local recurrence and lymph node metastasis. J Plast Reconstr Aesthetic Surg. 2018;71(8):1153–8.
84. Connolly SM, Baker DR, Coldiron BM et al. AAD/ACMS/ASDSA/ASMS 2012 appropriate use criteria for Mohs micrographic surgery: a report of the American academy of dermatology, American college of Mohs surgery, American Society for dermatologic surgery association, and the American society for Mohs surgery. J Am Acad Dermatol. 2012;67(4):531–50.
85. Council ML, Alam M, Gloster HM et al. Identifying and defining complications of dermatologic surgery to be tracked in the American college of Mohs surgery (ACMS) registry. J Am Acad Dermatol. 2016;74(4):739–45.
86. Cook JL, Perone JB. A prospective evaluation of the incidence of complications associated with Mohs micrographic surgery. Arch Dermatol. 2003;139(2):143–52.
87. Alam M, Ibrahim O, Nodzenski M et al. Adverse events associated with mohs micrographic surgery: multicenter prospective cohort study of 20 821 Casesat 23 centers. JAMA Dermatol. 2013;149(12):1378–5.
88. Basu P, Goldenberg A, Cowan N, Eilers R, Hau J, Jiang SIB. A 4-year retrospective assessment of postoperative complications in immunosuppressed patients following Mohs micrographic surgery. J Am Acad Dermatol. 2019;80(6):1594–601.
89. Brewer JD, Colegio OR, Phillips PK et al. Incidence of and risk factors for skin cancer after heart transplant. Arch Dermatol. 2009;145(12):1391–6.
90. Garrett GL, Blanc PD, Boscardin J et al. Incidence of and risk factors for skin cancer in organ transplant recipients in the United States. JAMA Dermatol. 2017;153(3):296–303.
91. Karia PS, Azzi JR, Heher EC, Hills VM, Schmults CD. Association of sirolimus use with risk for skin cancer in a mixed-organ cohort of solid-organ transplant recipients with a history of cancer. JAMA Dermatology. 2016;152(5):533–40.
92. Huang CC, Boyce SM. Surgical margins of excision for basal cell carcinoma and squamous cell carcinoma. Semin Cutan Med Surg. 2004;23(3):167–73.
93. Veness MJ, Harris D. Role of radiotherapy in the management of organ transplant recipients diagnosed with non-melanoma skin cancers. Australas Radiol. 2007;51(1):12–20.
94. Babington S, Veness MJ, Cakir B, Gebski VJ, Morgan GJ. Squamous cell carcinoma of the lip: is there a role for adjuvant radiotherapy in improving local control following incomplete or inadequate excision? ANZ J Surg. 2003;73(8):621–5.
95. Geist DE, Garcia-Moliner M, Fitzek MM, Cho H, Rogers GS. Perineural invasion of cutaneous squamous cell carcinoma and basal cell carcinoma: raising awareness and optimizing management. Dermatologic Surg. 2008;34(12):1642–51.
96. Immerman SC, Scanlon EF, Christ M, Knox KL. Recurrent squamous cell carcinoma of the skin. Cancer. 1983;51(8):1537–40.
97. Ballantyne AJ, Cottel WI, Saal B, Shelley WB, Shelley ED, Z MC. Perineural invasion by SCC. J Dermatol Surg Oncol. 1984;10(7):502–6.
98. Carter JB, Johnson MM, Chua TL, Karia PS, Schmults CD. Outcomes of primary cutaneous squamous cell carcinoma with perineural invasion an 11-year cohort study. JAMA Dermatol. 2013;149(1):35–42.
99. Ross AS, Schmults CD. Sentinel lymph node biopsy in cutaneous squamous cell carcinoma: a systematic review of the English literature. Dermatol Surg. 2006;32(11):1309–21.
100. O'Bryan K, Sherman W, Niedt GW et al. An evolving paradigm for the workup and management of high-risk cutaneous squamous cell carcinoma. J Am Acad Dermatol. 2013;69. Mosby Inc.
101. Jambusaria-Pahlajani A, Miller CJ, Quon H, Smith N, Klein RQ, Schmults CD. Surgical monotherapy versus surgery plus adjuvant radiotherapy in high-risk cutaneous squamous cell carcinoma: a systematic review of outcomes. Dermatologic Surg. 2009;35(4):574–85.
102. Han A, Ratner D. What is the role of adjuvant radiotherapy in the treatment of cutaneous squamous cell carcinoma with perineural invasion? Cancer. 2007;109(6):1053–59.
103. Tanvetyanon T, Padhya T, McCaffrey J et al. Postoperative concurrent chemotherapy and radiotherapy for high-risk cutaneous squamous cell carcinoma of the head and neck. Head Neck. 2015;37(6):840–5.

104. Fu T, Aasi SZ, Hollmig ST. Management of high-risk squamous cell carcinoma of the skin. Curr Treat Options Oncol. 2016;17(7).
105. Koyfman SA, Joshi N, Vidimos A. Adjuvant radiotherapy in high-risk cutaneous squamous cell cancer of the head and neck in immunosuppressed patients. JAAD Case Rep. 2015;1(6):S5–7.
106. Warren TA, Panizza B, Porceddu SV et al. Outcomes after surgery and postoperative radiotherapy for perineural spread of head and neck cutaneous squamous cell carcinoma. Head Neck. 2016;38(6):824–31.
107. Harris BN, Pipkorn P, Nguyen KNB et al. Association of adjuvant radiation therapy with survival in patients with advanced cutaneous squamous cell carcinoma of the head and neck. JAMA Otolaryngol—Head Neck Surg. 2019;145(2):153–8.
108. Balamucki CJ, Mancuso AA, Amdur RJ et al. Skin carcinoma of the head and neck with perineural invasion. Am J Otolaryngol—Head Neck Med Surg. 2012;33(4):447–54.
109. Mendenhall WM, Amdur RJ, Hinerman RW, Cognetta AB, Mendenhall NP. Radiotherapy for cutaneous squamous and basal cell carcinomas of the head and neck. Laryngoscope. 2009;119(10):1994–9.
110. Ruiz ES, Koyfman SA, Que SKT, Kass J, Schmults CD. Evaluation of the utility of localized adjuvant radiation for node-negative primary cutaneous squamous cell carcinoma with clear histologic margins. J Am Acad Dermatol. 2019 July.
111. Sapir E, Tolpadi A, McHugh J et al. Skin cancer of the head and neck with gross or microscopic perineural involvement: patterns of failure. Radiother Oncol. 2016;120(1):81–6.
112. Lott DG, Manz R, Koch C, Lorenz RR. Aggressive behavior of nonmelanotic skin cancers in solid organ transplant recipients. Transplant. 2010;90(6):683–7.
113. Manyam B V, Garsa AA, Chin RI et al. A multi-institutional comparison of outcomes of immunosuppressed and immunocompetent patients treated with surgery and radiation therapy for cutaneous squamous cell carcinoma of the head and neck. Cancer. 2017;123(11):2054–60.
114. Kaplan AL, Cook JL. Cutaneous squamous cell carcinoma in patients with chronic lymphocytic leukemia. Skinmed. 2005;4(5):300–4.
115. Oddone N, Morgan GJ, Palme CE et al. Metastatic cutaneous squamous cell carcinoma of the head and neck: the immunosuppression, treatment, extranodal spread, and margin status (ITEM) prognostic score to predict outcome and the need to improve survival. Cancer. 2009;115(9):1883–91.
116. Thompson AK, Kelley BF, Prokop LJ, Murad MH, Baum CL. Risk factors for cutaneous squamous cell carcinoma recurrence, metastasis, and disease-specific death: a systematic review and meta-analysis. JAMA Dermatol. 2016;152(4):419–28.
117. Veness MJ, Morgan GJ, Palme CE, Gebski V. Surgery and adjuvant radiotherapy in patients with cutaneous head and neck squamous cell carcinoma metastatic to lymph nodes: combined treatment should be considered best practice. Laryngoscope. 2005;115(5):870–5.
118. Ebrahimi A, Clark JR, Lorincz BB, Milross CG, Veness MJ. Metastatic head and neck cutaneous squamous cell carcinoma: Defining a low-risk patient. Head Neck. 2012;34(3):365–70.
119. Taylor BW, Brant TA, Mendenhall NP et al. Carcinoma of the skin metastatic to parotid area lymph nodes. Head Neck. 1991;13(5):427–33.
120. Czarnecki D, Staples M, Mar A, Giles G, Meehan C. Metastases from squamous cell carcinoma of the skin in Southern Australia. Dermatology. 1994;189(1):52–4.
121. Joseph MG, Zulueta WP, Kennedy PJ. Squamous cell carcinoma of the skin of the trunk and limbs: the incidence of metastases and their outcome. Aust N Z J Surg. 1992;62(9):697–701.
122. Peat B, Insull P, Ayers R. Risk stratification for metastasis from cutaneous squamous cell carcinoma of the head and neck. ANZ J Surg. 2012;82(4):230–3.
123. Allen JE, Stolle LB. Utility of sentinel node biopsy in patients with high-risk cutaneous squamous cell carcinoma. Eur J Surg Oncol. 2015;41(2):197–200.
124. Durham AB, Lowe L, Malloy KM et al. Sentinel lymph node biopsy for cutaneous squamous cell carcinoma on the head and neck. JAMA Otolaryngol Head and Neck Surg. 2016;142:1171–1176. American Medical Association.
125. Gore SM, Shaw D, Martin RCW et al. Prospective study of sentinel node biopsy for high-risk cutaneous squamous cell carcinoma of the head and neck. In: Head and neck. Vol 38. John Wiley and Sons Inc.; 2016, p. e884–9.
126. Kwon S, Dong ZM, Wu PC. Sentinel lymph node biopsy for high-risk cutaneous squamous cell carcinoma: clinical experience and review of literature. World J Surg Oncol. 2011;9.
127. Takahashi A, Imafuku S, Nakayama J, Nakaura J, Ito K, Shibayama Y. Sentinel node biopsy for high-risk cutaneous squamous cell carcinoma. Eur J Surg Oncol. 2014;40(10):1256–62.

128. Michl C, Starz H, Bachter D, Balda BR. Sentinel lymphonodectomy in nonmelanoma skin malignancies. Br J Dermatol. 2003;149(4):763–9.
129. Eastman AL, Erdman WA, Lindberg GM, Hunt JL, Purdue GF, Fleming JB. Sentinel lymph node biopsy identifies occult nodal metastases in patients with Marjolin's ulcer. J Burn Care Rehabil. 25(3):241–5.
130. Nouri K, Rivas MP, Pedroso F, Bhatia R, Civantos F. Sentinel lymph node biopsy for high-risk cutaneous squamous cell carcinoma of the head and neck. Arch Dermatol. 2004;140(10):1284.
131. Hatta N, Morita R, Yamada M, Takehara K, Ichiyanagi K, Yokoyama K. Implications of popliteal lymph node detected by sentinel lymph node biopsy. Dermatologic Surg. 2006;31(3):327–30.
132. Reséndiz-Colosia JA, Valenzuela-Flores AA, Torres-Nuñez G et al. Lymphatic mapping and sentinel lymph node biopsy in patients with high risk squamous cell carcinoma of the skin. Gac Med Mex. 143(3):209–14 [cited 2019 Nov 17]. Available from: www.ncbi.nlm.nih.gov/pubmed/17722449
133. Cecchi R, Buralli L, De Gaudioc C. Sentinel lymphonodectomy in non-melanoma skin cancers. Chir Ital. 2006;58(3):347–51.
134. Renzi C, Caggiati A, Mannooranparampil TJ et al. Sentinel lymph node biopsy for high risk cutaneous squamous cell carcinoma: case series and review of the literature. Eur J Surg Oncol. 2007;33(3):364–9.
135. Rastrelli M, Soteldo J, Zonta M et al. Sentinel node biopsy for high-risk cutaneous nonanogenital squamous cell carcinoma: a preliminary result. Eur Surg Res. 2010;44(3–4):204–8.
136. Krediet JT, Beyer M, Lenz K et al. Sentinel lymph node biopsy and risk factors for predicting metastasis in cutaneous squamous cell carcinoma. Br J Dermatol. 2015;172(4):1029–36.
137. Ahmed MM, Moore BA, Schmalbach CE. Utility of head and neck cutaneous squamous cell carcinoma sentinel node biopsy: a systematic review. Otolaryngology—Head and Neck Surgery (United States). 2014;150:180–7.
138. Navarrete-Dechent C, Veness MJ, Droppelmann N, Uribe P. High-risk cutaneous squamous cell carcinoma and the emerging role of sentinel lymph node biopsy: a literature review. J Am Acad Dermatol. 2015;73(1):127–37.
139. Wu MP, Sethi RK V, Emerick KS. Sentinel lymph node biopsy for high-risk cutaneous squamous cell carcinoma of the head and neck. Laryngoscope. 2019 Mar.
140. Tejera-Vaquerizo A, Cañueto J, Llombart B, Martorell-Calatayud A, Sanmartín O. Predictive value of sentinel lymph node biopsy in cutaneous squamous cell carcinoma based on the AJCC-8 and Brigham and women's hospital staging criteria. Dermatologic Surg. 2019 Sep:1.
141. Chabrillac E, Lusque A, Cavallier Z et al. Cutaneous squamous cell carcinoma tumour size is associated with sentinel lymph node metastasis in a cohort of 69 patients. Acta Derm Venereol. 2019.
142. Navarrete-Dechent C, Veness MJ, Droppelmann N, Uribe P. Cutaneous squamous cell carcinoma and the emerging role of sentinel lymph node biopsy. G Ital di Dermatologia e Venereol. 2018;153(3):403–18.
143. Fukushima S, Masuguchi S, Igata T et al. Evaluation of sentinel node biopsy for cutaneous squamous cell carcinoma. J Dermatol. 2014;41(6):539–41.
144. Altinyollar H, Berberoğlu U, Çelen O, Mah K. Lymphatic mapping and sentinel lymph node biopsy in squamous cell carcinoma of the lower lip. Eur J Surg Oncol. 2002;28(1):72–4.
145. Wagner JD, Evdokimow DZ, Weisberger E et al. Sentinel node biopsy for high-risk nonmelanoma cutaneous malignancy. Arch Dermatol. 2004;140(1):75–9.
146. Reschly MJ, Messina JL, Zaulyanov LL, Cruse W, Fenske NA. Utility of sentinel lymphadenectomy in the management of patients with high-risk cutaneous squamous cell carcinoma. Dermatologic Surg. 2003;29(2):135–40.
147. Maruyama H, Tanaka R, Fujisawa Y, Nakamura Y, Ito S, Fujimoto M. Availability of sentinel lymph node biopsy for cutaneous squamous cell carcinoma. J Dermatol. 2017;44(4):431–7.
148. Gershenwald JE, Coit DG, Sondak VK, Thompson JF. The challenge of defining guidelines for sentinel lymph node biopsy in patients with thin primary cutaneous melanomas. Ann Surg Oncol. 2012;19(11):3301–3.
149. Wong SL, Faries MB, Kennedy EB et al. Sentinel lymph node biopsy and management of regional lymph nodes in Melanoma: American society of clinical oncology and society of surgical oncology clinical practice guideline update. J Clin Oncol. 2018;36(4):399–13.
150. Morton DL, Thompson JF, Cochran AJ et al. Final trial report of sentinel-node biopsy versus nodal observation in melanoma. N Engl J Med. 2014;370(7):599–609.
151. Quinn PL, Oliver JB, Mahmoud OM, Chokshi RJ. Cost-effectiveness of sentinel lymph node biopsy for head and neck cutaneous squamous cell carcinoma. J Surg Res. 2019;241:15–23.
152. Tomaszewski JM, Lau E, Corry J. Utility of positron emission tomography/computed tomography for nodal staging of cutaneous squamous cell carcinoma in patients with chronic lymphocytic leukemia. Am J Otolaryngol—Head Neck Med Surg. 2014;35(1):66–9.

153. Wysong A, Newman JG, Covington KR et al. Validation of a 40-gene expression profile test to predict metastatic risk in localized high-risk cutaneous squamous cell carcinoma. J Am Acad Dermatol. 2020.
154. Litchman GH, Fitzgerald AL, Kurley SJ, Cook RW, Rigel DS. Impact of a prognostic 40-gene expression profiling test on clinical management decisions for high-risk cutaneous squamous cell carcinoma. Curr Med Res Opin. 2020;36(8):1295–300.

Merkel Cell Carcinoma in Solid Organ Transplant Recipients

11

Liang Ding, Nathalie C. Zeitouni, and Michael Bax

INTRODUCTION

Merkel cell carcinoma (MCC) is a rare and aggressive skin cancer of neuroendocrine origin and is associated with a higher mortality rate than that of cutaneous melanoma.[1] It predominantly affects older men with Fitzpatrick skin type I and II and has a propensity for local recurrence and metastases.[2] At the time of presentation, approximately 40% of patients have regional or distant metastatic disease.[2] A subset of patients (3%–20%) can also present with metastases without a known primary MCC.[3] Immunosuppressed individuals are at an increased risk of developing MCC and have a relatively poor prognosis relative to their immunocompetent counterparts.[4,5] Solid organ transplant recipients (SOTRs) are an important subset of the immunosuppressed population. As we learn more about the role of the immune system in the development and treatment of MCC, it will be more important than ever to better understand how this malignancy affects this vulnerable population.

EPIDEMIOLOGY

In the immunocompetent population, MCC predominantly affects light skinned individuals, typically in their 7th or 8th decade of life, with a mean age at diagnosis of 74–76 years.[6] Approximately 95% of MCC diagnosed from 1973 to 2006 occurred in the white population. According to the Surveillance, Epidemiology, and End Results (SEER-18) Program database, the incidence of MCC was 0.7 per 100,000 people per year in the United States in 2013.[7] Aging plays a pivotal role in the development of MCC as the incidence increases by 98-fold from age 40 to >85 years. A decline in immune function occurs as one ages. Because of the aging of the "baby boomer" generation, the MCC incidence in the United States is predicted to increase to 3284 cases in 2025.[7]

Among patients with solid organ transplants, the overall risk of developing MCC is high. In a large US transplant and cancer data registry study, the risk of posttransplant MCC was increased 23.8-fold compared with that in the general population.[8] In a multicenter retrospective cohort, the incidence rate of posttransplant MCC was found to be 2 per 100,000 person-years.[9] In contrast to immunocompetent patients, MCC

 DOI: 10.1201/9781003001461-11

occurs at a younger age in organ transplant recipients with a mean age between 53 years and 59.1 years.[4] In a study of 189,498 SOTRs in the United States from 1987 to 2009, Clarke and colleagues[8] found that the incidence rate correlated with the age at transplantation (20–34 years old = 4.5%, 35–49 years old = 7.2%, 50–64 years old = 19.7%, and >65 = 25.7%). MCC incidence rates also increase significantly with time since transplant, with the highest incidence occurring ≥10 years after transplantation. On average, post-transplant MCC occurs 7.6 years after transplantation.[10] Similar to the general population, MCC risk is higher with male sex and in white individuals.[6] Posttransplant MCC can arise in atypical locations, but the majority of MCCs are found on the head and neck area similar to immunocompetent patients.[6] The incidence of MCC was not significantly different when comparing by the type of organ transplanted.[8] However, the type of immunosuppressive medication did affect the MCC incidence. Patients receiving cyclosporine, azathioprine, or mammalian target of rapamycin (mTOR) inhibitors had a higher risk of MCC compared with that of the patients not taking these medications. Patients who were taking tacrolimus or mycophenolate mofetil were found to have a lower risk of MCC. The highest risk of MCC development was found in those patients receiving both cyclosporine and azathioprine for maintenance immunosuppression.

Immunosuppressed patients constitute about 10% of the MCC patient population, with a higher incidence compared with that of their immunocompetent counterparts.[10] Patients with human immunodeficiency virus (HIV) have a 13-fold increased risk of developing MCC when compared with that of the general population.[11–13] Moreover, patients with organ transplantation or HIV tend to have MCC onset at an earlier age than that of other immunosuppressed individuals.[10,12,13] They also develop MCC in atypical locations. The average period from the time of HIV diagnosis to the time of MCC diagnosis was 9.5 years.[13] AIDS patients with poorly controlled HIV infection had higher Merkel cell polyomavirus (MCPyV) viral loads than that in those with well-controlled HIV infection, suggesting that severe immunosuppression may facilitate MCPyV infection.[14]

CLINICAL COURSE IN SOLID ORGAN TRANSPLANT RECIPIENTS

It is well established that MCC is more common in immunosuppressed patients with a 13.4-fold increased risk in the HIV-positive population and a 10-fold increased risk in SOTRs when compared with the risk in the immunocompetent population.[12] SOTRs have a significant reduction in MCC-specific, overall, and progression-free survival (PFS) when compared with results in immunocompetent patients.[4] In this study, Arron and colleagues compared 8 SOTRs with 89 immunocompetent patients with MCC. They found that SOTRs with MCC presented at a younger age (59 vs. 72 years) and also had a worse stage of disease at presentation. When their data was adjusted for sex, age, and stage at presentation, they found that SOTRs had a 4-fold increased hazard for progression of disease, 10-fold increased hazard for death from MCC, and 10-fold increased hazard for death from all causes. Stage of disease at presentation was a significant predictor for all three outcomes. When compared with immunocompetent hosts at 1 year, SOTRs with MCC had significantly worse PFS (12.5% vs. 69.6%), disease-specific survival (56.2% vs. 97.4%), and overall survival (46.8 vs. 88.6%). This data made it clear that SOTRs with MCC have much worse outcomes than those of other immunosuppressed patients with MCC, such as those with HIV or hematologic malignancies, and that SOTRs with MCC should be considered a special subset of immunosuppressed patients with MCC.

A similar study was performed by Cook and colleagues,[15] which retrospectively evaluated the differential outcomes of 89 immunosuppressed patients with nonmetastatic MCC; 21% of these immunosuppressed patients were SOTRs. Time to recurrence was similar among all of the immunosuppression types, but there was a discrepancy when it came to MCC-specific and overall survival. This study found that patients with HIV/AIDS and SOTRs had the worst MCC-specific survival and overall survival compared with those of all other forms of immunosuppression. The authors concluded from this that there were subsets of immunosuppressed patients who may respond better to salvage treatments. However, in the case of SOTRs, there are often less salvage treatment options such as immunotherapy available.

PATHOGENESIS

MCC was first described as trabecular carcinoma of the skin by Cyril Toker in 1972.[16] The name was later changed because the tumor cells resembled the Merkel cell, which is present in the basal epidermis surrounding hair follicles and is now known to be involved in gentle touch reception.[17] The exact cell of origin still remains unclear. Merkel cell precursors such as pre-B cells, pro-B cells, and dermal fibroblasts are potential cells of origin based on results of gene expression profiling and molecular studies.[18,19]

Similar to other skin cancers, the link between MCC and ultraviolet (UV) radiation is well established.[20,21] Specifically, it is the MCPyV– MCC that is most directly linked with exposure to UV radiation. With the help of DNA sequencing, researchers have been able to identify important differences between MCPyV+ and MCPyV– tumors. The identification of numerous signature UV mutations (C-to-T pyrimidine dimers) in MCPyV– tumors explains how UV-induced damage accumulates and leads to uncontrolled cell proliferation.[22] Exome sequencing on 49 MCC tumors showed that MCPyV– tumors had a median of 1121 somatic single nucleotide variants per exome with frequent mutations in *RB1* and p53. This is in contrast to a median of 12.5 somatic single nucleotide variants per tumor in MCPyV+ tumors.[23] In another study, 86% of MCPyV– MCC displayed a high mutation burden associated with signature UV-mediated DNA damage.[24] MCPyV– MCC harbored mutations in *RB1*, *TP53*, *NOTCH1*, and *FAT1*.

In contrast to UV radiation-induced MCC, MCPyV+ tumors are driven by integration of the virus into the host genome. The high incidence of MCC in the immunosuppressed population as well as the elderly population led researchers to believe that an infectious etiology could be responsible for carcinogenesis. Analysis of MCC tumors utilizing whole-transcriptome sequencing detected a 5387 base-pair genome of the previously undescribed MCPyV that was present in 80% of MCC tumors and only 8% of control tissues.[25] Two oncoproteins, large T-antigen (LT) and small T-antigen (ST) are produced by the virus once it is integrated into the host genome at a nonspecific binding site.[26] The truncated LT oncoprotein targets the retinoblastoma tumor suppressor gene, which can result in unregulated cell proliferation.[27] The ST oncoprotein acts on the FBXW7-binding domain and is believed to be responsible for the initiation of tumorigenesis in MCC.[28] The interplay of LT and ST oncoproteins in MCC carcinogenesis is still not fully understood but may be potential therapeutic targets in the treatment of MCC.[29]

Although MCC is a rare malignancy, MCPyV is believed to be ubiquitous in humans with up to 80% of the population thought to be infected with the virus.[30,31] Under very rare circumstances, it is believed that UV radiation may produce specific mutations in the viral genome that can drive oncogenesis and lead to evasion of the immune response.[32]

Published data showed a high frequency of detection of MCPyV in patients with solid organ transplantation. Husseiny and colleagues[33] assessed the MCPyV viral load in the serum and urine from immunosuppressed kidney transplant patients and healthy volunteers using Quantitative real-time polymerase chain reaction (q-PCR). They found that MCPyV viruria was detected in 30% of kidney transplant patients (vs. 15% of healthy donors), although the urine viral load of MCPyV was similar between the two groups. MCPyV viruria was not detectable in kidney transplant patients with clinical BK virus (BKV) reactivation.[34] In pediatric kidney transplant recipients, MCPyV DNA was more frequently detected (36.9% of the recipients) than the JC virus (8.7%), BK Virus (6.5%), and lymphotropic polyomavirus (2.2%). Higher frequency of detection of MCPyV was also observed in lung transplant recipients. MCPyV DNA was detected in 33.8% of transbronchial biopsies from 66 lung transplant recipients, whereas KI virus DNA was only discovered in 9.2% of the specimens and WU polyomavirus in 12.3% of the samples.[35]

In organ transplant recipients, immunosuppressants are administered to prevent graft rejection resulting in iatrogenic immunosuppression. Immunosuppressants like calcineurin inhibitors cause a 200-fold higher risk of skin cancer and promote tumorigenesis by hindering the nucleotide excision repair pathway.[36] Partial regression of metastatic MCC was reported in a patient after the withdrawal of azathioprine.[37] There have also been several cases of spontaneous regression of MCC. The first case of complete spontaneous regression of MCC was reported by O'Rourke and Bell in 1986.[38] In addition to regression of the primary tumor, there have also been reports of spontaneous regression of metastatic MCC.[39] The exact mechanism of this regression is unknown. Interestingly, many of the aforementioned cases of regression occurred immediately following some sort of intervention such as a skin biopsy or fine-needle aspiration of a regional lymph node. Paulson and colleagues[40,41] investigated the inflammatory response of tumors that underwent spontaneous resolution and found that a robust intratumoral CD8+ infiltrate was associated with a better prognosis.

Koba et al.[42] attempted to gain insight into exactly what happens after a skin biopsy of MCC to determine if the biopsy itself was enough to produce an immune reaction that might be responsible for regression of the cancer. Unfortunately, they were unable to prove that diagnostic biopsy is enough to induce a CD8+ intratumoral infiltration and immune recognition.

CLINICAL FEATURES

MCC usually appears as a firm, often painless dome-shaped nodule and can be red, purple, violet, or skin colored (Figure 11.1). Typically, the tumor develops rapidly and can have a nonspecific appearance mimicking basal cell carcinomas or subcutaneous cysts. In a review of 195 patients, 56% of lesions were presumed to be benign at the time of biopsy.[11] Cutaneous metastatic MCC or in transit disease can present as multiple erythematous nodules or indurated subcutaneous plaques (Figure 11.2).[43]

The most common anatomic locations for the primary MCC are the head and neck region (43%–53% of MCC cases), followed by the upper limbs and shoulder (24%), legs and hip (15%), trunk (11%), and other regions such as the oral and genital mucosa (9%).[44]

The most significant clinical features of MCC were summarized in an acronym: AEIOU. A for asymptomatic/lack of tenderness; E for expanding rapidly (<3 months); I for immunosuppression; O for older than age 50; and U for UV-exposed sites (location). In a study of 195 MCC patients, Heath and colleagues[11] found that approximately 32% of the patients met ≥4 criteria of AEIOU, and around 89% of patients met ≥3 criteria of AEIOU.

HISTOLOGY

Tissue sampling is compulsory at obtaining the diagnosis of MCC. The tumor typically resides in the dermis with frequent involvement of the overlying epidermis and underlying subcutis. Standard hematoxylin and eosin (H&E) stains reveal sheets and nests of densely packed basaloid cells with a finely granular chromatin pattern.[45] Frequent mitoses and areas of necrosis are commonly seen (Figure 11.3). Other features may include lymphovascular invasion, perineural invasion, and pagetoid spread within the epidermis.

MCC may occasionally show squamous, sarcomatous, eccrine, glandular, and melanocytic differentiation. Pulitzer and colleagues[46] reported that unlike pure MCC, combined squamous and Merkel cell tumors were negative for MCPyV, and they had about 38-fold higher mutations per megabase by

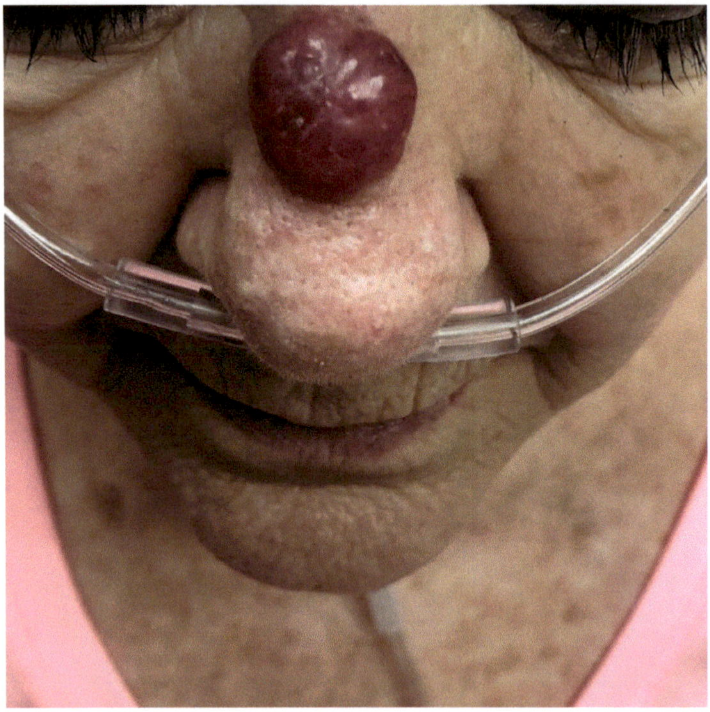

FIGURE 11.1 Primary Merkel cell carcinoma on the nasal dorsum.

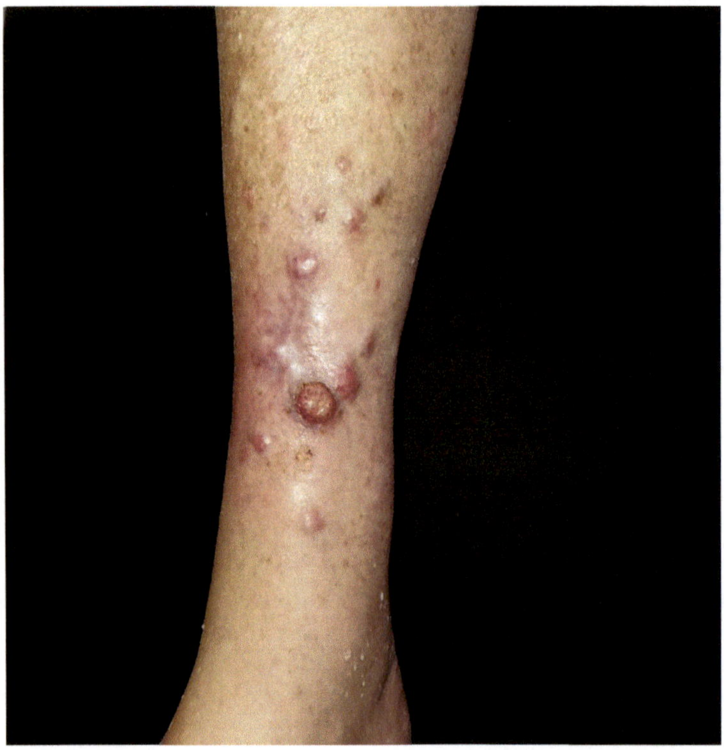

FIGURE 11.2 Cutaneous Merkel cell carcinoma metastases on the lower leg.

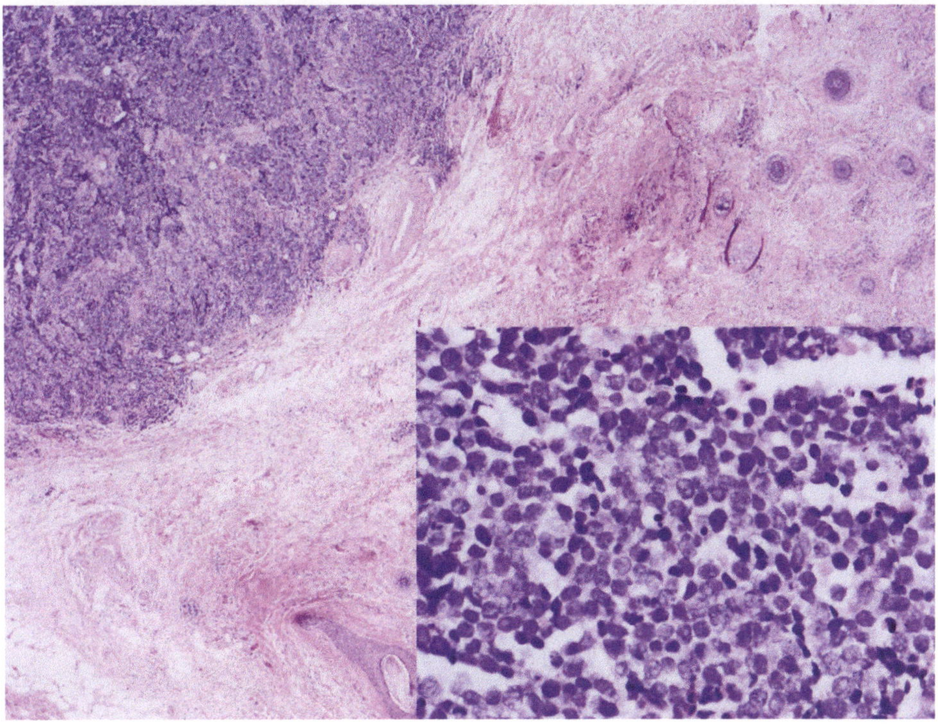

FIGURE 11.3 Histology of Merkel cell carcinoma (H&E).

next-generation sequencing. An additional 12 cases of combined MCCs with squamous, follicular, sarcomatous, glandular, or neuroblastic differentiation were all negative for MCPyV by PCR analysis.[47]

The differential diagnosis of the "small, round, blue cell tumor" is broad. Given the implications for prognosis and management, immunohistochemical stains are often utilized to confirm the diagnosis of MCC.[26] The tumor cells of MCC are positive for pan-cytokeratin, CK20, CAM 5.2, AE1 / AE3, and CK903 (34 beta E12), EMA (epithelial membrane antigen), Ber-EP4, and neuroendocrine markers.[48] CK20 immunostaining is a relatively specific and sensitive marker for MCC. It is positive in 90% of MCC with a classic dot-like paranuclear pattern (Figure 11.4). Generally speaking, MCC is negative for CK7, CDX2, TTF1 (thyroid transcription factor-1), CD45, vimentin, S100, and other melanoma markers. It is worth noting that MCPyV– MCC exhibits a more aberrant immunohistochemical profile than MCPyV+ tumors.[49]

MCC needs to be distinguished from other small blue cell tumors such as small cell carcinoma of the lung, Ewing's sarcoma, small cell melanoma, and lymphoma. The "classical" IHC profile of these tumors are listed as follows:

- MCC: CK20+ (dot-like), CK7–, NSE+, S100–, CD45–, CD99 rarely +
- Small cell carcinoma of the lung: CK20–, CK7+, NSE+, TTF-1+
- Ewing's sarcoma: CK20–, CD99+
- Small cell melanoma: CK20–, S100+, other melanoma markers
- Lymphoma: CK20–, NSE–, CD20+, CD3+, CD43+, CD45+[48]

In addition to immunohistochemistry studies, the diagnosis of MCC can also be confirmed by electron microscopy. The electron microscopy view of MCC is similar to that of Merkel cells. The most characteristic findings are perinuclear bundles of tightly packed intermediate filaments (10 nm), electron-dense neurosecretory granules, and well-developed desmosomes.[50]

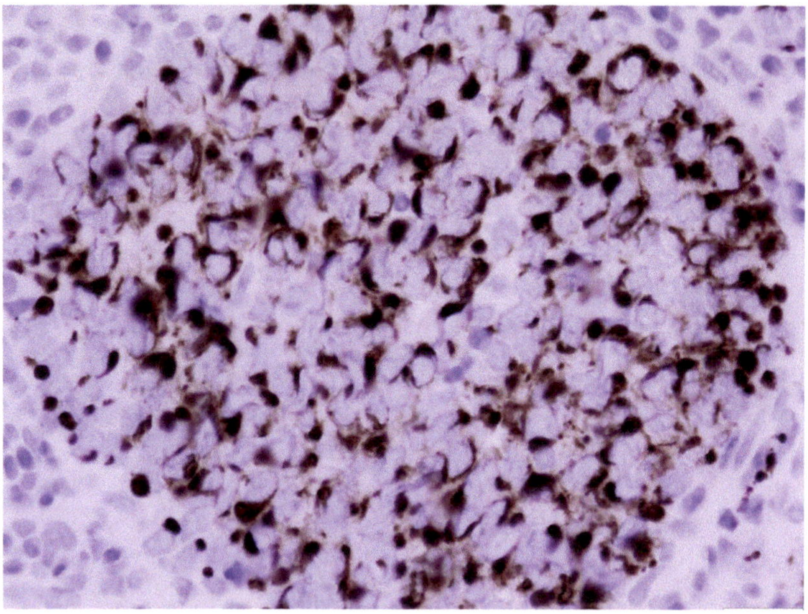

FIGURE 11.4 MCC with CK20+ staining in a paranuclear dot-like pattern.

Multiple chromosomal abnormalities have been reported in MCC. Chromosomes 1, 4, 5, 6, 8, 13, and 20 are the frequently affected ones.[51] Inactivating mutation of *RB1* occurs in nearly all MCPyV– MCCs. Mutations in genes encoding regulatory proteins of the tyrosine kinase signaling (*PIK3CA*, *KIT*, and *PDGFR*) have also been reported.[52] However, the connection between these cytogenetic alternations and pathogenesis and clinical outcomes is unclear. To date, none of the findings provided sufficient clinical information to justify its routine application.

STAGING SYSTEM

The TNM staging system is the most widely applied system for cancer staging. It is recommended by both the American Joint Committee on Cancer (AJCC) and the Union for International Cancer Control (UICC). The 2017 AJCC eighth edition tumor, node, metastasis (TNM) staging system of MCC is the latest edition that plays a pivotal role in patient management and prognosis. This staging system was validated upon an analysis of 9387 patients from the National Cancer Database who had MCC diagnosed between 1998 and 2012.[44] In contrast to the previous edition, the eighth edition has separate criteria for clinical and pathologic staging. It is important to point out that the staging system for MCC does not take into account if the patient is immunosuppressed. Studies have demonstrated that MCC in the immunosuppressed, specifically SOTRs, has a tendency to behave more aggressively when compared with MCC in immunocompetent individuals.[4,15] For this reason, it will be important for future MCC staging systems to consider taking into account the immune status of the patient.

At the time of presentation, 65% of the 9387 MCC patients had localized disease (stage I or II), 26% had nodal involvement (stage III), and 8% of patients had distant metastases (stage IV).[44] The estimated 5-year overall survival of these groups was 51% for stage I and II, 35% for stage III, and 14% for stage IV disease. Of note, patients who presented with nodal disease and an unknown primary lesion had an improved prognosis compared with that of patients who presented with nodal disease and a concurrent primary tumor (42% vs. 27%, respectively).

TABLE 11.1 8th Edition AJCC Staging System

CLINICAL STAGE	*PRIMARY TUMOR (T)*	*LYMPH NODE (N)*	*METASTASIS (M)*
0	**In situ**	**No regional lymph node metastasis**	**No distant metastasis**
I	≤2 cm maximum tumor dimension	Nodes negative by clinical exam*	No distant metastasis
IIA	>2 cm maximum tumor dimension	Nodes negative by clinical exam*	No distant metastasis
IIB	Primary tumor invades bone, muscle, fascia, or cartilage	Nodes negative by clinical exam*	No distant metastasis
III	Tumor with any size and depth	Nodes positive by clinical exam*	No distant metastasis
IV	Any	Regional lymph nodes positive or negative	Distant metastasis detected by clinical exam

**No pathological exam performed*

PATHOLOGICAL STAGE	*PRIMARY TUMOR (T)*	*LYMPH NODE (N)*	*METASTASIS (M)*
0	In situ, within the epidermis only	No regional lymph node metastasis	No distant metastasis
I	≤2 cm maximum tumor dimension	Nodes negative by pathological exam	No distant metastasis
IIA	>2 cm maximum tumor dimension	Nodes negative by pathological exam	No distant metastasis
IIB	Primary tumor invades bone, muscle, fascia, or cartilage	Nodes negative by pathological exam	No distant metastasis
IIIA	Tumor with any size and depth OR	Nodes positive by pathological exam only**	No distant metastasis
	Unknown primary	Nodes positive by clinical exam, and confirmed by pathological exam	No distant metastasis
IIIB	Tumor with any size and depth	Nodes positive by clinical exam, and confirmed by pathological exam or in-transit metastasis	No distant metastasis
IV	Any	Regional lymph nodes positive or negative	Distant metastasis detected by pathological exam

Abbreviation: AJCC, American Joint Committee on Cancer.

*** Nodal involvement not apparent on clinical exam, occult lymph node involvement*

Source: Modified from Table 2 from Harms et al.[44]

MANAGEMENT

The low incidence of MCC makes prospective randomized clinical trials difficult. Therefore, much of the basis for treatment recommendations comes from small case series, retrospective reviews, and expert opinion. Even more scarce is the amount of evidence that exists for managing MCC in SOTRs. Knowing that MCC behaves more aggressively and has worse outcomes in SOTRs, special consideration should be given to this subset of patients to be more aggressive during the initial treatment of their disease. It is also of utmost importance to provide patient education regarding early detection of recurrence and maintain close clinical follow up of these patients. Additional patient information can be found on the website *merkelcell.org*.

The management of MCC requires multidisciplinary care as defined by the National Comprehensive Cancer Network (NCCN) clinical practice guidelines.[53] After a biopsy confirms the diagnosis of MCC, initial staging should be performed with a baseline positron emission tomography/computed tomography (PET/CT) scan. The goal of imaging is primarily to detect regional nodal or distant metastases.[2] A prospective study performed in 2018 investigated the utility of a pretreatment PET scan in 58 patients diagnosed with MCC.[54] This study found that the PET scan influenced the treatment decision in 27% of patients, and that 26% of the patients were upstaged based on the results of the scan.

At the time of diagnosis, patients should also have a baseline MCPyV antibody test to assess for the presence of seropositivity. A 2017 study of 219 patients from the University of Washington demonstrated that 1% of healthy controls are positive for MCPyV antibodies; however, 52% of patients with MCC have positive MCPyV titers.[55] Interestingly, immunosuppressed patients (n = 23) were less likely to produce detectable antibodies. Seropositivity was found to be independently associated with a decreased risk of recurrence. The risk of recurrence in seronegative patients was 42% higher than that in their seropositive counterparts. Monitoring the titers of seropositive patients throughout treatment was also beneficial for detecting early recurrence when tumor burden is lower. A rising oncoprotein titer had a 66% positive predictive value for recurrence whereas a falling titer had a 97% negative predictive value. Seropositive patients can be reliably followed with serology, whereas seronegative patients should be followed with serial imaging to detect early recurrence. In some cases, the antibody test was able to outperform imaging at detecting early recurrence.[56] In practice, a combination of serial imaging and antibody titers in seropositive patients should be used to follow patients with MCC.

Definitive treatment is primarily surgical for localized disease and should consist of a wide local excision with 1–3 cm margins.[57] Mohs surgery, or modified Mohs surgery utilizing rush permanent sections with 100% margin control, can also be considered in certain anatomic locations.[58] The main goal of the excision is to obtain histologically negative margins. The size of the margin should be balanced with the morbidity of the procedure and the anatomic location as the local recurrence rate after wide local excision ranges from 25% to 40%.[57–59] Retrospective studies comparing Mohs micrographic surgery and wide local excision have demonstrated reduced recurrence rates with Mohs (5%–22%), but prospective studies have not been performed and follow-up data is limited.[29]

Sentinel lymph node biopsy (SLNB) should be considered for most patients with clinically node negative disease. If a SLNB is planned, it is imperative that it be performed prior to surgical excision of the primary tumor, taking care not to disrupt the draining lymphatics. Studies have shown that up to 30% of patients with clinically negative nodal disease will have pathologically positive nodal disease.[60,61] Tumor size tends to correlate with likelihood of positive nodal disease, but small tumors (<0.5 cm) still carry up to a 14% risk of occult nodal disease.[44,62,63]

The cost-effectiveness of SLNB is often debated. However, patients proven to have a negative SLNB at initial diagnosis have a 76% 5-year survival compared with 59% for those that only undergo clinical nodal evaluation.[64]

Assessing nodal status is important for prognostic purposes. The 5-year survival for patients with a positive SLNB ranges from 50% to 62% versus 60%–80% in those with a negative SLNB.[61,65] SLNB is also useful for selecting which patients would benefit from regionally directed treatments such as completion dissection or regional radiation therapy. Patients with clinically positive nodal disease at the time of diagnosis should have fine-needle or core biopsy confirming metastatic disease.

MCC is a radiation-sensitive malignancy. Radiation can be used as monotherapy in patients who are poor surgical candidates or in situations where surgery would result in significant functional morbidity.[66–69] Monotherapy can provide effective local control of the primary site, but rates of distant recurrence and MCC-specific survival are increased in patients treated with radiation as monotherapy compared with results in those treated with complete surgical resection.[66,69–70] Higher doses (60–66 Gy) and a wider treatment field are necessary when radiation is used as monotherapy to improve survival.[53]

Adjuvant radiation to the primary site in the setting of negative surgical margins and negative SLNB is a controversial subject. More recent evidence demonstrated improved outcomes when adjuvant radiation to the primary site was administered. Two of the larger, more recent, retrospective studies showed a survival benefit for adjuvant radiation to the primary site after surgery in early, localized disease. However, this survival benefit diminished when more advanced/regional disease was present.[71,72] Prophylactic radiation to the regional draining lymph node basin in the setting of a negative SLNB can be performed in high-risk individuals, when lymphovascular invasion is present in the primary tumor, or if a SLNB is not performed.[73] Given the high recurrence risk and poor overall survival for SOTRs, strong consideration should be given to elect for adjuvant radiation to the primary site as well as the regional nodal basin.

When a positive SLNB is encountered, treatment options consist of completion node dissection, definitive radiation therapy to the nodal basin, or a combination of both treatments. Unfortunately, few studies have investigated the differences among those three options. The two studies that have retrospectively reviewed these treatment options failed to show a difference in survival benefit or rates of regional recurrence.[29,74] The NCCN does recommend adjuvant radiation to the lymph node basin after completion dissection if there are multiple nodes involved or if there is extracapsular extension present.[53]

Evidence also suggests that the immune system plays a critical role in the response to radiation therapy. Immunosuppressed patients with metastatic MCC were shown to have worse rates of PFS and worse local control than those in their immunocompetent counterparts when treated with standard-dose radiation therapy with curative intent.[75]

Regardless of the treatment pursued, close surveillance is critical. Patient education regarding sun protection and self-skin and lymph node examination is recommended. Complete physical examinations paying special attention to the primary tumor site and the regional draining lymph node basin should be performed regularly by the clinician with a low threshold for diagnostic biopsy. The highest risk for recurrence is within the first 2 years, with the draining nodal basin the most likely location of recurrent disease. Full skin and lymph node examinations should be performed every 3–4 months for 2 years; they can then be spaced to every 6 months.[76] Guidelines for routine imaging have not been established. Follow-up imaging is dependent on the individual patient risk factors and symptoms. PET/CT is the modality of choice to detect regional recurrence or distant metastases.

Management of recurrent disease or patients with distant metastases is highly individualized and consultation should be sought with a multidisciplinary tumor board. Altering or decreasing immunosuppression in SOTRs should strongly be considered and could potentially improve the clinical course in those with MCC. Early and frequent communication with the transplant team is critical. Unfortunately, the scarcity of the data prevents conclusions from being made regarding specific immunosuppression regimens. Much of the guidance is based off of data from the cutaneous squamous cell carcinoma literature. There is likely a benefit from avoidance or reduction of cyclosporine and azathioprine in addition to transitioning to an mTOR inhibitor such as sirolimus.[4] However, the modification of immunosuppressants must be balanced against the possible risk of organ rejection.

In patients with oligometastatic disease, short-course radiation therapy is a viable option. In 2015, a study retrospectively evaluating 93 metastatic MCC tumors treated with palliative single fraction radiation therapy was performed.[77] Radiation therapy (8 Gy) was applied to the MCC lesions, and 94% of the tumors had an objective response and 45% of the tumors had a complete response. This in-field response was durable with no progression seen in 77% of the tumors at a median time of 277 days. Unfortunately, immunosuppressed patients had a higher rate of in-field progression compared with that of their immunocompetent counterparts.

Chemotherapy has mainly been used for palliation, with platinum-based agents and etoposide being the most commonly utilized treatment. The initial response to chemotherapy is rarely sustained with progressive disease developing in 90% of patients at 10 months.[78]

In organ transplant recipients with advanced disease, clinical trials should be considered whenever possible. Immunotherapy is emerging as the most promising and first-line treatment for advanced MCC in immunocompetent patients.

The recent approval of immune checkpoint inhibitors (ICIs) for advanced and metastatic MCC has given hope to many patients (see Chapter 13). Early trial data with the use of pembrolizumab in immunocompetent patients showed an objective response rate (ORR) of 56% and an estimated PFS of 67% at 6 months.[79] These results led to pembrolizumab being incorporated in the treatment options for advanced MCC in the NCCN guidelines.[79] Nivolumab, in a different study, showed an ORR of 68% and a PFS of 82% at 3 months. In 2017, avelumab was the first FDA-approved drug for advanced MCC based on the results of an international clinical trial. This study showed an ORR of 32% with a PFS of 40% at 6 months.[80] ICIs also were found to be effective in both MCPyV+ and MCPyV− tumors. Despite these encouraging results, there remains a need to improve outcomes. Ongoing clinical trials include the use of adjuvant or neoadjuvant ICIs, adding CTLA-4 blockade, or combining with intratumoral injections of the oncolytic virus talimogene laherparepvec (TVEC).[79]

SOTRs have been excluded from immunotherapy trials, and currently ICIs are not recommended in transplant patients because of the risk of organ rejection. Most of the data on immunotherapy in transplant patients comes from literature reviews of case reports and small series, especially in melanoma and squamous cell carcinoma. ICIs seem to be effective in SOTRs with advanced disease, and most of the deaths seen in these patients were related to disease progression and not graft loss or rejection.[81,82] However, a multidisciplinary team consultation with the patient remains paramount in weighting the risks and benefits of any immunotherapy in SOTRs. Early phase trials are underway to assess the safety and efficacy of ICIs in immunosuppressed patients.[82]

PROGNOSIS

Tumor staging and assessment of the nodal involvement at the time of diagnosis is the most important prognostic factor for MCC. Overall, 5-year survival for patients with localized disease is 51%, whereas the survival for those with nodal or distant metastases decreases to 35% and 14%, respectively.[44] SOTRs have a poorer outcome compared with that of immunocompetent patients, with higher overall mortality as well as an elevated MCC-specific mortality rate.[83]

Patients with MCPyV+ MCC have a better prognosis than those with MCPyV− tumors. In a cohort study of 219 MCC patients, those with MCPyV oncoprotein seropositivity at diagnosis had a decreased risk of recurrence.[55] An additional study by Moshiri and colleagues[84] corroborated these findings. Fifty-three of the 282 patients in this cohort were negative for MCPyV. This virus-negative subset was found to have an increased risk of disease progression (hazard ratio [HR]: 1.77) and MCC-specific death (HR: 1.85).[84] Published data suggest that surrogate markers such as antibodies against MCPyV oncoproteins can serve as prognostic factors.[85] Therefore, the 2018 NCCN guidelines for MCC have recommended the incorporation of MCPyV oncoprotein antibody titer tests into the initial workup of MCC.[53] Specifically, antibody titers to the LT oncoprotein can be measured at baseline and if present can be used as surveillance to assess response to treatment and potentially detect early recurrence. This assay (AMERK test) is currently available in the United States through the University of Washington in Seattle. In Europe, it is available through la Faculte de Pharmacie de Tours, in France (*merkelcell.org*).

The programmed death-ligand 1 (PD-L1) immunosuppressive pathway is upregulated in MCC, and several trials of PD-L1 inhibitors have shown promising results.[86–88] Lipson and colleagues[89] studied PD-L1 expression and MCPyV DNA in 49 patients with MCC. Approximately half of the MCPyV+ specimens were PD-L1 positive, whereas none of MCPyV− specimens showed PD-L1 expression, suggesting that MCPyV could induce PD-L1 expression during immune response.[89]

Several histologic metrics have been identified as having potential prognostic significance. The presence of intratumoral CD3+ cells was independently associated with better overall survival and improved MCC-specific survival.[90] An additional study of 181 MCC tumors demonstrated that intratumoral CD8+ cell count is an independent prognostic factor of MCC.[41] Increased intratumoral CD8+ infiltration correlates with improved MCC-specific survival. There was no relationship established between the presence of intratumoral lymphocytes and MCPyV status. The traditional histologic tumor-infiltrating lymphocytes (TILs) are defined as lymphocytes present at the tumor-to-stroma interface. In contrast to intratumoral CD3+ or CD8+ cells, traditional histologic TILs have negligible independent prognostic value in the evaluation of survival in MCC patients.[41,91]

Other histologic features that have been associated with worse prognosis include expression of p63 in early stage (stage I--II) MCC tumors, as well as the presence of lymphovascular invasion.[92–94]

WAIT TIME BEFORE TRANSPLANTATION FOR MCC

Solid organ transplantation has made great advancement in recent years, allowing patients who would have previously died from organ failure to live longer than ever before. However, the scarcity of organ donations makes the task of organ stewardship extremely challenging. Pretransplantation history of cutaneous malignancy is correlated with the development of posttransplantation cutaneous malignancy. This results in significant morbidity and mortality in these patients. MCC has a high rate of local recurrence, distant metastasis, and poor 5-year overall survival rates, particularly in the immunosuppressed population. In an effort to decrease the risk in patients with a history of cutaneous malignancy, a consensus opinion from the International immunosuppression and Transplant Skin Cancer Collaborative (ITSCC) was released in 2016 and provided expert recommendations for pretransplantation wait times for MCC, cutaneous squamous cell carcinoma, and malignant melanoma.[95] These recommendations were based on the likelihood of tumor recurrence and disease-specific death. Survival rates for MCC are highly dependent on nodal status with the survival curves flattening and stabilizing between 2 and 3 years.[64] In patients with small tumors (<2 cm) and negative nodal status, 5-year survival rates approach 70%, whereas in patients with positive nodal status, the 5-year survival rate is 42%. Based on these findings, the committee advised against solid organ transplantation in patients with stage III or higher disease (positive nodal status). For patients with stage IIb or less, the recommendation was for a minimum pretransplantation wait time of 2 years after MCC treatment.

SUMMARY OF KEY POINTS

- MCC is an aggressive cutaneous malignancy with a propensity for locoregional recurrence and metastatic disease.
- The immunosuppressed population is particularly susceptible to developing MCC.
- SOTRs are a subset of this group that are known to have poor outcomes from this disease.
- Patient education, early diagnosis, multidisciplinary care, and aggressive initial treatment are paramount to improve overall outcomes.
- Additional research dedicated to this topic and emerging therapies provide hope for improved outcomes in SOTRs with MCC.

REFERENCES

1. Lemos B, Nghiem P. Merkel cell carcinoma: more deaths but still no pathway to blame. J Invest Dermatol. 2007;127(9):2100–3.
2. Akaike G, Akaike T, Fadl SA, Lachance K, Nghiem P, Behnia F. Imaging of Merkel cell carcinoma: what imaging experts should know. Radiographics. 2019;39(7):2069–84.
3. Pulitzer MP, Amin BD, Busam KJ. Merkel cell carcinoma: review. Adv Anat Pathol. 2009;16(3):135–44.
4. Arron ST, Canavan T, Yu SS. Organ transplant recipients with Merkel cell carcinoma have reduced progression-free, overall, and disease-specific survival independent of stage at presentation. J Am Acad Dermatol. 2014;71(4):684–90.
5. Paulson KG, Iyer JG, Blom A, Warton EM, Sokil M, Yelistratova L et al. Systemic immune suppression predicts diminished Merkel cell carcinoma-specific survival independent of stage. J Invest Dermatol. 2013;133(3):642–6.
6. Albores-Saavedra J, Batich K, Chable-Montero F, Sagy N, Schwartz AM, Henson DE. Merkel cell carcinoma demographics, morphology, and survival based on 3870 cases: a population based study. J Cutan Pathol. 2010;37(1):20–7.
7. Paulson KG, Park SY, Vandeven NA, Lachance K, Thomas H, Chapuis AG et al. Merkel cell carcinoma: current US incidence and projected increases based on changing demographics. J Am Acad Dermatol. 2018;78(3):457–63, e452.
8. Clarke CA, Robbins HA, Tatalovich Z, Lynch CF, Pawlish KS, Finch JL et al. Risk of Merkel cell carcinoma after solid organ transplantation. J Natl Cancer Inst. 2015;107(2).
9. Garrett GL, Blanc PD, Boscardin J, Lloyd AA, Ahmed RL, Anthony T et al. Incidence of and risk factors for skin cancer in organ transplant recipients in the United States. JAMA Dermatol. 2017;153(3):296–303.
10. Ma JE, Brewer JD. Merkel cell carcinoma in immunosuppressed patients. Cancers (Basel). 2014;6(3):1328–50.
11. Heath M, Jaimes N, Lemos B, Mostaghimi A, Wang LC, Penas PF et al. Clinical characteristics of Merkel cell carcinoma at diagnosis in 195 patients: the AEIOU features. J Am Acad Dermatol. 2008;58(3):375–81.
12. Engels EA, Frisch M, Goedert JJ, Biggar RJ, Miller RW. Merkel cell carcinoma and HIV infection. Lancet. 2002;359(9305):497–8.
13. Izikson L, Nornhold E, Iyer JG, Nghiem P, Zeitouni NC. Merkel cell carcinoma associated with HIV: review of 14 patients. AIDS 2011;25(1):119–21.
14. Wieland U, Silling S, Scola N, Potthoff A, Gambichler T, Brockmeyer NH et al. Merkel cell polyomavirus infection in HIV-positive men. Arch Dermatol. 2011;147(4):401–6.
15. Cook M, Baker K, Redman M et al. Differential outcomes among immunosuppressed patients with Merkel cell carcinoma: impact of immunosuppression type on cancer-specific and overall survival. Am J Clin Oncol. 2019;42(1):82–8.
16. Toker C. Trabecular carcinoma of the skin. Arch Dermatol. 1972 Jan;105(1):107–10.
17. Maricich SM, Wellnitz SA, Nelson AM, Lesniak DR et al. Merkel cells are essential for light-touch responses. Science. 2009 Jun 19;324(5934):1580–2.
18. Zur Hausen A, Rennspiess D, Winnepenninckx V, Speel EJ, Kurz AK. Early B-cell differentiation in Merkel cell carcinomas: clues to cellular ancestry. Cancer Res. 2013 Aug 15;73(16):4982–7.
19. Tilling T, Wladykowski E, Failla AV, Houdek P, Brandner JM, Moll I. Immunohistochemical analyses point to epidermal origin of human Merkel cells. Histochem Cell Biol. 2014 Apr;141(4):407–21.
20. Agelli M, Clegg LX, Becker JC, Rollison DE. The etiology and epidemiology of merkel cell carcinoma. Curr Probl Cancer. 2010 Jan–Feb;34(1):14–37.
21. Robertson JP, Liang ES, Martin RC. Epidemiology of Merkel cell carcinoma in New Zealand: a population-based study. Br J Dermatol. 2015 Sep;173(3):835–7.
22. Starrett GJ, Marcelus C, Cantalupo PG, Katz JP et al. Merkel cell polyomavirus exhibits dominant control of the tumor genome and transcriptome in virus-associated Merkel cell carcinoma. mBio. 2017 Jan 3;8(1):e02079–16.
23. Goh G, Walradt T, Markarov V, Blom A et al. Mutational landscape of MCPyV-positive and MCPyV-negative Merkel cell carcinomas with implications for immunotherapy. Oncotarget. 2016 Jan 19;7(3):3403–15.
24. Wong SQ, Waldeck K, Vergara IA, Schroder J, Madore J, Wilmott JS et al. UV-associated mutations underlie the etiology of MCV-negative Merkel cell carcinomas. Cancer Res. 2015;75(24):5228–34.
25. Feng H, Shuda M, Chang Y, Moore PS. Clonal integration of a polyomavirus in human Merkel cell carcinoma. Science. 2008;319(5866):1096–100.

26. Coggshall K, Tello TL, North JP, Yu SS. Merkel cell carcinoma: an update and review: pathogenesis, diagnosis, and staging. J Am Acad Dermatol. 2018 Mar;78(3):433–42.
27. Houben R, Adam C, Baeurle A, Hesbacher S et al. An intact retinoblastoma protein-binding site in Merkel cell polyomavirus large T antigen is required for promoting growth of Merkel cell carcinoma cells. Int J Cancer. 2012 Feb 15;130(4):847–56.
28. Verhaegen ME, Mangelberger D, Harms PW, Eberl M et al. Merkel cell polyomavirus small T antigen initiates Merkel cell carcinoma-like tumor development in mice. Cancer Res. 2017 Jun 15;77(12):3151–7.
29. Tello TL, Coggshall K, Yom SS, Yu SS. Merkel cell carcinoma: an update and review: current and future therapy. J Am Acad Dermatol. 2018 Mar;78(3):445–54.
30. Chen T, Hedman L, Mattila PS, Jartti T et al. Serological evidence of Merkel cell polyomavirus primary infections in childhood. J Clin Virol. 2011 Feb;50(2):125–9.
31. Tolstov YL, Pastrana DV, Feng H, Becker JC et al. Human Merkel cell polyomavirus infection II MCV is a common human infection that can be detected by conformational capsid epitope immunoassays. Int J Cancer. 2009 Sep 15;125(6):1250–6.
32. Church CD, Nghiem P. How does the Merkel polyomavirus lead to a lethal cancer? Many answers, many questions, and a new mouse model. J Invest Dermatol. 2015 May;135(5):1221–4.
33. Husseiny MI, Anastasi B, Singer J, Lacey SF. A comparative study of Merkel cell, BK and JC polyomavirus infections in renal transplant recipients and healthy subjects. J Clin Virol. 2010;49(2):137–40.
34. Signorini L, Belingheri M, Ambrogi F, Pagani E, Binda S, Ticozzi R et al. High frequency of Merkel cell polyomavirus DNA in the urine of kidney transplant recipients and healthy controls. J Clin Virol. 2014;61(4): 565–70.
35. Bergallo M, Costa C, Terlizzi ME, Astegiano S, Curtoni A, Solidoro P et al. Quantitative detection of the new polyomaviruses KI, WU and Merkel cell virus in transbronchial biopsies from lung transplant recipients. J Clin Pathol. 2010;63(8):722–5.
36. Kuschal C, Thoms KM, Schubert S, Schafer A, Boeckmann L, Schon MP et al. Skin cancer in organ transplant recipients: effects of immunosuppressive medications on DNA repair. Exp Dermatol. 2012;21(1):2–6.
37. Muirhead R, Ritchie DM. Partial regression of Merkel cell carcinoma in response to withdrawal of azathioprine in an immunosuppression-induced case of metastatic Merkel cell carcinoma. Clin Oncol (R Coll Radiol). 2007;19(1):96.
38. O'Rourke MG, Bell JR. Merkel cell tumor with spontaneous regression. J Dermatol Surg Oncol. 1986 Sep;12(9):994, 996, 1000.
39. Wooff JC, Trites JR, Walsh NM, Bullock MJ. Complete spontaneous regression of metastatic Merkel cell carcinoma: a case report and review of the literature. Am J Dermatopathol. 2010 Aug;32(6):614–17.
40. Paulson KG, Iyer JG, Simonson WT, Blom A, Thibodeau RM, Schmidt M et al. CD8+ lymphocyte intratumoral infiltration as a stage-independent predictor of merkel cell carcinoma survival: a population-based study. Am J Clin Pathol. 2014 Oct;142(4):452–8.
41. Paulson KG, Iyer JG, Tegeder AR, Thibodeau R, Schelter J, Koba S et al. Transcriptome-wide studies of merkel cell carcinoma and validation of intratumoral CD8+ lymphocyte invasion as an independent predictor of survival. J Clin Oncol. 2011 Apr 20;29(12):1539–46.
42. Koba S, Paulson KG, Nagase K, Tegeder A, Thibodeau R, Iyer JG et al. Diagnostic biopsy does not commonly induce intratumoral CD8 T cell infiltration in Merkel cell carcinoma. PLoS One. 2012;7(7):e41465.
43. Zeitouni NC, Giordano CN, Kane JM. In-transit Merkel cell carcinoma treated with isolated limb perfusion or isolated limb infusion: a case series of 12 patients. Dermatol Surg. 2011;37(3):357–64.
44. Harms KL, Healy MA, Nghiem P, Sober AJ, Johnson TM, Bichakjian CK et al. Analysis of prognostic factors from 9387 Merkel cell carcinoma cases forms the basis for the new 8th edition AJCC staging system. Ann Surg Oncol. 2016;23(11):3564–71.
45. Weedon D. Neural and neuroendocrine tumors. Philadelphia, PA: Churchill Livingstone, Elsevier; 2010.
46. Pulitzer MP, Brannon AR, Berger MF, Louis P, Scott SN, Jungbluth AA et al. Cutaneous squamous and neuroendocrine carcinoma: genetically and immunohistochemically different from Merkel cell carcinoma. Mod Pathol. 2015;28(8):1023–32.
47. Martin B, Poblet E, Rios JJ, Kazakov D, Kutzner H, Brenn T et al. Merkel cell carcinoma with divergent differentiation: histopathological and immunohistochemical study of 15 cases with PCR analysis for Merkel cell polyomavirus. Histopathology. 2013;62(5):711–22.
48. Wong HH, Wang J. Merkel cell carcinoma. Arch Pathol Lab Med. 2010 Nov;134(11):1711–16.
49. Pasternak S, Carter MD, Ly TY, Doucette S, Walsh NM. Immunohistochemical profiles of different subsets of Merkel cell carcinoma. Hum Pathol. 2018;82:232–8.

50. Warner TF, Uno H, Hafez GR, Burgess J, Bolles C, Lloyd RV, Oka M. Merkel cells and Merkel cell tumors: ultrastructure, immunocytochemistry and review of the literature. Cancer. 1983 Jul 15;52(2):238–45.
51. Erstad DJ, Cusack JC. Mutational analysis of merkel cell carcinoma. Cancers (Basel). 2014;6(4):2116–36.
52. Swick BL, Srikantha R, Messingham KN. Specific analysis of KIT and PDGFR-alpha expression and mutational status in Merkel cell carcinoma. J Cutan Pathol. 2013;40(7):623–30.
53. Bichakjian CK, Olencki T, Aaso AZ et al. NCCN clinical practice guidelines in oncology for Merkel cell carcinoma. National Comprehensive Cancer Network; 2016. Available from: https://www.researchgate.net/publication/325704358_Merkel_Cell_Carcinoma_Version_12018_NCCN_Clinical_Practice_Guidelines_in_Oncology.
54. Poulsen M, Macfarlane D, Veness M et al. Prospective analysis of the utility of 18-FDG PET in Merkel cell carcinoma of the skin: a trans tasman radiation oncology group study, TROG 09:03. J Med Imaging Radiat Oncol. 2018;62(3):412–19.
55. Paulson KG, Lewis CW, Redman MW et al. Viral oncoprotein antibodies as a marker for recurrence of Merkel cell carcinoma: a prospective validation study. Cancer. 2017;123(8):1464–74.
56. Lachance K, Akaike T, Cahill K et al. 590 detecting Merkel cell carcinoma recurrence using a blood test: outcomes from 774 patients. J Invest Dermatol. 2019;139:s101.
57. Ratner D, Nelson BR, Brown MD, Johnson TM. Merkel cell carcinoma. J Am Acad Dermatol. 1993;29(2 Pt 1):143–56.
58. Singh B, Qureshi MM, Truong MT, Sahni D. Demographics and outcomes of stage I and II Merkel cell carcinoma treated with Mohs micrographic surgery compared with wide local excision in the national cancer database. J Am Acad Dermatol. 2018 Jul;79(1):126–34.
59. Haag ML, Glass LF, Fenske NA. Merkel cell carcinoma: diagnosis and treatment. Dermatol Surg. 1995;21(8):669–83.
60. Gunaratne DA, Howle JR, Veness MJ. Sentinel lymph node biopsy in Merkel cell carcinoma: a 15-year institutional experience and statistical analysis of 721 reported cases. Br J Dermatol. 2016;174(2):273–81.
61. Allen PJ, Bowne WB, Jaques DP, Brennan MF, Busam K, Coit DG. Merkel cell carcinoma: prognosis and treatment of patients from a single institution. J Clin Oncol. 2005;23(10):2300–9.
62. Iyer JG, Storer BE, Paulson KG et al. Relationships among primary tumor size, number of involved nodes, and survival for 8044 cases of Merkel cell carcinoma. J Am Acad Dermatol. 2014;70(4):637–43.
63. Smith FO, Yue B, Marzban SS et al. Both tumor depth and diameter are predictive of sentinel lymph node status and survival in Merkel cell carcinoma. Cancer. 2015;121(18):3252–60.
64. Lemos BD, Storer BE, Iyer JG, Phillips JL, Bichakjian CK, Fang LC et al. Pathologic nodal evaluation improves prognostic accuracy in Merkel cell carcinoma: analysis of 5823 cases as the basis of the first consensus staging system. J Am Acad Dermatol. 2010;63(5):751–61.
65. Mehrany K, Otley CC, Weenig RH, Phillips PK, Roenigk RK, Nguyen TH. A meta-analysis of the prognostic significance of sentinel lymph node status in Merkel cell carcinoma. Dermatol Surg. 2002;28(2):113–17.
66. Pape E, Rezvoy N, Penel N et al. Radiotherapy alone for Merkel cell carcinoma: a comparative and retrospective study of 25 patients. J Am Acad Dermatol. 2011;65(5):983–90.
67. Leonard JH, Ramsay JR, Kearsley JH, Birrell GW. Radiation sensitivity of Merkel cell carcinoma cell lines. Int J Radiat Oncol Biol Phys. 1995;32(5):1401–7.
68. Harrington C, Kwan W. Outcomes of Merkel cell carcinoma treated with radiotherapy without radical surgical excision. Ann Surg Oncol. 2014;21(11):3401–5.
69. Veness M, Foote M, Gebski V, Poulsen M. The role of radiotherapy alone in patients with Merkel cell carcinoma: reporting the Australian experience of 43 patients. Int J Radiat Oncol Biol Phys. 2010;78(3):703–9.
70. Fang LC, Lemos B, Douglas J, Iyer J, Nghiem P. Radiation monotherapy as regional treatment for lymph node-positive Merkel cell carcinoma. Cancer. 2010;116(7):1783–90.
71. Bhatia S, Storer BE, Iyer JG et al. Adjuvant radiation therapy and chemotherapy in Merkel cell carcinoma: survival analyses of 6908 cases from the national cancer data base. J Natl Cancer Inst. 2016 May 31;108(9):djw042.
72. Mojica P, Smith D, Ellenhorn JDI. Adjuvant radiation therapy is associated with improved survival in Merkel cell carcinoma of the skin. J Clin Oncol. 2007;25:1043–7.
73. Jouary T, Leyral C, Dreno B et al. Adjuvant prophylactic regional radiotherapy versus observation in stage I Merkel cell carcinoma: a multicentric prospective randomized study. Ann Oncol. 2012;23:1074–80.
74. Fields RC, Busam KJ, Chou JF et al. Recurrence after complete resection and selective use of adjuvant therapy for stage I through III Merkel cell carcinoma. Cancer. 2012;118(13):3311–20.
75. Tseng YD, Nguyen MH, Baker K et al. Effect of patient immune status on the efficacy of radiation therapy and recurrence-free survival among 805 patients with Merkel cell carcinoma. Int J Radiat Oncol Biol Phys. 2018;102(2):330–9.

76. Garrett GL, Zargham H, Schulman JM, Jafarian F, Yu SS, Arron ST. Merkel cell carcinoma in organ transplant recipients: case reports and review of the literature. JAAD Case Rep. 2015 Nov 24;1(6):S29–32.
77. Iyer JG, Parvathaneni U, Gooley T et al. Single-fraction radiation therapy in patients with metastatic Merkel cell carcinoma. Cancer Med. 2015;4(8):1161–70.
78. Tai PT, Yu E, Winquist E et al. Chemotherapy in neuroendocrine/Merkel cell carcinoma of the skin: case series and review of 204 cases. J Clin Oncol. 2000;18(12):2493–9.
79. Colunga A, Pulliam T, Nghiem P. Merkel cell carcinoma in the age of immunotherapy: facts and hopes. Clin Cancer Res. 2018 May 1;24(9):2035–43.
80. Kaufman HL, Russell J, Hamid O, Bhatia S, Terheyden P, D'Angelo SP et al. Avelumab in patients with chemotherapy-refractory metastatic Merkel cell carcinoma: a multicentre, single-group, open-label, phase 2 trial. Lancet Oncol. 2016 Oct;17(10):1374–5.
81. Fisher J, Zeitouni N, Fan W, Samie FH. Immune checkpoint inhibitor therapy in solid organ transplant recipients: a patient-centered systematic review. J Am Acad Dermatol. 2020 Jun;82(6):1490–500.
82. d'Izarny-Gargas T, Durrbach A, Zaidan M. Efficacy and tolerance of immune checkpoint inhibitors in transplant patients with cancer: a systematic review. Am J Transplant. 2020 Sep;20(9):2457–65.
83. Asgari MM, Sokil MM, Warton EM, Iyer J, Paulson KG, Nghiem P. Effect of host, tumor, diagnostic, and treatment variables on outcomes in a large cohort with Merkel cell carcinoma. JAMA Dermatol. 2014;150(7):716–23.
84. Moshiri AS, Doumani R, Yelistratova L et al. Polyomavirus-negative Merkel cell carcinoma: a more aggressive subtype based on analysis of 282 cases using multimodal tumor virus detection. J Invest Dermatol. 2017;137(4):819–27.
85. Paulson KG, Carter JJ, Johnson LG, Cahill KW, Iyer JG, Schrama D et al. Antibodies to Merkel cell polyomavirus T antigen oncoproteins reflect tumor burden in Merkel cell carcinoma patients. Cancer Res. 2010;70(21):8388–97.
86. Nghiem PT, Bhatia S, Lipson EJ, Kudchadkar RR, Miller NJ, Annamalai L et al. PD-1 blockade with pembrolizumab in advanced Merkel-cell carcinoma. N Engl J Med. 2016;374(26):2542–52.
87. Nghiem P, Bhatia S, Lipson EJ, Sharfman WH, Kudchadkar RR, Brohl AS et al. Durable tumor regression and overall survival in patients with advanced Merkel cell carcinoma receiving pembrolizumab as first-line therapy. J Clin Oncol 2019;37(9):693–702.
88. Topalian SL, Bhatia S, Amin A, Kudchadkar RR, Sharfman WH, Lebbe C et al. Neoadjuvant nivolumab for patients with resectable Merkel cell carcinoma in the checkmate 358 trial. J Clin Oncol. 2020;38(22):2476–87.
89. Lipson EJ, Vincent JG, Loyo M, Kagohara LT, Luber BS, Wang H et al. PD-L1 expression in the Merkel cell carcinoma microenvironment: association with inflammation, Merkel cell polyomavirus and overall survival. Cancer Immunol Res. 2013;1(1):54–63.
90. Sihto H, Joensuu H. Tumor-infiltrating lymphocytes and outcome in Merkel cell carcinoma, a virus-associated cancer. Oncoimmunology. 2012;1(8):1420–1.
91. Feldmeyer L, Hudgens CW, Ray-Lyons G, Nagarajan P, Aung PP, Curry JL et al. Density, distribution, and composition of immune infiltrates correlate with survival in Merkel cell carcinoma. Clin Cancer Res. 2016;22(22):5553–63.
92. Stetsenko GY, Malekirad J, Paulson KG, Iyer JG, Thibodeau RM, Nagase K. p63 expression in Merkel cell carcinoma predicts poorer survival yet may have limited clinical utility. Am J Clin Pathol. 2013 Dec;140(6):838–44.
93. Fields RC, Busam KJ, Chou JF, Panageas KS, Pulitzer MP, Allen PJ et al. Five hundred patients with Merkel cell carcinoma evaluated at a single institution. Ann Surg. 2011;254(3):465–73; discussion 473–65.
94. Asioli S, Righi A, de Biase D, Morandi L, Caliendo V, Picciotto F et al. Expression of p63 is the sole independent marker of aggressiveness in localised (stage I-II) Merkel cell carcinomas. Mod Pathol. 2011;24(11):1451–61.
95. Zwald F, Leitenberger J, Zeitouni N, Soon S, Brewer J, Arron S et al. Recommendations for solid organ transplantation for transplant candidates with a pretransplant diagnosis of cutaneous squamous cell carcinoma, Merkel cell carcinoma and melanoma: a consensus opinion from the international transplant skin cancer collaborative (ITSCC). Am J Transplant. 2016;16(2):407–13.

Rare Skin Cancers *Kaposi's Sarcoma, Sebaceous Carcinoma, Atypical Fibroxanthoma, and Dermatofibrosarcoma Protuberans*

12

Kimberly L. Brady

INTRODUCTION

The skin cancers discussed in previous chapters occur relatively frequently in both the immunocompetent and the solid organ transplant recipient (SOTR) populations. Therefore, there is substantially more data and evidence-based literature regarding these tumors. In contrast, the malignancies discussed in this chapter are uncommonly or rarely encountered in both immunocompetent patients and immunocompromised SOTRs. Consequently, data are lacking and much of the literature relies on individual case reports and summaries of cases. Although infrequent, these cutaneous malignancies are still important considerations in the differential diagnosis of cutaneous neoplasms in the setting of organ transplantation. This chapter discusses rare skin cancers in SOTRs including Kaposi's sarcoma (KS), sebaceous carcinoma (SC), atypical fibroxanthoma (AFX), and dermatofibrosarcoma protuberans (DFSP).

KAPOSI'S SARCOMA

Epidemiology

The incidence of KS is increased by 84- to 500-fold in SOTRs compared with that in non-SOTRs.[1–3] The prevalence of posttransplant KS varies by geographic area and seems to be related to the geographic

 DOI: 10.1201/9781003001461-12

distribution of human herpesvirus type 8 (HHV-8) infection.[4] The prevalence of KS specifically in the renal transplant population has been reported to occur in up to 11.8% of patients, with higher rates seen in Africa, the Middle East, and Mediterranean regions.[5–12] According to the Collaborative Transplantation Research Group of Ile de France (GCIF) registry, which contains European data, prevalence is significantly higher among liver transplant recipients (1.24%) compared with that in kidney transplant recipients (0.45%) and heart transplant recipients (0.41%).[13] The Cincinnati Transplant Tumor Registry (CTTR), now known as the Israel Penn International Transplant Tumor Registry, showed that KS represented 5.7% of neoplasms occurring as de novo malignancies in 8191 organ transplant patients.[14] In a registry-based study in the United States (US), Cahoon et al.[15] found a significantly increased risk of KS in SOTRs associated with male sex, non-white race, non-US citizens, lung transplant recipients, and older age at the time of transplant. KS risk appears to decrease with time since transplant and also with recent calendar year.[15]

There are differences in the patterns of presentation between the US and the international SOTR populations who develop KS.[16] In one of the largest studies of posttransplant KS, Woodle et al.[16] analyzed data from 63 US patients and 305 international patients from the Israel Penn Transplant Tumor Registry. They found posttransplant KS in US patients was diagnosed at a mean age of 46.9 years and the median time to diagnosis was 19.3 months. In contrast, international patients had a mean age at diagnosis of 41.9 years and a shorter median time from transplant to diagnosis of 12.2 months.[16] Worldwide, the male to female ratio was about 3:1.[12,14,16]

Clinical Presentation

KS occurs as one of four forms: the classical form, the endemic form, the epidemic form in acquired immunodeficiency syndrome (AIDS) patients, and the posttransplant form in SOTRs. Each form of KS presents with different clinical patterns and can occur as cutaneous lesions, visceral lesions, or mixed cutaneous and visceral lesions.[4,17] Classical KS, which typically affects elderly men of Mediterranean descent, presents with slowly progressive, bluish-red, well-demarcated, painless macules, plaques, and nodules mostly on the lower extremities, as well as lymph node involvement.[4,17,18] Visceral involvement is uncommon. Endemic KS occurs in sub-Saharan Africa and predominantly affects men of a younger age group.[4,17] Nodules on the feet and legs may grow rapidly and ulcerate. Epidemic KS is an AIDS-related illness that tends to have extensive skin and visceral involvement.[17] Posttransplant KS may occur in immunocompromised SOTRs.[4,17] KS typically occurs in the early posttransplant period, with the highest incidence in the first year and the majority of cases occurring within the first 3 years.[15]

Posttransplant KS has a similar clinical appearance to that of classical KS. Cutaneous lesions begin as multifocal, dark blue or purplish macules and progress to become coalescent nodules and plaques on the feet and lower extremities[4,9,19] (Figure 12.1a, b). Approximately 90% of transplant recipients with KS have cutaneous and/or mucosal lesions.[14,18,20] Visceral disease predominantly affects the lymph nodes, gastrointestinal tract, and lungs.[19] The frequency of visceral involvement can vary depending on the type of allograft and geographic location. Visceral involvement occurs in up to 25% to 30% of renal transplant recipients and 50% of heart and liver transplant recipients.[13,20,21] In the US, patients present primarily with only cutaneous involvement and have visceral involvement (either visceral alone or mixed pattern) in 27% of cases, whereas international patients have a higher rate of visceral involvement (47%).[16]

KS is a tumor of lymphatic endothelial cell origin.[22] Several factors contribute to the development of posttransplant KS, including immunosuppression and HHV-8 seropositivity.[4] Administration of immunosuppressive medications may lead to the reactivation of HHV-8 in patients who were seropositive prior to transplantation.[4] More than 80% of SOTRs with posttransplant KS are seropositive for HHV-8 prior to undergoing transplantation.[23] Transplant patients with antibodies against HHV-8 have an increased risk of developing KS. Italian studies of renal transplant recipients have demonstrated 15%–28% of patients with antibodies to HHV-8 antigen prior to transplantation.[23–25] Of the seropositive group, 15%–23% developed

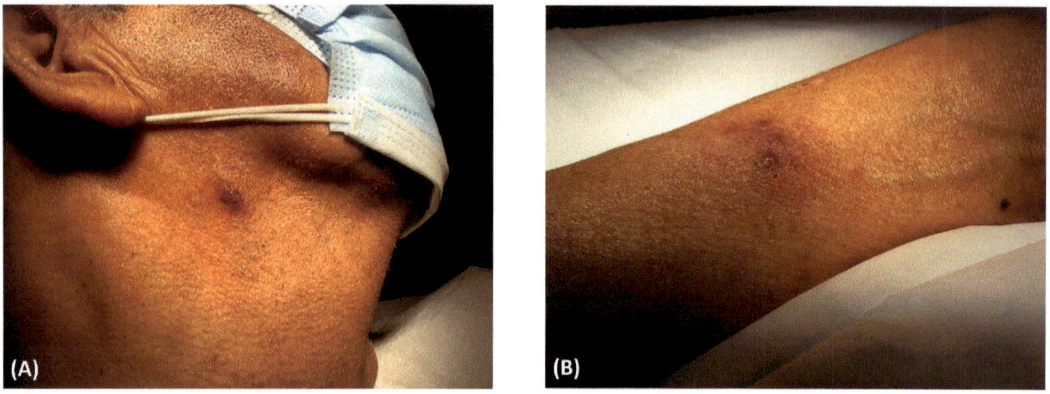

FIGURE 12.1 Several Kaposi's sarcoma lesions that developed within the first-year post lung (**a, b**) transplantation. (Nathalie C. Zeitouni, MDCM.)

posttransplant KS, whereas only 0.7%–1.1% of the seronegative patients developed posttransplant KS.[23,24] Alternatively, patients can acquire a new HHV-8 infection, either from the donated organ, as a primary infection, or rarely through blood.[4] The seroconversion rate after transplantation is 16%–25%.[23–25]

Histology

The clinical diagnosis of KS should be confirmed with histology. In the early patch stage, KS histology is characterized by irregular, jagged vascular channels surrounding preexisting blood vessels. As the tumor evolves, diffuse vascular and cellular infiltrates are seen in the dermis and extend into the subcutaneous fat. Infiltrating cells arranged in fascicles become more spindled and are observed in close proximity to slit-like vessels (Figure 12.2a, b). Spindled cells show variable nuclear pleomorphism and reveal occasional mitotic figures (Figure 12.2c). An inflammatory infiltrate consisting of predominantly lymphocytes and plasma cells, in addition to extravasated red blood cells and hemosiderin deposits, can be found in the dermis.[9,19,26] CD31 and D2–40, which are markers for lymphatic endothelium, as well as CD34 and factor VIII-related antigen can be identified by immunohistochemical stains[21,26] (Figure 12.2d). Demonstration of HHV-8 in the tissue using LNA-1 antigen can confirm the diagnosis of KS[21,26] (Figure 12.2e).

Management

Like other skin cancers in SOTRs, KS can be significantly affected by the level and type of immunosuppression. Patients who are treated with calcineurin inhibitor-based immunosuppression regimens, such as

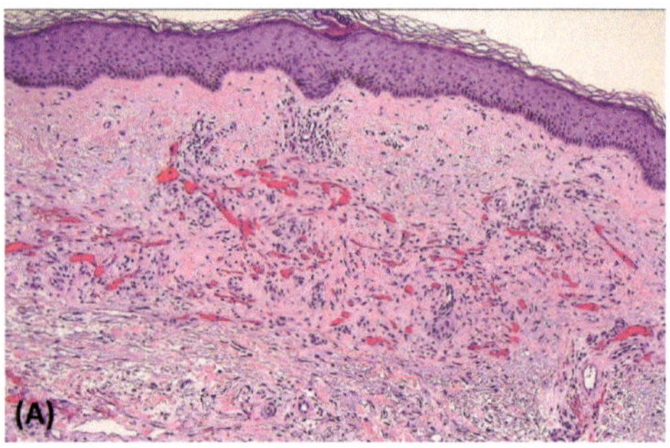

FIGURE 12.2A (40×) Neoplastic blood vessels and spindle cells surround preexisting blood vessels and adnexal structures. (David Glembocki, MD.)

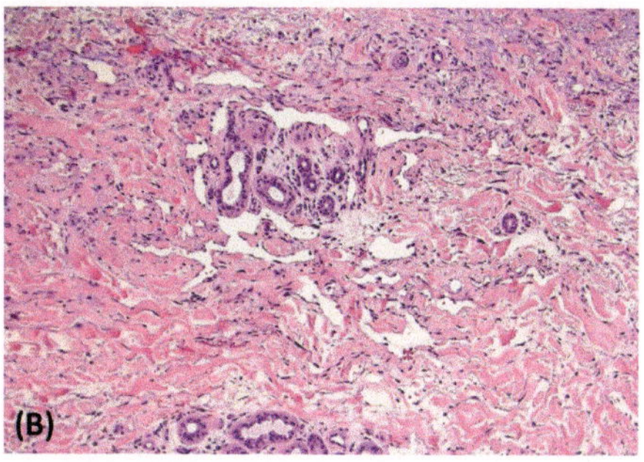

FIGURE 12.2B (100×) Thin-walled neoplastic blood vessels dissecting between collagen bundles and around eccrine glands. (David Glembocki, MD.)

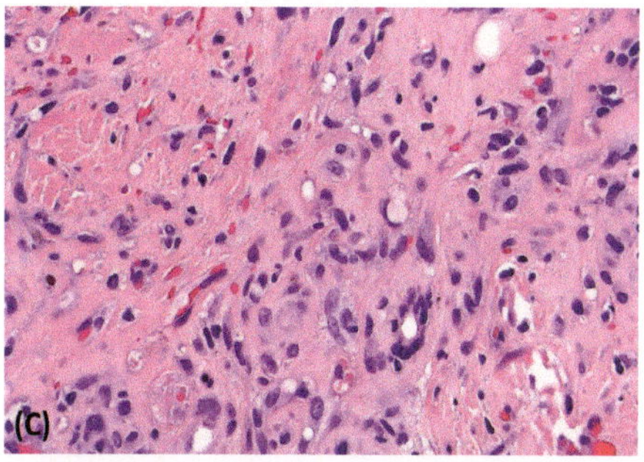

FIGURE 12.2C (400×) Neoplastic blood vessels lined by atypical hyperchromatic endothelial cells are accompanied by atypical spindle cells with cytoplasmic eosinophilic hyaline globules. (David Glembocki, MD.)

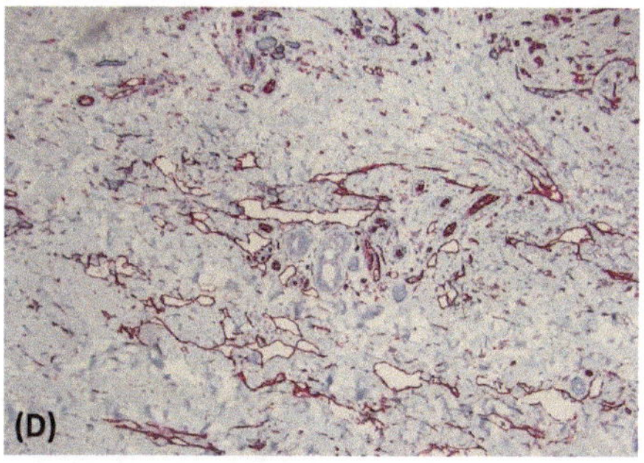

FIGURE 12.2D (100×) CD31 highlights the infiltrative growth pattern of the neoplastic blood vessels. (David Glembocki, MD.)

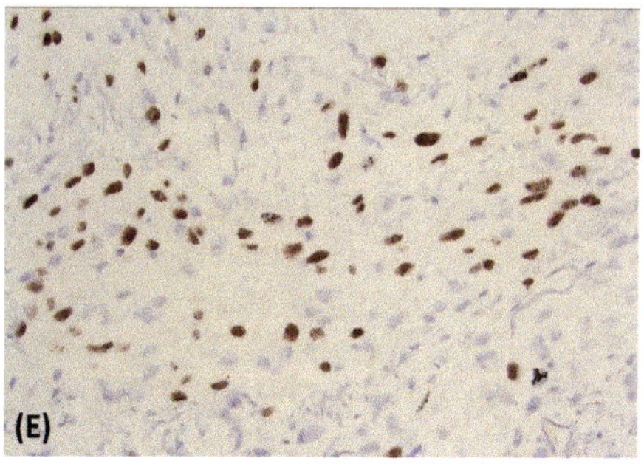

FIGURE 12.2E (100×) IHC for HHV-8 demonstrates nuclear positivity. (David Glembocki, MD.)

cyclosporine and tacrolimus, are at higher risk for development of KS.[4] The initial management strategy for posttransplant KS is decreasing the intensity of immunosuppression.[4,14,17,18,22,27] Another option is to switch the immunosuppression from calcineurin inhibitors to mammalian target of rapamycin (mTOR) inhibitors, such as sirolimus or everolimus.[4,6,22,27]

Otherwise, KS in SOTRs is managed similarly to classical KS.[4,14,17,18,22] Localized disease can be treated with surgical excision, cryotherapy, or laser ablation.[4,17,18,21,22] Topical treatments, such as imiquimod 5% and alitretinoin 0.1%, have been shown to be of benefit in some patients with KS.[4,22] Also, partial responses have been seen with intralesional chemotherapy with vinblastine and intralesional interferon.[17,22] Patients should be initially evaluated for the extent of disease with imaging such as positron emission tomography/computed tomography (PET/CT). Patients who have visceral disease or more extensive disease may require systemic chemotherapy. A variety of systemic chemotherapy agents can be used alone or in combination and can include doxorubicin (pegylated, liposomal), vinblastine (±bleomycin), paclitaxel, etoposide, vinorelbine, and gemcitabine.[22,27–29] Some authors have reported treatment of KS with radiotherapy and/or interferon,[14] but others have suggested avoidance because of the increased risk of other cutaneous malignancies from radiation and the potential allograft rejection from systemic interferon.[4,18,21] Antiviral drugs have not shown *in vivo* effect on KS.[21]

HHV-8 screening of organ donors and/or recipients is still debated. Some authors have proposed HHV-8 serologic screening those from highly HHV-8 endemic areas in order to identify and monitor patients who are at increased risk for posttransplant HHV-8-related disease.[25] However, the preferred nucleic acid test, the frequency of monitoring, and a clinically relevant viral load threshold have not yet been established.[30]

Prognosis

The course of KS is chronic and tends to be rather indolent. According to the CTTR, treatment by various means and combinations (including immunosuppression reduction, radiation, surgery, chemotherapy, alpha-interferon, and antivirals) led to complete remission in 53% of those with non-visceral disease and in 27% of those with visceral disease.[14] In a recently published multicenter retrospective cohort study, Delyon et al.[27] reported that 83% of patients had a response to treatment at 6 months, including 40% with complete responses and 43% with partial responses. Complete response was more frequent in patients with non-visceral disease (47%) than in those with visceral disease (30%), but partial response was more frequent in patients with visceral disease (51%) than in those with non-visceral disease (31%). At 6 months, 11% of patients had progression of disease.

An increase in immunosuppression may lead to disease progression, and a reduction in the level of immunosuppression can lead to a reduction or complete remission of lesions. The CTTR demonstrated that reduction of immunosuppression alone led to complete remission in 16.6% of total cases, including those with visceral disease (16.9%) and non-visceral disease (16.1%).[14] A more recent study by Cattaneo et al.[12] determined that 45% of patients experienced regression when immunosuppression was reduced, although some of these patients had other treatments in conjunction with immunosuppression reduction. In a multicenter retrospective cohort study, Delyon et al.[27] found that immunosuppression was minimized in almost all patients, and 50% of complete responses were obtained by a decrease in immunosuppression alone.

A potential risk in decreasing immunosuppression is loss of the allograft to rejection or impaired function. According to the CTTR, in 34 renal transplant patients with reduction or cessation of immunosuppression, 20 lost their allograft to rejection, 2 had impaired renal function, and 12 maintained stable renal function.[14] Cattaneo et al.[12] demonstrated that 4 of 20 patients lost their grafts because of end-stage renal disease. Delyon et al.[27] reported that 34 of 145 grafts were lost, but noted that the hazard ratio of graft rejection did not differ for conversion to mTOR inhibitors versus no conversion to mTOR inhibitors. It is possible for renal transplant recipients to return to hemodialysis in the case of end-stage renal disease. However, immunosuppression reduction in nonrenal transplant recipients is more difficult to manage because loss of the allograft, such as a heart or liver, results in death unless another transplant can be performed.

In the cohort presented by Delyon et al.,[27] less than 20% of patients received chemotherapy for KS with visceral involvement and/or rapid progression. Patients with visceral disease who were treated with chemotherapy showed complete response in 28% of cases and partial response in 44% of cases. In those with visceral disease who were not treated with chemotherapy, 55% had complete responses and 32% had partial responses.[27]

The estimated survival rate is 69%–82% at 5 years and 64% at 10 years but varies with the extent of disease.[16,27] Death can occur from infection, rejection, or KS itself. Patients with visceral involvement have a significant reduction in survival compared with that in those with only cutaneous disease. International and US patients with only cutaneous disease have a survival rate of 90% and 92% at 1 year, respectively.[16] In comparison, international and US patients with visceral forms of the disease have a survival rate of 70% and 83% at one year, respectively.[16] Additionally, patients with heart transplants appear to have a shorter survival compared with that of those with kidney transplants.[16]

SEBACEOUS CARCINOMA

Epidemiology

SC is an uncommon adnexal tumor that can present sporadically or in association with Muir-Torre Syndrome (MTS). According to two large retrospective analyses, first, at the Mayo Clinic in Rochester, MN, by Hoss et al.,[31] and second, at the Barts and London National Health Service Trust by Harwood et al.,[32] the prevalence of sebaceous carcinoma among SOTRs was estimated to be 0.6%—0.9%. The study by Harwood et al. revealed that in transplant recipients, appendageal tumors occurred with increased frequency, the tumors were more commonly malignant, and sebaceous carcinoma and other sebaceous tumors in particular were significantly increased.[32] More recently, a population study of SC among SOTRs in the United States, from 1987–2017, found a 25-fold increase in the incidence of SC. The incidence was particularly elevated in lung transplant patients and after a cutaneous squamous cell carcinoma diagnosis.[33]

Clinical Presentation

SCs can occur in any skin containing sebaceous glands, especially those with a higher density of sebaceous glands, such as the eyelids, face, scalp, and neck.[34] In the general population, SC presents as a painless pink or yellow nodule, although the clinical features can vary.[34] Although the periorbital region is a common location for sebaceous carcinoma, about 60.7% are extraorbital[34] (Figure 12.3).

In SOTRs, the mean age at diagnosis of SC is 64–66 years old,[31,32] and the median time from transplantation to diagnosis is 6.0 years.[31] The majority of SCs in SOTRs are located in extraocular sites.[31,32,35–38] According to Hoss et al.,[31] the mean tumor size was 1.67 cm. Immunosuppression regimens varied among the patients and included prednisone, mycophenolate mofetil, tacrolimus, azathioprine, or cyclosporine.[31,32]

It is unclear why appendageal tumors and specifically SC are overrepresented in transplant recipients. However, it is thought that immunosuppressive medications, ultraviolet radiation, genetic factors, and human papillomavirus infection are possible factors contributing to tumor growth.[32] Immunosuppressive medications can reduce immune surveillance, and it is hypothesized that they could also exert direct carcinogenic effects.[32] In particular, azathioprine may have a more prominent role in SC development.[36]

MTS is a variant of Lynch syndrome and is characterized by a sebaceous neoplasm or keratoacanthoma in association with visceral malignancy.[34] The affected genes are *MLH1*, *MSH2*, and *MSH6*, which play a role in DNA mismatch repair. Ineffective mismatch repair results in microsatellite instability (MSI), which then leads to tumor formation. Immunosuppression associated with solid organ

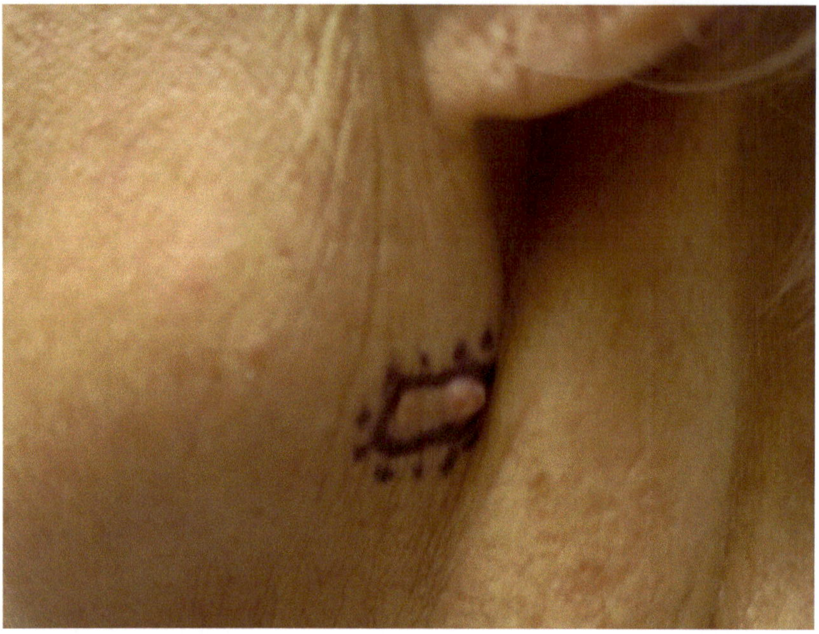

FIGURE 12.3 A pink-yellow papule along the jawline of a renal transplant recipient was diagnosed as a sebaceous carcinoma. (Kimberly L. Brady, MD.)

transplantation can lead to an unmasking phenomenon of a latent MTS phenotype, which may partially account for the increased frequency of sebaceous tumors with MSI in immunosuppressed patients.[36] This unmasking phenomenon has been demonstrated in cases of SOTRs who developed benign and malignant sebaceous tumors and later have genetic testing for systemic germline mutations to confirm a diagnosis of MTS.[37,38,42]

Hoss et al.[31] found that three of six SCs in transplant recipients had loss of at least one mismatch repair protein in their biopsied tumor, and two of the patients were suspected of having MTS. Harwood et al.[36] confirmed the presence of MSI in three of six sebaceous carcinomas from renal transplant recipients, one of whom fulfilled MTS criteria. However, not all SOTRs with sebaceous tumors with MSI have MTS, and this suggests that there is an alternative mechanism whereby SCs develop outside of the context of MTS.

Histology

SC can be diagnosed by histologic examination.[39] Sebocytes with cytologic atypia and variable degrees of differentiation are arranged in lobules or sheets that are separated by a fibrovascular stroma. The cells may appear foamy or vacuolated. Periorbital SC shows pagetoid growth in 24%–50% Staining for oil-red-O and Sudan black reveals lipids in vacuolated cells. SC has an immunohistochemistry profile positive for nuclear factor XIIIa, androgen receptor, adipophilin, perilipin, and ± Ber-EP4.[40]

Management

Certain individuals diagnosed with SC may benefit from screening for MTS. Genetic testing is recommended for patients with extraocular SC with a Mayo Muir-Torre syndrome risk score of at least 2.[40] The Mayo Muir-Torre syndrome risk score is based on the following clinical criteria: age <60 years, at least two sebaceous neoplasms, personal medical history of Lynch-related cancer, and family history of Lynch-related cancer.[41] MTS screening is not recommended for patients with periocular SC.[40] Young patients age <50 years old with their first SC may benefit from genetic testing if they have loss of mismatch repair (MMR) protein staining on the tumor and otherwise do not meet the Mayo Muir-Torre syndrome risk score threshold.[40] Patient who are diagnosed with MTS should undergo routine preventive cancer screening.[40] Surgical resection is the mainstay of treatment for SC.[34] Wide local excision (WLE) historically has been the standard of care; however, Mohs micrographic surgery (MMS) offers the advantage of complete tumor resection with clear margins while maximizing the preservation of healthy tissue, especially in cosmetically sensitive areas such as the eyelids and face. Although use of sentinel lymph node biopsy is not routinely recommended for extraocular SC, it can be considered for periocular SC tumors stage T2c or higher of the eighth edition of the American Joint Committee on Cancer (AJCC) staging system.[40]

Radiation therapy and systemic chemotherapy are generally reserved for patients who are poor surgical candidates or those with recurrent or metastatic disease.[34]

Oral isotretinoin may be used as a prophylactic treatment to prevent the development of sebaceous neoplasms in MTS patients.[37] Also, changing immunosuppressive agents from calcineurin inhibitors to sirolimus may be an effective management strategy, as in the case of one patient with MTS who had a marked reduction of new sebaceous neoplasm formation after switching from tacrolimus to sirolimus.[42]

Prognosis

Overall mortality is increased in SOTR with SC compared to immunocompetent patients, although few deaths are attributed to SC.[33] (The overall prevalence of sebaceous carcinoma in SOTRs is low, and therefore accurate assessments of prognosis are difficult. However, in general, outcomes are good after complete surgical excision.[31,32]) In the study by Hoss et al., none of the nine patients (all of whom had extraorbital disease) had recurrence after WLE or MMS, although one patient died of metastatic disease from sebaceous carcinoma, which was likely present at the time of initial biopsy.[31] None of the transplant recipients described by Harwood et al. had recurrence of their sebaceous carcinoma at a mean follow-up time of 3.5 years.[32] The increased SC risk in SOTR highlights the importance of immunosuppression. Close clinical surveillance is recommended at least every 6 months following a diagnosis of sebaceous carcinoma, and the frequency can be tailored to the individual patient depending on their risk for additional cutaneous malignancies.[40]

ATYPICAL FIBROXANTHOMA

Epidemiology

AFX is an uncommon, spindle cell cutaneous malignancy. Histologically, AFX is similar to undifferentiated pleomorphic sarcoma (UPS), which was previously known as malignant fibrous histiocytoma (MFH), and therefore many consider AFX to be a less aggressive, superficial variant of UPS.

Hafner et al.[43] reported a higher incidence of AFX and MFH in renal transplant recipients and suggested that the risk for AFX may be increased in immunosuppressed patients. Among 642 renal transplant recipients over a 2-year period, there was one case of AFX, which is equivalent to an incidence of 78/100,000 persons per year and a prevalence of 0.16%.

In a multicenter retrospective chart review combined with a literature search by McCoppin et al.,[44] 16 SOTRs were identified to have either AFX (12 tumors) or UPS/MFH (4 tumors). The mean age of the SOTRs with AFX at the time of presentation was 62 years, and the average time from transplantation to diagnosis of AFX or UPS/MFH was 10.5 years. All the patients in this study were male, which is consistent with the male predominance among immunocompetent AFX and UPS/MFH patients.

Clinical Presentation

Often, AFX presents as a solitary, pink to red, asymptomatic nodule on sun-exposed areas. (Figures 12.4 and 12.5) It may bleed or ulcerate. According to cases series and reports, AFX tumors in SOTRs predominantly present on the head and neck.[43–48] Tumors tend to be larger in immunosuppressed patients. The majority of patients were immunosuppressed with cyclosporine and azathioprine, but regimens also included mycophenolate mofetil, tacrolimus, sirolimus, and methotrexate. The transplanted organs included kidney, heart, and liver.

Histology

AFX is characterized by a well-circumscribed, non-encapsulated dermal tumor that is either contiguous with the epidermis or separated from the epidermis by a grenz zone.[49] The cellular proliferation consists of plump spindle cells with prominent nuclei in poorly arranged fascicles, haphazardly arranged large polyhedral cells, and mononucleated, multinucleated, or osteoclast-like giant cells. Atypical mitoses and cellular pleomorphism are seen (Figure 12.6).

Immunohistochemistry is important for differentiating AFX from other spindle cell tumors.[49] Most cases of AFX stain positively for CD10 and procollagen 1. Cytokeratin and p63 are negative in AFX, whereas they are positive in spindle cell cutaneous squamous cell carcinoma. S100 is negative in AFX and positive in desmoplastic melanomas. It may be difficult to histologically distinguish AFX from UPS. Characteristics that favor UPS include involvement of the deep subcutis, penetration of the fascia or muscle, tumor necrosis, and vascular invasion.[50] If clinically suspicious for AFX, deep or excisional biopsies are recommended to assess the depth of invasion whenever possible.

Management

Treatment of AFX involves surgical removal with negative margins either by WLE or MMS. In immunocompetent patients, MMS offers a lower recurrence rate compared with that of WLE and maximizes healthy tissue preservation.[44,51–53] Similarly, in SOTRs, there are lower recurrence rates of AFX treated with MMS compared with that of those treated with excision as demonstrated by McCoppin et al.[44] They

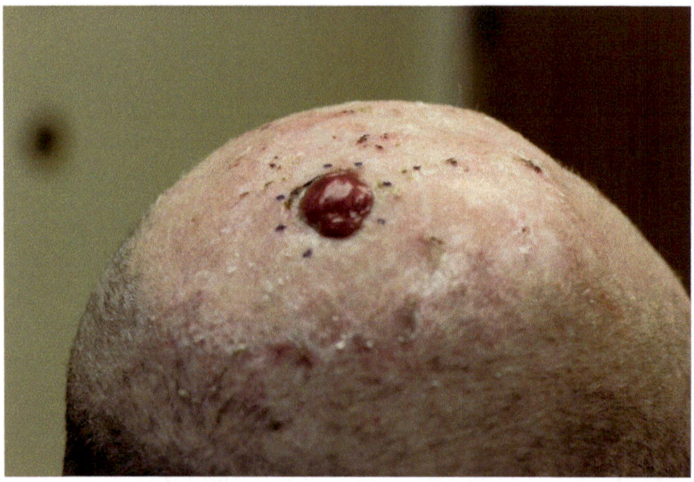

FIGURE 12.4 The vertex of the scalp of a renal transplant patient developed a bleeding, friable, nodular atypical fibroxanthoma. (M. Laurin Council, MD.)

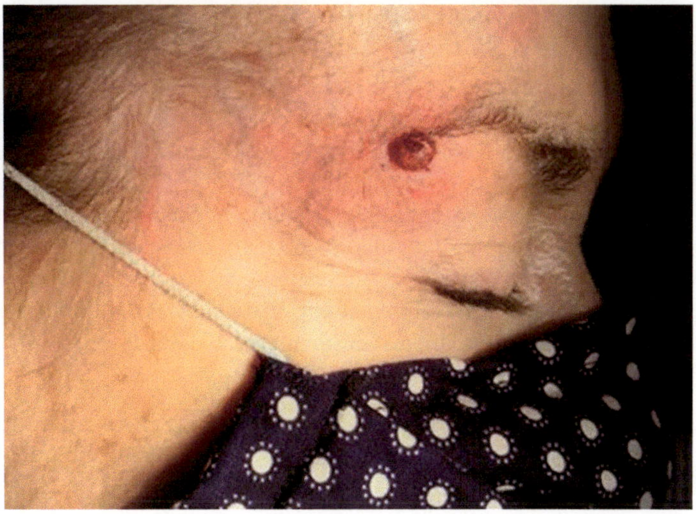

FIGURE 12.5 Atypical fibroxanthoma of the right lateral eyebrow in a lung transplant patient. (Nathalie C. Zeitouni, MDCM.)

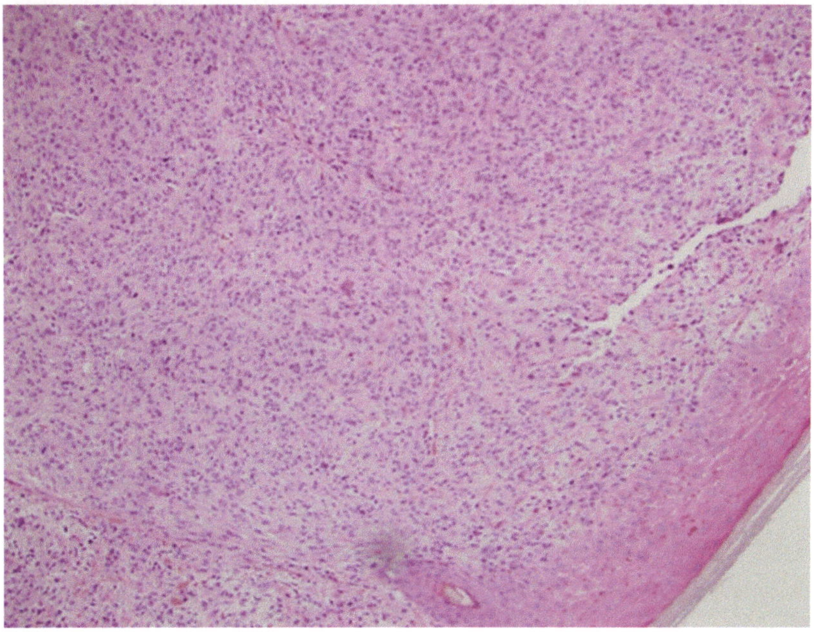

FIGURE 12.6 The dermis contains a cellular proliferation of plump spindle cells with prominent nuclei poorly arranged in fascicles and admixed with multinucleated giant cells consistent with atypical fibroxanthoma. (Marc D. Brown, MD.)

found that none of the six AFX tumors treated with MMS recurred or metastasized, whereas three of the five AFXs treated with WLE recurred or metastasized.

If possible, reduction of immunosuppression should be considered because greater immunosuppression results in decreased immune surveillance.[44] Radiation treatment is usually reserved for recurrent or metastatic tumors.[44]

Prognosis

Typically, a diagnosis of AFX carries a good prognosis, as there is a low incidence of recurrence (2.4%–9%) or metastasis (0%–4%) in the immunocompetent population.[44] Metastatic AFX tends to be associated with vascular or deep tissue invasion, tumor necrosis, and impaired host immunity, and some believe these cases are actually metastatic UPS.[44,50] In the immunocompromised SOTR population, patients with AFX are at greater risk for local recurrence, metastasis, and mortality compared with risks in the immunocompetent population.[44] In the cases tabulated by McCoppin et al.,[44] recurrence occurred in three of the 12 patients with AFX (25%) and metastasis occurred in one (8%) (Figure 12.7), and the single patient with recurrent and metastatic AFX died from his disease. The elevated recurrence and metastatic rates suggest more aggressive behavior in SOTRs.

DERMATOFIBROSARCOMA PROTUBERANS

Epidemiology

DFSP is a rare, low-grade sarcoma with a tendency for local recurrence and rare metastatic spread. In the general population, the estimated incidence is 0.8 to 5 per million.[54] Because of the rarity of this tumor and the few reports in the literature of posttransplant DFSP, there is not enough data to determine whether DFSP is overrepresented in the SOTR population.

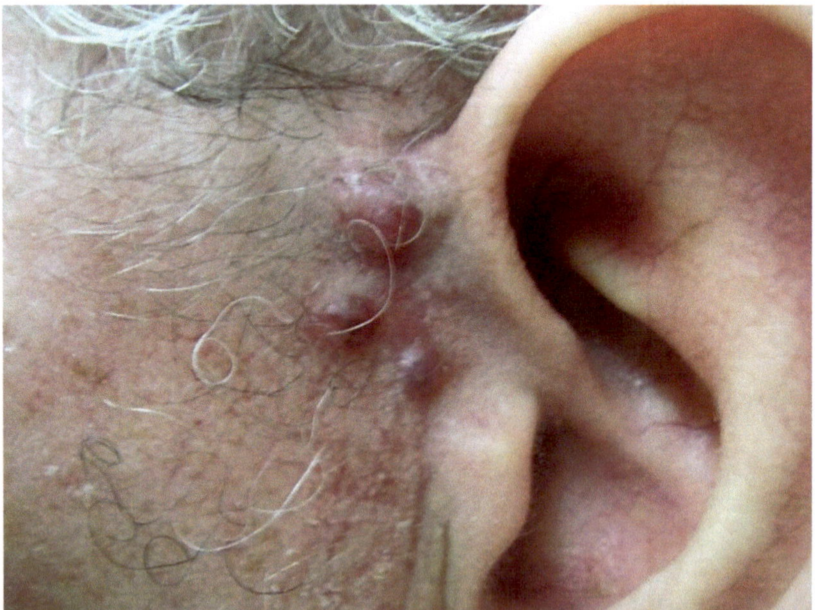

FIGURE 12.7 The left preauricular cheek demonstrates three metastatic papules arising from a primary atypical fibroxanthoma on the temple of a liver transplant patient. (Marc D. Brown, MD.)

Clinical Presentation

In the general population, DFSP typically presents as an asymptomatic, indurated plaque that slowly enlarges over months to years. The most common locations are the trunk and proximal extremities.

There have been three reports of DFSP occurring in SOTRs.[55–57] All reported cases were in men aged 34–61 years who were 3–16 years post renal transplant. The men were of varying ethnicity: Chinese, Caucasian, and Mauritian. The tumors appeared as firm, asymptomatic, slowly enlarging nodules and plaques on the chin, shoulder, and arm. The DFSP on the arm was within the scar at the site of an arteriovenous fistula. The clinical descriptions of the tumors were similar to those of DFSPs that presented in immunocompetent individuals. Two of the men were immunosuppressed with cyclosporine and azathioprine; one of those additionally took prednisone. The immunosuppressive regimen of the third patient was not discussed.

Histology

The characteristic histology of DFSP is proliferation of monomorphic, dermal spindle cells arranged in a whorled or storiform pattern.[54] It is an infiltrative tumor involving both the dermis and subcutis with tentacle-like projections forming a honeycomb appearance.[54] Immunohistochemical staining is mostly negative, except for vimentin and CD34, which are almost always positive.[55] DFSP can be differentiated from benign dermatofibroma, which is positive for Factor XIIIa and negative for CD34.[54]

In the three cases mentioned previously, the histologic appearance of the tumors was consistent with the classic histologic characteristics in immunocompetent patients. Each of the tumors demonstrated infiltrative, spindle cells arranged in a storiform pattern with uniform cellularity and low mitotic activity.[55–57] In two of the cases, the authors reported positive immunostaining with CD34.[55,57]

More than 90% of DFSP are characterized by a translocation between chromosomes 17 and 22 [t(17;22)(q22;q13)].[58] This translocation fuses the strongly expressed collagen type 1 alpha 1 (*COL1A1*) gene with the platelet-derived growth factor B-chain (*PDGFB*) gene resulting in overexpression of PDGFB.[58] PDGFB is a ligand for the tyrosine kinase PDGF receptor (PDGFR), and therefore constant stimulation leads to continual generation and proliferation of tumor cells.[58] Imatinib mesylate inhibits the tyrosine kinase PDGFR in DFSP cells causing downregulation of this enzyme activity. This accounts for the clinical benefit and therapeutic efficacy against DFSP.[58]

Management

Imaging studies are not required for every DFSP but may be helpful in certain cases. Magnetic resonance imaging (MRI) can help determine the extent of large or recurrent lesions. Computed tomography (CT) scanning may be useful if underlying bone involvement is suspected. Although guidelines for imaging are not included in the National Comprehensive Cancer Network (NCCN) guidelines, some authors suggest ruling out pulmonary metastases with chest CT for those with locally advanced, recurrent or fibrosarcomatous DFSP, or chest radiograph for all other DFSP patients.[58]

SOTRs with DFSP are managed according to the same guidelines for nontransplant patients. Surgical excision with negative margins is the treatment of choice. Varied approaches include traditional excision with 2–4 cm margins to investing fascia, MMS, or complete circumferential and peripheral deep margin assessment performed as a meticulous en face permanent section examination of all surgical margins.[59,60] A systematic review found that compared with wide excision, MMS potentially has lower recurrence rates.[54] In contrast, a retrospective review of 48 patients demonstrated similar rates of local recurrence, although positive margins were more common in patients treated with wide excision compared with those treated with MMS.[61]

Imatinib has been used for unresectable, recurrent, or metastatic DFSP, and radiation therapy may also be an option for very large or recurrent tumors or those with positive resection margins.[54,59]

Prognosis

DFSP tends to follow an indolent course, growing slowly over several years. It has a high tendency for local recurrence and low risk of metastatic spread (0.5%–5%).[54] In the general population, more recent data have shown a local recurrence rate of 7.3% with WLE using wide margins (i.e., 2–4 cm).[54] Tumors located on the head/neck and extremities tend to have a higher local recurrence rate compared with that of tumors located on the trunk.[54] Most reported recurrences tended to occur within 3 years of excision.[54] Pooled data from studies suggested that the local recurrence rate of DFSP after MMS is about 1%.[54] Of the three cases of DFSP reported in renal transplant recipients, none had reported recurrence or metastases after WLE.[55–57]

CONCLUSION

SOTRs are surviving longer with the advances in immunosuppressive management. However, these patients may proceed to develop secondary skin cancers that stem from lifelong immunosuppression. Although data is limited, cutaneous neoplasms that are rare in the immunocompetent population may occur with increased frequency in the immunosuppressed SOTR population. It is also possible that these tumors behave more aggressively with an increased tendency to locally recur or metastasize. Regardless, SOTRs require close monitoring for all types of skin cancers, and they should remain vigilant about skin cancer prevention and sun protective measures.

SUMMARY OF KEY POINTS

- KS is a tumor of endothelial cell origin that occurs with increased frequency in the SOTR population. It occurs more commonly in geographic areas with a high HHV-8 prevalence. The cutaneous lesions are similar to those seen in classical KS and often consist of multifocal purplish, reddish-blue nodules. The viscera can be affected as well, and this tends to be associated with a worse prognosis. Decreasing immunosuppression or switching to an mTOR inhibitor can lead to regression of KS. However, a change in the immunosuppression regimen can also put that patient at risk for allograft rejection or impaired function.
- SC is an uncommon adnexal tumor that can occur sporadically or in association with MTS, and its prevalence appears to be increased in SOTRs. The majority of sebaceous carcinoma cases described in SOTRs were in extraorbital locations. Tumors should be screened for loss of MMR proteins, and patients may require genetic testing for MTS if MSI is detected. First line treatment of sebaceous carcinoma is surgical resection.
- AFX is an uncommon, spindle cell tumor that has been reported in SOTRs. All tumors have been reported to be in male patients in the head and neck locations. Compared with immunocompetent patients, SOTRs with AFX appear to have more aggressive tumors with higher rates

of local recurrence and metastasis, although the total number of reported cases is relatively low. Surgical excision is the primary treatment option, and MMS has demonstrated lower rates of local recurrence.

- DFSP is a rare, low-grade sarcoma that has only been reported three times in SOTRs. All patients were male renal transplant recipients, but otherwise other demographics including age, tumor location, race, time from transplant to diagnosis, and immunosuppressive regimens varied among them. Although none of these cases recurred, DFSP in the general population has a tendency to recur locally. Surgical excision is the primary mode of treatment, and MMS may offer lower recurrence rates.

REFERENCES

1. Harwood AR, Osoba D, Hofstader SL, Goldstein MB et al. Kaposi's sarcoma in recipients of renal transplants. Am J Med. 1979;67:759–65.
2. Jensen P, Hansen S, Moller B, Leivestad T et al. Skin cancer in kidney and heart transplant recipients and different long-term immunosuppressive therapy regimens. J Am Acad Dermatol. 1999;40:177–86.
3. Serraino D, Angeletti C, Carrieri MP, Longo B et al. Kaposi's sarcoma in transplant and HIV-infected patients: an epidemiologic study in Italy and France. Transplant. 2005;80:1699–704.
4. Hosseini-Moghaddam SM, Soleimanirahbar A, Mazzulli T, Rotstein C et al. Post renal transplantation Kaposi's sarcoma: a review of its epidemiology, pathogenesis, diagnosis, clinical aspects, and therapy. Transplant Infect Dis. 2012;14:338–45.
5. Dudderidge TJ, Khalifa M, Jeffery R, Amlot P et al. Donor-derived human herpes virus 8-related Kaposi's sarcoma in renal allograft ureter. Transpl Infect Dis. 2008;10:221–6.
6. Yaich S, Charfeddine K, Zaghdane S, El Aoud N et al. Sirolimus for the treatment of Kaposi Sarcoma after renal transplantation: a series of 10 cases. Tranplant Proc. 2012;44:2824–6.
7. Zavos G, Moris D, Vernadakis S, Bokos J et al. Incidence and management of Kaposi Sarcoma in renal transplant recipients: the Greek experience. Transplant Proc. 2014;46:3199–202.
8. Einollahi B, Lessan-Pezeshki M, Nourbala MH, Simforoosh N, et al. Kaposi's sarcoma following living donor kidney transplantation: review of 7,939 recipients. Int Urol Nephrol. 2009;41:679–85.
9. Zmonarski SC, Boratynska M, Puziewicz-Zmonarska A, Kazimierczak K et al. Kaposi's sarcoma in renal transplant recipients. Ann Transplant. 2005;10:59–65.
10. Lessan-Pezeshki M, Einollahi B, Khatami MR, Mahdavi M. Kidney transplantation and Kaposi's sarcoma: review of 2050 recipients. Transplant Proc. 2001;33:2818.
11. Shahbazian H. Kaposi sarcoma in kidney transplanted patients. Urol J. 2004;2:111–14.
12. Cattaneo D, Gotti E, Perico N, Bertolini G et al. Cyclosporine formulation and Kaposi's sarcoma after renal transplantation. Transplant. 2005;80:743–8.
13. Farge D. Kaposi's sarcoma in organ transplant recipients: the collaborative transplantation research group of Ile de France. Eur J Med. 1993;2:339–43.
14. Penn I. Sarcomas in organ allograft recipients. Transplant. 1995;60:1485–91.
15. Cahoon EK, Linet MS, Clarke CA, Pawlisk KS et al. Risk of Kaposi Sarcoma after solid organ tranplantation in the United States. Int J Cancer. 2018;143:2741–8.
16. Woodle ES, Hanaway M, Buell J, Gross T, et al. Kaposi Sarcoma: an analysis of the US and international experiences from the Israel Penn international transplant tumor registry. Transplant Proc. 2001;33:3660–1.
17. Penn I. Kaposi's sarcoma in transplant recipients. Transplant. 1997;64:669–73.
18. Euvard S, Kanitakis J, Claudy A. Skin cancers after organ transplantation. N Eng J Med. 2003;348:1681–91.
19. Ponticelli C, Cucchiara D, Bencini P. Skin cancer in kidney transplant recipients. J Nephrol. 2014;27:285–94.
20. Moosa MR. Kaposi's sarcoma in kidney transplant recipients: a 23-year experience. Q J Med. 2005;98:205–14.
21. Euvard S, Kanitakis J. Kaposi's sarcoma in organ transplant recipients. In: Otley CC, Stasko T, editors. Skin disease in organ transplantation. New York: Cambridge University Press; 2008; p. 195–8.
22. Mittal A, Colegio OR. Skin cancers in organ transplant recipients. Am J of Transplant. 2017;17:2509–30.
23. Cattani P, Capuano M, Graffeo R, Ricci R et al. Kaposi's sarcoma associated with previous human herpesvirus 8 infection in kidney transplant recipients. J Clin Microbiol. 2001;39:506–8.

24. Diociaiuti A, Nanni G, Cattani P, Lesnoni La Parola I et al. HHV8 in renal transplant recipients. Transplant Int. 2000;13:S410–12.
25. Chiereghin A, Barozzi P, Petrisli E, Piccirilli G et al. Multicenter prospective study for laboratory diagnosis of HHV8 infection in solid organ donors and transplant recipients and evaluation of the clinical impact after transplantation. Transplant. 2017;101:1935–44.
26. Patterson JW. Vascular tumors. In: Weedon's skin pathology. 5th ed. London: Elsevier Limited; 2021; p. 1121–67.
27. Delyon J, Rabate C, Euvard S, Harwood CA et al. Management of Kaposi sarcoma after solid organ transplantation: a European retrospective study. J Amer Acad Dermatol. 2019;81:448–55.
28. Zustovich F, Ferro A, Toso S. Gemcitabine for the treatment of classic Kaposi's Sarcoma: a case series. Anticancer Res. 2013;33:5531–4.
29. Brambilla L, Recalcati S, Tourlaki A. Vinorelbine therapy in classic Kaposi's sarcoma: a retrospective study of 20 patients. Eur J Dermatol. 2015;25:535–8.
30. Razonable RR. Progress toward HHV-8 prevention after transplantation: In search for optimal diagnostic strategies. Transplant. 2017;101:1751–2.
31. Hoss E, Nelson SA, Sharma A. Sebaceous carcinoma in solid organ transplant recipients. Int J Dermatol. 2017;56:746–9.
32. Harwood CA, McGregor JM, Swale VJ, Proby CM et al. High frequency and diversity of cutaneous appendageal tumors in organ transplant recipients. J Am Acad Dermatol. 2003;48:401–8.
33. Sargen MR, Cahoon EK, Lynch CF, Tucker MA, et al. Sebaceous carcinoma incidence and survival among solid organ transplant recipients in the United States, 1987–2017. JAMA Dermatol. Advance online publication.
34. Kyllo RL, Brady KL, Hurst EA. Sebaceous carcinoma: review of the literature. Dermatol Surg. 2015;41:1–15.
35. Seo BF, Jung HW, Choi IK, Rhie JW. Sebaceous carcinoma of the suprapubic area in a liver transplant patient. Ann Dermatol. 2014;26:395–8.
36. Harwood CA, Swale VJ, Bataille VA, Quinn AG et al. An association between sebaceous carcinoma and microsatellite instability in immunosuppressed organ transplant recipients. J Invest Dermatol. 2001;116:246–53.
37. Landis MN, Davis CL, Bellus GA, Wolverton SE. Immunosuppression and sebaceous tumors: a confirmed diagnosis of Muir-Torre syndrome unmasked by immunosuppressive therapy. J Am Amer Dermatol. 2011;65:1054–8.
38. Tomonari M, Shimada M, Nakada Y, Yamamoto I et al. Muir-Torre syndrome: sebaceous carcinoma concurrent with colon cancer in a kidney transplant recipient; a case report. BMC Nephrol. 2019;20:394–9.
39. Patterson JW. Tumors of cutaneous appendages. In: Weedon's skin pathology. 5th ed. London: Elsevier Limited; 2021;p. 951–1015.
40. Owen JL, Kibbi N, Worley B, Kelm RC et al. Sebaceous carcinoma: evidence-based clinical practice guidelines. Lancet. 2019;20:e699–714.
41. Roberts ME, Riegert-Johnson DL, Thomas BC, Rumilla KM et al. A clinical scoring system to identify patients with sebaceous neoplasms at risk for the Muir-Torre variant of Lynch syndrome. Genet Med. 2014;16:711–6.
42. Levi Z, Hazazi R, Kedar-Barnes I, Hodak E et al. Switching from tacrolimus to sirolimus halts the appearance of new sebaceous neoplasms in Muir-Torre syndrome. Am J Transplant. 2007;7:476–9.
43. Hafner J, Kunzi W, Weinreich T. Malignant fibrous histiocytoma and atypical fibroxanthoma in renal transplant recipients. Dermatol. 1999;198:29–32.
44. McCoppin HH, Christiansen D, Stasko T, Washington C et al. Clinical spectrum of atypical fibroxanthoma and undifferentiated pleomorphic sarcoma in solid organ transplant recipients: a collective experience. Dermatol Surg. 2012;38:230–9.
45. Kanitakis J, Euvard S, Montazeri A, Garnier A, Garnier JL et al. Atypical fibroxanthoma in a renal graft recipient. J Am Acad Dermatol. 1996;35:262–4.
46. Perrett CM, Cerio R, Proby CM, Harwood CA. Atypical fibroxanthoma in a renal transplant recipient. Histopathology. 2005;47:326–7.
47. Ferri E, Iaderosa GA, Armato E. Atypical fibroxanthoma of the external ear in a cardiac transplant recipient: case report and the causal role of the immunosuppressive therapy. Auris Nasus Larynx. 2008;35:260–3.
48. Kovach BT, Sams HH, Stasko T. Multiple atypical fibroxanthomas in a cardiac transplant recipient. Dermatol Surg. 2055;31:467–70.
49. Patterson JW. Tumors and tumor-like proliferations of fibrous and related tissues. In: Weedon's skin pathology. 5th ed. London: Elsevier Limited; 2021;p. 1017–1065.
50. Iorizzo LJ, Brown MD. Atypical fibroxanthoma: a review of the literature. Dermatol Surg. 2011;37:146–57.
51. Ang GC, Roenigk RK, Otley CC, Phillips PK. More than 2 decades of treating atypical fibroxanthoma at Mayo Clinic: what have we learned from 91 patients? Dermatol Surg. 2009;35:765–72.

52. Davis JL, Randle HW, Zalla MJ et al. A comparison of Mohs micrographic surgery and wide local excision for the treatment of atypical fibroxanthoma. Dermatol Surg. 1997;23:105–10.
53. Huether MJ, Zitelli JA, Brodland DG. Mohs micrographic surgery for the treatment of spindle cell tumors of the skin. J Amer Acad Dermatol. 2001;44:565–9.
54. Bogucki B, Neuhaus I, Hurst EA. Dermatofibrosarcoma protuberans: a review of the literature. Dermatol Surg. 2012;38:537–51.
55. Brown VL, Proby CM, Harwood CA, Cerio R. Dermatofibrosarcoma protuberans in a renal transplant recipient. Histopathology. 2003;42:195–203.
56. Lai KN, Lai FM, King WWK, Li PKT et al. Dermatofibrosarcoma protuberans in a renal transplant patient. Aust NZ J Surg. 1995;65:900–2.
57. Picciotto F, Basolo B, Massara C, Caliendo V et al. Dermatofibrosarcoma protuberans at the site of arteriovenous fistula in a renal transplant recipient. Transplant. 1999;68:1074–5.
58. Lemm D, Mügge LO, Mentzel T, Höffken K. Current treatment options in dermatofibrosarcoma protuberans. J Cancer Res Clin Oncol. 2009;135:653–65.
59. National Comprehensive Cancer Network (NCCN). NCCN clinical practice guidelines in oncology (2020 Aug 6). Available from: www.nccn.org/professionals/physician_gls
60. Farma JM, Ammori JB, Zager JS, Marzban SS et al. Dermatofibrosarcoma protuberans: how wide should we resect? Ann Surg Oncol. 2010;17:2112–18.
61. Meguerditchian AN, Wang J, Lema B, Kraybill WG et al. Wide excision or Mohs micrographic surgery for the treatment of primary dermatofibrosarcoma protuberans. Am J Clin Oncol. 2010;33:300–3.

Immunotherapy in Organ Transplant Recipients

13

Maressa C. Criscito and John A. Carucci

INTRODUCTION

The number of solid organ transplants performed in the United States has tripled since the 1980s and continues to increase at a substantial rate. In 2019, almost 40,000 organ transplants from both living and deceased donors were performed, marking an 8.7% increase from 2018 and a seventh consecutive annual record of organ transplantation in the United States.[1]

With the rapid increase in solid organ transplants and the advent of highly effective immunosuppressive medications, solid organ transplant recipients (SOTRs) have experienced significant improvement in survival rates.[2] Yet, as improvements in organ transplantation prolongs patients' lives, posttransplant malignancies have become an increasing threat to long-term survival. SOTRs have a 2- to 4-fold increased risk of malignancy compared with that of the general population, a risk that is thought to be because of a state of immune tolerance induced by the immunosuppressive medications necessary to maintain the graft.[3,4] Specifically, increased rates of malignancies such as skin cancer, lymphoma, kidney, head and neck cancer, colorectal cancer, and lung cancer have been reported in the organ transplant population.[5,6]

Skin cancer is the most common posttransplant malignancy, with an incidence rate in SOTRs nearly 5 times that of all cancers combined in the general United States population.[7] Cutaneous malignancies account for up to 50% of all malignancies in SOTRs and include keratinocyte carcinomas (KC; cutaneous squamous cell carcinoma (cSCC) and basal cell carcinoma [BCC]), malignant melanoma (MM), Merkel cell carcinoma (MCC), and Kaposi sarcoma. KC comprise 90%–95% of cutaneous malignancies in the transplant population, with SOTRs having a 65- to 250-fold increased risk of developing cSCC compared with that in the general population.[2,4–10] Additionally, compared with age-matched controls, SOTRs have an estimated 2- to 8-fold higher risk of developing MM.[9] Although the exact pathogenesis of skin cancer development in SOTRs is not fully understood, it is generally accepted that immunosuppressive medications play an important role. Proposed mechanisms through which immunosuppression may contribute to the development of skin cancer include reduced immune surveillance, direct or indirect carcinogenic effects of immunosuppressive agents, and the proliferation of oncogenic viruses in the setting of immunosuppression.[11–17]

A number of risk factors for posttransplant skin cancer have been identified, which include the duration of immunosuppression (Table 13.1).[10–16] The cumulative incidence of cutaneous malignancies increases with time from transplantation, likely related to the duration of immunosuppression, with the posttransplant incidence rate of cSCC as high as 70% after 20 years.[15] In addition to age at transplantation and duration

 DOI: 10.1201/9781003001461-13

TABLE 13.1 Risk Factors Associated with the Development of Posttransplant Cutaneous Malignancies

Patient specific	Older age Male sex Fair skin (Fitzpatrick skin type I-III) History of significant UV exposure History of skin cancers or precancerous lesions prior to transplant
Transplant associated	Older age at transplantation Lung, heart, or pancreas-kidney > kidney > liver transplant Degree of immunosuppressive therapy: Three-drug regimen associated with significantly greater incidence of cSCC in SOTRs than two-drug regimen Treatment with cyclosporine and azathioprine Voriconazole use HPV infection: High beta-HPV viral load in the eyebrow hairs found to be associated with a greater risk of cSCC in SOTRs

Abbreviations: cSCC, cutaneous squamous cell carcinoma; HPV, human papillomavirus; SOTRs, solid organ transplant recipients; UV, ultraviolet.

of immune suppression, additional risk factors for the development of cutaneous malignancies include the degree and type of immunosuppressive regimen.[9,16] Treatment with cyclosporine or azathioprine is associated with a greater risk of development of posttransplant cutaneous malignancies. In contrast, immunosuppression with mycophenolate mofetil or the mammalian target of rapamycin (mTOR) inhibitors sirolimus and everolimus are associated with a lower risk of skin malignancies in SOTRs.[18] Additionally, thoracic transplantation is also associated with a greater risk of skin cancer development, although this is likely related to the greater degree of immunosuppression necessary to support graft viability.[17] Furthermore, increased age, white race, and male sex are also associated with a greater risk of posttransplant skin cancer, with additional risk factors of personal or family history of skin cancer, skin phototype, sun exposure, and history of sunburns to be considered in determining an individual risk as well.[4,9]

Malignancies in the transplant population tend to be more aggressive than those in the general population, with cancer being the second leading cause of death in transplant patients.[3] Recently, cancer immunotherapy has transformed the oncologic landscape, demonstrating potential for successful and durable response in various cancer types, including cutaneous malignancies. Cancer immunotherapies utilize T cells as the anticancer drug, with T cell activation obtained through 1) use of immune checkpoint inhibitors (ICIs); 2) adoptive transfer of anticancer T cells; and 3) induction *in vivo* by vaccination or endogenous delivery of neoantigens subsequent to other anticancer therapies.[17,19]

Although cancer immunotherapies promote T cell activation against neoantigens on tumor cells, T cell stimulation is also implicated as one of the major mediators of allograft rejection.[4,6,19] Because of this substantial risk, SOTRs were excluded in prior clinical trials investigating the safety and efficacy of cancer immunotherapies. Thus, SOTRs represent a largely neglected population within the field of cancer immunotherapy and would greatly benefit from further research, especially given the increased malignancy risk of this population. Although there is limited data regarding the use of cancer immunotherapy in the transplant population, the use of ICIs and intralesional oncolytic virotherapy have received the most attention and will be highlighted herein.

IMMUNE CHECKPOINT INHIBITORS

In 1893, William Coley first reported effective immunotherapy in the treatment of malignant tumors when he described tumor shrinkage after the injection of bacteria into sites of sarcoma.[20] Almost 120 years later, cancer immunotherapy in the form of ICIs began to revolutionize cancer treatment with the advent of cytotoxic T-lymphocyte-associated protein 4 (CTLA-4), programmed cell death protein-1 (PD-1), and programmed death-ligand 1 (PD-L1) inhibitors.[21] By blocking checkpoint proteins from binding with their partner proteins, ICIs allow T cells to target tumor cells, eliciting an immunologic response.

In 2011, the United States Food and Drug Administration (FDA) approved the first ICI, ipilimumab, a monoclonal human CTLA-4 antibody, for the treatment of metastatic melanoma based on the results of overall improved survival seen in treated patients.[21–22] Shortly afterwards, PD-1 inhibitors gained approval for MM, non-small cell lung cancer, and head and neck squamous cell carcinoma, along with other metastatic cancers. More recently, the PD-1 inhibitor cemiplimab was approved for the treatment of locally advanced or metastatic cSCC and in June 2020, pembrolizumab was approved for patients with recurrent or metastatic cSCC not curable by surgery or radiation.[23] Furthermore, the PD-L1 inhibitor avelumab has recently gained approval for MCC, further broadening the treatment armamentarium for cutaneous malignancies (Table 13.2).[21,22] Indications for ICIs continue to expand to include several other cancer types, substantially increasing the number of patients receiving these therapies.

The Tumor Microenvironment and Immune Checkpoint Inhibitors

As the indications for ICIs continue to grow, their use for the treatment of advanced malignancies in SOTRs remain unclear. Given the need for chronic immunosuppression and the risk of allograft rejection, SOTRs with advanced malignancies have largely been excluded from original clinical trials on the safety and efficacy of ICIs.[24] In the tumor microenvironment, tumor cells and surrounding tumor-infiltrating lymphocytes inhibit T cell-mediated immunosurveillance in several ways. For one, upregulation of inhibitory checkpoint molecules, such as PD-L1 and PD-L2, may occur. When PD-1, as expressed on CD8 T cells, interacts with the ligand PD-L1 on tumor cells or antigen presenting cells (APCs), an inhibitory signal results that decreases effective T cell activity in the tumor microenvironment (Figure 13.1).[24–27] Another inhibitory T cell protein, CTLA-4, competes with activating proteins of CD28 for its ligands, CD80 and CD86, on APCs (Figure 13.2). Blockade of checkpoint molecules results in activation and enhancement of T cell activity, stimulating both the cell-mediated and humoral antitumor immune responses. Specifically, CTLA-4 inhibitors modulate T cell activation during the antigen priming phase, whereas the PD-1/PD-L1 inhibitors function during the effector phase of tumor-specific T cell response.[28]

Importantly, both CTLA-4 and PD-1/PD-L1 have demonstrated critical roles in the immune tolerance required for graft survival, mostly through the interaction with regulatory T cells (Tregs).[29,30] Tregs comprise 5%–10% of circulating CD4 T cells and play a critical role in immune tolerance to self-antigens. Tregs are able to suppress immune function and autoreactivity via a combination of mechanisms, including cell contact-dependent suppression, cell contact-independent suppression, direct induction of apoptosis, and cytokine release.[29,30] Thus, Tregs may play a particularly important role in suppressing T cell activation after exposure to allo-antigens in SOTRs. Although the blockade of both CTLA-4 and PD-1 pathways results in decreasing T cell activation, the precise mechanisms of each pathway are fundamentally different and thus each method produces a distinct cellular phenotype.[29,30]

The interaction of CTLA-4 on Tregs and B7 ligands on APCs promote Treg-mediated suppression of both effector T cell activation as well as APC maturation, leading to the recognition of the APC-presented antigen and upregulation of the indoleamine 2,3-dioxygenase (IDO) pathway on APCs. The IDO pathway may be critical in establishing and maintaining Treg-mediated immune suppression and peripheral tolerance.[31,32] Thus, the use of CTLA-4 inhibitors in SOTRs may prevent Treg-induced immunosuppression and promote alloreactivity via increased stimulation and activation of effector T cells. In fact, blocking the CTLA-4 pathway in mice transplant models has demonstrated enhanced

TABLE 13.2 United States Food and Drug Administration (FDA) Approved Immune Checkpoint Inhibitors (ICIs) for Cutaneous Malignancies[22]

CUTANEOUS MALIGNANCY	*ICI CLASS*	*MEDICATION NAME*	*FDA APPROVED INDICATION*	*APPROVAL YEAR*
Malignant melanoma	CTLA-4	Ipilimumab (Yervoy)	Surgically unresectable stage 3 or 4 malignant melanoma previously treated or untreated in adults and pediatric patients >12 years	2011, 2017
			In combination with nivolumab for *BRAF* V600 wild-type unresectable or metastatic melanoma	2015
			In combination with nivolumab for unresectable or metastatic melanoma across *BRAF* status	2016
			Adjuvant treatment of cutaneous melanoma stage IIIA, IIIB, and IIIC after complete resection along with total lymphadenectomy	2015
	Programmed cell death protein-1 (PD-1)	Nivolumab (Opdivo)	Unresectable or metastatic melanoma that progressed following treatment with ipilimumab or a BRAF inhibitor in *BRAF* mutation-positive patients	2014
			In combination with ipilimumab for unresectable or metastatic melanoma regardless of *BRAF* status	2016
			Lymph node-positive or metastatic melanoma patients who had undergone complete resection	2017
			First-line therapy in patients with recurrent or metastatic melanoma regardless of *BRAF* V600-mutation status	2017
	Programmed cell death protein-1 (PD-1)	Pembrolizumab (Keytruda)	Metastatic melanoma refractory to ipilimumab and BRAF inhibitor with *BRAF* mutation	2014
			Previously untreated advanced melanoma regardless of *BRAF* mutation status	2015
			Adjuvant treatment of lymph node(s)-positive melanoma following complete resection	2019
			Metastatic melanoma with limited resectability, if there is no disease after resection, as an adjuvant therapy	2019

(*Continued*)

TABLE 13.2 United States Food and Drug Administration (FDA) Approved Immune Checkpoint Inhibitors (ICIs) for Cutaneous Malignancies[22] (Continued)

CUTANEOUS MALIGNANCY	ICI CLASS	MEDICATION NAME	FDA APPROVED INDICATION	APPROVAL YEAR
Cutaneous squamous cell carcinoma	Programmed cell death protein-1 (PD-1)	Cemiplimab (Libtayo)	Metastatic or locally advanced cutaneous squamous cell carcinoma patients who are not candidates for curative surgery or radiation	2018
	Programmed cell death protein-1 (PD-1)	Pembrolizumab (Keytruda)	Recurrent or metastatic cutaneous squamous cell carcinoma that is not curable by surgery or radiation	2020
Merkel cell carcinoma	Programmed death-ligand 1 (PD-L1)	Avelumab (Bavencio)	Metastatic Merkel cell carcinoma of adults and pediatric patients >12 years including those who have not received prior chemotherapy	2017
	Programmed cell death protein-1 (PD-1)	Pembrolizumab	First-line therapy for adult and pediatric patients with recurrent or locally advanced or metastatic Merkel cell carcinoma	2018

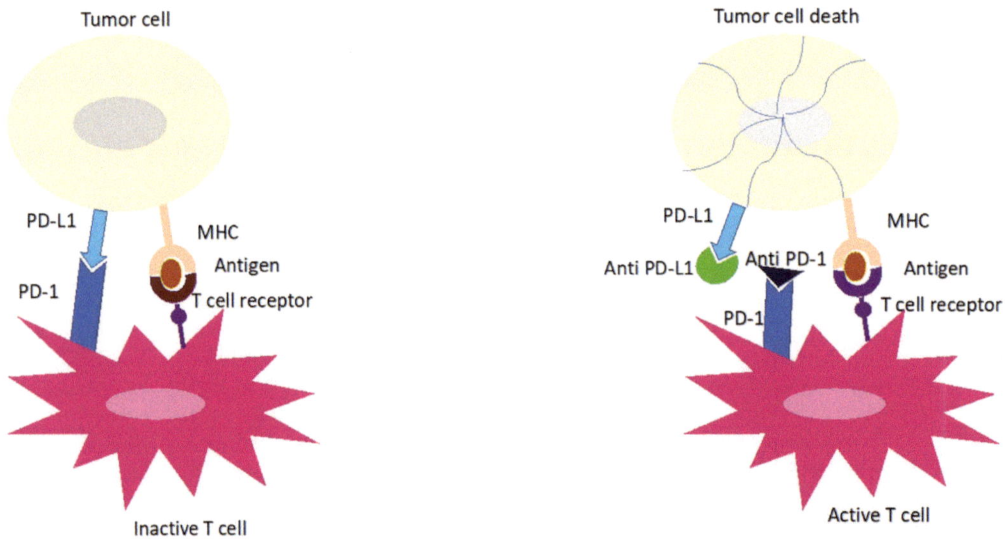

FIGURE 13.1 PD-L1 binds with PD-1 and inhibits T cell activation, preventing T cell killing of the tumor cell. Blocking PD-L1 or PD-1 stimulates T cell activation, allowing for a T cell-mediated antitumor response.

acute cellular rejection.[29,30] Additionally, the PD-1/PD-L1 axis has demonstrated importance in maintaining allograft tolerance in transplant recipients, as PD-L1 signaling is critical for Treg induction, suppression of effector T cell function and expansion, and, ultimately, allograft acceptance.[33] Thus, the upregulation of PD-L1 in the allograft promotes T regulatory cell activity and enhances the inhibitory signaling to alloreactive T cell activity.

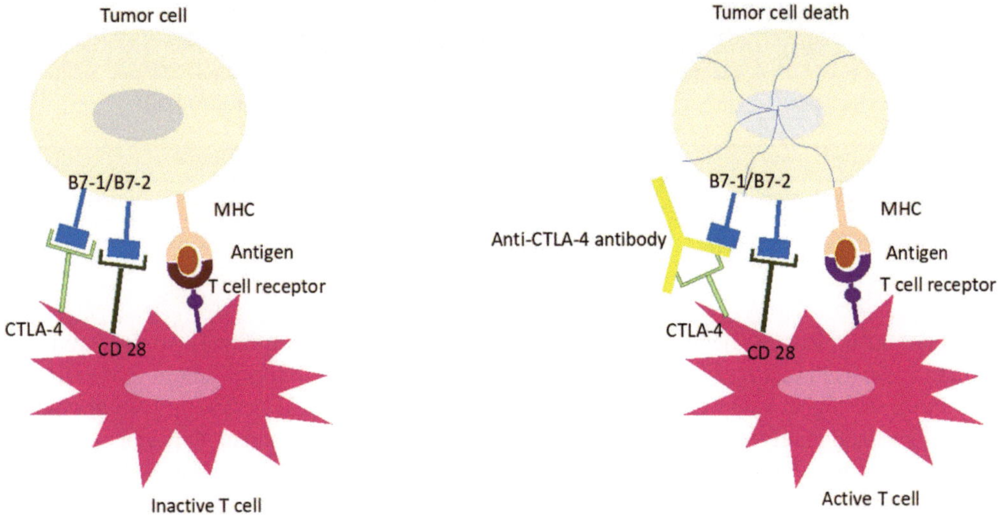

FIGURE 13.2 CTLA-4/B7 binding inhibits T cell activation. Blocking of CTLA-4 with an anti-CTLA-4 antibody stimulates a T cell antitumor immune response.

Use of Immune Checkpoint Inhibitors in Solid Organ Transplant Recipients

It is imperative to consider the careful balance of immunosuppression with immune activation in the treatment of malignancies in SOTRs. At present, there is a paucity of data regarding the safety and efficacy of ICIs in the organ transplantation population, with the majority of the current literature consisting of case reports, case series, and systematic reviews, although prospective clinical studies are underway. Existing data on the risk of graft rejection and malignancy response in transplant patients receiving ICIs for the treatment of advanced malignancies is outlined following.[3,4,34–39]

Risk of Graft Rejection and Graft Loss in SOTRs Receiving ICIs

Pooled analyses of existing publications demonstrate high rates (~40%) of graft rejection in SOTRs with malignancies treated with ICIs.[3,4,34–39] In most cases, rejection may be halted by withdrawing immunotherapeutic agents and increasing the immunosuppressive regimen, specifically with high-dose corticosteroids and occasionally other aggressive immunosuppressive therapies. The feared complication of graft rejection is graft loss, which is a life-threatening event in recipients of heart, lung, and liver, as these patients will not be eligible for re-transplant. In contrast, kidney recipients who experience graft rejection or loss may be maintained on dialysis. Importantly, death secondary to complications from allograft loss or rejection have been reported to range from 14% to 46% of patients.[3,4] The risk of graft rejection and loss may be related to the type of ICI, the type of organ transplant, the immunosuppressive regimen, and the time since transplantation, further discussed in the sections following (Table 13.3).

Type of Immune Checkpoint Inhibitor

Upon review of the literature, the highest rate of allograft rejection may be associated with PD-1 inhibitors, although further study is necessary to confirm this finding. Specifically, it has been suggested that

TABLE 13.3 Risk Factors Associated with Allograft Rejection in SOTRs Who Received ICIs

RISK FACTOR	*PROPOSED ASSOCIATION*
Type of immune checkpoint inhibitor	PD-1 inhibitors (nivolumab > pembrolizumab)
Type of organ transplant	Kidney transplant
Immunosuppressive regimen	Immunosuppressive regimen that includes low-dose prednisone

Abbreviations: ICIs, immune checkpoint inhibitors; PD-1, programmed cell death protein 1; SOTRs, solid organ transplant recipients.

the highest risk of transplant rejection is associated with the PD-1 inhibitor nivolumab, followed by pembrolizumab, and was lowest for patients who received the CTLA-4 inhibitor ipilimumab.[3,4,34] It has been speculated that the higher rate of rejection with the PD-1/L1 blockade is because of alloimmunity that largely relies on an alloantigen-mediated response that resembles the mechanism of tumor immune rejection. Additionally, anti-PD-1/L1 has higher antitumor response rates than that of anti-CTLA-4, with the differing allograft rejection rates possibly reflecting that discrepancy.[34,35] However, one must also consider that patients treated with PD-1/L1 inhibitors may have previously been treated with the CTLA-4 inhibitor ipilimumab, raising the possibility of combined dual effects from both classes of ICIs in these patients.[3] Additionally, the risk of immune-related adverse events with ICIs may further complicate a patient's clinical picture, as potential complications of ICIs, such as autoimmune pneumonitis and colitis, may be difficult to distinguish from frank rejection.

Type of Organ Transplant and Immunosuppressive Regimen

With regards to the type of organ transplantation, the highest rejection rates seemingly occur in patients with a kidney transplant, followed by liver and then heart transplant, although additional research is necessary to confirm this finding.[4,36,37] Additionally, the rates of death secondary to graft rejection are highest among liver transplant patients compared with rates in those with kidney or heart transplants.[4]

The type of immunosuppressive regimen may also be correlated with graft rejection after ICIs. It has been suggested that patients who receive immunosuppression with low-dose prednisone have higher rates of allograft rejection compared with rates in those who receive other immunosuppressive therapies.[3,4] Additionally, patients who receive tacrolimus-based regimens or combination immunosuppressive therapy also have demonstrated lower rates of allograft rejection. Interestingly, mTOR inhibitors have been shown to decrease the risk of developing KCs and may further have a dual action of immunosuppression and cancer-directed treatment via the PI3-K/Akt/mTOR pathway. It was suggested that mTOR inhibitors may play a critical role in managing the immune tumor environment by regulating the expression of PD-L1, an area that requires additional study.[38] At present, it is speculated that premedicating with a higher dose of systemic immunosuppression may be an effective method to decrease the risk of acute cellular rejection in patients receiving ICIs, although this balance must be pursued with caution.[3,4,39]

Time Since Transplantation

It remains unclear whether prior episodes of rejection before ICI use are associated with allograft rejection or loss. Furthermore, there does not appear to be a correlation between the time of transplantation and the rate or timing of ICI-induced allograft rejection. Biopsies of rejected organs have demonstrated an acute T lymphocyte-mediated process in half of the patients who received ICIs, even at 25 years after transplantation.[3] A mixed cellular- and antibody-mediated rejection may also be observed, suggesting that a secondary phenomenon induced by T cell activation accompanying the ICI therapy may occur, further triggering a humoral response. These findings stand at odds with the general understanding that T cell-mediated rejection rarely occurs beyond 10 years after transplantation, unlike antibody-mediated rejection.[3] Additionally, the positive expression of PD-1 and PD-L1 in some of the biopsies suggests that the PD-1 pathway likely contributes to the pathogenesis of allograft tolerance and rejection.[34,35] PD-L1 expression on allograft lymphocytes has been suggested as a marker of rejection after treatment with ICIs. However, further larger studies are necessary to validate this finding.

Tumor Response

Importantly, in SOTRs who receive ICIs, most deaths are not related to graft failure but instead to progression of metastatic disease or death secondary to an underlying condition.[4,38] It has been estimated that 51% to 64% of transplant patients eventually succumb to their malignancy. In fact, of the patients who experienced any response to therapy or had stable disease, 35% experienced rejection.[4]

Rates of progression or death secondary to malignancy were highest for those who receive ipilimumab, followed by nivolumab, and then pembrolizumab, albeit a statistically nonsignificant finding. The overall response rate (ORR) was highest for pembrolizumab (53%), with nivolumab demonstrating a 26% ORR in SOTRs who received ICIs and ipilimumab showing a 20% ORR.[4]

The type of immunosuppression regimen may also influence tumor response in SOTRs receiving ICIs. The ORR for transplant patients who received single-agent immunosuppression, defined as prednisone, tacrolimus, sirolimus, or cyclosporine, was 46% compared with the ORR of 29% for those who received combined immunosuppression.[4]

The literature currently suggests a trend towards positive clinical responses in SOTRs who receive ICIs for the treatment of cutaneous malignancies. In fact, the response rate of ipilimumab for transplant recipients with melanoma has been demonstrated to be similar to the ORR of ipilimumab in prior clinical trials.[4] The same was true for the use of nivolumab and pembrolizumab in SOTRs with MM. Furthermore, positive clinical responses in SOTRs who received ICIs for the treatment of cSCC and MCC have also been suggested.[4] However, further research is necessary to provide more concrete findings regarding the preceding given the small sample sizes of the current data.

Prospective Trials

The efficacy of ICIs among SOTRs is controversial, with prospective clinical trials necessary to further investigate. The only prospective study reported to date is a phase I clinical trial testing the safety of nivolumab in 4 renal transplant recipients with multiple myeloma, head and neck SCC, renal cell carcinoma, and bladder cancer.[39] In this study, the patients were required to have a serum creatinine level of <180 μmol/L and absence of human leukocyte antigen donor-specific antibodies (DSAs). The patients received one, two, three, and nine doses of nivolumab, respectively. None of the patients had a graft rejection and only one patient (who received nine doses) experienced a partial response.[39] Although the study was small, the safety profile of nivolumab among select patients with renal transplants without DSA appears to be encouraging and warrants testing in a larger-scale trial. Another phase I trial is open and accruing patients with a history of a renal transplant who had unresectable or metastatic cutaneous melanoma or MCC diagnosed.[40] Patients in this study will receive prednisone, tacrolimus, and nivolumab, with the addition of ipilimumab in those who experience progression of disease. The primary end point of the study is response rate at 16 weeks among patients without allograft loss.[40]

The use of immunotherapy poses particular challenges in transplant patients as modulating the immune environment can lead to allograft rejection. Thus, when considering immunotherapy in patients with a history of transplant, it is important to balance the risk of graft rejection and the potential benefit of effective and durable tumor response.[41] In the case of renal transplantation, the expectation of allograft failure and use of hemodialysis may be an acceptable outcome with limited other options and significant disease. However, acute allograft rejection may not be acceptable in many cases—such as heart and lung transplant—where measures like dialysis with graft failure are not an option. At present, use of these therapies in SOTRs is generally not recommended and advised with caution given the risk for allograft rejection.[41] In fact, SOTRs with malignancies treated with ICIs require multidisciplinary management with active involvement of transplant and oncology teams, amongst many others. Future research is necessary to explore the safety and efficacy of immunotherapy in the SOTR population in an effort to develop guidelines to assist clinical care.

INTRALESIONAL IMMUNOTHERAPIES IN SOTRS

SOTRs are often not eligible for systemic immunotherapies because of the potential risk of allograft rejection. This makes SOTRs with advanced malignancies a challenging population to treat, as systemic immunotherapy may not be considered safe and most local treatments may not offer durable responses. Intralesional (or intratumoral) therapies, most commonly with oncolytic viruses, offer exciting potential in cancer treatment and involve the direct injection of agents to promote local and systemic antitumor immune response while minimizing systemic toxicities.[42] Currently, there are several clinical trials investigating the use of intralesional immunotherapies, both as monotherapy as well as in combination with ICIs, for the treatment of metastatic or unresectable cutaneous malignancies in immunocompetent patients. Importantly, the use of these agents in the organ transplant population is largely unexplored and SOTRs remain excluded from these clinical trials at present.

Intralesional Immune Checkpoint Inhibitors

In 2018, the PD-1 inhibitor cemiplimab was approved for the treatment of metastatic or unresectable cSCC. This approval was based on the results from phase II clinical trial with systemic cemiplimab, which demonstrated an ORR of 50% in locally advanced and 47% in metastatic disease with systemic cemiplimab.[43] Currently, a phase I study investigating the utility of preoperative intralesional cemiplimab for patients with recurrent cSCC is underway.[44] Although SOTRs are notably excluded from this clinical study, the potential benefit of intralesional immunotherapy should be considered in the transplant population and further investigation is warranted.

Intralesional Therapy with Oncolytic Virus

Talimogene laherparepvec (T-VEC) is the only intralesional oncolytic virotherapy approved by the United States FDA for the treatment of stage IIIB, IIIC, and IVM1a melanoma with cutaneous, subcutaneous, or lymph node metastases.[45,46] It is a genetically modified double-stranded DNA herpes simplex virus type 1 that induces tumor-specific T cell responses by stimulating viral pathogenicity, enhancing tumor-selective replication, and reducing virally mediated suppression of antigen presentation.[47,48] T-VEC selectively replicates in and lyses tumor cells, promoting regional antitumor immunity and inducing a systemic immune response with abscopal effects noted.[48]

In the phase III Oncovex (GM-GSF) Pivotal Trial in Melanoma (OPTiM), T-VEC demonstrated a higher durable response rate (16%), ORR (26%), complete remission (11%), and median overall survival (23.3 months) compared with results for granulocyte-macrophage colony-stimulating factor.[45,48] Patients also demonstrated a 50% reduction in the size of 34% of noninjected nonvisceral lesions and a 15% reduction in the size of visceral lesions. Final long-term analysis confirmed that T-VEC was associated with durable responses and prolonged survival.[49] Based on these findings, T-VEC was believed to be a good option as monotherapy in patients with localized disease who may not require or have failed systemic treatments.[45,49,50]

Importantly, T-VEC may be associated with relatively mild side effects, which include self-limiting flu-like symptoms and injection-site reactions,[45] making T-VEC monotherapy a considerably less toxic alternative to systemic immunotherapies. However, the combination of T-VEC with systemic therapies is currently being investigated, with promising early results, as T-VEC has demonstrated synergistic effects with other systemic ICIs.[51,52] It is hypothesized that oncolytic viruses may transform the tumor microenvironment from immune-suppressed to immune-activated, promoting a proinflammatory milieu and antitumor immunity in the setting of systemic therapy.[51,52]

At present, the use of T-VEC in SOTRs is limited to case reports, as SOTRs remain excluded from previous and current clinical trials. One published case highlighted the successful treatment of a heart transplant patient with recurrent locally advanced cutaneous melanoma who received salvage T-VEC therapy. The patient achieved complete remission after 5 cycles of therapy, with no evidence of graft rejection.[48] An additional case highlights the successful use of intralesional T-VEC for the treatment of in-transit melanoma metastases in a patient with stage IIIC MM in the setting of a heart and kidney transplant.[47] The patient received 11 cycles of T-VEC over an 8-month period and remained relapse-free at 13 months without any evidence of graft rejection.[47] Finally, the use of T-VEC in combination with topical imiquimod should be considered for SOTRs with locally advanced disease given the potential for complete clearance of cutaneous in-transit metastases without signs of organ rejection.[53]

Additional oncolytic virus therapies under investigation include CAVATEK (coxsackievirus A21) and HF 10 (spontaneously mutated herpes simplex virus-1 [HSV-1]).[42] However, these therapies have not been utilized in the transplant population.

Although intralesional therapies may be promising for the treatment of malignancies in SOTRs because of limited systemic effects, additional research is necessary to explore the safety and efficacy in the transplant population. Regardless, a multidisciplinary approach with the transplant and oncology teams is of high importance when considering these therapies for SOTRs.

CONCLUSION

Cancer immunotherapy is revolutionizing the treatment of advanced and metastatic cancers, with ICIs and oncolytic virotherapy, amongst others, becoming integral components in the therapeutic armamentarium. Although the use of cancer immunotherapy has demonstrated positive data in the general population, these therapeutic agents must be utilized with caution in the solid organ transplant population until additional prospective, randomized clinical trials are performed. In the interim, physicians must exercise caution when administering immunotherapy, balancing the risk of graft rejection with progression of oncologic disease.

SUMMARY OF KEY POINTS

- SOTRs are at higher risk of developing posttransplant malignancies, with cutaneous neoplasms being the most common.
- There is a paucity of data regarding the use of immunotherapy for the treatment of malignancies in SOTRs as this population is largely excluded from clinical trials because of the risk of allograft rejection.

- Risk of graft rejection and graft loss in transplant recipients receiving ICIs may be associated with the type of ICI, type of organ transplant, immunosuppressive regimen, and time since transplantation.
- Importantly, in SOTRs who receive ICIs, most deaths were related to the progression of metastatic disease or secondary to underlying condition, rather than graft rejection or graft loss.
- The use of intralesional immunotherapies in the transplant population may be beneficial given the limited systemic side effects, although clinical trials are necessary to confirm their safety and efficacy.

REFERENCES

1. Organ procurement and transplantation network. U.S. Department of Health & Human Services. 2020. Available from: https://optn.transplant.hrsa.gov/data/
2. Euvrard S, Kanitakis J, Claudy A. Skin cancers after organ transplantation. N Engl J Med. 2003 Apr 24;348(17):1681–91.
3. Abdel-Wahab N, Safa H, Abudayyeh A et al. Checkpoint inhibitor therapy for cancer in solid organ transplantation recipients: an institutional experience and a systematic review of the literature. J Immunother Cancer. 2019 Apr 16;7(1):106.
4. Fisher J, Zeitouni N, Fan W et al. Immune checkpoint inhibitor therapy in solid organ transplant recipients: a patient-centered systematic review. J Am Acad Dermatol. 2019 Jul 11;82(6).
5. Engels EA, Pfeiffer RM, Fraumeni JF et al. Spectrum of cancer risk among US solid organ transplant recipients. JAMA. 2011 Nov 2;306(17):1891–901.
6. Smedman TM, Line PD, Guren TK et al. Graft rejection after immune checkpoint inhibitory therapy in solid organ transplant recipients. Acta Oncol. 2018 Oct;57(10):1414–18.
7. Garrett GL, Blanc PD, Boscardin J et al. Incidence of and risk factors for skin cancer in organ transplant recipients in the United States. JAMA Dermatol. 2017;153(3):296–303.
8. Krynitz B, Olsson H, Lundh Rozell B et al. Risk of basal cell carcinoma in Swedish organ transplant recipients: a population-based study. Br J Dermatol. 2016 Jan;174(1):95–103.
9. Fattouh K, Ducroux E, Decullier E et al. Increasing incidence of melanoma after solid organ transplantation: a retrospective epidemiological study. Transpl Int. 2017 Nov;30(11):1172–80.
10. Tessari G, Girolomoni G. Nonmelanoma skin cancer in solid organ transplant recipients: update on epidemiology, risk factors, and management. Dermatol Surg. 2012 Oct;38(10):1622–30.
11. Hiesse C, Rieu P, Kriaa F et al. Malignancy after renal transplantation: analysis of incidence and risk factors in 1700 patients followed during a 25-year period. Transplant Proc. 1997 Feb–Mar;29(1–2):831–3.
12. Greenberg JN, Zwald FO. Management of skin cancer in solid-organ transplant recipients: a multidisciplinary approach. Dermatol Clin. 2011 Apr;29(2):231–41.
13. Penn I. Post-transplant malignancy: the role of immunosuppression. Drug Saf. 2000 Aug;23(2):101–13.
14. Athar M, Walsh SB, Kopelovich L, Elmets CA. Pathogenesis of nonmelanoma skin cancers in organ transplant recipients. Arch Biochem Biophys. 2011 Apr 15;508(2):159–63.
15. Bouwes Bavnick JN, Euvrard S, Naldi L et al. Keratotic skin lesions and other risk factors are associated with skin cancer in organ-transplant recipients: a case-control study in The Netherlands, United Kingdom, Germany, France, and Italy. J Invest Dermatol. 2007 Jul;127(7):1647–56.
16. Naldi L, Venturuzzo A, Invernizzi P. Dermatological complications after solid organ transplantation. Clin Rev Allergy Immunol. 2018 Feb;54(1):185–212.
17. Nagarajan P, Asgari MM, Green AC et al. Keratinocyte carcinomas: current concepts and future research priorities. Clin Cancer Res. 2019 Apr 15;25(8):2379–91.
18. Euvrard S, Morelon E, Rostaing L et al. Sirolimus and secondary skin-cancer prevention in kidney transplantation. N Engl J Med. 2012 Jul;367(4):329–39.
19. Liu M, Guo W, Zhang S. Cancer immunotherapy in patients with new or recurrent malignancies after liver transplantation. Int J Surg Oncol (NY). 2017 Dec;2(11):e49.
20. Coley WB. The treatment of malignant tumors by repeated inoculations of erysipelas: with a report of ten original cases. 1893. Clin Orthop Relat Res. 1991 Jan;262:3–11.

21. Hodi FS, O'Day SJ, McDermott DF et al. Improved survival with ipilimumab in patients with metastatic melanoma. N Engl J Med. 2010 Aug 19;363(8):711–23.
22. Vaddepally RK, Kharel P, Pandey R, Garje R, Chandra AB. Review of indications of FDA-approved immune checkpoint inhibitors per NCCN guidelines with the level of evidence. Cancers (Basel). 2020 Mar 20;12(3):738.
23. Grob JJ, Gonzalez R, Basset-Seguin N et al. Pembrolizumab monotherapy for recurrent or metastatic cutaneous squamous cell carcinoma: a single-arm phase II trial (KEYNOTE-629). J Clin Oncol. 2020 Sep 1; 38(25):2916–25.
24. Chae TK, Galvez C, Anker JF et al. Cancer immunotherapy in a neglected population: the current use and future of T-cell-mediated checkpoint inhibitors in organ transplant patients. Cancer Treat Rev. 2018 Feb;63:116–21.
25. Wong K, Shen J, D'Ambruoso S et al. Safety and efficacy of immune checkpoint inhibitors in patients with metastatic cancer post solid organ transplantation: a case report and review of the literature. Transplant Proc. 2019 Nov;51(9):3053–8.
26. McCoy KD, Le Gros G. The role of CTLA-4 in the regulation of T cell immune responses. Immunol Cell Biol. 1999 Feb;77(1):1–10.
27. Postow MA, Callahan MK, Wolchok JD. Immune checkpoint blockade in cancer therapy. J Clin Oncol. 2015 Jun 10;33(17):1974–82.
28. Johnson DB, Sullivan RJ, Menzies AM. Immune checkpoint inhibitors in challenging populations. Cancer. 2017 Jun 1;123(11):1904–11.
29. Ingulli E. Mechanism of cellular rejection in transplantation. Pediatr Nephrol. 2010 Jan;25(1):61–74.
30. Riella LV, Paterson AM, Sharpe AH et al. Role of the PD-1 pathway in the immune response. Am J Transplant. 2012 Oct;12(10):2575–87.
31. Munn DH. Indoleamine 2,3-dioxygenase, tregs and cancer. Curr Med Chem. 2011;18(15):2240–6.
32. Furukara A, Wisel SA, Tang Q. Impact of immune-modulatory drugs on regulatory T cell. Transplant. 2016 Nov;100(11):2288–300.
33. Kean LS, Turka LA, Blazar BR. Advances in targeting co-inhibitory and co-stimulatory pathways in transplantation settings: the Yin to the Yang of cancer immunotherapy. Immunol Rev. 2017 Mar;276(1):192–212.
34. Kumar V, Shinagare AB, Rennke HG et al. The safety and efficacy of checkpoint inhibitors in transplant recipients: a case series and systematic review of literature. Oncologist. 2020 Feb 11;25(6).
35. DeLeon TT, Salomao MA, Aqel BA et al. Pilot evaluation of PD-1 inhibition in metastatic cancer patients with a history of liver transplantation: the Mayo clinic experience. J Gastrointest Oncol. 2018 Dec;9(6):1054–62.
36. Halloran PF, Famulski KS, Chang J. A probabilistic approach to histologic diagnosis of antibody-mediated rejection in kidney transplant biopsies. Am J Transplant. 2017 Jan;17(1):129–39.
37. Friend BD, Venick RS, McDiarmid SV et al. Fatal orthotopic liver transplant organ rejection induced by a checkpoint inhibitor in two patients with refractory, metastatic hepatocellular carcinoma. Pediatr Blood Cancer. 2017 Dec;64(12).
38. O'Donnell JS, Massi D, Teng MWL et al. PI3K-AKT-mTOR inhibitor in cancer immunotherapy, redux. Semin Cancer Biol. 2018 Feb;48:91–103.
39. d'Izarny-Gargas T, Durrbach A, Zaidan M. Efficacy and tolerance of immune checkpoint inhibitors in transplant patients with cancer: a systematic review. Am J Transplant. 2020 Feb 6;20(9).
40. Tacrolimus, nivolumab, and ipilimumab in treating kidney transplant recipients with selected unresectable or metastatic cancers. NCT03816332. Available from: https://clinicaltrials.gov/ct2/show/NCT03816332
41. Stevenson ML, Carucci J, Colegio OR. Skin cancer in transplant recipients: scientific retreat of the international immunosuppression and transplant skin cancer collaborative and skin cancer in organ transplant patients-Europe. Clin Transplant. 2019 Dec;33(12):e13736.
42. Hamid O, Ismail R, Puzanov I. Intratumoral immunotherapy-update 2019. Oncologist. 2019 Nov 29;25(3).
43. Migden MR, Rischin D, Schmults CD et al. PD-1 blockade with cemiplimab in advanced cutaneous squamous-cell carcinoma. N Engl J Med. 2018 Jul 26;379(4).
44. Pre-operative cemiplimab administered intralesionally for patients with recurrent cutaneous squamous cell carcinoma. NCT03889912. Available from: https://clinicaltrials.gov/ct2/show/NCT03889912
45. Andtbacka RH, Kaufman HL, Collichio F et al. Talimogene laherparepvec improves durable response rate in patients with advanced melanoma. J Clin Oncol. 2015 Sep 1;33(25):2780–8.
46. Franke V. Talimogene laherparepvec monotherapy, an elegant alternative to systemic immunotherapy for the treatment of early metastatic melanoma. Br J Dermatol. 2019 Jul;181(1):20–.
47. Ressler J, Silmbrod R, Stepan A et al. Talimogene laherparepvec (T-VEC) in advanced melanoma: complete response in a heart and kidney transplant patient, a case report. Br J Dermatol. 2019 Jul;181(1):186–9.
48. Schvartsman G, Perez K, Flynn JE et al. Safe and effective administration of T-VEC in a patient with heart transplantation and recurrent locally advanced melanoma. J Immunother Cancer. 2017 Jun 20;5:45.

49. Andtbacka RHI, Collichio F, Harrington KJ et al. Final analyses of OPTiM: a randomized phase III trial of talimogene laherparepvec versus granulocyte-macrophage colony-stimulating factor in unresectable stage III-IV melanoma. J Immunother Cancer. 2019 Jun 6;7(1):145.
50. Queen D, Samie FH, Zeitouni NC. Future directions and challenges facing intralesional immunotherapy with talimogene laherparepvec for advanced melanoma. Dermatol Surg. 2019 Sep 30;47(1).
51. Long GV, Dummer R, Ribas A et al. A phase I/III, multicenter, open-label trial of talimogene laherparepvec (T-VEC) in combination with pembrolizumab for the treatment of unresected, stage IIIb-IV melanoma (MASTERKEY-265). J Immunotherapy Cancer. 2015;3:181.
52. Chesney J, Puzanov I, Collichio F et al. Randomized, open-label phase II study evaluating the efficacy and safety of talimogene laherparepvec in combination with ipilimumab versus ipilimumab alone in patients with advanced, unresectable melanoma. J Clin Oncol. 2018 Jun 10;36(17):1658–67.
53. Sunshine JC, Sosman J, Shetty A, Choi JN. Successful treatment of in-transit metastatic melanoma in a renal transplant patient with combination T-VEC/imiquimod immunotherapy. J Immunother. 2020 May;43(4):149–52.

14 Bacterial, Fungal, and Viral Skin Infections in Organ Transplant Recipients

Alexandra Geusau

INTRODUCTION

One of the major problems in immunocompromised patients after solid-organ transplantation is infection, often also a major determinant of the outcome of transplantation (TX). The skin and the mucous membranes occupy a central position in infections in these patients. First, the skin is the first barrier against infections and any disturbance of this barrier can contribute to a change in skin flora or facilitate the entrance of pathogens. Second, skin infections may be a sign or the cause of systemic infection and therefore call for a high index of suspicion. In organ transplant recipients (OTRs), classical skin infections such as cellulitis due to group A streptococci, wound infections caused by staphylococci, as well as superficial fungal infections or herpes reactivations may differ with regard to clinical signs, severity, incidence, or course of the disease. For dermatophytes, so-called non-virulent fungi frequently diagnosed in immunocompetent individuals, there may be widespread infection or scalp involvement and even local invasion into the dermis. Common infections with human papilloma viruses (HPV) may lead to extensive cutaneous involvement and be difficult to eradicate.

The skin may also be the site of infections with opportunistic pathogens generally without pathogenic potency for humans. Most commonly, these infections are either due to fungi occurring on the surface of the skin and mucous membranes as saprophytes, such as *Candida* spp., or descend from the environment. Relevant organisms in this scenario also include *Aspergillus* spp. and *Cryptococcus neoformans*, and bacteria such as *Nocardia* spp. or nontuberculous mycobacteria (NTM). Infections due to so-called endemic fungi, *Histoplasma capsulatum* or *Coccidioides*, are distributed geographically and very rarely diagnosed. Generally, cutaneous lesions may also represent disseminated systemic infection metastatic to the skin from a non-cutaneous portal of entry.[1]

The incidence and risk of infections in OTRs varies and depends on various factors, including the type of organ transplanted, the degree and type of immunosuppression (IS), the need for additional antirejection therapy, and the occurrence of surgical complications connected with the transplant procedure; it is also determined by interaction between the patient's epidemiological exposures and net state of IS.[1–4] Antifungal

DOI: 10.1201/9781003001461-14

and antiviral prophylaxis also influences the expression pattern and the frequency of respective skin infections.[5] Recently, microbiota changes/disruption under IS after TX have been associated not only with chronic rejection but also infection; however, there is no data on the impact of this observation on skin infections.[6,7]

Nevertheless, there is a similar pattern of infection in all forms of organ TX and a consistent timetable for the occurrence of different infections after TX[1,3,8] with different time points according to the pathogen. There is also a typical chronology of infections when the skin and mucous membranes are involved and a particular time line of skin infections following organ TX.[3,8,9] This time line represents three overlapping periods of risk. The first is the perioperative period to approximately 30 days after TX; the main problems come from bacterial wound infections because of the surgical procedure, pyoderma or reactivation of herpes viruses being the major problems as well as *Candida* infections. In the second period, from 1 to 6–12 months after TX, opportunistic skin infections classically associated with IS become manifest. Beyond 6–12 months, the clinical course of skin infections is largely determined by the presence or absence of chronic rejection and whether additional antirejection therapy is required. As usually IS is reduced after 6 months, the spectrum of causative organisms approaches that of the general population and comprises mycoses or HPV infections. Patients with frequent episodes of rejection who are maintained on a higher baseline level of IS remain at risk for the opportunistic agents more classically seen in the second to sixth months posttransplantation (Figure 14.1).[3,9]

Skin infections have been shown to be highly prevalent in OTRs, with 55%–97% of the patients having some type of infection.[10] In a single center study on registered skin diseases of >1700 kidney transplant recipients (KTRs) over a 12-year observation period, skin infections were the most commonly

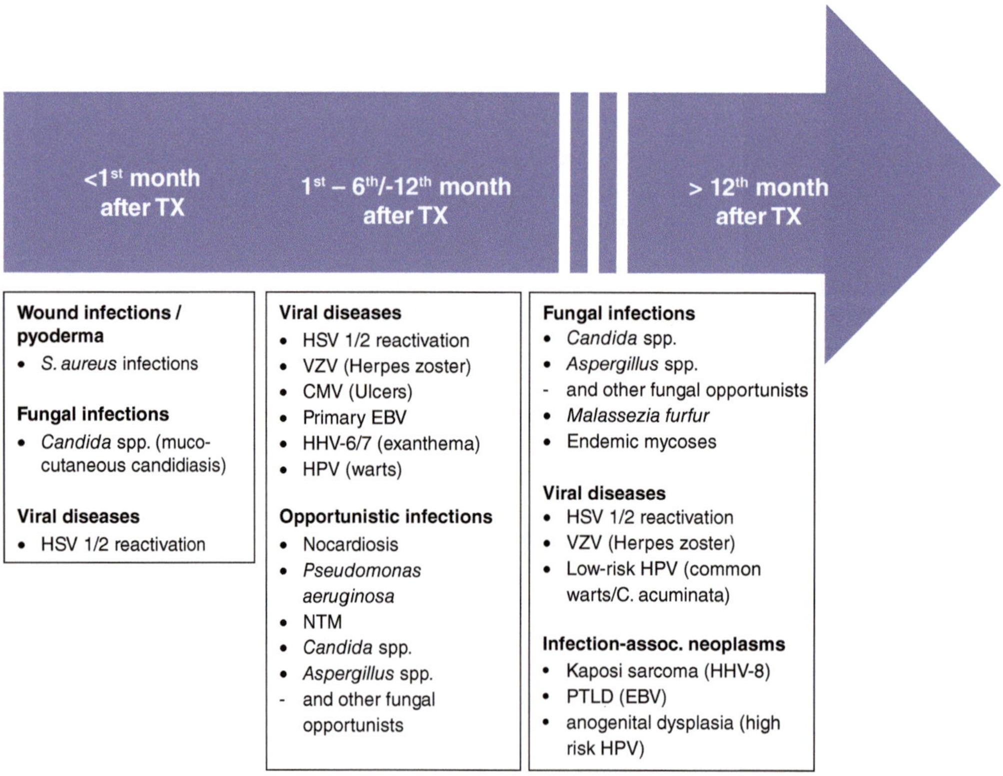

FIGURE 14.1 The time line of cutaneous infections following organ transplantation. C.acuminata, condylomata acuminata; CMV, cytomegalovirus; EBV, Epstein-Barr virus; HHV, human herpes virus; HPV, human papillomavirus; HSV, herpes simplex virus; NTM, nontuberculous mycobacteria; PTLD, posttransplant lymphoproliferative disorder; spp, species; TX, transplantation; VZV, varicella zoster virus. (Modified from references 3, 4, and 9.)

recorded diagnosis. The overall contribution of skin infections to the relative distributions of skin disease decreased with time after transplantation, whereas the contribution of keratinocyte cancers (KC) strongly increased.[10] In this study, viral infections, particularly due to herpes simplex virus (HSV) and varicella zoster virus (VZV), as well as yeast infections, namely candidiasis occurred relatively early, at a median of 2 years after TX. The median time to the occurrence/diagnosis of bacterial and other fungal infections was considerably longer. Of the bacterial infections, bacterial folliculitis was more common during the first years after transplantation, at a median of 4.4 years, whereas cellulitis was registered after longer post-TX time periods.[10] Accordingly, regardless of the post-TX period, the skin and soft tissue infections were frequent contributors to morbidity and mortality in the immunocompromised host, which underlines why cutaneous symptoms and their clarification require careful attention in OTRs.

BACTERIAL SKIN INFECTIONS

Cutaneous lesions in combination with fever in patients under IS present a diagnostic challenge; they may indicate fungal, mycobacterial, or viral infections or lymphoproliferative diseases, as well as bacterial skin infections (BSIs) (Table 14.1). The clinical presentation of BSIs in OTRs is not necessarily different compared with that in the immunocompetent population, but atypical or more severe clinical manifestations may occur.[11] The prevalence of BSIs is increased: according to a case-control study, BCI was diagnosed in 42.4% of KTR compared with 14.2% of the controls.[12]

BSIs most commonly are associated with species of *Streptococcus* or *Staphylococcus* (Figure 14.2) and comprise impetigo contagiosa, which are thin-walled vesicles and pustules, ecthyma, an ulcerative skin manifestation commonly seen on the shins or dorsal feet, furuncles, abscesses, or folliculitis. The latter is reported to be the most prevalent cutaneous manifestation of *S. aureus* infection in the first 6 months following kidney transplantation as asserted by Hogewoning and coworkers.[13] The same authors found that 6.7% of the KTR developed impetigo of some form in their posttransplantation period.[11] Bullous impetigo is associated strictly with staphylococcal infection, particularly with strains that produce exfoliative toxin A, which targets the protein desmoglein 1.[14]

S. aureus colonization of the anterior nares, frequently also involving methicillin-resistant *S. aureus* (MRSA), has been identified as a risk factor for the development of infections in various settings. As it may be the source of bacteremia, proper eradication with intranasal mupirocin prior to transplantation is recommended in selected patients by some authors, because according to a prospective study in 323 liver transplant recipients (LTRs) screened prior to TX, multivariate analysis revealed that MRSA and methicillin-sensitive *S. aureus* nasal carriage, as well as alcoholic cirrhosis, were independent predictors of *S. aureus* infections including bacteremia, pneumonia, intra-abdominal abscesses, and wound infections.[15] In contrast to this report, no association could be found between nasal *S. aureus* colonization and cutaneous staphylococcal infections according to a small study in KTRs, challenging screening for nasal *S. aureus* carriage as a preventive measure for *S. aureus* infections in OTRs, in particular OTRs other than LTRs.[12]

Staphylococcal species can also cause necrotizing fasciitis, although commonly also because of polymicrobial infection, representing a devastating cutaneous infection. Apart from other factors, IS is one of the risk factors. The infection spreads through the superficial and deep fascia, most commonly on the extremities and abdominal wall, and requires emergent surgical debridement along with broad-spectrum antimicrobial therapy.[16] According to a literature review, OTRs with necrotizing fasciitis were more than twice as likely to present with shock when compared with rates in a control group.[17]

Infection with *Pseudomonas aeruginosa*, a gram-negative rod-shaped ubiquitous bacterium, is considered opportunistic, insofar as serious infection often occurs during existing diseases or under IS. The most common cutaneous manifestation of *P. aeruginosa* infection is ecthyma gangrenosum, characterized by rapidly spreading ulcers,[18] which are often regarded as a sign of underlying

TABLE 14.1 Clinical Criteria for the Diagnosis of Bacterial and Viral Skin Lesions in Transplant Recipients

	ORGANISM	*CUTANEOUS SYMPTOMS*
Bacterial skin infections	*Staphylococcus aureus*	Local infections (folliculitis, furuncles, carbuncles, abscess, impetigo contagiosa, bullous impetigo, ecthyma), wound infections, soft-tissue infections (cellulitis), necrotizing fasciitis, staphylococcal scalded-skin syndrome (SSSS), MRSA infection
	Group A streptococcus *(Streptococcus pyogenes)*	Impetigo contagiosa, ecthyma, cellulitis
	Group B streptococcus	Primary skin and soft-tissue infections
	Pseudomonas aeruginosa and other gram-negative rods (e.g., *E. coli, P. mirabilis, K. pneumoniae* (opportunistic pathogens)	Necrotizing fasciitis, ecthyma gangrenosum, soft-tissue infections, abscess formation, necrosis, ulceration
	Streptococcus pneumoniae	Soft-tissue infections
	Nocardia (opportunistic pathogen)	Primary cutaneous nocardiosis: soft-tissue infections (cellulitis), abscesses, lymphocutaneous infection, mycetoma; eventually systemic dissemination
	Mycobacteria	Infections with typical mycobacteria: primary cutaneous inoculation with sporotrichoid or verrucous appearance OR spread from local deep tissue (scrophuloderma). Infections with nontuberculous mycobacteria: ulcerating or suppurative nodules, tumors, inflammatory papules, verrucous plaques
	Bartonella henselae/quintana	Bacillary angiomatosis: localized or disseminated red-violaceous vascular nodules, plaques, tumors)
Viral skin infections	Human herpesviruses (HHV)	
	HSV-1, 2	Vesicles, pustules, chronic large ulcers (orofacial, anogenital), widespread local or disseminated infection, eczema herpeticum
	VZV	Varicella, herpes zoster, disseminated cutaneous infection, chronic herpes zoster, chronic ecthymatous varicella
		Infectious mononucleosis (morbilliform exanthema, ulcers, purpuric eruptions, papules, vesiculobullous eruption), oral hairy leukoplakia/oral papulosis (hyperkeratotic lesions with corrugated appearance of lateral tongue/coalescing papules on the surface of the tongue), posttransplant lymphoproliferative disorder (PTLD)

(*Continued*)

TABLE 14.1 Clinical Criteria for the Diagnosis of Bacterial and Viral Skin Lesions in Transplant Recipients (Continued)

	ORGANISM	*CUTANEOUS SYMPTOMS*
	CMV	Maculopapular rash, ulcers, purpuric eruptions, necrotic papules, vesiculobullous eruptions, petechiae
	HHV-8	Kaposi's sarcoma (reddish macules, vascular tumors)
	Human papilloma viruses (HPV)	Warts, condylomata acuminata, HPV-associated penile/vulvar/cervical/anal intraepithelial neoplasia (PIN, VIN, CIN, AIN)
	Molluscum contagiosum virus (a Poxvirus)	Mollusca contagiosa

Abbreviations: CMV, cytomegalovirus; HHV, human herpesvirus; HSV, herpes simplex virus; MRSA, methicillin-resistant *Staphylococcus aureus*; PTLD, posttransplant lymphoproliferative disorder; SSSS, staphylococcal scalded skin syndrome; VZV, varicella-zoster virus.

Source: Adapted from Ilyas et al.[11] and Pettit et al.[16]

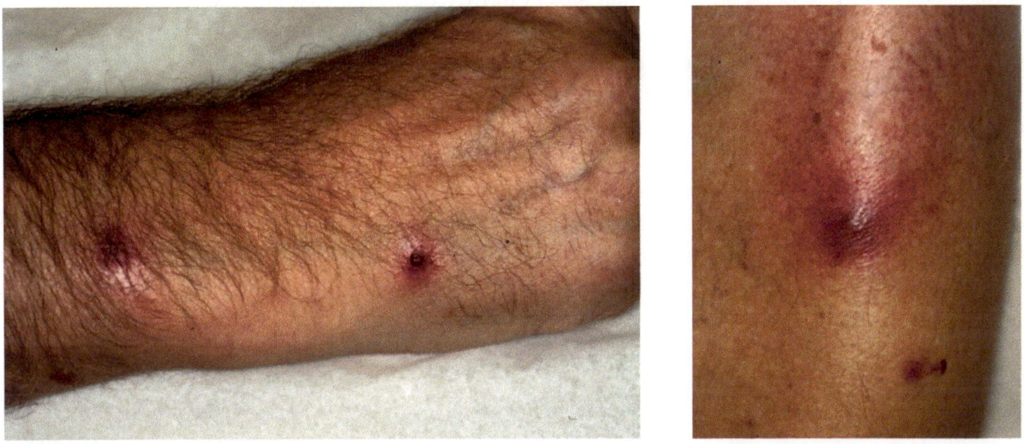

FIGURE 14.2 *S. aureus*-associated deep inflammatory lesions mimicking "vasculitis" on the extremities of a heart transplant recipient; broad-spectrum PCR revealed *S. aureus.*

septicemia.[11] In the scenario of OTRs, *P. aeruginosa* and other gram-negatives or anaerobes may also be responsible for cellulitis.

Nocardiosis is a rare localized—pulmonary, central nervous system, and cutaneous—or systemic suppurative disease caused by several species of bacteria in the genus *Nocardia*, a group of aerobic, gram-positive bacteria that belong to the Actinomycetaceae family.[19] Infection occurs either by direct inoculation or inhalation.[20] The clinical presentation on the skin is nonspecific and includes ulcers, abscess formation, granulomas, soft tissue infection, and lymphocutaneous infection. Disseminated *Nocardia* infection in immunocompromised patients is a rare but life-threatening disease.[21,22] Although *Nocardia* usually causes pulmonary infections, there are case reports on primary cutaneous nocardiosis in OTRs, usually because of direct inoculation, most commonly caused by *N. brasiliensis*.[23] For diagnosis, both microbiological and histological testing on biopsy specimens should be performed with attempts to culture *Nocardia*.[24]

Actinomycosis is a rare and heterogeneous infection involving gram-positive anaerobic bacteria, which are commensals in the oral cavity and digestive tract. Unlike nocardiosis, actinomycosis is mainly reported in immunocompetent patients, although both diseases are due to bacteria that belong to the same order, Actinomycetales. According to a retrospective analysis of seven cases, the prevalence of actinomycosis in OTRs was very low, namely 0.02%.[25]

Bacillary angiomatosis (BA) or so-called "cat-scratch disease" is a rare vasculoproliferative disorder due to *Bartonella henselae* or *Bartonella quintana*,[26] which usually presents as red or violaceous lesions that resemble hemangiomas (Figure 14.3). An important differential diagnosis is Kaposi sarcoma or pyogenic granuloma. The lesions may be solitary or widespread, preferentially on the face and extremities. Additional symptoms may include fever, lymphadenopathy, and vascular nodules within the organs.[26] Exposure to the bacterium is most commonly through cats, which might help explain why a staggering 25% of cases of BA in OTRs were in the pediatric or adolescent population, despite only 3%–4% of OTRs being in this age range.[26,27] BA mainly has been reported in patients infected with HIV. *Bartonella* species are difficult to identify in culture, and the diagnosis eventually relies on the demonstration of the pathogen within the lesions. Nowadays, a polymerase chain reaction (PCR)-based assay is an accurate method for the detection of *Bartonella*. Antibiotic therapy includes long-term application of doxycycline or ciprofloxacin.[26]

Skin infections caused by mycobacteria (MB), which are acid-fast, nonmotile, weakly gram-positive rods, may be due to "typical" MB, *M. tuberculosis* (TB) or nontuberculous mycobacteria (NTM) (Table 14.2). The latter are ubiquitous environmental organisms with generally no attributable pathogenicity; however, they may affect both immunocompromised and—under certain circumstances—immunocompetent patients. Infections with MB are not necessarily a sign of immunosuppression, but particularly for NTM, depend on individual susceptibility or, in the case of cutaneous infections, may result from a minor, often unrecognized trauma to the skin. Approximately 90% of NTM infections involve the pulmonary system; the rest affect lymph nodes, skin and soft tissue, as well as bones.[28]

TB is acquired primarily by inhalation of aerosolized droplets containing the organisms, leading to respiratory tract infection with subsequent dissemination. Typical MB infections seem to be rare in OTRs, particularly in populations with low prevalence of the disease. The occurrence of early post-TX reactivation of TB disease at an estimated rate of 2.1% among OTRs despite treatment for a latent TB infection may be a concern. In OTRs living in TB-endemic regions, exposure to TB with a potential for infection or reinfection is possible.[29] According to a retrospective study in 2500 KTRs, infections with TB were mainly pulmonary, whereas NTM infections were located in the skin, tendons, and joints. In this survey, the prevalence of MB disease was estimated to be 0.56%, with 0.36% TB and 0.20% NTM infections. The total dose of corticosteroids was found to be the major risk factor for infection.[30]

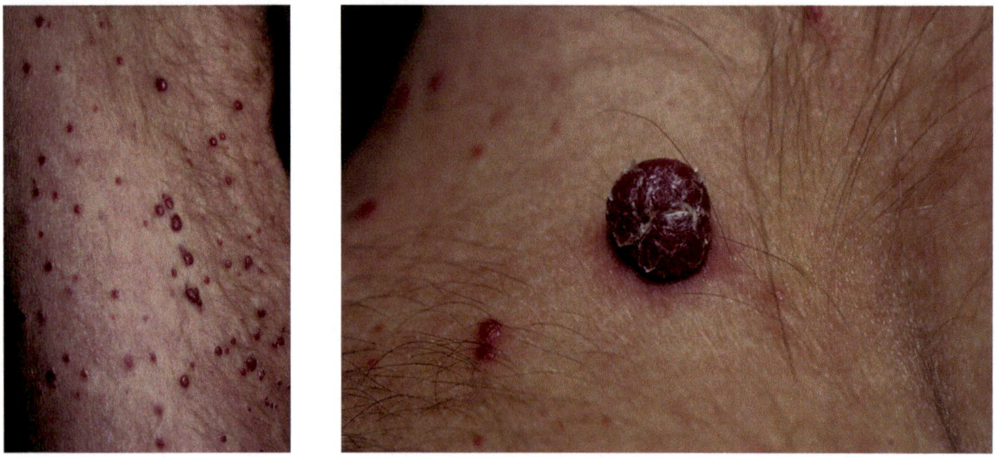

FIGURE 14.3 Bacillary angiomatosis due to *B. henselae* in an AIDS patient; hundreds of hemangioma-like lesions were distributed on the entire surface of his body. The skin lesions were accompanied by fever, weight loss, and lymphadenopathy.

TABLE 14.2 Classification of Nontuberculous Mycobacteria (NTM) Commonly Causing Human Disease (Pulmonary and Extrapulmonary)

PATHOGEN	*CLASSIFICATION OF NTM COMMONLY CAUSING HUMAN DISEASE*	*DISEASE*
M. avium complex (MAC)	RG III, SGB	Pulmonary disease
M. abscessus complex	RG IV, RGB	
M. kansasii	RGI, SGB	
M. malmoense	RG III, SGB	
M. xenopi	RG III, SGB	
M. avium complex (MAC)	RG III, SGB	Lymphadenitis
M. scrofulaceum	RG II, SGB	
M. malmoense	RG III, SGB	
M. haemophilum	RG III, SGB	
M. abscessus complex	RG IV; RGB	Skin, soft tissue, fish tank granuloma, "swimming pool granuloma"
M. chelonae	RG IV, RGB	
M. fortuitum complex	RG IV, RGB	
M. marinum	RG I, SGB	
M. ulcerans	RG III, SGB	
M. avium complex (MAC)	RG III, SGB	Bone infection
M. xenopi	RG III, SGB	
M. marinum	RG I, SGB	
M. kansasii	RG I, SGB	
M. abscessus complex	RG IV, RGB	
M. fortuitum complex	RG IV, RGB	

Abbreviations: NTM, nontuberculous mycobacteria; RG I, Runyon group I; RG II, Runyon group II; RG III, Runyon group III; RG IV, Runyon group IV; RGB, rapidly growing bacteria; SGB, slowly growing mycobacteria.

Source: Adapted from Koh, W.-J. Nontuberculous Mycobacteria—Overview. Microbiol Spectr. 2017 Jan;5(1). doi: 10.1128/microbiolspec.TNMI7-0024-2016).

Cutaneous infections with MB may either be primary due to direct inoculation of the pathogen, endogenous due to spread of pulmonary tuberculosis by hematogenous or lymphatic dissemination, or due to penetration of a tuberculous process from underlying tissue, so-called scrofuloderma (Figure 14.4).[31] Approximately 30% of TB cases after TX are extrapulmonary and 16% are disseminated. Atypical presentations were often observed, including pyomyositis, cutaneous ulcers, tenosynovitis, gastrointestinal disease, and lymphadenitis.[32]

The clinical spectrum of cutaneous and subcutaneous TB and NTM infections can be quite diverse and may mimic acute bacterial infections or tumors, presenting as inflammatory papules, suppurative nodules, or verrucous plaques.[29,31] NTM infections may also manifest as osteoarticular disease, pleuropulmonary or bloodstream infection, lymphadenitis, and multi-organ disease.[33] Therefore, MB disease has to be considered with any unexplained febrile illness, surgical site or bone infection, nonhealing wound or cutaneous lesion, especially when routine bacterial cultures are nondiagnostic.[34]

According to a case-control single-center study,[34] lung transplant recipients are at a higher risk for NTM disease compared with that of the other types of OTRs. Structural abnormalities, potential exposure of the transplanted lung to environmental pathogens, and the advanced state of IS in lung transplant recipients are considered to contribute to this higher risk. There was wide diversity in the causative NTM species observed in this study, but *M. abscessus* was the most common, followed by *M. avium* complex. The sites of infection also varied from pleuro-pulmonary disease to cutaneous and deep tissue, intra-abdominal, and disseminated infections.[34] *M. marinum* causes fish tank and

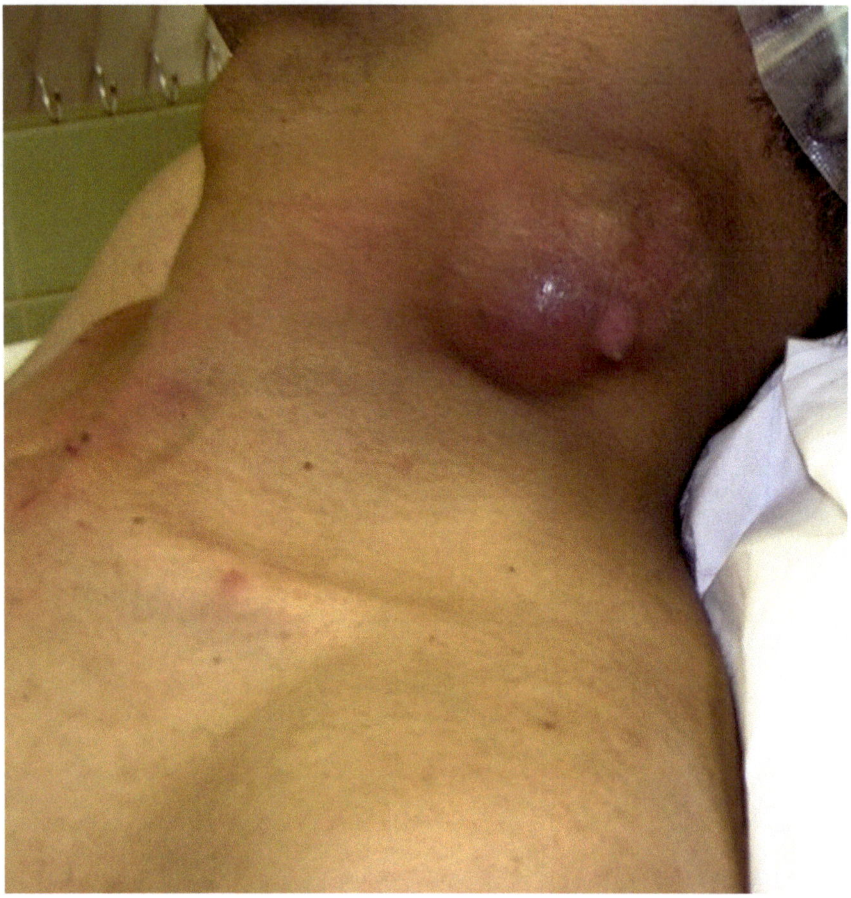

FIGURE 14.4 Scrofuloderma: Involvement of the skin with *Mycobacteria tuberculosis* due to penetration from underlying tuberculous lymphadenitis in an immunocompetent patient. (Prof Stefan Winkler, Vienna.)

swimming pool granuloma, not that infrequently observed in immunocompetent patients. A few cases of these infections have been reported in OTRs; usually they are more severe when compared with NTM infections in immunocompetent hosts.[35]

The diagnosis of cutaneous MB infections is made from skin biopsy findings that include special stains demonstrating acid-fast bacilli in clusters; however, diagnosis is often impossible to make because of the pauci-bacillary nature of the illness. Mycobacterial cultures used to be the "gold standard" for the diagnosis; however, DNA PCR should be used in preference over culture for the diagnosis, particularly with inconclusive histopathology.[32] Although granulomas on histopathology are suggestive of possible MB disease, the absence of granulomatous lesions does not necessarily negate the diagnosis in OTRs who have attenuated immune responses.[33] In addition, NTM cultures need proper media selection and specific growth requirements.[33] For prognostic and therapeutic considerations, it is necessary to identify the NTM to the level of the species and even the subspecies; this can be accomplished by molecular probes and 16S rDNA sequencing.[36] The use of a quantitative test, e.g. γ-interferon release assays (IGRA), a sensitive and specific detection method for the diagnosis of latent tuberculosis, is unreliable in active disease, has a significantly reduced sensitivity in patients with moderate or severe immunosuppression, and is useless in the diagnosis of NTM infections, as only *M. kansasii*, *M. szulgai*, *M. gordonae*, *M. flavescens*, and *M. marinum* produce positive IGRA test results.[37,38] As a rule, each patient with active MB skin disease should undergo a CT scan of the lungs to exclude active pulmonary disease.

The therapy of cutaneous MB infections in OTRs is the same as in the nontransplant population, although often more complicated given the potential drug interactions between antimycobacterial and IS agents. The choice of drugs and the duration of therapy is dependent on the specific isolate, the extent of the disease, and the degree of IS.[33] For the treatment of TB infections, a combination of at least three of the following agents is used: isoniazid, rifampicin, pyrazinamide, and ethambutol and streptomycin. In case of multidrug-resistant TB infection, a combination of these agents with quinolones and clarithromycin has to be considered.[32,39]

Cutaneous lesions due to NTM such as *M. marinum* are often superficial in immunocompetent patients, may regress spontaneously or after antibiotic monotherapy with e.g., clarithromycin, trimethoprim-sulfamethoxazole, or doxycycline.[35] In immunocompromised OTRs, the infection is usually more severe and treatment with at least two antibiotics is advised (e.g., clarithromycin and trimethoprim-sulfamethoxazole). Doxycycline may be combined with rifampicin or ethambutol in severe cases. Particularly for deep cutaneous infections, surgical excision is essential in order to reduce the bacterial load. Besides surgical debridement or excision, the reduction of IS therapy may be pivotal for a successful treatment of any MB disease.

FUNGAL SKIN INFECTION

In general, the rates, timing, and type of fungal infections in OTRs vary by the type of transplant received, LTRs, for instance, are more likely to have early fungal infection, often due to *Candida* spp. In OTRs, preemptive antifungal therapy may also lead to the emergence of unusual fungal pathogens. The level of IS therapy plays a pivotal key role in fungal infections: OTR with chronic rejection kept on higher dosages of IS therapy are more prone to late fungal infections due to *Aspergillus* or *Cryptococcus*.[40] This finding is supported by the resolution of fungal lesions after discontinuation of IS and antifungal therapy with voriconazole.[41] Fungal skin infections in OTRs include classical dermatomycoses, opportunistic infections, and infections with rare fungal pathogens (Table 14.3). For diagnosis of all forms of fungal infections, the isolation of etiologic agent from clinical samples is required. Direct microscopic examination is a suitable method for early diagnosis; *Candida* spp. and *Mucorales* appear as pseudohyphae and blastospores and broad non-septate and ribbon-like hyphae, respectively. In the case of deep cutaneous infections, skin biopsy for histopathologic investigation involving special staining is necessary. Increasingly, apart from cultures, molecular methods are being used for the detection of fungal agents.

In OTRs compared with immunocompetent individuals, **classical fungal skin infections** may differ with regard to the clinical signs, severity, or course of the disease. Dermatophytes, belonging to the genera *Trichophyton, Microsporum* and *Epidermophyton* are filamentous fungi characterized by their ability to grow in the presence of keratin substrates. Anthropophilic dermatophytes only infect humans; zoophilic dermatophytes infect animals and, occasionally, humans. Dermatophytes account for the largest group of pathogens responsible for benign skin mycoses limited to the stratum corneum or keratinized adnexal structures such as nails, affecting 20%–25% of the population. *Trichophyton* infections in OTRs, however, may be widespread (Figure 14.5) or with scalp involvement, or local invasion into the dermis.[42] These deep dermatophytoses are rarely described in case reports as a late complication in OTRs, usually preceded by superficial dermatophytosis; they might be prevented by prompt treatment of the early manifestation.[42] Clinically, deep dermatophytosis is characterized by discrete nodules in proximity to a superficial dermatophyte infection,[43] but the presentation of the lesions may be polymorphic.[42] Most infections may be treated with topical antifungals, but more aggressive infection may require systemic therapy. There is no consensus on treatment; systemic antifungals such as terbinafine and azoles are effective, but drug interactions between antifungal and immunosuppressive agents have to be respected.

TABLE 14.3 Classification and Clinical Criteria for the Diagnosis of Fungal Skin Lesions in Transplant Recipients

	CLASS	*FUNGAL PATHOGENS*	*CUTANEOUS SYMPTOMS*
Classical dermatomycoses	Dermatophytes	Anthropophilic species: *Trichophyton rubrum, T. interdigitale, Epidermophyton floccosum, T. tonsurans* Zoophilic species: *Microsporum canis, T. mentagrophytes, T. verrucosum*	Tinea pedis, manum, and corporis, tinea capitis, palmoplantar keratoderma, deep dermal (granulomatous) skin infection, erythematous papules, proximal subungual white onychomycosis
	Molds	*Scopulariopsis* spp.	Onychomycosis, subcutaneous infiltration
	Yeasts	*Malassezia furfur*	Pityriasis versicolor, folliculitis
Opportunistic fungal skin infections	Yeasts	*Candida* spp., mostly *C. albicans*, also *C. tropicalis, C. krusei, C. glabrata, C. parapsilosis*	Oropharyngeal infection ("thrush"), mucocutaneous candidiasis, glossitis, pseudomembranous and erythematous stomatitis, perlèche, paronychial, nail and skin fold infection, *Candida* balanitis, vulvovaginal candidiasis, folliculitis, pustules, "*Candida* granuloma"
		Cryptococcus spp. (mostly *C. neoformans*)	Papulopustular lesions, molluscum contagiosum-like small umbilicated papules, pustules, nonhealing (vegetative ulcers), cellulitis, subcutaneous nodules
	Molds	*Aspergillus* spp. (*A. niger, A. fumigatus, A. Flavus*)	Inflammatory skin infiltrates, erythematous/purpuric papules, edematous plaques, nodules, bullae, ulcers, necrotic would infection
		Mucorales spp. (*Rhizopus, Rhizomucor, Lichtheimia, Absidia, Mucor* spp.)	Inflammatory infiltration of the nasal mucous membranes and paranasal sinuses, rhinocerebral mucormycosis, wound infection, hemorrhagic subcutaneous nodules, and cellulitis, pustules, plaques, ulcers
	Dematiaceous fungi (molds or yeasts)	*Bipolaris, Exophiala jeanselmei, Cladosporium, Alternaria, Curvularia* spp., *Nattrassia mangiferae*	Clinically, three different types of infections, i.e., phaeohyphomycosis, chromoblastomycosis, and mycetoma, which are subcutaneous and deep-seated infections,

(*Continued*)

TABLE 14.3 Classification and Clinical Criteria for the Diagnosis of Fungal Skin Lesions in Transplant Recipients (Continued)

	CLASS	FUNGAL PATHOGENS	CUTANEOUS SYMPTOMS
			single cysts, and nodes evolving into abscesses with/without sinus tracts (sometimes without local or systemic signs of inflammation), plaques, ulcerating nodules, crusted/hemorrhagic lesions
	Non dematiaceous fungi (molds or yeasts)	*Fusarium, Penicillium, Paecilomyces, Acremonium, Scopulariopsis, Scedosporium* spp.	Hyalohyphomycosis: Nodules, necrotic, ulcerating nonhealing skin lesions, purpuric papules, lymphocutaneous, subcutaneous infections, pustules, molluscum contagiosum-like central necrotic papules (*Penicillium marneffei)*
Rare fungal infections	Dimorphic fungi	*Sporotrichosis schenckii*	Sporotrichosis: Nodules, papules, pustules, ulcerated plaques with erythematous borders, subcutaneous nodules, lymph node involvement, lymphocutaneous and mucocutaneous infection, bone or joint involvement
	Yeasts	*Trichosporon* spp.	Tinea-like lesions, papules, nodules, necrotic ulcers
Endemic mycoses	Dimorphic fungi	*Histoplasma capsulatum* (South America, Mississippi and Ohio river valleys)	Usually sign of systemic disease. Inflammatory tumors, papules, nodules, erythematous macules, pustules, ulcers, cellulitis, vegetative plaques, oral lesions (ulcers, nodules, mimicking squamous cell carcinoma)
		Coccidioides immitis (Central America, Southwest United States), Mexico)	Usually sign of systemic disease. Verrucous, crusted papules and plaques, subcutaneous cold abscesses, ulcers, disseminated papules, lymphadenopathy, papulopustules, necrotizing cellulitis
		Blastomyces dermatitidis (south-central, Midwestern United States, central Canada, Africa)	Usually sign of systemic disease. Disseminated papulopustules

(Continued)

TABLE 14.3 Classification and Clinical Criteria for the Diagnosis of Fungal Skin Lesions in Transplant Recipients (Continued)

CLASS	FUNGAL PATHOGENS	CUTANEOUS SYMPTOMS
	Penicillium marneffei (South East Asia)	Usually sign of systemic (pulmonary) disease. Umbilicated papules, nodules, ulcers
	Paracoccidioides brasiliensis (Latin America)	Pulmonary form, mucocutaneous form (granulomas, ulcers, scarring), lymphatic form.

Source: Geusau A and Presterl E, Skin Disease in Organ transplantation, edt. Otley and Stasko, 2008, Cambridge University Press; with permission.

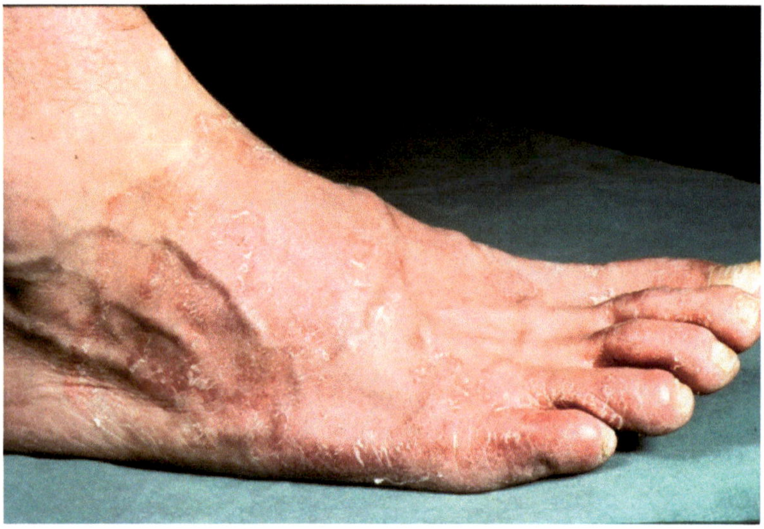

FIGURE 14.5 Tinea pedis presenting as chronic moccasin-type tinea in an immunocompromised patient. Erythematous, scaly plaques covering the sole, lateral, and plantar surfaces of the arch.

The non-dermatophyte yeast *Malassezia furfur,* commonly found in normal human skin presenting as pityriasis versicolor, may also cause infection of the hair follicles or folliculitis (Figure 14.6), particularly when the patient is under IS therapy. In a Turkish study in 400 KTRs, the most common infectious skin condition identified was pityriasis versicolor, affecting 23.7% of the patients. Eventually, the high prevalence of this superficial fungal infection in the study performed in individuals living in a humid, Mediterranean climate reflected an environmental influence on the prevalence of particular skin infections.[44] In the same study, the most commonly seen dermatophyte infection was tinea pedis (5%), followed by tinea corporis (4.2%). Under normal conditions, the mold *Scopulariopsis brevicaulis* causes onychomycosis and subcutaneous infiltration. Invasive disease was described in lung transplant patients in a few reports and was associated with increased mortality as this fungus is highly resistant to the current antifungal agents.[45]

Opportunistic fungal infections are caused by fungal saprophytes or fungi of the environment; in a severely immunocompromised host, virtually any fungal saprophyte generally without pathogenic potency may lead to infection. The most commonly isolated organisms (>80%) in the scenario of opportunistic infections include *Candida albicans, Cryptococcus neoformans*, and *Aspergillus fumigatus. Candida* spp. is the “classical opportunist” occurring on the surface of mucous membranes as saprophytes.[46,47] Candidiasis is the most common opportunistic fungal infection of the oral cavity (Figure 14.7), affecting

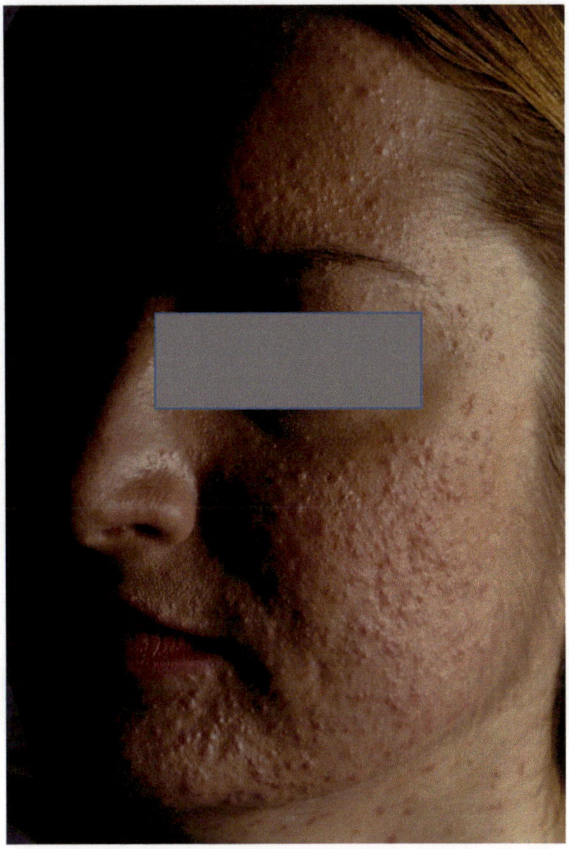

FIGURE 14.6 Steroid acne in a young lung-transplant recipient who was receiving high-dose steroids 2 months after transplantation; a tape stripping of the skin surface stained with methylene blue also revealed spores and hyphae indicating superficial *Malassezia furfur* infection, i.e., pityrosporum folliculitis.

up to 64% of patients and may clinically present as the atrophic or pseudomembranous type.[48] Other authors report on a prevalence of about 4% to 25.5% in KTRs; the difference in the frequency may result from differences in methodology among studies.[44] Oropharyngeal candidiasis is highly prevalent during the first 3 posttransplant months, gradually tapering off in the subsequent months of the first posttransplant year.[13,49] The most common representative of the genus *Candida* is *C. albicans*, but other *Candida* spp. Also have been described, among them the most prevalent *C. tropicalis*, *C. krusei*, which possesses an intrinsic resistance to azoles, *C. glabrata*, which has shown high-levels of acquired resistance to fluconazole, and *C. parapsilosis*. Regardless of the transplanted organ, there is a statistically significant decrease in the number of positive culture results as well as of symptomatic candidiasis and an increase of isolated non-*albicans Candida* species corresponding to length of the posttransplantation period.[50,51]

Cutaneous candidiasis has a wide variety of presentations, including superficial dermatitis, intertrigo, folliculitis and balanitis, may involve the paronychial region (Figure 14.8), and may present as granulomatous skin infection—so-called Majocchi's granuloma—or as cellulitis; an even wider variety of fungal infections can occur in the immunosuppressed host. However, primary *Candida* spp. infections of the deep skin and soft tissue are extremely rare.[51] In the scenario of IS, colonization with *Candida* spp. may not only cause direct infection of the skin and mucous membranes, but the skin lesions may also be indicative of disseminated, systemic disease associated with a high mortality rate.[46,47]

The second most frequent opportunistic fungal infection in OTRs, particularly in lung transplant patients, is caused by *Aspergillus spp.*, a ubiquitous dimorphic fungus. Skin lesions usually indicate generalization of the disease (Figure 14.9) associated with high mortality rate; however, rare cases of primary

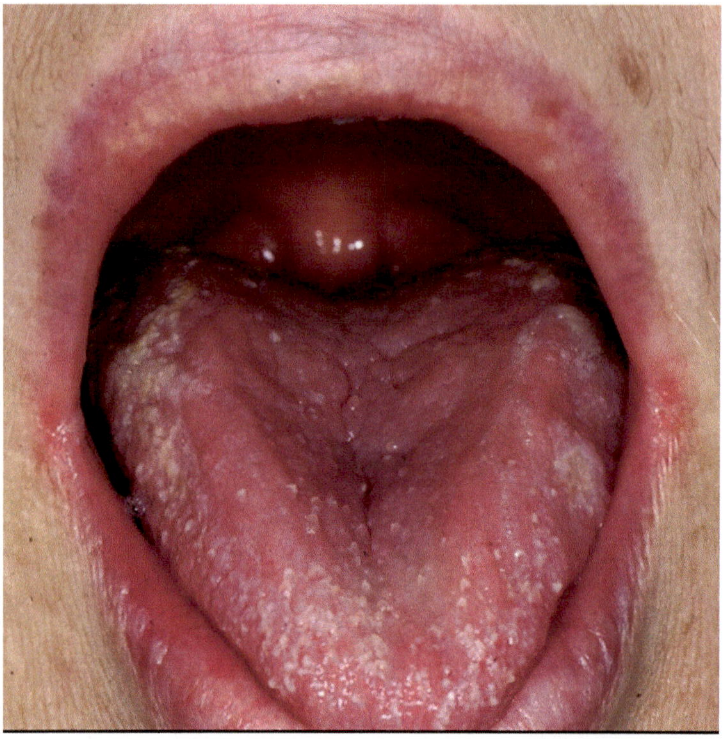

FIGURE 14.7 Candidiasis in an immunocompromised patient; white patches on the tongue.

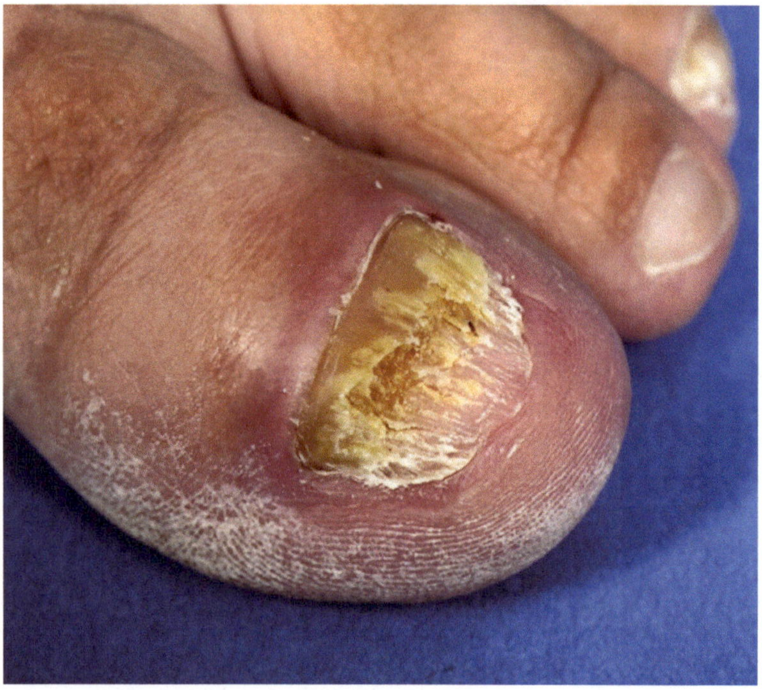

FIGURE 14.8 Candida paronychia of the right bunion (apart from onychomycosis) in a 70-year-old lung transplant recipient, with a painful inflammation of the nail bed. Wet mount preparation of a smear with potassium hydroxide (KOH) showed numerous pseudo-hyphae. Fungal culture revealed infection with *Candida guillermonii.*

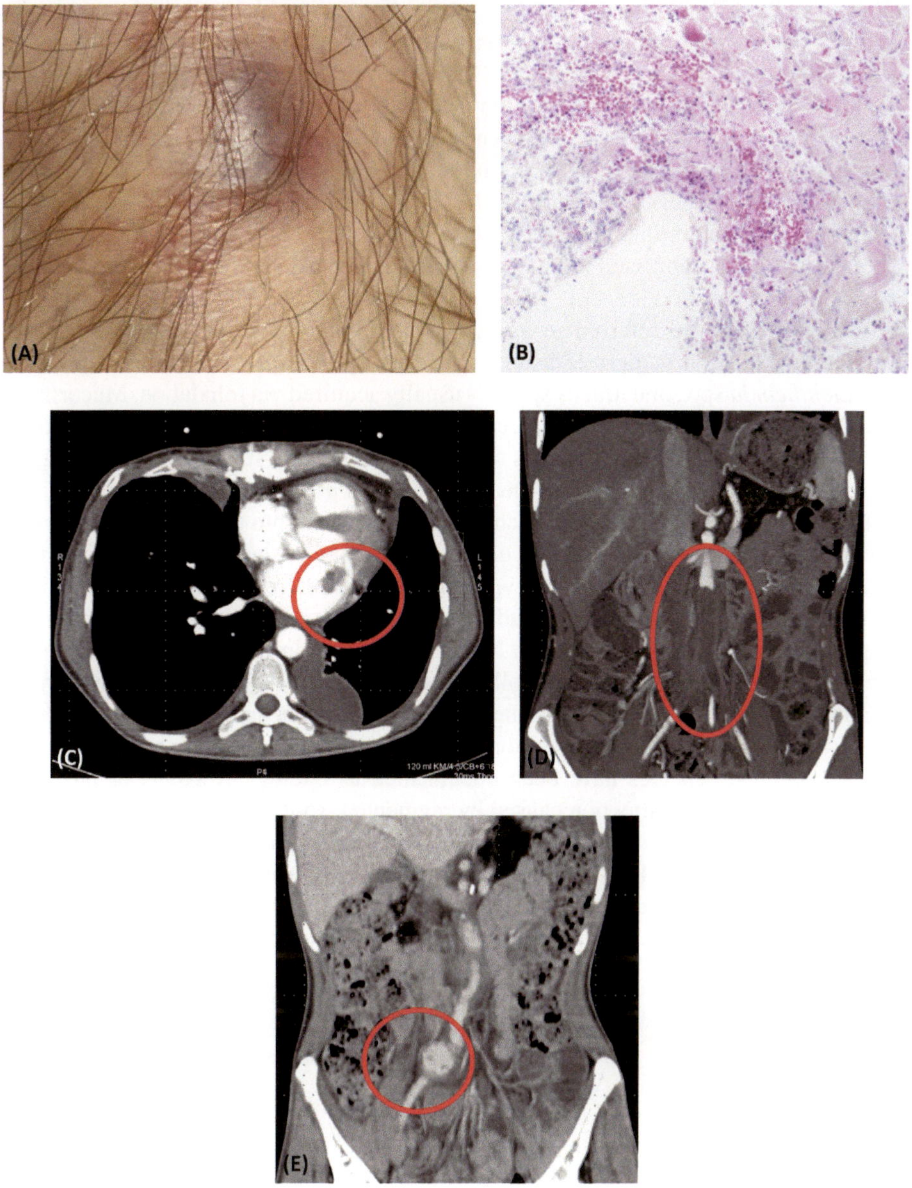

FIGURE 14.9 Invasive aspergillosis with metastatic spread to the skin in a 27-year-old lung transplant recipient. Three months after TX, the patient presented with a single, painful, inflammatory subcutaneous nodule on the right lower leg (**a**), suspicious for (bacterial) soft tissue infection. However, histology of a biopsy of this skin lesion revealed deep granulomatous inflammation and fungal elements (PAS-staining) (**b**). *Aspergillus fumigatus* was isolated by culture and Amphotericin B in lipid formulation was initiated. Shortly, the patient complained about headaches, which were due to fungal infection of the paranasal sinuses. He developed conjunctival inflammation in the right eye as a sign of fungal endophthalmitis requiring vitrectomy. Within 1 week, the patient's condition deteriorated. CT scan revealed an atrioventricular (fungal) tumor (**c**). An ultrasound indicated endocarditis involving the mitral valve (image not shown). Fungal aortitis causing thrombosis of the distal aorta abdominalis and the bifurcation as well as abscess formation (**d**) required urgent surgical intervention employing autologous bifurcation replacement. In the further course, the patient developed an aneurism of the right *A. iliaca communis* (**e**) and mesenteric arteries, splenetic mycotic abscess formation, plugging of the *A. poplitea dexter*, and fungal endocarditis with aortic valve insufficiency due to vegetations. A further attempt to restore his cardiac situation failed and the patient died.

cutaneous infections have been reported in OTRs, arising for instance in a surgical wound, presenting as necrotic ulcers or skin nodules e.g., due to *Aspergillus niger* or *fumigatus*.[52,53]

Cutaneous involvement due to *Cryptococcus* spp., mainly *Cryptococcus neoformans,* is reported in up to 15% of OTRs with disseminated disease diagnosed. Therefore, in the case of cutaneous cryptococcosis, investigation for disseminated disease, even in the absence of other symptoms or signs, is mandatory.[54] The skin may also be the primary site of infection because of direct inoculation of the pathogen, presenting for instance as cellulitis[55] (Figure 14.10). *C. neoformans* is a ubiquitous encapsulated yeast commonly found in soil contaminated by bird feces. It may cause disease when inhaled from environmental sources by immunosuppressed individuals, with the central nervous system and lungs being the organs most frequently involved.[56]

Infections that used to be referred to as zygomycosis are now better named mucormycosis, as *Zygomycota* is not included in modern fungal classification systems. The most common representatives are *Rhizopus, Lichtheimia* spp., and *Mucor* spp.,[57,58] usually acquired via inhalation. Mucormycoses occur in the nose and paranasal sinuses and may spread into the orbit and brain. Spores are ubiquitous in the environment and can also be found in cultures of swabs from healthy subjects. Occasionally, direct skin inoculation or contamination of wounds may lead to localized primary skin disease.[57] There are several key signs that point towards mucormycosis, such as fungal invasion into the blood vessels resulting in the formation of blood clots followed by necrosis of the surrounding tissue due to the loss of blood supply. According to a case series of 10 OTRs with "zygomycosis" and 106 reviewed cases in the literature published in 2006,[59] the clinical presentation included not only rhino-sino-orbital disease but rhinocerebral, pulmonary, gastrointestinal, cutaneous, renal, and disseminated disease. The most frequently isolated genera were *Rhizopus* in 73% of the cases, followed by *Mucor* (13%), then called mucormycosis. The overall mortality was high, namely 49%.[59] A favorable outcome was associated with limited, surgically accessible disease and early surgical intervention along with the administration of amphotericin B.

More than 100 fungal species have been documented as etiological agents of phaeohyphomycosis—a term used to describe an infection caused by pigmented, so-called dematiaceous fungi, including *Bipolaris, Exophiala, Cladosporium, Alternaria* spp., and *Nattrassia mangiferae*, which are environmental molds or yeasts (Figures 14.11–13). They cause a broad spectrum of disease, not only affecting the skin and subcutaneous tissue because of accidental inoculation into the skin after minor trauma but also are associated with pneumonia, central nervous system infection, and disseminated disease.[60] A 20-year

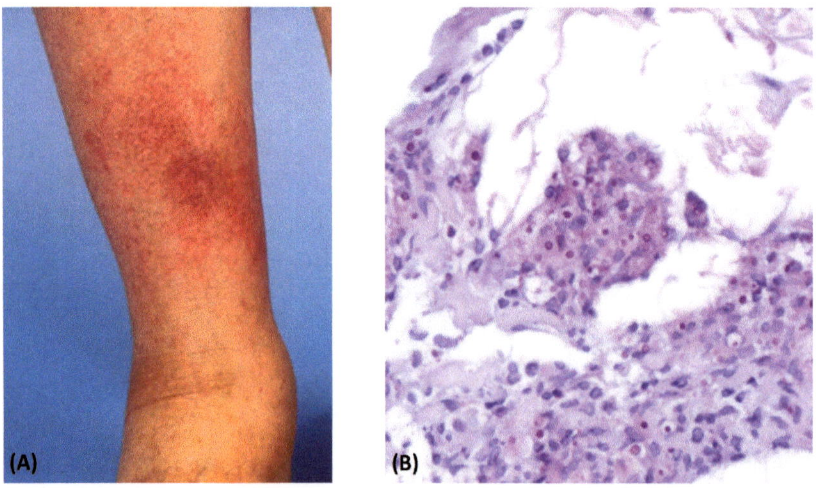

FIGURE 14.10 Cryptococcal cellulitis in a long-term lung transplant patient who exhibited erythematous tender subcutaneous plaques on the right lower leg resembling cellulitis (**a**). Skin lesion biopsy showed a granulomatous inflammation in the subcutaneous tissue; hematoxylin and eosin staining of the specimen revealed masses of spores with nonstaining capsules (**b**).

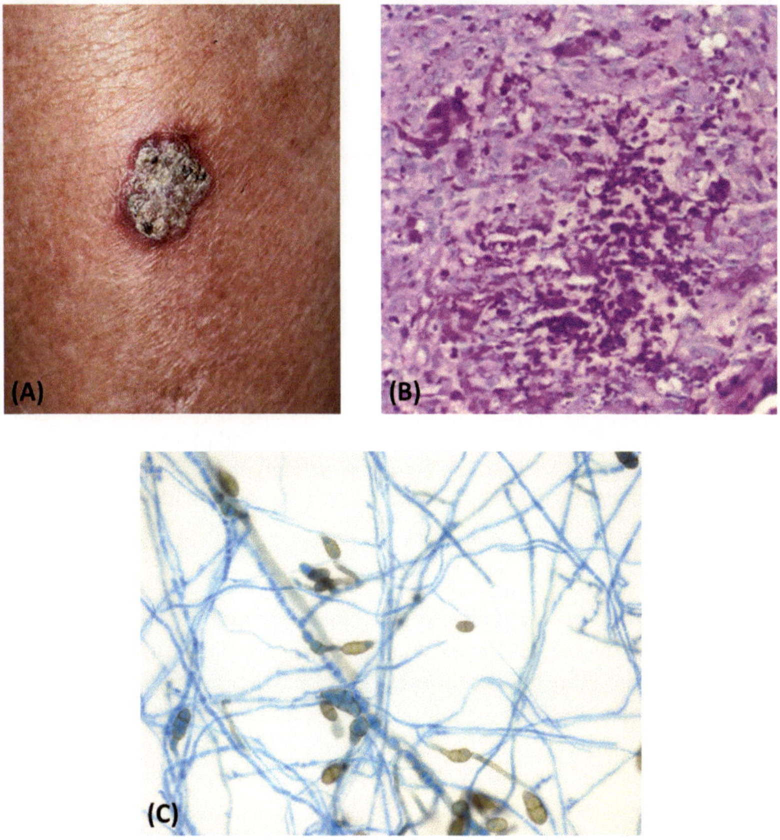

FIGURE 14.11 Cutaneous alternariosis in 67-year-old, otherwise healthy lung transplant recipient. He exhibited a scaly, firm erythematous plaque on the skin (**a**). Histology (PAS staining) showed fungal elements (**b**); *Alternaria infectoria* E. Simmon was cultured, with the characteristic macroconidia (**c**).

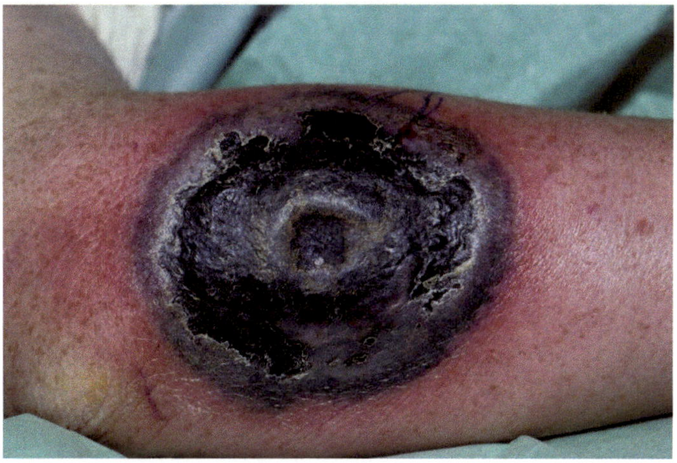

FIGURE 14.12 Phaeohyphomycosis in an immunosuppressed patient who was still in the neutropenic phase following bone marrow transplantation. The patient exhibited a huge, deep-seated inflammatory black plaque; fungal culture revealed an invasive mold infection due to *Hormographiella aspergillata,* which is an anamorphic (asexual) form of *Coprinus cinereus*, a principally edible mushroom growing in the forest. Under normal conditions it is harmless to human and animal health. The patient had also pulmonary involvement which led to her death.

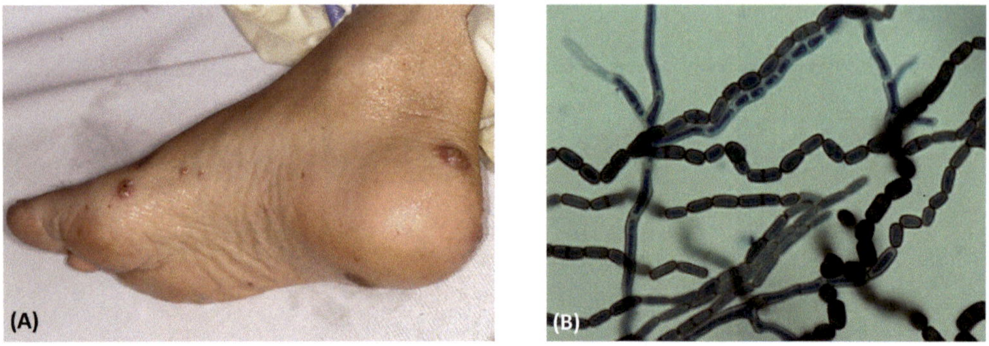

FIGURE 14.13 Disseminated infection with *Nattrassia mangiferae*. The patient, a 62-year-old kidney transplant recipient, developed disseminated black granulomatous skin lesions (**a**) accompanied by L2/L3-spondylodiscitis, moderate swelling of the paraspinal soft tissues, and pulmonary infiltrates. Culture from a skin biopsy and an L2/L3 aspirate proved infection with *Nattrassia mangiferae*, a dematiaceous fungus. (**b**) *N. mangiferae*: lactophenol blue stain; broad hyphae forming non-septate conidia (Prof. Dr. Birgit Willinger and Prof. Dr. Stefan Winkler, Vienna.)

retrospective observational study on the characteristics and outcome of deep fungal skin infections in 46 OTRs asserted phaeohyphomycoses as the most common cause. In the vast majority of cases—namely 89%—primary infection of the skin had occurred. The clinical presentation comprised nodules and/or papules in half of the patients, abscess formation in 15%, and cellulitis/panniculitis or inflammatory plaques in 13% of the cases, as well as ulcerated or necrotic lesions.[61] According to a large study in 56 OTRs and stem cell transplant patients with phaeohyphomycosis, the most frequent causative pathogen was *Alternaria* spp., isolated in 32% of the cases. Lungs, skin, and sinuses were the most common sites of infection, but in more than half of the cases dissemination occurred. Bone marrow transplant recipients had a higher rate of pulmonary infection, whereas OTRs had a higher rate of cutaneous disease. In this study there was a 25% overall mortality rate, significantly higher in the stem cell transplant patients (42%) compared with 10% in the OTRs.[60]

Hyalohyphomycosis refers to subcutaneous and systemic infections caused by non-dematiaceous hyaline molds or yeasts (e.g., *Fusarium, Penicillium, Paecilomyces, Acremonium*, and *Scopulariopsis* spp.). *Scedosporium apiospermum* is also a common etiological agent of this group. Infections of the skin usually manifest as pustules or subcutaneous nodules. Immunosuppressed patients, especially the patients with hematological malignancies, prolonged neutropenia, and patients in the aftermath of hematopoietic stem cell TX may suffer from disseminated disease with pulmonary and cerebral abscesses associated with a high mortality rate.[62]

Rare fungal infections comprise dimorphic fungi like *Sporothrix schenckii* or yeasts such as *Trichosporon* spp. (Figure 14.14) as well as endemic mycoses, which are potential differential diagnoses in OTRs who have had contact with the causative organism in a particular geographic area (see Table 14.3).[63] These infections comprise coccidioidomycosis, histoplasmosis, and blastomycosis, caused respectively by the primary pathogens *Coccidioides immitis, Histoplasma capsulatum*, and *Blastomyces dermatitidis*, all acquired by inhalation any time after TX. Other endemic mycoses are paracoccidioidomycosis, penicilliosis, and sporotrichosis. Dermatological manifestations may appear as the consequence of disseminated fungal disease.[64] Treatment of endemic mycoses in OTRs has traditionally required prolonged therapy with conventional antifungal agents that have a number of serious drawbacks: low efficacy, side effects, toxicities, and potentially severe drug–drug interactions. During the past decade, however, there have been many treatment advances including the development of lower-toxicity lipid-based formulations of amphotericin B and the development of a new generation of azole antifungals such as voriconazole and posaconazole.[63]

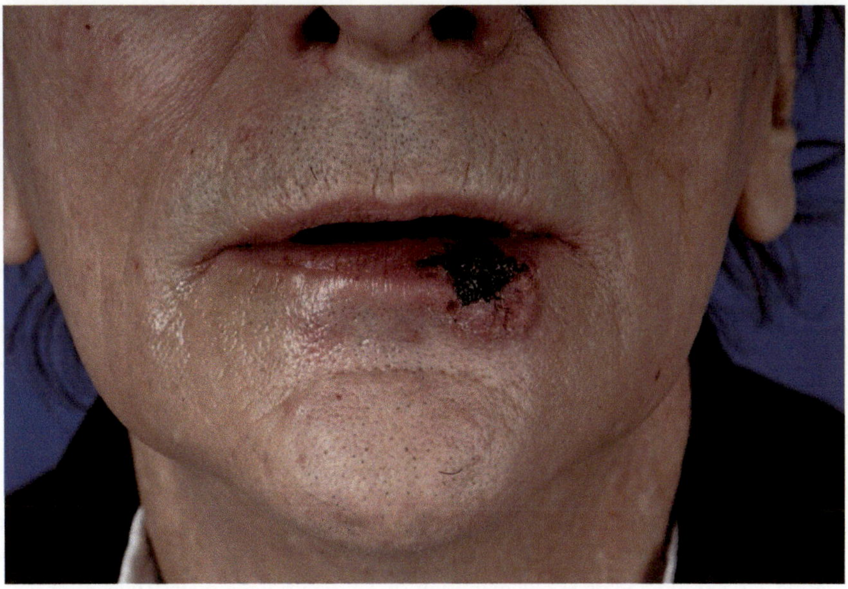

FIGURE 14.14 A scaly tumor on the lower lip of an OTR mimicking squamous cell carcinoma. *Trichosporon beigelii* infection was detected; *T. beigelii*, synonymously called *Trichosporon cutaneum*, is a rare yeast causing tinea-like lesions, papules, nodules, or necrotic ulcers.

VIRAL SKIN INFECTION

In the great majority of cases, viruses affecting the skin in OTRs are simply reactivation of latent infections, primarily of the human herpesviruses (HHVs) family, proliferation of subclinical infection with human papilloma viruses (HPVs), or superficial *Molluscum contagiosum virus* (MCV). HHVs comprise herpes simplex virus (HSV) types 1 and 2, varicella-zoster virus (VZV), cytomegalovirus (CMV), Epstein-Barr virus (EBV), and HHV-6, -7, and -8; the latter is associated with the development of Kaposi sarcoma (KS) (Table 14.1). They all share several characteristics, such as latency after primary infection, cell association, and potential oncogenicity. They can reactivate during IS, leading to adverse effects in the OTR including severe organ dysfunction as well as allograft rejection.[65] Infection with multiple viruses simultaneously is also common in immunocompromised individuals.[66]

HUMAN HERPESVIRUS (HHV) FAMILY

Of the HHVs, HSV, VZV, CMV, and to a lesser extent EBV cause a variety of infections that involve mucocutaneous surfaces of the oropharynx or anogenital regions in OTRs, but apart from that they cause a wide variety of clinical syndromes. Manifestations in the affected regions are characterized by painful, ulcerating vesicles of the skin and the mucous membranes. HSV manifestations occur in up to 60% of OTRs, mostly because of reactivation during the first 3 months after TX or under antirejection therapy, respectively, commonly presenting as herpes labialis.[67]

HSVs are the most common viral pathogen causing oral ulcers,[68] whereas oral CMV infections are uncommon in OTRs and have only been reported in 1.3% of KTRs, for instance.[69] Occasionally, VZV or EBV have been reported as causative agents of oral ulcers.[66,70] Under IS, lesions associated with HSV and CMV may be atypical, presenting as recurrent stomatitis[66] or progressively enlarging, vegetative chronic ulcers (Figures 14.15 and 14.16) or as hypertrophic pseudotumor forms, eventually resistant to acyclovir.[71] The infection may also present as herpetic whitlow, a chronic, painful HSV-associated lesion typically affecting the fingers or thumbs. Dissemination and generalized disease as well as neurologic syndromes also were described.[71–73] The identification of the presumed pathogen, i.e., the type of HHV by PCR for a timely and accurate diagnosis is imperative in order to prevent deterioration, particularly in the immunocompromised host, eventually amended by tissue biopsy and immunohistochemistry.[66,74]

Skin disease due to VZV is expected to occur in about 22% of OTRs, generally as reactivation of the latent virus, presenting as herpes zoster (HZ), which tends to occur later than HSV infection, more than 3 months after TX.[75–77] The incidence of HZ is estimated at 8%–11% during the first 4 years after TX.[75] In the scenario of organ-TX, reinfection with VZV may occur, or recurrent or necrotic HZ (Figure 14.17), as well as a spread of the initial dermatome mimicking varicella or HZ duplex bilateralis.[78] Reactivation may also result in dissemination with life-threatening visceral disease, with an estimated mortality of 30% as reported in KTRs.[75,77] Preventive measures include antiviral prophylaxis and pretransplant vaccination in VZV seronegative TX candidates or HZ-vaccination in TX candidates over 50 years of age; live attenuated HZ vaccine posttransplant is currently contraindicated.[79,80] In a large phase III trial, early vaccination of autologous haemopoietic stem-cell transplant recipients—not OTRs—during their peritransplant period with a recently licensed inactivated VZV vaccine was shown to be effective for the prevention of herpes zoster.[81]

Treatment of HSV and VZV diseases includes acyclovir, a guanosine analog, as well as oral valacyclovir, a prodrug of acyclovir, and famciclovir. They have in common that phosphorylation by viral thymidine kinase is required for the receipt of the active drug. Occasionally, resistant thymidine kinase-negative strains are induced in immunocompromised patients. Alternative drugs are foscarnet and cidofovir, which act through direct inhibition of viral DNA polymerase activity.[82]

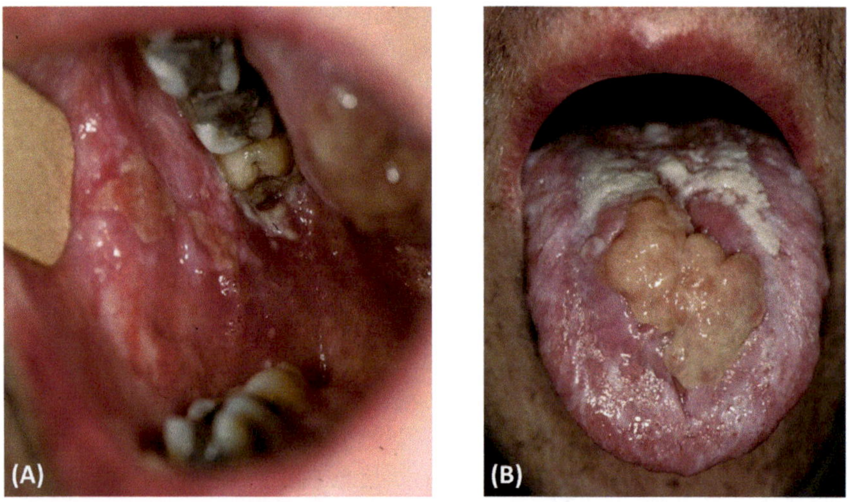

FIGURE 14.15 Herpes vegetans clinically presenting as (**a**) chronic, persistent ulceration of the oral mucosa in a heart transplant recipient (**b**) or as a vegetating tumor on the tongue in a kidney transplant patient; in both cases, herpes simplex virus type 1 could be isolated by PCR.

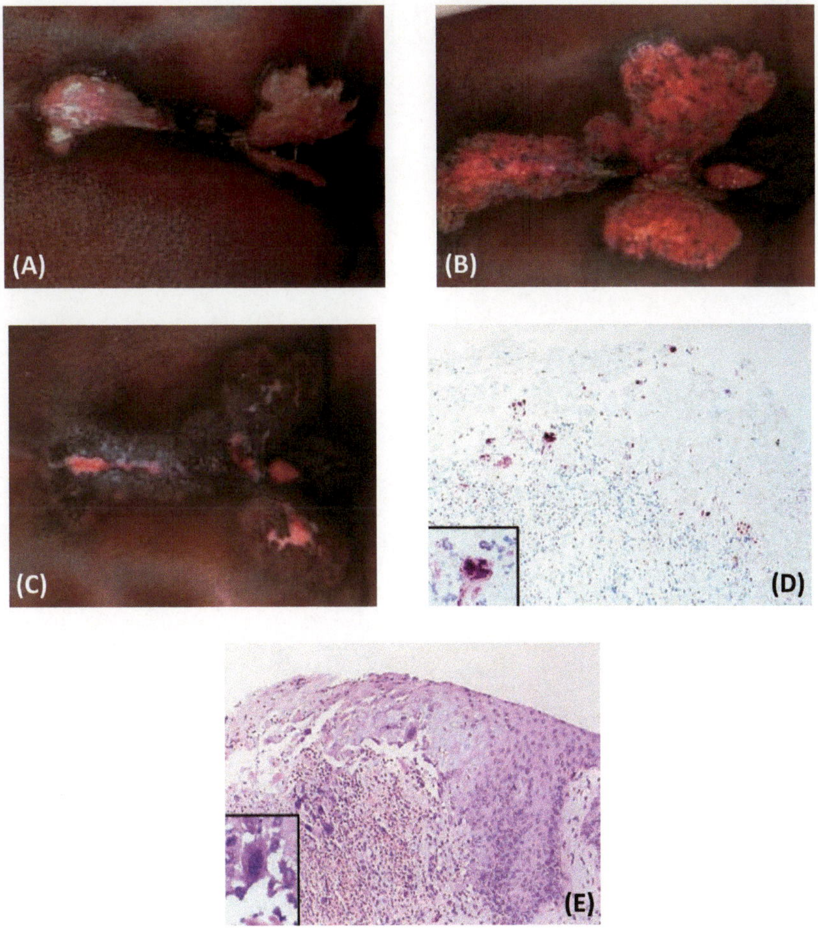

FIGURE 14.16 Herpes vegetans: Chronic HSV-2 associated perianal ulceration in an AIDS-patient that was HSV-2 positive by PCR analysis (**a**), which appeared and progressed (**b**) during treatment of a cytomegalovirus pneumonitis with ganciclovir, indicating an acyclovir-resistant herpes simplex virus type 2 strain. Almost complete healing after the third IV cidofovir treatment (**c**). Histologic exam revealed ballooning degeneration of epidermal cells with enlarged round nuclei on the dermo-epidermal junction at the marginal part of the ulcer (**d**) and *in situ* hybridization was positive for herpes simplex virus in a multinucleated nucleus of an infected cell (inset) (**e**) (T. Kopp, A. Geusau, A. Rieger, G. Stingl. Successful treatment of an aciclovir-resistant herpes simplex type 2 infection with cidofovir in an AIDS patient. British Journal of Dermatology 2002; 147: 134–138, with permission.).

Cutaneous findings with CMV infection were reported in 10%–20% of patients with systemic infection; unrelated to systemic infection, CMV may also present as a nonhealing ulcer in the perineal area.[72] According to a recent review of 58 cases in the literature with cutaneous CMV infection/reactivation under various circumstances, the most common manifestations were perianal ulcers followed by oral ulcers; rashes, vesiculo-bullous eruptions, necrotic papules, nodules and morbilliform patches, petechiae, as well as CMV reactivation after drug-induced hypersensitivity syndrome were less common.[70] The standard of care for treatment of CMV infection and disease is intravenous ganciclovir or its oral prodrug, valganciclovir.[65]

Systemic infection with EBV may present with a diffuse morbilliform eruption along with fever, pharyngitis, lymphadenopathy, and fatigue and is associated with the majority of posttransplant

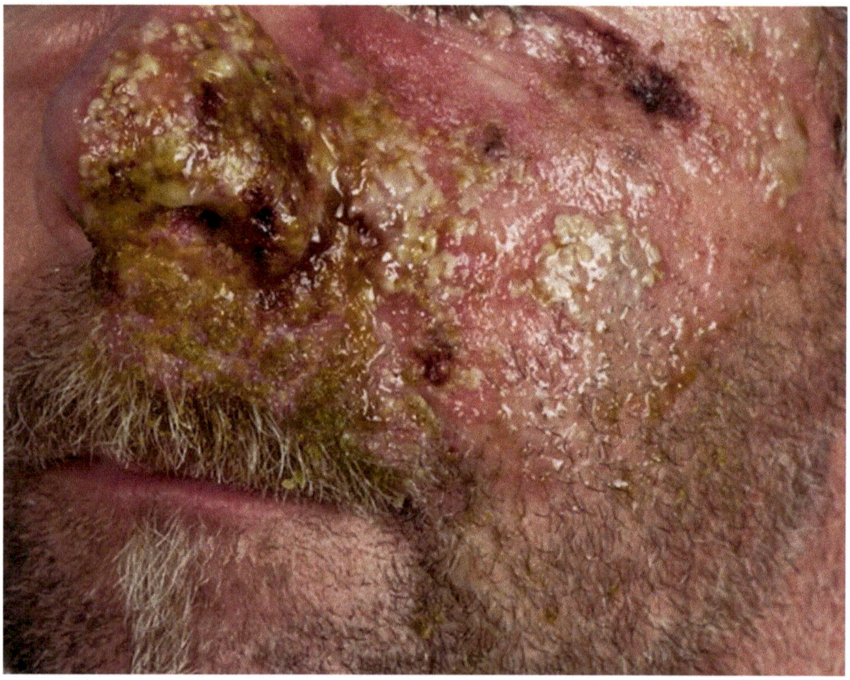

FIGURE 14.17 Necrotic herpes zoster in an otherwise healthy heart transplant recipient.

lymphoproliferative disorders, while one-third are EBV-negative; OTRs have a 50%–120% increased risk compared with that in the general population.[83] A cutaneous manifestation associated with EBV infection in immunosuppressed patients is oral hairy leukoplakia, which presents with poorly demarcated "hairy" lesions on the lateral tongue and responds to acyclovir (Figure 14.18).[72]

HHV-6 is the primary cause of exanthema subitum—a macular rash that spreads from the trunk to the neck and extremities and is usually present in children; however, in OTRs, reactivation may occur, causing fever and a CMV-like syndrome or a syndrome of rash, hepatitis, or aseptic meningitis. When recognized, HHV-6 is often a co-pathogen with CMV.[72]

HHV-8 is a lymphotropic HHV associated with KS. Skin lesions usually present with reddish-blue macules evolving to tumors; they can occur singularly, in a limited area, or be widespread (Figure 14.19). In OTRs, a prevalence of 0.5%–5% depending on the patient's country of origin was reported; the incidence of KS in OTRs was reportedly 500-times greater than that in the immunocompetent population.[84,85] Reduction of IS has been shown to be efficacious in inducing remission of KS in KTRs, therefore tapering down the IS regimen is the cornerstone of KS management, preferentially accompanied by conversion to an mTOR inhibitor.[86,87]

HUMAN PAPILLOMA VIRUSES

The most common viral cause of cutaneous lesions in OTRs are HPVs, which affect up to 50% of KTRs and causing warts or condylomata that eventually evolve into giant lesions (Figure 14.20), the Buschke-Lowenstein tumor, and HPV-associated cancers.[88] In OTRs, warts may be more extensive and more difficult to eradicate compared with those in immunocompetent patients; OTRs may never

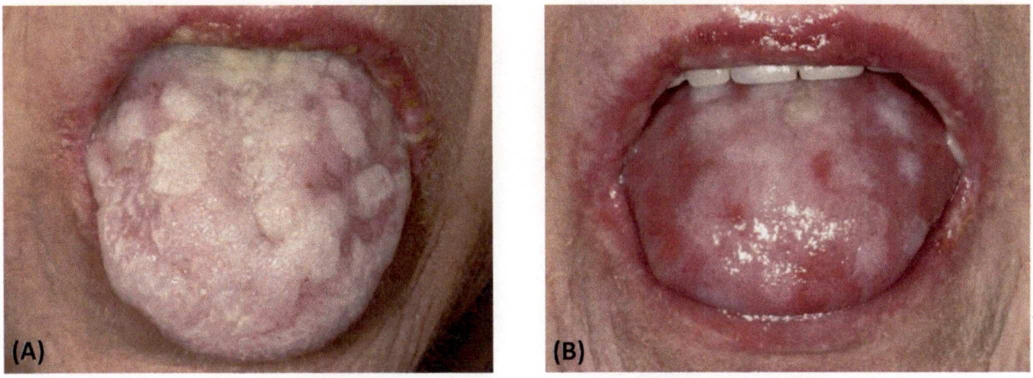

FIGURE 14.18 Oral papulosis in graft-versus-host disease, presenting as painful broad-based whitish papules at the edges and surface of the tongue (**a**) was positive for Epstein-Barr Virus by PCR analysis; improvement after 2 weeks of valaciclovir therapy (**b**). (G. Stary, A. Geusau, H. Greinix, L. Vormittag, G. Stingl, W. Rabitsch. Epstein-Barr Virus-associated Oral Papulosis in Graft-versus-host Disease, Acta Derm Venereol. 2010 Sep;90(5):542–3, with permission.)

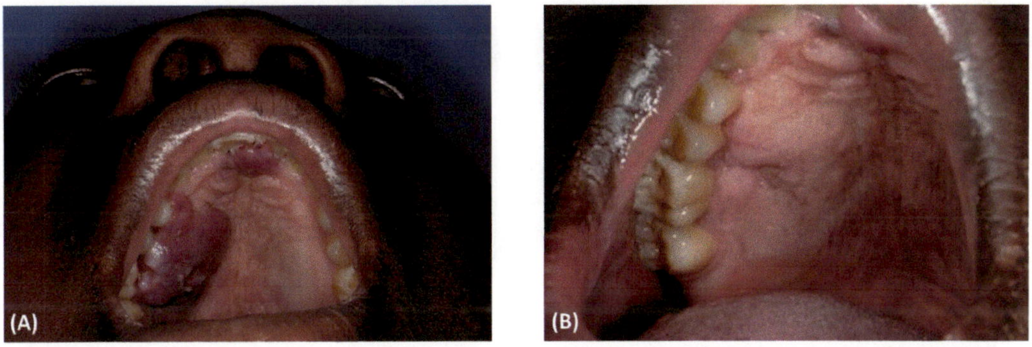

FIGURE 14.19 Kaposi's sarcoma in a kidney transplant recipient presenting as a tumor on the hard palate (**a**). The patient had also intestinal involvement, and he had a complete response under 9-months' treatment with thalidomide 100 mg/day as shown in (**b**).

topically clear HPV infections (Figure 14.21). Treatment includes cryotherapy, electrosurgery, or agents such as 5-fluorouracil, imiquimod, or podophyllotoxin[88,89]; however, OTRs often require a multimodal approach to management.[90] Several studies, including a large meta-analysis on 31,977 subjects[91] and an extensive registry study (n = 187,649),[92] showed an increased risk of HPV-associated cancers of the anogenital as well as the oropharyngeal region in OTRs compared with that in the general population. Therefore, it is very important to carefully monitor OTRs with regard to the presence and progression of high-risk HPVs (especially HPV 16 and 18).[93] Also, consider biopsy of nonresponding lesions to evaluate for malignancy.[78] Despite limited data on the efficacy of HPV vaccination in OTRs for prevention of HPV-related cancers, there is a convincing argument for the vaccination of OTRs to be made, based on three cohort studies, which also evaluated immunogenicity in this cohort.[94,95] A consistent increase in the risk of cervical neoplasia and invasive cervical cancer in female OTRs emphasizes the need for screening throughout a woman's lifetime.[96]

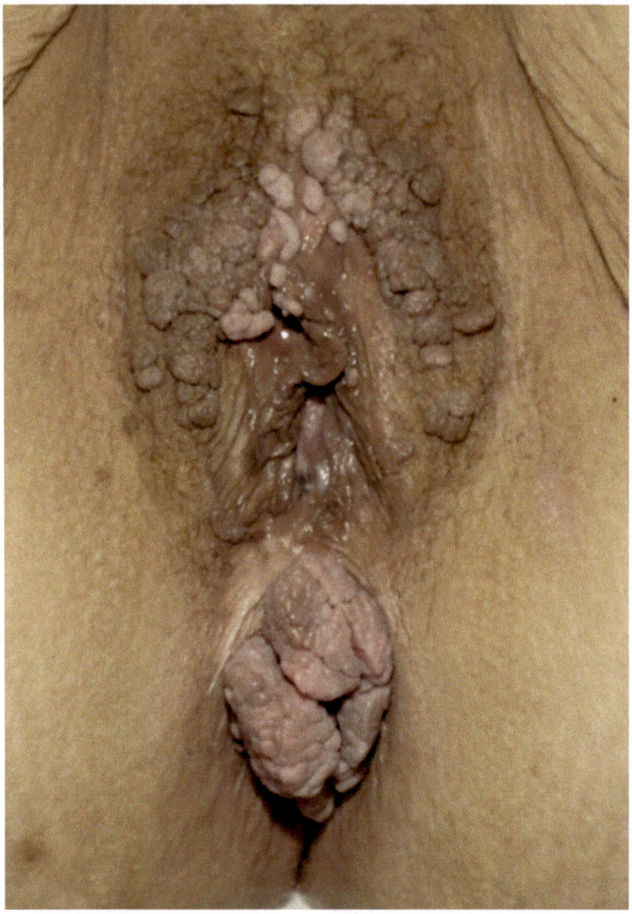

FIGURE 14.20 Giant condylomata acuminata (Buschke-Löwenstein tumor) in a transplant patient who had undergone three kidney transplantations, positive for HPV 6 and 11 (hybrid capture analysis).

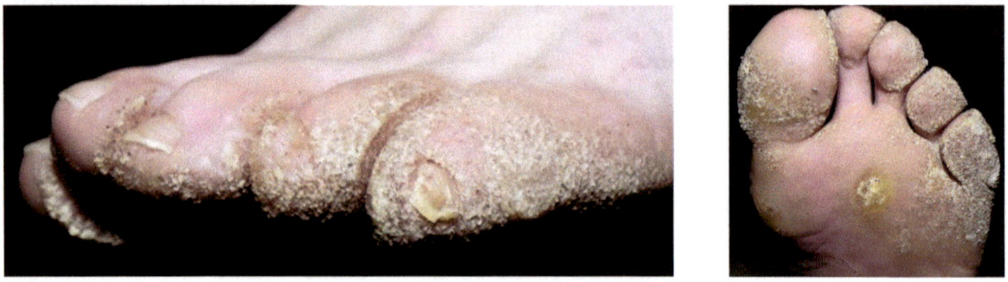

FIGURE 14.21 Verrucae vulgares on the feet of a young kidney transplant recipient.

MOLLUSCUM CONTAGIOSUM

The characteristic small, firm, umbilicated papules of mollusca contagiosa (MC), a poxvirus infection, often become very large and numerous and may even present as giant lesions in OTRs (Figure 14.22), affecting approximately 7% of these patients.[72] As with HPV-associated lesions, it can be difficult for

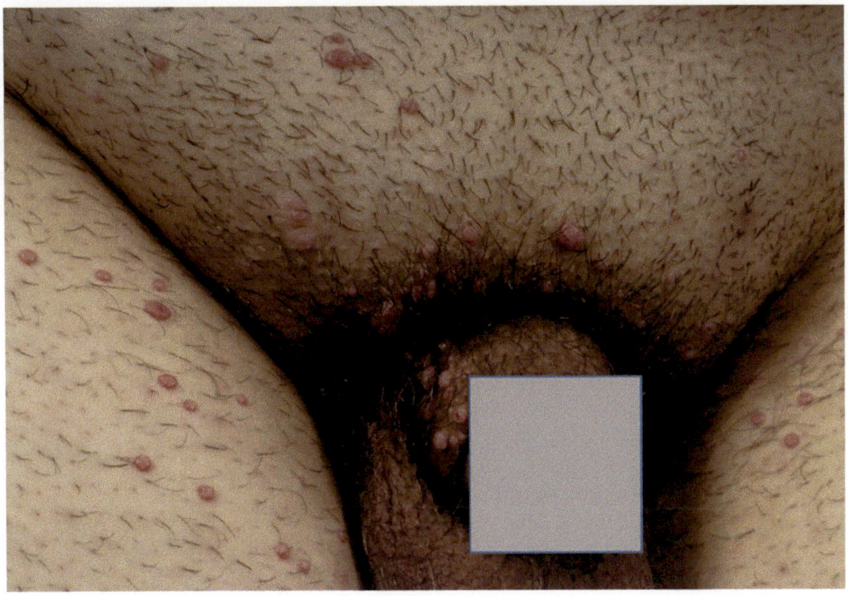

FIGURE 14.22 Mollusca contagiosa in the genital area of a kidney transplant recipient.

OTRs to clear MC, which becomes a severe and chronic infection.[72] Treatment includes localized destruction and, in rare cases, interferon alpha or cidofovir or imiquimod.[97]

TRICHODYSPLASIA SPINULOSA-ASSOCIATED POLYOMAVIRUS (TSPYV)

A rare dermatologic entity in the scenario of IS is trichodysplasia spinulosa (TS), a cutaneous eruption of spiny papules predominantly affecting the face associated with the human *Trichodysplasia spinulosa*-associated polyomavirus (TSPyV). TS is associated with a distinctive histologic picture of abnormally maturing anagen follicles, characterized by excessive inner root sheath cell proliferation and folliculocentric papular eruption that can progress to disfiguring leonine facies when left untreated.

TS was first described in 1999 by Haycox and colleagues in an OTR.[98] Treatment proved difficult and the lesions tend to persist with ongoing immunosuppression; there were some reports on treatment success with topical cidofovir 1–3% cream.[99]

INVESTIGATIONS AND PREVENTIVE MEASURES OF SKIN INFECTIONS IN OTRS

The diagnosis of any skin infection in OTRs must be confirmed by strict identification of the presumed pathogen. The investigations should cover the full spectrum of bacteria, fungi, parasites, and viruses, as in the scenario of IS, multiple and concomitant infections may develop in the same patient, even within the same lesion. Therapeutic and preventive strategies may also include the modification of the IS regimen.[2,4,8]

Ideally, a biopsy should be obtained not only for histopathology, but also for bacterial and fungal broad-spectrum PCR.

Antimicrobial prophylaxis for skin infections is generally not recommended for those who have already been transplanted. Appropriate treatment should be initiated according to the type of infection. Preventive measures include sufficient moistening of the skin as well as protection when manual work is carried out. Any preemptive and prophylactic antiviral regimens should be based on the epidemiology and pathogenesis of the viral disease. As domestic animals can transmit a whole host of pathogens, patients should have as little contact as possible. In addition to the search for active preexisting infection in the transplant candidate, immunization remains a cornerstone of preventive strategy.[3]

Overall, the accompanying use of immunosuppressive agents in OTRs calls for a high index of suspicion for skin infections, appropriate diagnosis, and early therapy; skin and soft-tissue infections in transplant recipients may be a sign of or a reason for systemic infection.

SUMMARY OF KEY POINTS

- Due to life-long immunosuppression, organ transplant recipients are at marked increased risk not only for skin cancer but also at risk of skin infections either of fungal, viral, or bacterial origin.
- Investigations should cover the full spectrum of these pathogens.
- One should always consider systemic infection.
- The overall contribution of skin infections to the relative distributions of skin disease decreases with time after transplantation, whereas the contribution of keratinocyte cancers strongly increases.
- There is a similar pattern of infection in all forms of OTR and a consistent timetable for the occurrence of different infections after transplantation.

REFERENCES

1. Patel R, Paya CV. Infections in solid-organ transplant recipients. Clin Microbiol Rev. 1997;10(1):86–124.
2. Fishman JA. Infection in solid-organ transplant recipients. N Engl J Med. 2007;357(25):2601–14.
3. Fishman JA. Infection in organ transplantation. Am J Transplant. 2017;17(4):856–79.
4. Fishman JA, Rubin RH. Infection in organ-transplant recipients. N Engl J Med. 1998;338(24):1741–51.
5. Welte T, Len O, Munoz P, Romani L, Lewis R, Perrella A. Invasive mould infections in solid organ transplant patients: modifiers and indicators of disease and treatment response. Infection. 2019;47(6):919–27.
6. Nellore A, Fishman JA. The microbiome, systemic immune function, and allotransplantation. Clin Microbiol Rev. 2016;29(1):191–9.
7. Sepulveda M, Pirozzolo I, Alegre ML. Impact of the microbiota on solid organ transplant rejection. Curr Opin Organ Transplant. 2019;24(6):679–86.
8. Fishman JA. Opportunistic infections-coming to the limits of immunosuppression? Cold Spring Harb Perspect Med. 2013;3(10):a015669.
9. Ulrich C, Hackethal M, Meyer T, Geusau A, Nindl I, Ulrich M et al. Skin infections in organ transplant recipients. J Dtsch Dermatol Ges. 2008;6(2):98–105.
10. Wisgerhof HC, Edelbroek JR, de Fijter JW, Feltkamp MC, Willemze R, Bouwes Bavinck JN. Trends of skin diseases in organ-transplant recipients transplanted between 1966 and 2006: a cohort study with follow-up between 1994 and 2006. Br J Dermatol. 2010;162(2):390–6.
11. Ilyas M, Maganty N, Ginsberg Z, Sharma A. Skin infections due to bacteria in solid organ transplant recipients: a review. Dermatology. 2017;233(5):358–65.

12. Ada S, Seckin D, Azap O, Budakoglu I, Haberal M. Prevalence of cutaneous bacterial infections and nasal carriage of staphylococcus aureus in recipients of renal transplants. Clin Exp Dermatol. 2009;34(2):156–60.
13. Hogewoning AA, Goettsch W, van Loveren H, de Fijter JW, Vermeer BJ, Bouwes Bavinck JN. Skin infections in renal transplant recipients. Clin Transplant. 2001;15(1):32–8.
14. Amagai M, Matsuyoshi N, Wang ZH, Andl C, Stanley JR. Toxin in bullous impetigo and staphylococcal scalded-skin syndrome targets desmoglein 1. Nat Med. 2000;6(11):1275–7.
15. Bert F, Bellier C, Lassel L, Lefranc V, Durand F, Belghiti J et al. Risk factors for staphylococcus aureus infection in liver transplant recipients. Liver Transpl. 2005;11(9):1093–9.
16. Green RJ, Dafoe DC, Raffin TA. Necrotizing fasciitis. Chest. 1996;110(1):219–29.
17. Sarani B, Strong M, Pascual J, Schwab CW. Necrotizing fasciitis: current concepts and review of the literature. J Am Coll Surg. 2009;208(2):279–88.
18. Nakai N, Takenaka H, Kishimoto S. Ecthyma gangrenosum without pseudomonas septicemia in a kidney transplant recipient. J Dermatol. 2008;35(9):585–9.
19. Ambrosioni J, Lew D, Garbino J. Nocardiosis: updated clinical review and experience at a tertiary center. Infection. 2010;38(2):89–97.
20. Baek JO, Kim JS, Lee SK, Jeong JH, Lee MJ, Seo IH. Two cases of primary cutaneous nocardiosis caused by intralesional injection. Dermatol Ther. 2019;32(1):e12775.
21. Herzog AL, Wanner C, Lopau K. Successful short-term intravenous treatment of disseminated nocardia farcinica infection with severe hyponatremia after kidney transplantation: a case report. Transplant Proc. 2016;48(9):3115–19.
22. Khadka P, Basnet RB, Khadka P, Shah DS, Pokhrel BM, Rijal BP et al. Disseminated Nocardiosis in renal transplant recipient under therapy for pulmonary tuberculosis: a case report. BMC Res Notes. 2017;10(1):83.
23. Lederman ER, Crum NF. A case series and focused review of nocardiosis: clinical and microbiologic aspects. Medicine (Baltimore). 2004;83(5):300–13.
24. Chikowski RE, Sprigle AM, Krishna SM, Nunley JR. Primary cutaneous Nocardia vinacea in a renal transplant recipient: report of a rare case and review of the literature. Clin Exp Dermatol. 2014;39(4):534–6.
25. Rousseau C, Piroth L, Pernin V, Cassuto E, Etienne I, Jeribi A et al. Actinomycosis: An infrequent disease in renal transplant recipients? Transpl Infect Dis. 2018;20(6):e12970.
26. Moulin C, Kanitakis J, Ranchin B, Chauvet C, Gillet Y, Morelon E et al. Cutaneous bacillary angiomatosis in renal transplant recipients: report of three new cases and literature review. Transpl Infect Dis. 2012;14(4):403–9.
27. Apalsch AM, Nour B, Jaffe R. Systemic cat-scratch disease in a pediatric liver transplant recipient and review of the literature. Pediatr Infect Dis J. 1993;12(9):769–74.
28. Koh WJ. Nontuberculous mycobacteria-overview. Microbiol Spectr. 2017;5(1).
29. Abad CLR, Deziel PJ, Razonable RR. Treatment of latent TB infection and the risk of tuberculosis after solid organ transplantation: comprehensive review. Transpl Infect Dis. 2019;21(6):e13178.
30. Vandermarliere A, Van Audenhove A, Peetermans WE, Vanrenterghem Y, Maes B. Mycobacterial infection after renal transplantation in a Western population. Transpl Infect Dis. 2003;5(1):9–15.
31. Coelho ID, Romaozinho C, Teixeira AC, Rodrigues L, Ferreira E, Santos L et al. A rare manifestation of tuberculosis in a renal transplant patient: a case report. Transplant Proc. 2019;51(5):1618–20.
32. Subramanian AK, Theodoropoulos NM. Infectious diseases community of practice of the American society of T mycobacterium tuberculosis infections in solid organ transplantation: guidelines from the infectious diseases community of practice of the American society of transplantation. Clin Transplant. 2019;33(9): e13513.
33. Abad CL, Razonable RR. Non-tuberculous mycobacterial infections in solid organ transplant recipients: an update. J Clin Tuberc Other Mycobact Dis. 2016;4:1–8.
34. Longworth SA, Vinnard C, Lee I, Sims KD, Barton TD, Blumberg EA. Risk factors for nontuberculous mycobacterial infections in solid organ transplant recipients: a case-control study. Transpl Infect Dis. 2014;16(1):76–83.
35. Assiri A, Euvrard S, Kanitakis J. Cutaneous mycobacterium marinum infection (Fish Tank Granuloma) in a renal transplant recipient: case report and literature review. Cureus. 2019;11(10):e6013.
36. Griffith DE, Aksamit T, Brown-Elliott BA, Catanzaro A, Daley C, Gordin F et al. An official ATS/IDSA statement: diagnosis, treatment, and prevention of nontuberculous mycobacterial diseases. Am J Respir Crit Care Med. 2007;175(4):367–416.
37. Chen G, Wang H, Wang Y. Clinical application of quantiFERON-TB gold in-tube in the diagnosis and treatment of tuberculosis. Eur J Clin Microbiol Infect Dis. 2019;39(4).
38. Kuznetcova TI, Sauty A, Herbort CP. Uveitis with occult choroiditis due to Mycobacterium kansasii: limitations of interferon-gamma release assay (IGRA) tests (case report and mini-review on ocular non-tuberculous mycobacteria and IGRA cross-reactivity). Int Ophthalmol. 2012;32(5):499–506.

39. van Zyl L, du Plessis J, Viljoen J. Cutaneous tuberculosis overview and current treatment regimens. Tuberculosis (Edinb). 2015;95(6):629–38.
40. Patterson JE. Epidemiology of fungal infections in solid organ transplant patients. Transpl Infect Dis. 1999;1(4):229–36.
41. Ahmed J, Ditmars DM, Sheppard T, del Busto R, Venkat KK, Parasuraman R. Recurrence of scedosporium apiospermum infection following renal re-transplantation. Am J Transplant. 2004;4(10):1720–4.
42. Rouzaud C, Hay R, Chosidow O, Dupin N, Puel A, Lortholary O et al. Severe dermatophytosis and acquired or innate immunodeficiency: a review. J Fungi (Basel). 2015;2(1).
43. Kershenovich R, Sherman S, Reiter O, Huss SR, Didkovsky E, Mimouni D et al. A unique clinicopathological manifestation of fungal infection: a case series of deep dermatophytosis in immunosuppressed patients. Am J Clin Dermatol. 2017;18(5):697–704.
44. Dicle O, Parmaksizoglu B, Gurkan A, Tuncer M, Demirbas A, Yilmaz E. Skin infections in 401 renal transplant recipients in southern Turkey. Exp Clin Transplant. 2009;7(2):133–6.
45. Huang L, Chen W, Guo L, Zhao L, Cao B, Liu Y et al. Scopulariopsis/microascus isolation in lung transplant recipients: a report of three cases and a review of the literature. Mycoses. 2019;62(10):883–92.
46. Badiee P, Kordbacheh P, Alborzi A, Zeini F, Mirhendy H, Mahmoody M. Fungal infections in solid organ recipients. Exp Clin Transplant. 2005;3(2):385–9.
47. Tsambaos D, Badavanis G. Skin manifestations in solid organ transplant recipients. Skin Pharmacol Appl Skin Physiol. 2001;14(5):332–43.
48. Gulec AT, Demirbilek M, Seckin D, Can F, Saray Y, Sarifakioglu E et al. Superficial fungal infections in 102 renal transplant recipients: a case-control study. J Am Acad Dermatol. 2003;49(2):187–92.
49. Santos SBD, Sabadin CES, Mario DN, Rigo L, Barbosa DA. Presence of Candida spp. and candidiasis in liver transplant patients. An Bras Dermatol. 2018;93(3):356–61.
50. Antoniewicz L, Relijc D, Poitschek C, Presterl E, Geusau A. Mucosal Candida infection and colonisation as well as associated risk factors in solid organ transplant recipients. Eur J Clin Microbiol Infect Dis. 2009;28(8):945–57.
51. Krishnan N, Patel B, Palfrey W, Isache C. Rapidly progressive necrotizing cellulitis secondary to Candida tropicalis infection in an immunocompromised host. IDCases. 2020;19:e00691.
52. Ramos A, Ussetti P, Laporta R, Lazaro MT, Sanchez-Romero I. Cutaneous aspergillosis in a lung transplant recipient. Transpl Infect Dis. 2009;11(5):471–3.
53. Thomas LM, Rand HK, Miller JL, Boyd AS. Primary cutaneous aspergillosis in a patient with a solid organ transplant: case report and review of the literature. Cutis. 2008;81(2):127–30.
54. Chakradeo K, Paul Chia YY, Liu C, Mudge DW, De Silva J. Disseminated cryptococcosis presenting initially as lower limb cellulitis in a renal transplant recipient—a case report. BMC Nephrol. 2018;19(1):18.
55. Geusau A, Sandor N, Messeritsch E, Jaksch P, Tintelnot K, Presterl E. Cryptococcal cellulitis in a lung-transplant recipient. Br J Dermatol. 2005;153(5):1068–70.
56. Marques S, Carmo R, Ferreira I, Bustorff M, Sampaio S, Pestana M. Cryptococcosis in renal transplant recipients: a single-center experience. Transplant Proc. 2016;48(7):2289–93.
57. Page AV, Evans AJ, Snell L, Liles WC. Primary cutaneous mucormycosis in a lung transplant recipient: case report and concise review of the literature. Transpl Infect Dis. 2008;10(6):419–25.
58. Vulsteke JB, Deeren D. Cutaneous mucormycosis. Transpl Infect Dis. 2019;21(2):e13039.
59. Almyroudis NG, Sutton DA, Linden P, Rinaldi MG, Fung J, Kusne S. Zygomycosis in solid organ transplant recipients in a tertiary transplant center and review of the literature. Am J Transplant. 2006;6(10):2365–74.
60. McCarty TP, Baddley JW, Walsh TJ, Alexander BD, Kontoyiannis DP, Perl TM et al. Phaeohyphomycosis in transplant recipients: results from the transplant associated infection surveillance network (TRANSNET). Med Mycol. 2015;53(5):440–6.
61. Galezowski A, Delyon J, Le Cleach L, Guegan S, Ducroux E, Alanio A et al. Deep cutaneous fungal infections in solid-organ transplant recipients. J Am Acad Dermatol. 2020;83(2).
62. Yu J, Chen Y, Fang J, Zhang K. Successful treatment of disseminated fusariosis in a patient with acute lymphoblastic leukemia: a case report and literature review. Medicine (Baltimore). 2019;98(26):e16246.
63. Malcolm TR, Chin-Hong PV. Endemic mycoses in immunocompromised hosts. Curr Infect Dis Rep. 2013;15(6):536–43.
64. Virgili A, Zampino MR, Mantovani L. Fungal skin infections in organ transplant recipients. Am J Clin Dermatol. 2002;3(1):19–35.
65. Reid GE, Lynch JP, Weigt S, Sayah D, Belperio JA, Grim SA et al. Herpesvirus respiratory infections in immunocompromised patients: epidemiology, management, and outcomes. Semin Respir Crit Care Med. 2016;37(4):603–30.

66. Ito K, Okuno T, Sawada A, Sakai K, Kato Y, Muro K et al. Recurrent aphthous stomatitis caused by cytomegalovirus, herpes simplex virus, and candida species in a kidney transplant recipient: a case report. Transplant Proc. 2019;51(3):993–7.
67. Balasubramaniam R, Kuperstein AS, Stoopler ET. Update on oral herpes virus infections. Dent Clin North Am. 2014;58(2):265–80.
68. Lopez-Pintor RM, Hernandez G, de Arriba L, de Andres A. Comparison of oral lesion prevalence in renal transplant patients under immunosuppressive therapy and healthy controls. Oral Dis. 2010;16(1):89–95.
69. Lopez-Pintor RM, Hernandez G, de Arriba L, Morales JM, Jimenez C, de Andres A. Oral ulcers during the course of cytomegalovirus infection in renal transplant recipients. Transplant Proc. 2009;41(6):2419–21.
70. Drozd B, Andriescu E, Suarez A, De la Garza Bravo MM. Cutaneous cytomegalovirus manifestations, diagnosis, and treatment: a review. Dermatol Online J. 2019;25(1).
71. Siqueira SM, Goncalves BB, Loss JB, Estrella RR. Vegetative chronic genital herpes with satisfactory response to imiquimod. An Bras Dermatol. 2019;94(2):221–3.
72. Ilyas M, Maganty N, Sharma A. Cutaneous infections from viral sources in solid organ transplant recipients. J Clin Virol. 2017;97:33–7.
73. Amenabar JJ, Duran MI, Montejo M, Lampreabe I. Herpes simplex virus encephalitis in a renal transplant patient. Nefrologia. 2006;26(2):270–3.
74. Mainville GN, Marsh WL, Allen CM. Oral ulceration associated with concurrent herpes simplex virus, cytomegalovirus, and Epstein-Barr virus infection in an immunocompromised patient. Oral Surg Oral Med Oral Pathol Oral Radiol. 2015;119(6):e306–14.
75. Fehr T, Bossart W, Wahl C, Binswanger U. Disseminated varicella infection in adult renal allograft recipients: four cases and a review of the literature. Transplant. 2002;73(4):608–11.
76. Helou E, Grant M, Landry M, Wu X, Morrow JS, Malinis MF. Fatal case of cutaneous-sparing orolaryngeal zoster in a renal transplant recipient. Transplant Infect Dis. 2017;19(4).
77. Rommelaere M, Marechal C, Yombi JC, Goffin E, Kanaan N. Disseminated varicella zoster virus infection in adult renal transplant recipients: outcome and risk factors. Transplant Proc. 2012;44(9):2814–17.
78. Gouveia AI, Borges-Costa J, Soares-Almeida L, Santana A, Guerra J. Atypical presentation of herpes zoster duplex bilateralis in a renal transplanted patient. Healthcare (Basel). 2013;2(1):20–6.
79. Danziger-Isakov L, Kumar D, Practice AICo. Vaccination of solid organ transplant candidates and recipients: guidelines from the American society of transplantation infectious diseases community of practice. Clin Transplant. 2019;33(9):e13563.
80. Rubin LG, Levin MJ, Ljungman P, Davies EG, Avery R, Tomblyn M et al. 2013 IDSA clinical practice guideline for vaccination of the immunocompromised host. Clin Infect Dis. 2014;58(3):e44–100.
81. Winston DJ, Mullane KM, Cornely OA, Boeckh MJ, Brown JW, Pergam SA et al. Inactivated varicella zoster vaccine in autologous haemopoietic stem-cell transplant recipients: an international, multicentre, randomised, double-blind, placebo-controlled trial. Lancet. 2018;391(10135):2116–27.
82. Fujii H, Harada S, Yoshikawa T, Yamada S, Omura N, Shibamura M et al. Differences in the likelihood of acyclovir resistance-associated mutations in the thymidine kinase genes of herpes simplex virus 1 and varicella-zoster virus. Antimicrob Agents Chemother. 2019;63(5).
83. Al-Mansour Z, Nelson BP, Evens AM. Post-transplant lymphoproliferative disease (PTLD): risk factors, diagnosis, and current treatment strategies. Curr Hematol Malig Rep. 2013;8(3):173–83.
84. Chang Y, Cesarman E, Pessin MS, Lee F, Culpepper J, Knowles DM et al. Identification of herpesvirus-like DNA sequences in AIDS-associated Kaposi's sarcoma. Science. 1994;266(5192):1865–9.
85. Mendez JC, Paya CV. Kaposi's sarcoma and transplantation. Herpes. 2000;7(1):18–23.
86. Delyon J, Rabate C, Euvrard S, Harwood CA, Proby C, Gulec AT et al. Management of Kaposi sarcoma after solid organ transplantation: a European retrospective study. J Am Acad Dermatol. 2019;81(2):448–55.
87. Montagnino G, Bencini PL, Tarantino A, Caputo R, Ponticelli C. Clinical features and course of Kaposi's sarcoma in kidney transplant patients: report of 13 cases. Am J Nephrol. 1994;14(2):121–6.
88. Rudlinger R, Smith IW, Bunney MH, Hunter JA. Human papillomavirus infections in a group of renal transplant recipients. Br J Dermatol. 1986;115(6):681–92.
89. Harwood CA, Perrett CM, Brown VL, Leigh IM, McGregor JM, Proby CM. Imiquimod cream 5% for recalcitrant cutaneous warts in immunosuppressed individuals. Br J Dermatol. 2005;152(1):122–9.
90. Varada S, Posnick M, Alessa D, Ramirez-Fort MK. Management of cutaneous human papillomavirus infection in immunocompromised patients. Curr Probl Dermatol. 2014;45:197–215.
91. Grulich AE, van Leeuwen MT, Falster MO, Vajdic CM. Incidence of cancers in people with HIV/AIDS compared with immunosuppressed transplant recipients: a meta-analysis. Lancet. 2007;370(9581):59–67.
92. Madeleine MM, Finch JL, Lynch CF, Goodman MT, Engels EA. HPV-related cancers after solid organ transplantation in the United States. Am J Transplant. 2013;13(12):3202–9.

93. Cistjakovs M, Sultanova A, Jermakova O, Sokolovska L, Chapenko S, Lesina-Korne B et al. Importance of high-risk human papillomavirus infection detection in female renal transplant recipients in the first year after transplantation. Infect Dis Obstet Gynecol. 2018:9231031.
94. Chin-Hong PV, Reid GE, Practice ASTIDCo. human papillomavirus infection in solid organ transplant recipients: guidelines from the American society of transplantation infectious diseases community of practice. Clin Transplant. 2019;33(9):e13590.
95. Vinkenes E, Nielsen MA, Blaakaer J. Is there evidence for efficacy of human papillomavirus vaccination in solid organ transplant recipients? Eur J Obstet Gynecol Reprod Biol X. 2019;4:100015.
96. Moscicki AB, Flowers L, Huchko MJ, Long ME, MacLaughlin KL, Murphy J et al. Guidelines for cervical cancer screening in immunosuppressed women without HIV infection. J Low Genit Tract Dis. 2019;23(2):87–101.
97. Calista D. Topical cidofovir for severe cutaneous human papillomavirus and molluscum contagiosum infections in patients with HIV/AIDS: a pilot study. J Eur Acad Dermatol Venereol. 2000;14(6):484–8.
98. Haycox CL, Kim S, Fleckman P, Smith LT, Piepkorn M, Sundberg JP, Howell DN, Miller SE. Trichodysplasia spinulosa-a newly described folliculocentric viral infection in an immunocompromised host. J Investig Dermatol Symp Proc. 1999;4(3):268–71. Epub 2000/02/16. PubMed PMID:10674379.
99. Matthews MR, Wang RC, Reddick RL, Saldivar VA, Browning JC. Viral-associated trichodysplasia spinulosa: a case with electron microscopic and molecular detection of the trichodysplasia spinulosa-associated human polyomavirus. J Cutan Pathol. 2011;38(5):420–31.

Direct Dermatologic Side Effects of Immunosuppressive Therapy in Solid Organ Transplant Recipients

15

Margaret Dowd, Nico Shary, Mike Wang, and Oscar R. Colegio

INTRODUCTION

Solid organ transplantation outcomes have steadily improved over the past several decades since the first successful kidney transplant in 1954, attributable to surgical advances as well as increasingly sophisticated immunosuppressive regimens. As a result, the direct dermatologic side effects of immunosuppressive agents (Figure 15.1) have become better characterized. In this chapter we will review non-malignant direct dermatologic sequelae of posttransplant immunosuppression.

INDUCTION THERAPY

During the induction phase, high-dose boluses of corticosteroids or immunosuppressive agents are administered perioperatively to patients undergoing transplantation to prevent early acute graft rejection (see Chapter 2).

Antithymocyte globulin (ATG) is given prior to organ transplant or during rejection episodes and can induce serum sickness. Serum sickness is an immune complex-mediated hypersensitivity reaction seen in 7–27% of patients.[1] The reaction can be seen within 7–14 days post initial exposure but can develop within

DOI: 10.1201/9781003001461-15

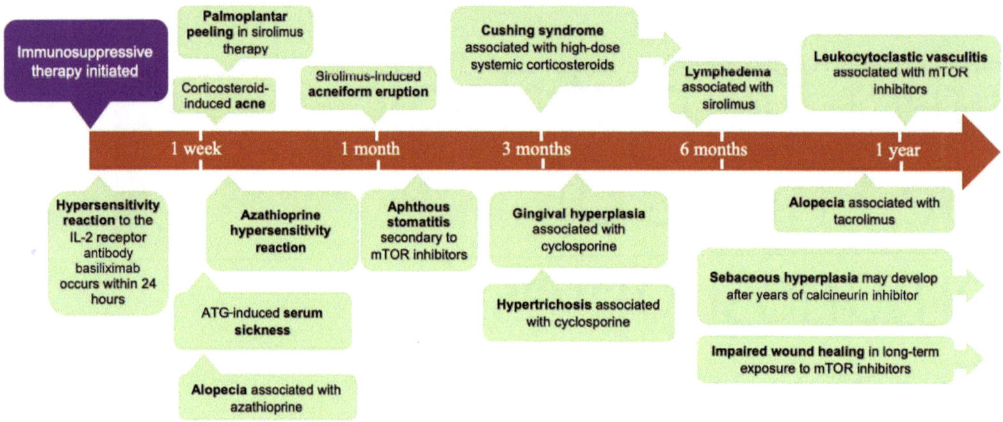

FIGURE 15.1 Timing of direct dermatologic manifestations associated with common immunosuppressive therapies in solid organ transplant recipients.

hours after reexposure.[2] Clinically, patients will present with an urticarial eruption, fever, arthralgias, and lymphadenopathy. The eruption will typically start centrally, on the abdomen, groin, or axillae prior to spreading to the trunk and extremities.[1,2] The diagnosis is made clinically, and the treatment involves high-dose steroids or plasma exchange in severe cases.[1,2]

Basiliximab is an IL-2 receptor monoclonal antibody that binds to the α chain (CD25) of the IL-2 receptor of T cells, preferentially inhibiting activated T cells, preventing proliferation and differentiation of the T cells responsible for acute graft rejection in transplant patients. Adverse reactions include acute hypersensitivity reactions, usually seen within the first 24 hours of drug administration and requiring immediate drug discontinuation. Development of cysts, herpes simplex, herpes zoster, hypertrichosis, pruritus, rash, or ulceration have been reported infrequently with the use of basiliximab.[3]

COMMON POSTTRANSPLANT IMMUNOSUPPRESSIVE AGENTS

Corticosteroids

Corticosteroids act directly on glucocorticoid receptors as both agonist and antagonist of gene transcription. The result is systemic effects on transcription factors, apoptosis, signal transduction, angiogenesis, and suppression of immunologic cells. Corticosteroids are a critical immunosuppressive agent in the initial posttransplant period. Initiated in high doses, this class of drugs is typically tapered or discontinued within the first year because of the risk of adverse systemic side effects. Common cutaneous manifestations of high-dose corticosteroid therapy include: steroid acne, Cushing syndrome, striae, dermal atrophy, skin fragility, and purpura.

Early Manifestations—1 to 2 Weeks Posttransplant

Steroid Acne

High-dose systemic corticosteroids can lead to the abrupt onset of monomorphic, papulopustular inflammatory eruption, often in the absence of comedones or inflammatory cysts, favoring the chest, upper back, and arms, but may also involve the face. It is differentiated from acne vulgaris by its abrupt onset, monomorphic appearance, and temporal relationship with the administration of corticosteroids. The eruption typically occurs within 1 week of systemic corticosteroid administration.[4]

Although a causal relationship between steroids and the development of acne has been definitively established,[5] the pathogenesis of steroid acne has not been well studied. One postulated mechanism is glucocorticoid induced Toll-like receptor 2 expression in epidermal keratinocytes, potentiating the inflammatory cascade activated by *Propionibacterium acnes*.[6] Treatment is tapering and/or eventual discontinuation of systemic corticosteroids, as well as the initiation of topical retinoids, benzoyl peroxide, or antibiotics.[5,7] Acneiform eruptions recalcitrant to therapy should raise suspicion of Pityrosporum folliculitis secondary to overgrowth of *Malassezia* spp. in the setting of immunosuppression.[8]

Late Manifestation—3 Months Posttransplant

Cushing Syndrome

Prolonged exposure to systemic corticosteroids, >2–3 months, leads to the development of Cushing syndrome, characterized by weight gain with redistribution of adipose tissue to truncal areas and the dorsocervical fat pad, as well as the classic "moon face." These changes are accompanied by dermal atrophy, which manifests with violaceous striae on the abdomen and proximal extremities (Figure 15.2), easy bruising, skin fragility, and poor wound healing.[9] Although the exact pathogenesis of Cushing syndrome is unclear, endogenous cortisol is known to be critical in maintaining normal blood glucose levels, and high levels of exogenous corticosteroids result in a catabolic state in which dermal connective tissue, bone, muscle, and vascular proteins are metabolized.[10] Hirsutism and acne vulgaris may also be present because of a subsequent elevation of systemic androgens.[11]

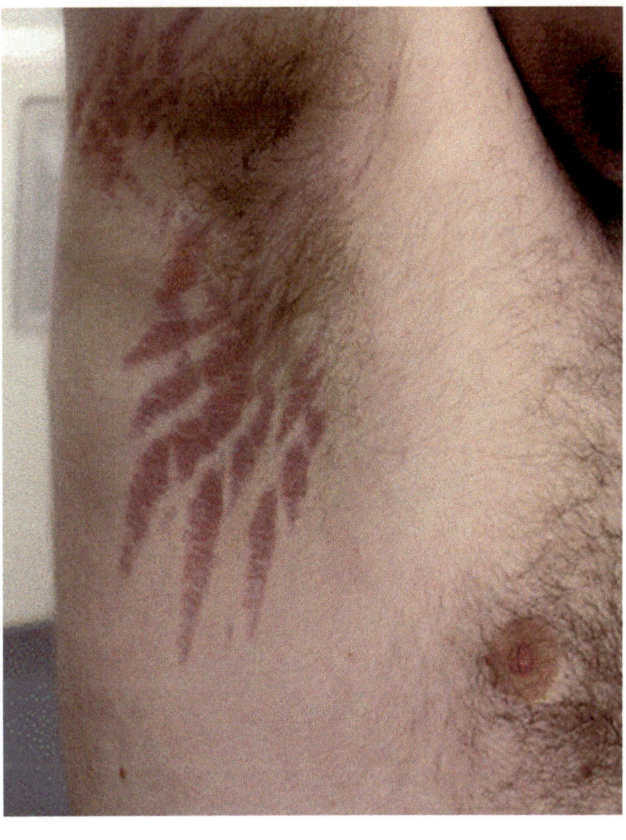

FIGURE 15.2 Striae rubrae. (From reference 18 with permission.)

Exogenous Cushing syndrome stigmata can be ameliorated with the withdrawal of corticosteroid therapy. However, withdrawal should be approached with caution as patients undergoing extended treatment with corticosteroids are at risk for exogenous steroid-induced hypothalamic-pituitary-adrenal axis suppression and consequent secondary adrenal insufficiency.[11,12] For these patients, complete discontinuation of steroids may not be possible. In these cases, alternative approaches to improve symptoms can be undertaken, such as diet and exercise in conjunction with dose reduction strategies to mitigate the effects of abnormal metabolism.

Calcineurin Inhibitors

Calcineurin inhibitors (CNIs) are widely used in solid organ transplant as steroid-sparing immunosuppressive agents and include tacrolimus and cyclosporine (see Chapter 2). These drugs bind to specific receptor proteins (FKBP and cyclophilin, respectively) resulting in inhibition of the intracellular enzyme calcineurin, preventing the dephosphorylation and activation of the transcription factor NFAT-1, ultimately reducing the transcription of IL-2 and the activity of T cells. The majority of dermatologic effects of CNIs are associated with cyclosporine and involve the pilosebaceous unit.[13] Tacrolimus has limited dermatologic side effects.

Early Manifestations—1 to 6 Months Posttransplant

Gingival Hyperplasia

In 25%–50% of adult SOTRs, gingival enlargement may occur within 3–6 months of initiating cyclosporine therapy.[14,15] The overgrowth typically begins in the interdental papillae (Figure 15.3) and may slowly extend to the facial and lingual aspects of the gingival margin. The tissue becomes friable and prone to bleeding. In some cases, gingival enlargement may impair speech, interfere with mastication, and lead to esthetic problems.[16,17] Gingival hyperplasia has also been reported in 70% of pediatric transplant patients,

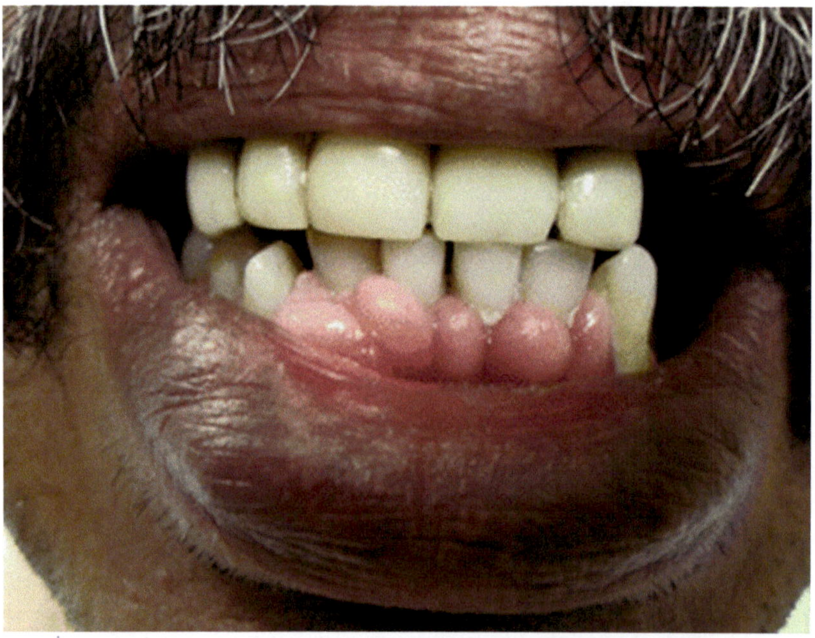

FIGURE 15.3 Gingival hyperplasia. (From reference 18 with permission.)

and men appear to be more susceptible than women.[18] Both phenytoin and nifedipine are also common causes of gingival enlargement. The combination of cyclosporine and nifedipine has been shown to result in an increased rate of gingival overgrowth.[19]

The upregulation of salivary inflammatory cytokines, such as interleukin (IL)-1a, IL-6, and IL-8, leading to increased proliferation of gingival fibroblasts and keratinocytes, has been implicated in the pathogenesis of cyclosporine-induced gingival hyperplasia.[14] Optimal oral hygiene is critical to the prevention of gingival hyperplasia, as plaque-induced gingival inflammation is likely the inciting event in the pathogenesis.[20] Once gingival hyperplasia has developed, modification of the immunosuppressive regimen is the most effective approach. Otherwise, professional debridement along with the use of antibacterial mouthwashes or chlorhexidine may reduce the severity of the overgrowth. Azithromycin 500 mg daily for 3 days has been reported to be of benefit.[13] Gingivectomy may be necessary in severe cases but recurrences can occur post-surgery.[19]

Hypertrichosis

Hypertrichosis is one of the most common cutaneous side effects of cyclosporine, affecting 70%–100% of patients within 6 months of initiation of cyclosporine therapy.[21–23] The reported hypertrichosis is dose-dependent and can affect patients of all ages. It may also be more prevalent in women and in those with dark hair[23,24] (Figure 15.4).

The pathophysiological basis of cyclosporine-induced hypertrichosis is unclear. Independent of its immunosuppressive effects, there are reports supporting cyclosporine prolonging the anagen phase and reducing the catagen phase of the hair growth cycle through modulation of calcineurin-associated cellular

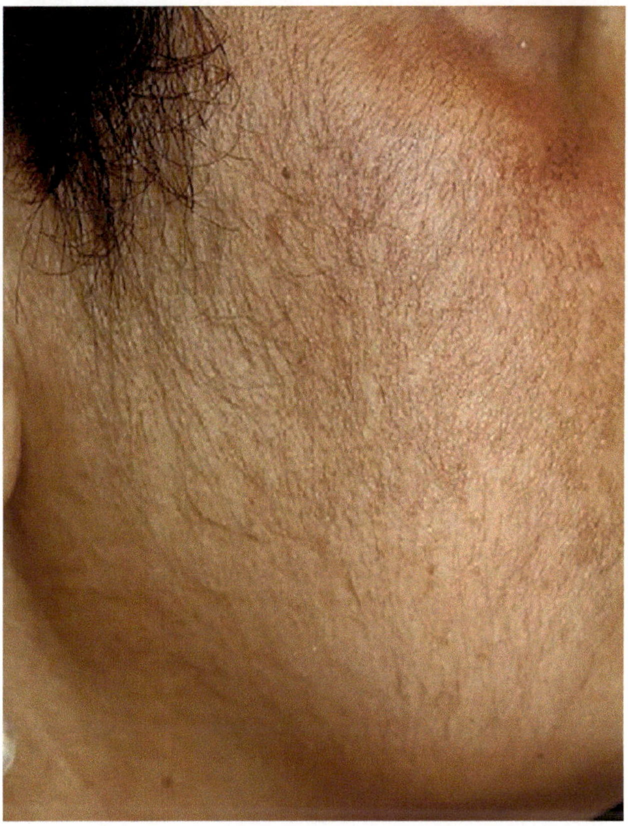

FIGURE 15.4 Hypertrichosis. (From reference 18 with permission.)

mechanisms in follicular keratinocytes.[25–27] Cyclosporine has also been shown to increase the cutaneous levels of 5α-dihydrotestosterone in a murine model, and may increase the level of serum testosterone metabolites in patients.[28,29] Cessation of cyclosporine, or substitution with tacrolimus, may resolve symptoms.[30,31] For patients who cannot alter their immunosuppressive regimen, laser hair removal has been shown to be a relatively safe treatment option with long-lasting results.[22]

Late—1 Year and Beyond Posttransplant

Alopecia

In contrast to cyclosporine, which can lead to an overgrowth of hair, tacrolimus can induce a diffuse, non-scarring, and often reversible alopecia in 10%–29% of patients.[32–34] Widespread thinning and hair shedding can be seen in patients.[13] The alopecia was reported more commonly in women and could occur as soon as 1 month after initiation of therapy or as late as after 1 year. The pathophysiology of tacrolimus-induced alopecia is unclear with some speculation as to possible drug-induced vasoconstriction.[13] The alopecia appears to be dose-dependent and not attributable to sex hormones, as the condition is reversible with dose-reduction of tacrolimus or with the administration of topical minoxidil.[35]

Sebaceous Hyperplasia

Sebaceous hyperplasia (SH) is a benign enlargement of the sebaceous gland that typically presents after years of cyclosporine therapy. Clinically, disseminated soft umbilicated skin-colored to yellow papules can be seen, mainly distributed on the face (Figure 15.5). SH affects predominantly middle-aged to elderly

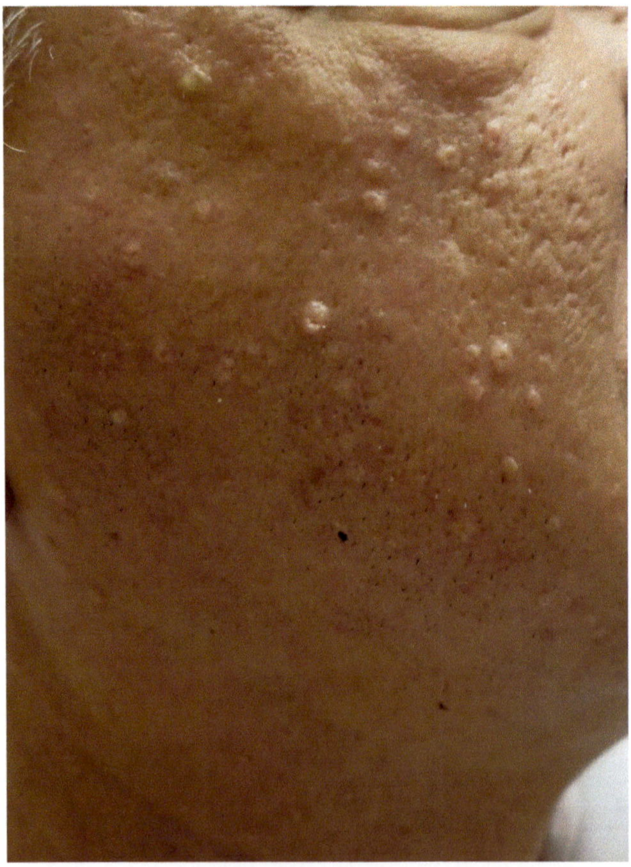

FIGURE 15.5 Sebaceous hyperplasia. (Gyorgy Paragh MD, PhD.)

men. Up to 30% of renal transplant patients on cyclosporine were reported to develop SH,[36] although other studies have reported variable rates of 6–16% in SOTRs.[37–39] In a study of 151 kidney transplant recipients who did not receive cyclosporine, none of these patients developed SH.[40] Although SH has been strongly linked to cyclosporine, other immunosuppressive medications including tacrolimus, mycophenolate mofetil, and prednisone were associated with a case of eruptive SH.[41]

As is the case for some of the other cutaneous reactions to immunosuppressive medication discussed in this chapter, the mechanism of cyclosporine-induced SH is not well understood. Cyclosporine may have a direct lipophilic effect on the pilosebaceous unit and may exert as well an occlusive follicular effect.[42] Another possible link between cyclosporine and SH may be dysplastic epithelial proliferation, which is supported by the correlation between the incidence of keratinocyte carcinomas and sebaceous hyperplasia in SOTRs.[36,37] The mainstay of treatment of SH is topical and systemic retinoids, or dose reduction of cyclosporine, but cryotherapy, electrodessication, pulse-dye laser therapy, and photodynamic therapy have been reported in the literature.[36,43–46] In a recent review of SH treatments, customizing therapy to different parameters was found to be the most effective approach.[42]

Mammalian Target of Rapamycin Inhibitors

The mammalian target of rapamycin (mTOR) inhibitors, which include sirolimus and everolimus, are relatively new and less frequently used immunosuppressive medications. Both agents inhibit mTOR, blocking transduction signaling of IL-2, leading to decreased T cell proliferation. They are often used in triple therapy in conjunction with a corticosteroid and may be selected as an alternative for patients with cyclosporine nephrotoxicity or for their antineoplastic activity. However, their use is often limited by intolerable adverse effects. The common mucocutaneous side effects of mTOR inhibitors include acneiform eruption, aphthous ulcers, lymphedema, and impaired wound healing.

Early Manifestations—1 to 6 Months Posttransplant

Acneiform Eruption

Between 15% and 45% of patients, more commonly males, treated with sirolimus will develop an acneiform eruption.[13,47,48] The morphology is non-comedonal inflammatory papules and pustules located on the face and trunk in a seborrheic distribution, often accompanied by folliculitis of the scalp.[13,47,48] This is considered separate and distinct from the inflammatory lesions of hidradenitis suppurativa (HS), which have also been observed in renal transplant patients treated with sirolimus but characteristically affect the axillary, perianal, and inguinal areas. The two are likely related to aberration in the differentiation of the pilosebaceous unit.

Sirolimus inhibition of mTOR, a central regulator of mammalian metabolism, leads to the downstream inhibition of epidermal growth factor (EGF).[48–50] EGF plays a key role in the differentiation of epidermal and adnexal cells, and the inhibition of EGF can result in the abnormal differentiation of the pilosebaceous unit.[51,52] This results in an acneiform eruption similar to that seen with direct inhibition of EGF by the EGF inhibitor drug class used in cancer chemotherapy. Spontaneous regression of the lesions may occur, whereas reported successful therapies include topical and systemic antibiotics as well as topical or systemic retinoids.[53] In the case of HS-like lesions, surgical excision has been used when antibiotic therapy fails.[47]

Aphthous Stomatitis

Oral stomatitis with aphthous ulcers manifests as small, superficial, discrete, and ovoid ulcers with a gray pseudomembrane over the labial and buccal mucosae, floor of the mouth, and the ventral tongue. Administration of mTOR inhibitors such as sirolimus and everolimus can lead to the rapid development of these ulcers, especially in cases of high loading doses.[54,55] Between 10% and 29% of newly transplanted SOTRs on sirolimus immunosuppression will develop stomatitis, whereas up to a 60% of renal transplant recipients who switched from tacrolimus and mycophenolate mofetil to sirolimus developed aphthae.[54–57]

The rapid development of aphthous ulcers after initiation of mTOR-inhibition therapy suggests a direct toxic insult to the oral mucosa.[47] However, cytomegalovirus (CMV) infection is postulated to contribute to the development of some of these lesions; therefore, viral etiology should be ruled out.[58] The ulcers were usually self-limited and resolve in 2 weeks or less. However, the lesions were associated with significant pain and may impede oral intake, which may result in significant morbidity.[53] Treatment is potent topical steroids, such as clobetasol 0.05% cream used twice a day.[59] In lesions in which CMV is detected, ganciclovir may be an effective therapy in select patients.

Lymphedema

Progressive lymphedema is a rare but debilitating side effect of sirolimus immunosuppressive therapy in SOTRs.[60,61] Patients typically present with lower extremity swelling, with a mean onset of 5 months after the initiation of sirolimus therapy. Approximately 25% of patients have bilateral involvement. Imaging by lymphoscintigraphy in patients with sirolimus-associated lymphedema reveals failure of either the superficial collecting lymphatic vessels or the entire lymphatic drainage system.[18]

The disruption of lymphatics is likely the result of impaired lymphangiogenesis. Sirolimus inhibits downstream vascular endothelial growth factor (VEGF) signaling, which is necessary for normal proliferation and migration of lymphatic endothelial cells.[62–64] As such, any insult to the lymphatic system, either by surgery, radiation, or other means will be inadequately repaired and lead to the development of lymphedema. Lymphedema is disfiguring and debilitating, and prompt cessation of sirolimus is necessary; however, it is not always reversible.[65]

Palmoplantar Peeling

Palmoplantar peeling is an extremely rare adverse reaction to sirolimus, observed within the first 2 weeks of initiating therapy. It presents as desquamation of the epidermal layer of the palms and soles with possible dry vesicles[66](Figure 15.6). The appearance closely resembles the desquamation seen during the resolution of the scarlatiniform rash of group A strep infections or the one seen with chemotherapy-mediated hand-foot syndrome. Unlike these forms of desquamation, however, sirolimus-induced palmoplantar peeling lacks preceding erythema and is limited to acral involvement. Patients do report tenderness in the areas of peeling.

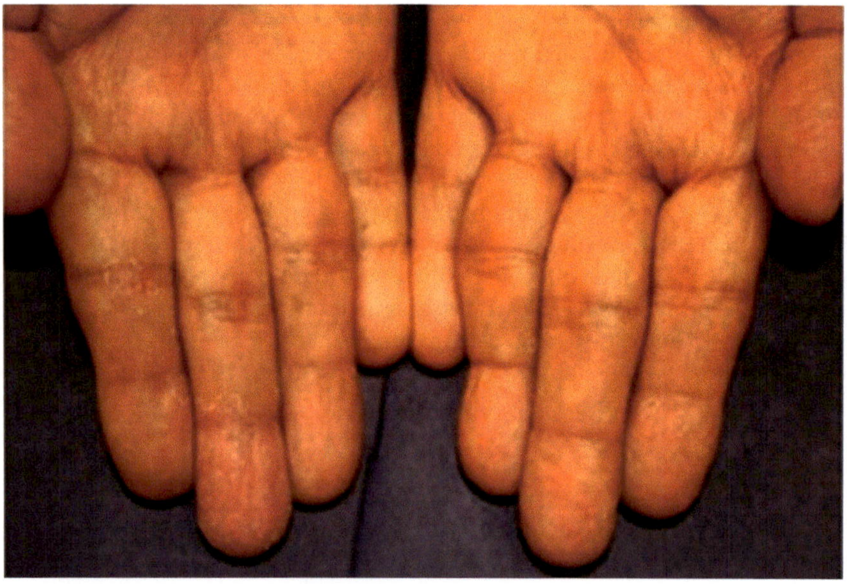

FIGURE 15.6 Palmoplantar peeling. (From reference 18 with permission.)

The underlying mechanism of desquamation is unclear. Although the condition is not life-threatening, it may lead to discomfort and functional impairment. Discontinuation of sirolimus leads to cessation of the peeling but may not be necessary as the peeling spontaneously resolves within 1–6 months.

Late Manifestations—One Year Posttransplant and Beyond

Leukocytoclastic Vasculitis

Leukocytoclastic vasculitis (LCV) is an extremely rare sequela of mTOR-inhibition therapy, with fewer than ten cases reported in the literature.[67–70] The condition generally presents over a year after initiation of therapy and manifests as palpable purpura of the extremities. Cutaneous lesions may herald systemic involvement, including the gastrointestinal tract, and can be associated with significant morbidity and mortality.

There is no clear pathoetiology, although activation of complement cascades and bradykinin have been implicated.[71] In reports of sirolimus-induced cutaneous LCV in SOTRs without systemic involvement, withdrawal of the mTOR inhibitor resulted in resolution.

Impaired Wound Healing

Compared with that of other immunosuppressive agents, mTOR inhibitors have a higher rate of wound healing complications.[13] Wound-related complications were observed in 43.2% of renal transplant patients taking sirolimus, compared with just 2.4% receiving mycophenolate mofetil.[72] These complications included superficial or fascial wound dehiscence, fluid collections, and infection.

Sirolimus and everolimus inhibit the activity of mTOR-mediated VEGF, which plays an essential role in wound healing. Inhibition of VEGF leads to decreased angiogenesis, fibroblast activity, and ultimately decreased wound tensile strength.[73] The effects of sirolimus and everolimus on wound healing are dose-dependent and can be minimized by reducing mTOR inhibition.[74,75] Discontinuation in patients with minor wound-healing complications is not necessary, and the majority of wound-healing complications can be managed in outpatient clinics.[13]

Nail Dystrophy

Onychopathy has been reported in up three-quarters of renal transplant patients on sirolimus, with pathology ranging from soft, brittle nails to yellow discoloration and fissuring.[47] Paronychia and pyogenic granulomas may also occur in SOTRs on mTOR inhibitors.[76] Paronychia has been successfully treated with topical steroids, whereas other onychopathy is resistant to topical therapy.[77]

Azathioprine

Azathioprine, a derivative of 6-mercaptopurine, is a purine analog. Its active metabolite, 6-thioguanine, is incorporated into DNA and RNA, inhibiting purine metabolism and cell division; impairment of the lymphocyte cell cycle results in profound immunosuppression.[10] One of the longest employed immunosuppressive agents, high-dose azathioprine bares a significant long-term risk of nonmelanoma skin cancer.[78] Other dermatologic manifestations of azathioprine immunosuppression include alopecia and azathioprine hypersensitivity syndrome.

Early Manifestations—1 Week to 1 Month Posttransplant

Alopecia

Alopecia has been seen in up to one-third of renal transplant patients undergoing therapy with azathioprine. It typically presents within a month of initiating treatment and is transient in nature.[79] It is difficult to determine if the alopecia that renal transplant patients experience is because of the transplant itself or is exacerbated by the azathioprine. However, in a case-controlled comparison of renal transplant and nontransplant patients treated with combination azathioprine and prednisone, there was no significant difference in the incidence of alopecia between the two groups, suggesting that the transplant alone didn't account for the incidence of azathioprine-induced alopecia.[79] The underlying pathogenesis is likely drug-induced disruption of the mitotic activity of the hair follicle resulting in an anagen effluvium.[80]

Azathioprine Hypersensitivity Syndrome

The most concerning immediate sequala of azathioprine is a rare but life-threatening hypersensitivity syndrome affecting approximately 2% of patients. It presents in the first to fourth week of therapy with fevers, hypotension, and oliguria.[13,81,82] When cutaneous lesions are present, they vary from morbilliform, vesicular, and erythema multiforme-like to erythema nodosum panniculitis-like lesions. The histologic results among the various morphologies are consistent, most commonly comprised of a dense neutrophilic infiltrate or leukocytoclastic vasculitis.[83] The underlying pathogenesis is a type IV hypersensitivity reaction, and prompt discontinuation of the medication is necessary.[81,82] Rechallenge with azathioprine is contraindicated and may result in life-threatening anaphylaxis.

Mycophenolate Mofetil

Mycophenolate mofetil (MMF) inhibits the enzyme inosine monophosphate dehydrogenase, disrupting *de novo* purine synthesis. Lymphocytes are preferentially impaired as they lack a purine salvage pathway and are thus dependent on the *de novo* purine pathway for DNA synthesis.[10] MMF is a known carcinogen, with long-term risk of lymphoproliferative malignancies as well as nonmelanoma skin cancer. It is associated with minimal dermatologic toxicities; however, aphthous stomatitis has been reported.

Aphthous Stomatitis

The incidence of aphthous ulcers associated with MMF therapy is controversial. In the rare reports of aphthae in SOTRs taking MMF, it has typically occurred in patients on combination immunosuppression with MMF and sirolimus or MMF and tacrolimus and has resolved with dose reduction of the calcineurin or mTOR inhibitor, questioning the role of MMF in the development of the ulcers.[57,84] One should be cautious in the setting of combination therapy with sirolimus, as the latter should be considered the more likely culprit. Nonetheless, it was reported in SOTRs receiving combination therapy with cyclosporine and prednisolone, resolving with discontinuation of MMF, and should be considered as a possible inciting factor.[85] The lesions present as discrete gray ulcers affecting the tongue and buccal mucosa. In SOTRs, these ulcers may become plaque-like and clustered, which can become painful and problematic for oral intake. First-line therapy is potent topical steroids, although in some cases oral colchicine, dapsone, or thalidomide may be necessary.[86] Viral examination for herpes simplex virus (HSV) and CMV should be performed, and these should be treated if present.

NEWER IMMUNOSUPPRESSIVE AGENT

Belatacept is a selective costimulation blocker that binds B7 family receptors (CD86 and CD80) to prevent costimulation and activation of T cells and is used for immunosuppressive maintenance with limited side effects.[87] Peripheral edema and hirsutism were described in one study of transplant patients taking belatacept.[88]

CONCLUSION

This chapter reviewed the direct dermatologic side effects of immunosuppressive medications in SOTRs, including their presentation, incidence, pathogenesis, and treatments. Awareness of these dermatologic complications may help in their recognition and management, improving outcomes for these patients.

SUMMARY OF KEY POINTS

- ATG is given prior to organ transplant or during rejection episodes and can induce serum sickness.
- Basiliximab is an IL-2 receptor monoclonal antibody used to prevent acute graft rejection. Adverse reactions include acute hypersensitivity reactions, as well as cysts, herpes simplex, herpes zoster, hypertrichosis, pruritus, rash, or ulceration.
- Corticosteroids act directly on glucocorticoid receptors as both agonist and antagonist of gene transcription. Common cutaneous manifestations of high-dose corticosteroid therapy include: steroid acne, Cushing syndrome, striae, dermal atrophy, skin fragility, and purpura.
- CNIs are used as steroid-sparing immunosuppressive agents and include tacrolimus and cyclosporine. These agents inhibit calcineurin and ultimately reduce the transcription of IL-2 and the activity of T cells. Cyclosporine dermatologic side effects include gingival hyperplasia, sebaceous hyperplasia, and hypertrichosis. Tacrolimus is associated with alopecia.
- mTOR inhibitors, which include sirolimus and everolimus, inhibit mTOR, blocking transduction signaling of IL-2, leading to decreased T cell proliferation. Adverse mucocutaneous side effects of mTOR inhibitors include acneiform eruption, aphthous ulcers, lymphedema, impaired wound healing, and nail changes.
- Azathioprine inhibits purine metabolism and cell division, leading to impairment of the lymphocyte cell cycle and profound immunosuppression. It is associated with a significant long-term risk of nonmelanoma skin cancer, alopecia, and azathioprine hypersensitivity syndrome.
- MMF inhibits the enzyme inosine monophosphate dehydrogenase, disrupting *de novo* purine synthesis. Lymphocytes are preferentially impaired as they lack a purine salvage pathway. It is associated with minimal dermatologic toxicities; however, aphthous stomatitis has been reported.
- Belatacept is a B7 ligand antagonist, with limited side effects. Peripheral edema and hirsutism have been reported.

REFERENCES

1. Tanriover B, Chuang P, Fishbach B et al. Polyclonal antibody-induced serum sickness in renal transplant recipients: treatment with therapeutic plasma exchange. Transplant. 2005;80(2):279–81.
2. Lundquist AL, Chari RS, Wood JH et al. Serum sickness following rabbit antithymocyte-globulin induction in a liver transplant recipient: case report and literature review. Liver Transpl. 2007;13(5):647–50.
3. Kahan BD, Rajagopalan PR, Hall M. Reduction of the occurrence of acute cellular rejection among renal allograft recipients treated with basiliximab, a chimeric anti-interleukin-2-receptor monoclonal antibody. United States Simulect Renal Study Group. Transplant. 1999;67(2):276–84.
4. Hurwitz RM. Steroid acne. J Am Acad Dermatol. 1989;21(6):1179–81.

5. Kazandjieva J, Tsankov N. Drug-induced acne. Clin Dermatol. 2017;35(2):156–62.
6. Shibata M, Katsuyama M, Onodera T, Ehama R, Hosoi J, Tagami H. Glucocorticoids enhance toll-like receptor 2 expression in human keratinocytes stimulated with propionibacterium acnes or proinflammatory cytokines. J Invest Dermatol. 2009;129(2):375–82.
7. Mills OH, Leyden JJ, Kligman AM. Tretinoin treatment of steroid acne. Arch Dermatol. 1973;108(3):381–4.
8. Yu HJ, Lee SK, Son SJ, Kim YS, Yang HY, Kim JH. Steroid acne vs. pityrosporum folliculitis: the incidence of pityrosporum ovale and the effect of antifungal drugs in steroid acne. Int J Dermatol. 1998;37(10):772–7.
9. Hopkins RL, Leinung MC. Exogenous cushing's syndrome and glucocorticoid withdrawal. Endocrinol Metab Clin North Am. 2005;34(2):371–84, ix.
10. Wolverton SE. Comprehensive dermatologic drug therapy. 3rd ed. Edinburgh: Saunders, Elsevier; 2013.
11. Mihailidis J, Dermesropian R, Taxel P, Luthra P, Grant-Kels JM. Endocrine evaluation of hirsutism. Int J Womens Dermatol. 2017;3(1 Suppl):S6–S10.
12. Livanou T, Ferriman D, James VH. Recovery of hypothalamo-pituitary-adrenal function after corticosteroid therapy. Lancet. 1967;2(7521):856–9.
13. Ilyas M, Colegio OR, Kaplan B, Sharma A. Cutaneous toxicities from transplantation-related medications. Am J Transplant. 2017;17(11):2782–9.
14. Ponnaiyan D, Jegadeesan V. Cyclosporine A: novel concepts in its role in drug-induced gingival overgrowth. Dent Res J (Isfahan). 2015;12(6):499–506.
15. Kumar S, Guliani A, Vinay K. Cyclosporine-induced gingival hypertrophy. JAMA Dermatol. 2019;155(4):487.
16. Sharma S, Dasroy SK. Images in clinical medicine: gingival hyperplasia induced by phenytoin. N Engl J Med. 2000;342(5):325.
17. Yu DS, Lee YB. Images in clinical medicine: medication-induced gingival hypertrophy. N Engl J Med. 2009;360(2):e2.
18. Colegio OR. Skin diseases in the immunosuppressed. Berlin: Springer; 2018.
19. Hallmon WW, Rossmann JA. The role of drugs in the pathogenesis of gingival overgrowth: a collective review of current concepts. Periodontol 2000. 1999;21:176–96.
20. Seymour RA, Thomason JM, Ellis JS. The pathogenesis of drug-induced gingival overgrowth. J Clin Periodontol. 1996;23(3 Pt 1):165–75.
21. Schena FP, Pascoe MD, Alberu J et al. Conversion from calcineurin inhibitors to sirolimus maintenance therapy in renal allograft recipients: 24-month efficacy and safety results from the CONVERT trial. Transplant. 2009;87(2):233–42.
22. Wysocki GP, Daley TD. Hypertrichosis in patients receiving cyclosporine therapy. Clin Exp Dermatol. 1987;12(3):191–6.
23. Imko-Walczuk B, Okuniewska A, Predota-Glowacka A et al. Benign cutaneous disease among polish renal transplant recipients. Transplant Proc. 2016;48(5):1660–6.
24. Berth-Jones J. The use of ciclosporin in psoriasis. J Dermatolog Treat. 2005;16(5–6):258–77.
25. Gafter-Gvili A, Kalechman Y, Sredni B, Gal R, Gafter U. Cyclosporin A-induced hair growth in mice is associated with inhibition of hair follicle regression. Arch Dermatol Res. 2004;296(6):265–9.
26. Gafter-Gvili A, Sredni B, Gal R, Gafter U, Kalechman Y. Cyclosporin A-induced hair growth in mice is associated with inhibition of calcineurin-dependent activation of NFAT in follicular keratinocytes. Am J Physiol Cell Physiol. 2003;284(6):C1593–603.
27. Taylor M, Ashcroft AT, Messenger AG. Cyclosporin A prolongs human hair growth in vitro. J Invest Dermatol. 1993;100(3):237–9.
28. Boudou P, Fiet J, Vexiau P, Villette JM, Hardy N, Dreux C. Greater conversion of testosterone to 5 alpha-dihydrotestosterone, reflecting increased peripheral 5 alpha-reductase activity in nude mice treated with high doses of cyclosporine A. J Steroid Biochem. 1990;36(6):597–601.
29. Cutolo M, Giusti M, Villaggio B et al. Testosterone metabolism and cyclosporin A treatment in rheumatoid arthritis. Br J Rheumatol. 1997;36(4):433–9.
30. Panicker VV, Mathew A, Dhamramaratnam A. Cosmetically disfiguring side effects of cyclosporine. Int J Trichology. 2012;4(1):50.
31. Thorp M, DeMattos A, Bennett W, Barry J, Norman D. The effect of conversion from cyclosporine to tacrolimus on gingival hyperplasia, hirsutism and cholesterol. Transplant. 2000;69(6):1218–20.
32. Kim HC, Hwang EA, Han SY, Park SB, Kim HT, Cho WH. Primary immunosuppression with tacrolimus in kidney transplantation: three-year follow-up in a single center. Transplant Proc. 2004;36(7):2082–3.
33. Tricot L, Lebbe C, Pillebout E, Martinez F, Legendre C, Thervet E. Tacrolimus-induced alopecia in female kidney-pancreas transplant recipients. Transplant. 2005;80(11):1546–9.
34. Chan AL, Wang HY. Reversibility of tacrolimus-induced alopecia: a case report and literature review. Clin Drug Investig. 2003;23(9):611–14.

35. Shapiro R, Jordan ML, Scantlebury VP et al. Alopecia as a consequence of tacrolimus therapy. Transplant. 1998;65(9):1284.
36. Salim A, Reece SM, Smith AG et al. Sebaceous hyperplasia and skin cancer in patients undergoing renal transplant. J Am Acad Dermatol. 2006;55(5):878–81.
37. de Berker DA, Taylor AE, Quinn AG, Simpson NB. Sebaceous hyperplasia in organ transplant recipients: shared aspects of hyperplastic and dysplastic processes? J Am Acad Dermatol. 1996;35(5 Pt 1):696–9.
38. Lugo-Janer G, Sanchez JL, Santiago-Delpin E. Prevalence and clinical spectrum of skin diseases in kidney transplant recipients. J Am Acad Dermatol. 1991;24(3):410–14.
39. Bencini PL, Montagnino G, Sala F, De Vecchi A, Crosti C, Tarantino A. Cutaneous lesions in 67 cyclosporin-treated renal transplant recipients. Dermatologica. 1986;172(1):24–30.
40. Taylor AE, Shuster S. Skin cancer after renal transplantation: the causal role of azathioprine. Acta Derm Venereol. 1992;72(2):115–19.
41. Levandoski KA, Girardi NA, Loss MJ. Eruptive sebaceous hyperplasia as a side effect of oral tacrolimus in a renal transplant recipient. Dermatol Online J. 2017;23(5).
42. Hussein L, Perrett CM. Treatment of sebaceous gland hyperplasia: a review of the literature. J Dermatolog Treat. 2020:1–12.
43. McDonald SK, Goh MS, Chong AH. Successful treatment of cyclosporine-induced sebaceous hyperplasia with oral isotretinoin in two renal transplant recipients. Australas J Dermatol. 2011;52(3):227–30.
44. Perrett CM, McGregor J, Barlow RJ, Karran P, Proby C, Harwood CA. Topical photodynamic therapy with methyl aminolevulinate to treat sebaceous hyperplasia in an organ transplant recipient. Arch Dermatol. 2006;142(6):781–2.
45. Burton CS, Sawchuk WS. Premature sebaceous gland hyperplasia: successful treatment with isotretinoin. J Am Acad Dermatol. 1985;12(1 Pt 2):182–4.
46. Jung HY, Kim M, Cho BK, Park HJ. A case of cyclosporine-induced sebaceous hyperplasia in a renal transplant patient successfully treated with isotretinoin. Ann Dermatol. 2016;28(2):271–2.
47. Mahé E, Morelon E, Lechaton S et al. Cutaneous adverse events in renal transplant recipients receiving sirolimus-based therapy. Transplant. 2005;79(4):476–2.
48. Mahé E, Morelon E, Lechaton S et al. Acne in recipients of renal transplantation treated with sirolimus: clinical, microbiologic, histologic, therapeutic, and pathogenic aspects. J Am Acad Dermatol. 2006;55(1):139–42.
49. Wipperman MF, Montrose DC, Gotto AM, Hajjar DP. Mammalian target of rapamycin: a metabolic rheostat for regulating adipose tissue function and cardiovascular health. Am J Pathol. 2019;189(3):492–501.
50. Nomura M, He Z, Koyama I, Ma WY, Miyamoto K, Dong Z. Involvement of the Akt/mTOR pathway on EGF-induced cell transformation. Mol Carcinog. 2003;38(1):25–32.
51. Dereure O. Skin reactions related to treatment with anticytokines, membrane receptor inhibitors and monoclonal antibodies. Expert Opin Drug Saf. 2003;2(5):467–73.
52. Laffitte E, Saurat JH. Kinase inhibitor-induced pustules. Dermatol. 2005;211(4):305–6.
53. Campistol JM, de Fijter JW, Flechner SM, Langone A, Morelon E, Stockfleth E. mTOR inhibitor-associated dermatologic and mucosal problems. Clin Transplant. 2010;24(2):149–56.
54. Kahan BD. Efficacy of sirolimus compared with azathioprine for reduction of acute renal allograft rejection: a randomised multicentre study, the rapamune US study group. Lancet. 2000;356(9225):194–202.
55. MacDonald AS. A worldwide, phase III, randomized, controlled, safety and efficacy study of a sirolimus/cyclosporine regimen for prevention of acute rejection in recipients of primary mismatched renal allografts. Transplant. 2001;71(2):271–80.
56. Toso C, Meeberg GA, Bigam DL et al. De novo sirolimus-based immunosuppression after liver transplantation for hepatocellular carcinoma: long-term outcomes and side effects. Transplant. 2007;83(9):1162–8.
57. van Gelder T, ter Meulen CG, Hené R, Weimar W, Hoitsma A. Oral ulcers in kidney transplant recipients treated with sirolimus and mycophenolate mofetil. Transplant. 2003;75(6):788–91.
58. Olczak-Kowalczyk D, Pawłowska J, Cukrowska B et al. Local presence of cytomegalovirus and Candida species vs oral lesions in liver and kidney transplant recipients. Ann Transplant. 2008;13(4):28–33.
59. Chuang P, Langone AJ. Clobetasol ameliorates aphthous ulceration in renal transplant patients on sirolimus. Am J Transplant. 2007;7(3):714–17.
60. Langer RM, Kahan BD. Incidence, therapy, and consequences of lymphocele after sirolimus-cyclosporine-prednisone immunosuppression in renal transplant recipients. Transplant. 2002;74(6):804–8.
61. Desai N, Heenan S, Mortimer PS. Sirolimus-associated lymphoedema: eight new cases and a proposed mechanism. Br J Dermatol. 2009;160(6):1322–6.
62. Kerjaschki D. How to control lymphangiogenesis: a novel role for rapamycin. Kidney Int. 2007;71(8):717–19.
63. Huber S, Bruns CJ, Schmid G et al. Inhibition of the mammalian target of rapamycin impedes lymphangiogenesis. Kidney Int. 2007;71(8):771–7.

64. Kobayashi S, Kishimoto T, Kamata S, Otsuka M, Miyazaki M, Ishikura H. Rapamycin, a specific inhibitor of the mammalian target of rapamycin, suppresses lymphangiogenesis and lymphatic metastasis. Cancer Sci. 2007;98(5):726–33.
65. Ardalan MR. Lymphedema attributed to sirolimus. J Nephropharmacol. 2013;2(2):35–6.
66. Liu LS, McNiff JM, Colegio OR. Palmoplantar peeling secondary to sirolimus therapy. Am J Transplant. 2014;14(1):221–5.
67. Hardinger KL, Cornelius LA, Trulock EP, Brennan DC. Sirolimus-induced leukocytoclastic vasculitis. Transplant. 2002;74(5):739–43.
68. Nagarajan S, Friedrich T, Garcia M, Kambham N, Sarwal MM. Gastrointestinal leukocytoclastic vasculitis: an adverse effect of sirolimus. Pediatr Transplant. 2005;9(1):97–100.
69. Pasqualotto AC, Bianco PD, Sukiennik TC, Furian R, Garcia VD. Sirolimus-induced leukocytoclastic vasculitis: the second case reported. Am J Transplant. 2004;4(9):1549–51.
70. Yee KW, Hymes SR, Heller L, Prieto VG, Welch MA, Giles FJ. Cutaneous leukocytoclastic vasculitis in a patient with myelodysplastic syndrome after therapy with the rapamycin analogue everolimus: case report and review of the literature. Leuk Lymphoma. 2006;47(5):926–9.
71. Kandalaft O, Samanani S, Aftab HB. Sirolimus associated pericarditis. J Am Coll Cardiol. 2018;71(Suppl 11):A2440.
72. Valente JF, Hricik D, Weigel K et al. Comparison of sirolimus vs. mycophenolate mofetil on surgical complications and wound healing in adult kidney transplantation. Am J Transplant. 2003;3(9):1128–34.
73. Ekici Y, Emiroglu R, Ozdemir H, Aldemir D, Karakayali H, Haberal M. Effect of rapamycin on wound healing: an experimental study. Transplant Proc. 2007;39(4):1201–3.
74. Dean PG, Lund WJ, Larson TS et al. Wound-healing complications after kidney transplantation: a prospective, randomized comparison of sirolimus and tacrolimus. Transplant. 2004;77(10):1555–61.
75. Klawitter J, Nashan B, Christians U. Everolimus and sirolimus in transplantation-related but different. Expert Opin Drug Saf. 2015;14(7):1055–70.
76. Raju DL, Bitzan M. Sirolimus-associated chronic pyogenic periungual infection. Kidney Int. 2007;71(6):476.
77. Mahé E, Morelon E, Lechaton S, Kreis H, De Prost Y, Bodemer C. Sirolimus-induced onychopathy in renal transplant recipients. Ann Dermatol Venereol. 2006;133(6–7):531–5.
78. Bottomley WW, Ford G, Cunliffe WJ, Cotterill JA. Aggressive squamous cell carcinomas developing in patients receiving long-term azathioprine. Br J Dermatol. 1995;133(3):460–2.
79. Zimmerman SW, Esch J. Skin lesions treated with azathioprine and prednisone: comparison of nontransplant patients and renal transplant recipients. Arch Intern Med. 1978;138(6):912–14.
80. Sonthalia S, Daulatabad D. Azathioprine-associated anagen effluvium. Indian J Dermatol Venereol Leprol. 2016;82(3):322–4.
81. Patel AA, Swerlick RA, McCall CO. Azathioprine in dermatology: the past, the present, and the future. J Am Acad Dermatol. 2006;55(3):369–89.
82. Knowles SR, Gupta AK, Shear NH, Sauder D. Azathioprine hypersensitivity-like reactions: a case report and a review of the literature. Clin Exp Dermatol. 1995;20(4):353–6.
83. Bidinger JJ, Sky K, Battafarano DF, Henning JS. The cutaneous and systemic manifestations of azathioprine hypersensitivity syndrome. J Am Acad Dermatol. 2011;65(1):184–91.
84. Philipone E, Rockafellow A, Sternberg R, Yoon A, Koslovsky D. Oral ulcerations as a sequela of tacrolimus and mycophenolate mofetil therapy. Oral Surg Oral Med Oral Pathol Oral Radiol. 2014;118(6):e175–8.
85. Garrigue V, Canet S, Dereure O et al. Oral ulcerations in a renal transplant recipient: a mycophenolate mofetil-induced complication? Transplant. 2001;72(5):968–9.
86. Letsinger JA, McCarty MA, Jorizzo JL. Complex aphthosis: a large case series with evaluation algorithm and therapeutic ladder from topicals to thalidomide. J Am Acad Dermatol. 2005;52(3 Pt 1):500–8.
87. Larsen CP, Pearson TC, Adams AB et al. Rational development of LEA29Y (belatacept), a high-affinity variant of CTLA4-Ig with potent immunosuppressive properties. Am J Transplant. 2005;5(3):443–53.
88. Grinyo J, Charpentier B, Pestana JM et al. An integrated safety profile analysis of belatacept in kidney transplant recipients. Transplant. 2010;90(12):1521–7.

Nail Disease and Nail Surgery in Solid Organ Transplant Recipients

16

Aleksandar L. Krunic
and Severin Laeuchli

INTRODUCTION

Nail disorders in the general population usually derive from different causes including but not limited to infections, inflammatory or metabolic conditions, malignancies, and pigment disturbances. In solid organ transplant recipients (SOTRs), nail changes can be seen in approximately 60% of individuals.[1] They are the result of a complex interplay of T-cell immune dysregulation, pretransplant condition (kidney, liver, or heart/lung failure), pretransplant comorbidities (actinic damage, human papilloma virus infection, fungal nail colonization, presence of precancerous lesions), the length of time posttransplantation as well as the type of immunosuppressive medications used to prevent the transplant rejection.

The proximal nail matrix presents an immunologically privileged area of the nail apparatus,[2] whereas the majority of T cells and Langerhans cells actually reside in the proximal and lateral nail fold and hyponychium. The cuticle at the proximal nail fold (PNF) and onychodermal band at the hyponychium present important "sealant" by prohibiting the penetration of bacteria, fungi, and other infectious agents in the nail apparatus and nail matrix proper. Hence, any damage to these structures can lead to disruption of this barrier and the development of infection.[3] Careful pretransplant history as well as consultations in the pretransplant and posttransplant periods should emphasize proper care of the fingernails and toenails, advise about pedicure/manicure as well as evaluate the risks of potential harmful exposures (environmental, professional) that could contribute to nail disease.[4]

We can roughly divide nail disease in SOTRs into the following four groups: 1) nail alterations (pigment changes and onychodystrophies), 2) nail apparatus infections, 3) nail neoplasia, and 4) immunosuppressive therapy-induced onychopathies. Although some nail changes could be only of cosmetic importance, others may serve as a clue for the diagnosis of the underlying systemic disease, metabolic effects, or drug toxicity or may present as a portal of entry/reentry of infectious agents into the organism, complicating already compromised immune surveillance in the affected individuals.

Therefore, careful examination of the nail apparatus and periungual area of the fingers and toes should be a mandatory part of dermatological consultation in the pretransplant period, as well as after the transplantation in order to recognize early and treat efficiently all nail conditions that can compromise, affect, or complicate the posttransplant course in SOTRs. Finally, the surgical approach should also be modified

DOI: 10.1201/9781003001461-16

in order to biopsy early, diagnose quickly, and treat all nail lesions in their early stage with proper antibiotic prophylaxis to avoid postoperative infections of the nail apparatus and subjacent bone infection in SORTs who have compromised cellular immunity and hitherto reduced protection from infective agents.

NAIL PLATE ALTERATIONS

Nail plate alterations (discolorations and onychodystrophies) affect approximately 40% of SORTs[1,5,6] (Table 16.1). The most common ones are: 1) absence of lunula, 2) splinter hemorrhage, 3) leukonychia (LKN), and 4) longitudinal ridging. Other nail plate abnormalities like koilonychia, clubbing, onycholysis, melanonychia, transverse ridging or Beau lines are not frequently reported and affect <5% of SOTRs. All nail plate abnormalities are multiple (polydactylous) and more often affect fingernails than toenails in the cohort of SOTRs.

Loss of Lunula

The absence of lunula is the most commonly observed nail abnormality, present in approximately 17.1%–29.8% of SOTRs.[1,5] The white color of the lunula results from two main anatomic factors: the keratogenous zone of the distal matrix with nuclear fragments that cause light diffraction and nail matrix capillaries that are less visible than nail bed capillaries because of the relative thickness of the nail matrix epithelium.[6] According to Abdelazziz et al.,[5] it is also found in 26.5% of healthy individuals. The loss of opacity and absence of lunula is probably caused by thinning of the nail matrix epithelium as well as slower keratinization of the nail matrix caused by anemia and malnutrition, especially in the pretransplant period. Saray et al.[4] reported a higher incidence of absent lunula in their cohort of hemodialysis patients (31.9%) in comparison with that in their renal transplant group, which actually improved in the posttransplant period affecting up to 17.1% individuals. Absent lunula has been reported in many other diseases[5] such as atherosclerosis, chronic obstructive pulmonary disease, and rheumatoid arthritis, in which the pallor of the nail could be produced by the vascular compromise present in these conditions. In addition, some individuals may have long PNFs and hence less visible lunula combined with the causes mentioned previously.[5]

Splinter Hemorrhage

Splinter hemorrhage (SH) (Figure 16.1) appears as filiform longitudinal lines of dark reddish color in the distal nail plate because of extravasation of blood from the parallel longitudinal vessels of the nail bed. The pathogenesis of SH is unclear but microtrauma, fragility of the blood vessels, and platelet disfunction

TABLE 16.1 Most Common Nail Plate Alterations in Solid Organ Transplant Recipients

TYPE	*PREVALENCE*
Absence of lunula	17.1%–29.8%
Splinter hemorrhage	11.0%–58.9%
Leukonychia	8.2%–27.4%
Longitudinal ridging	6.0%–11%
Other (koilonychia, clubbing, onycholysis, melanonychia, transverse ridging [Beau lines])	<5%

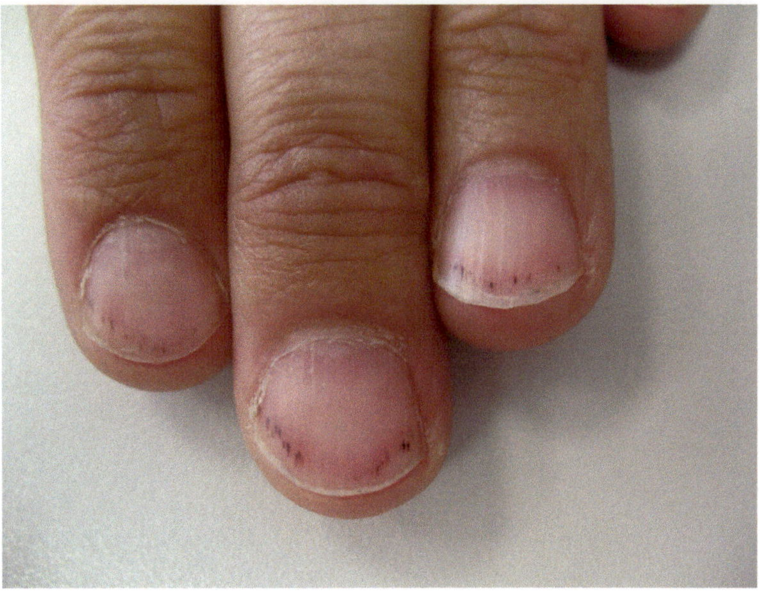

FIGURE 16.1. Splinter hemorrhage. (Prof. Dr. Eckart Haneke, Freiburg, Germany.)

may contribute to their development. They are described in 11%–58.9% of patients with renal failure (RF)[4,6] but also in other conditions like antiphospholipid antibody syndrome, subacute bacterial endocarditis, liver cirrhosis, rheumatoid arthritis, ischemic heart disease, diabetes mellitus, and hyperthyroidism.[6] The visibility of SH tends to improve after transplantation with the observed decreased incidence of 3.4% in SOTRs, probably because of the improvement of the local circulation by the presence of the functional newly transplanted organ (kidney, heart, or liver).[4,5]

Leukonychia

Different forms of LKN have been reported in approximately a quarter of SOTRs (8.2%–27.4%).[4,5] LKN is a white discoloration of the nail and may be caused by nail plate abnormalities (true LKN and pseudoLKN) or by nail bed abnormalities (apparent LKN).[7]

True LKN has been classified into four main types depending on the morphology of the white discoloration[8]: LKN totalis, LKN partialis, LKN striata, and LKN punctata and is produced by parakeratosis of the onychocytes, trauma, or fungal invasion of the nail plate (pseudoLKN), resulting in loss of nail plate transparency. It is persistent, i.e., does not disappear with vertical pressure applied to the nail plate, and it moves distally with the growth of the nail plate. True LKN of noninfectious origin is less common in SOTRs and is usually partial or punctate.[4,5] The cause of abnormal keratinization is not clear, but the direct effect of immunosuppressive medications and/or the immunosuppressive state itself can contribute to its development as described by Cribier et al.[9]

Apparent LKN (Figure 16.2), which is more common in SOTRs, actually derives from vascular changes in the nail bed most likely caused by edema with subsequent pressure on the dermal vasculature and hence, disappearance of pink color.[7,8] The most common form is Muehrcke's nails (Figure 16.3a), which present as paired transverse white lines on the nail plate. A state of hypoalbuminemia and anemia precedes the development of Muehrcke's nails and is often described in renal and cardiac transplant patients. They are seen more often when cyclosporine is part of the immunosuppressive regimen and are less likely when patients are not receiving corticosteroid medications.[5] Multiple transversal white and

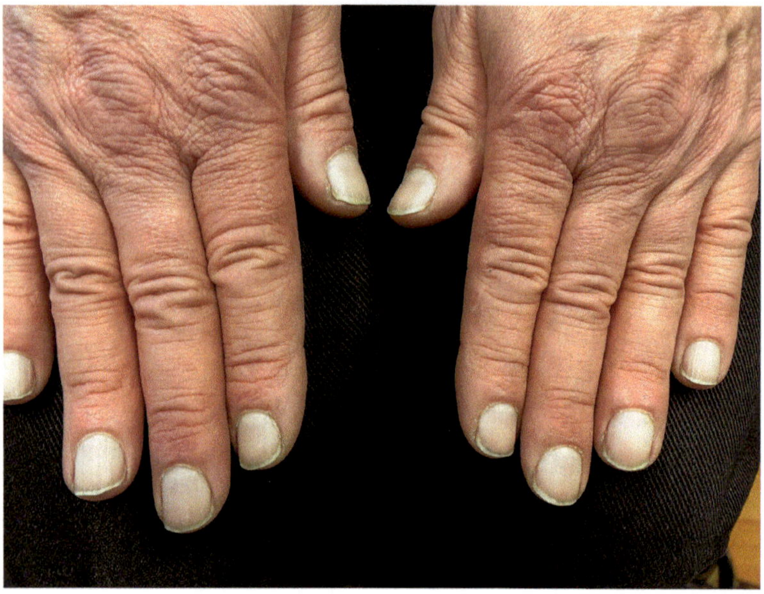

FIGURE 16.2 Total leukonychia.

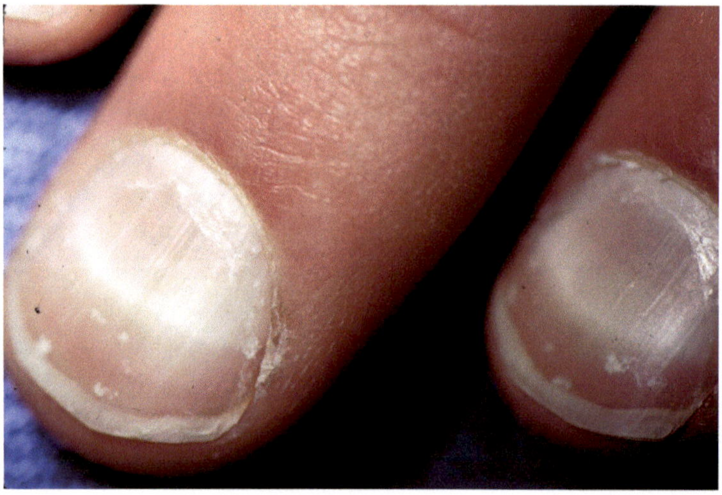

FIGURE 16.3A Muehrcke lines. (Phoebe Ritch MD, Oregon Health Sciences University, Portland, OR, USA.)

pink alternating streaks similar to Muehrcke's lines are reported as "nail flag" sign (Figure 16.3b) and are seen in cardiac transplants.[10] Half-and-half nails in which the proximal part is white and the distal is pink are a hallmark of RF (incidence 30%) and also are seen in SOTRs, but tend to improve and disappear after the transplantation.[5,8] Terry's nails, with the proximal two-thirds white and the distal third of the nail plate pink, are seen often in cirrhosis of the liver and also tend to improve after successful transplantation and restoration of the liver function.[11]

All forms of LKN described could also be seen in other conditions as well as healthy individuals, although less often. Different forms of LKN in SORTs are presented in Table 16.2.

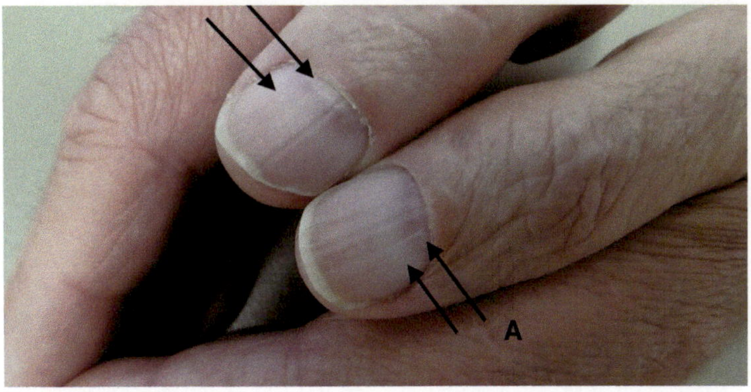

FIGURE 16.3B Nail flag sign. Note: A(arrow) points to lunula. The other arrow points to flag sign. (From reference 10. Published with permission from Philip M. Cohen MD, Sacramento, CA, USA.)

Longitudinal Ridging

Longitudinal ridging (Figure 16.4) is reported in 6%–11% of SOTRs.[4,5] They present as longitudinal indentations or projections in the relief of the nail plate. They are usually the result of trauma, nail plate fragility caused by preexisting peripheral vascular disease, or other conditions like lichen planus, Darier's disease, or rheumatoid arthritis, or can also be idiopathic. Some authors report a much higher prevalence of longitudinal ridging in RF patients (40%) with the tendency to improve after transplantation.[4] The transplant immunosuppressive regimen medications can also suppress and improve nail abnormalities like longitudinal ridging and LKN associated with psoriasis because of the synergistic suppressive effect on immune dysregulation present in this condition.[5]

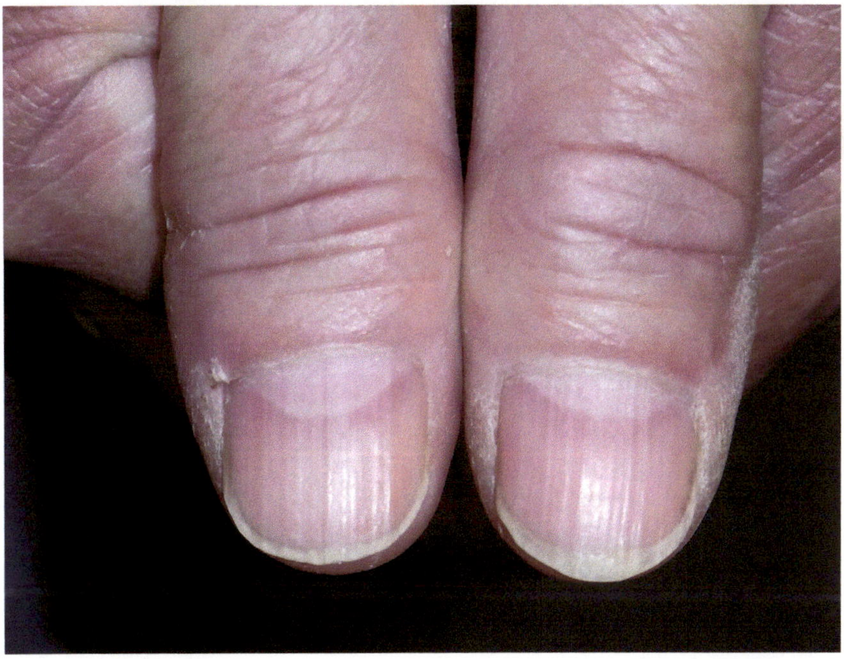

FIGURE 16.4 Longitudinal ridging of the nail. (Prof. Dr. Eckart Haneke, Freiburg, Germany.)

TABLE 16.2 Classification of Leukonychia in Solid Organ Transplant Recipients

TYPE OF LEUKONYCHIA	*CLINICAL PRESENTATION*	*PROPOSED ETIOLOGY IN SOTRS*	*OTHER ASSOCIATED CONDITIONS*
True leukonychia • (Abnormal keratinization of the nail plate) • Persists on vertical pressure • Moves distally with the growth of the nail plate	Partial, punctate, total, and striate (less common)	Immunocompromised state Immunosuppressive regimen Trauma Idiopathic Proximal subungual onychomycosis	Heavy metal poisoning (Mee's lines); acute illness (psoriasis, cardiac insufficiency, myocardial infarction, acute and chronic renal failure, pleural empyema, systemic infections, sickle cell anemia, systemic lupus erythematous, and pellagra)
Apparent leukonychia • Edema of the subepidermal perivascular space in the nail bed • Disappears on vertical pressure • Does not move with the nail plate, but may become transient as soon as condition improves	Meuhrcke's nails (increased incidence); renal and cardiac transplants	Immunocompromised state Immunosuppressive regimen (cyclosporine ↑; systemic steroids ↓) Anemia, hypoalbuminemia	Anemia, hypoalbuminema (<2.2 g/100 mL)
	Half-and-half nails (decreased after successful renal transplantation)		Chronic renal failure, Behcet's disease, Kawasaki disease, liver disease, Crohn's disease, zinc deficiency, and pellagra
	Terry's nails (decreased after successful liver transplantation)		Liver disease, adult-onset diabetes, and congestive heart failure
	"Nail flag" sign		Leprosy, diabetes, vitiligo
Pseudoleukonychia • Invasion of the dorsal nail plate with fungal hyphae • Keratin degranulation	Whitish macules in the nail plate	n/a	• White superficial onychomycosis • Manicure/pedicure Nail plate keratin damage due to nail polish

Abbreviation: SOTRs, solid organ transplant recipients.

NAIL APPARATUS INFECTIONS IN SOLID ORGAN TRANSPLANT RECIPIENTS

Infections of the nail apparatus can be caused by bacteria, fungi, viruses, and parasites. Human papillomavirus (HPV) infections of the periungual and subungual area and onychomycoses predominate as the most common infections in SORTs.[4,5] Bacterial infections of the nail and perionychium are less common but need to be recognized, because they become the source for infection of the soft tissues (cellulitis, necrotizing fasciitis), bones (osteomyelitis), and tendons (tenosynovitis).[13] Often there can be the presence of several infectious agents, i.e., combined bacterial and fungal nail infection, or some typical wart-like lesions could represent cutaneous foci of deep fungal infections like histoplasmosis.[14] The presence of concomitant bacterial infection of the nail plate could potentially interfere with the isolation of dermatophytes or other fungi from the nail plate because of the suppressive effect of bacteria on fungal growth (e.g., *Pseudomonas aeruginosa* and *Trichophyton rubrum* nail infection).[13] Finally, the use of acitretin or sirolimus can compromise wound healing and contribute to the development of painful paronychia and periungual granulations that can further complicate the diagnostic process and identification of the causative agent.[14–17] If we add herpetic whitlow and *Candida* spp. as other common causes of acute and chronic paronychia, respectively, we can easily understand why one should always bear in mind multifactorial origin and complex etiology of ungual/periungual infections in the scope of chronic and prolonged immunosuppression. Apart from isolation of infectious agent (direct fungal examination of nail clippings [KOH], bacterial culture, fungal culture, or molecular methods [PCR]), nail apparatus biopsy should be strongly considered in any presumably infectious ungual/periungual lesions not responding to therapy in order to obtain timely diagnosis, avoid confusion, and start appropriate treatment.[13]

Bacterial Infections of the Nail Unit

The incidence of bacterial skin infections in SOTRs is estimated to be from 5.7% to 18%.[12,18,19] Prior to transplantation, *Staphylococcus aureus* colonization of the anterior nares is estimated to be 67%.[20] In the majority of these cases, *S. aureus* is methicillin-resistant (MRSA) and was not properly eradicated in the pretransplantation period. Bacterial infection with *S. aureas*, which can spread under the nail, develops usually from acute or chronic paronychia. Apart from *S. aureus*, *Streptococcus pyogenes*, coagulase-negative staphylococci and *Peptostreptococcus* (oral mucosa anaerobes) are other isolated causative agents.[18,19] Acute paronychia[13] (Figure 16.5a and b) is an inflammation of a nail fold with or without abscess formation, usually affects single digits, and presents with erythema, edema, and tenderness of the lateral or PNF, with pallor, fluctuance, and purulent discharge. Chronic paronychia is usually polydactylous, lasts a minimum of 6 weeks, and is often related to chemical irritants. In SOTRs, the former can be coinfected with herpes simplex virus (HSV), and the latter with *Candida* spp.[13,19] Although immunosuppression and diabetes are very well-known general risk factors for its development, local conditions like repetitive minor trauma, nail psoriasis, artificial nails, manicure, nail biting (onychotillomania), thumb-sucking, and manipulation of a hangnail are additional causes of entry for the infection.[13] Felon is a subcutaneous infection of the distal digital pulp that presents with throbbing pain, tense swelling, and redness of the finger pad that does not spread proximally to the distal interphalangeal joint, because the process is confined with the septal compartments of the distal digit.[13] Common etiologic factors are puncture wounds at the distal digit (splinters, finger stick) or spread of untreated paronychia. Treatment of paronychia[13,21] includes elevation, splint of the affected finger/toe, warm soaks, topical antibiotics (gentamicin, mupirocin, topical nadifloxacin), and incision and drainage when obvious fluid collection is present.[13] Because SOTRs are immunocompromised, systemic therapy like cephalexin, trimethoprim/sulfamethoxazole, amoxicillin/clavulanate or clindamycin[13] is recommended to avoid regional (lymphangitis) or systemic dissemination (sepsis, bacterial endocarditis). Green nail syndrome or chloronychia[14] (Figure 16.6) is a classic triad of

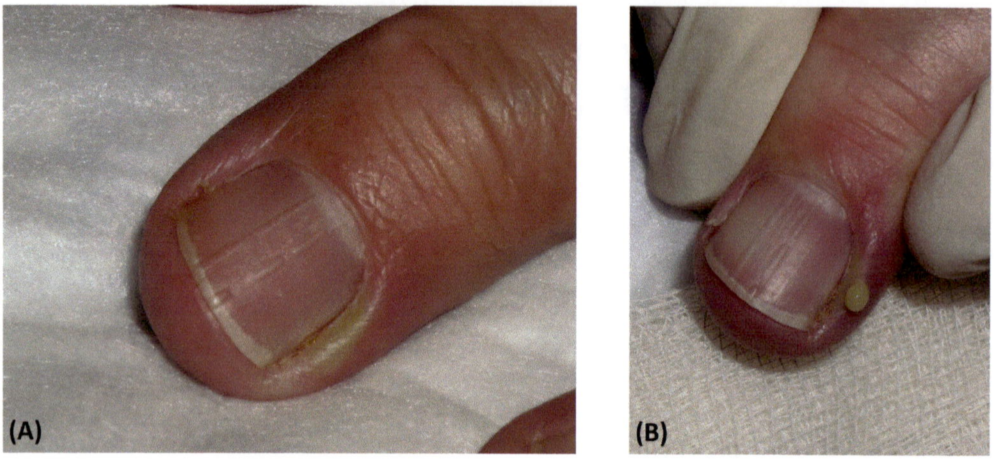

FIGURE 16.5 Acute paronychia with (**a**) edema of lateral nail fold and (**b**) purulent discharge after drainage. (Nathaniel Jelinek MD, Warwick, RI, USA.)

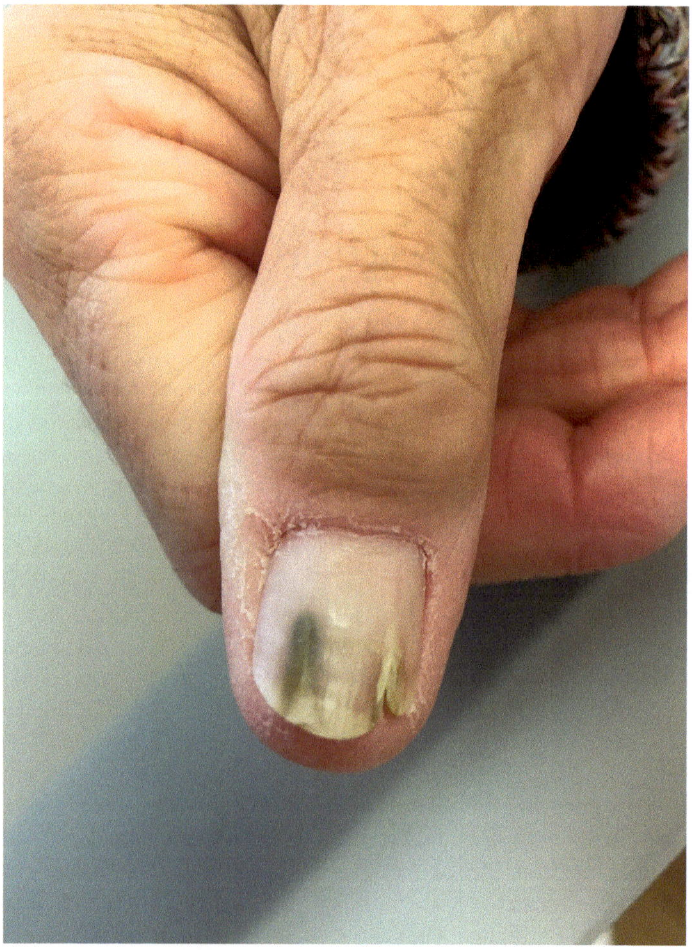

FIGURE 16.6 Green nail syndrome caused by *Pseudomonas aeruginosa* combined with onychomycosis. (Prof. Dr. Eckart Haneke, Freiburg, Germany.)

proximal paronychia, dorsolateral onycholysis, and green discoloration of the nail plate occurring because of infection by *Pseudomonas aeruginosa*. The green color occurs as a result of the diffusion of blackish-green pyocyanin and yellowish-green pyoverdine into the nail tissue and bacterial invasion of the nail plate.[14] In addition to the risk factors for paronychia mentioned previously, working in damp environments and prolonged exposure to water, soap, and detergents are contributing factors for green nail syndrome. Treatment of green nail syndrome is focused on the use of antibiotics with antipseudomonal activity, like topical antiseptics (chlorhexidine, 1% acetic acid, 0.1% octenidine dihydrochloride solution), topical antibiotics (gentamicin, ophthalmic ciprofloxacin, or ophthalmic tobramycin eyedrops), as well as systemic fluroquinolones (ciprofloxacin, levofloxacin), carbapenems, or antipseudomonal penicillins (piperacillin, ticarcillin).[14,22] The treatment should last a minimum of 2–3 weeks in order to avoid dissemination and the development of necrotizing fasciitis or ecthyma gangrenosum (*Pseudomonas* sepsis) in immunocompromised individuals.[14,22] The use of artificial nails should be discouraged in SOTRs because there is heavy colonization by both bacteria (mainly gram-negative) and fungi (*Candida* spp.), which can promote infection and complicate the attempts to eradicate pathogenic bacteria.[13,14,22] Nail parlors have recently been reported to harbor in the footbaths and sink drains different mycobacteria,[19,23] like *Mycobacterium cheloneae/abscessus*, *M. fortuitum* and *M. cosmeticum*,[24] which could cause a felon-like condition or furuncles on the toes. The skin lesions usually develop 4 weeks after the exposure. These infections carry the risk of dissemination and hematogenous spread in immunocompromised individuals. Treatment requires a combination of agents like ciprofloxacin and clarithromycin.[19] More complicated infection may require the use of other macrolides, amikacin, clofazimine, or imipenem.[23,24] Last but not least, nail apparatus could be a portal of entry for *Bartonella henseale*,[25] which is usually associated with cat bite and can present as paronychia with throbbing pain. Lesions can be vascular and bleed profusely. Typical clumped and solitary rods in the intercellular space could be detected by using an electron microscope or Whartin–Starry stain. The condition can mimic periungual Kaposi sarcoma (KS) or pyogenic granuloma, hence potential delay in the diagnosis and treatment. Untreated, it can lead to fever, lymphadenopathy, hemophagocytic syndrome, and renal graft rejection.[25] The recommended treatment is ciprofloxacin or doxycycline for 3 months.[14,25]

Fungal Infections of the Nail Apparatus in SOTRs

Fungal infections are the most common infections among SOTRs and are detected in about 34%–60% of individuals.[12,18,26] The prevalence of onychomycosis (OM) in SOTRs varies in different reports from 7.6%–29%.[4,5,18]

OM is an infection of the nails caused by dermatophytes (tinea ungium), non-dermatophyte filamentous fungi (molds), or yeast (*Candida* spp.). The majority of OMs appear in the first 3–6 months post-transplantation in more than half of SOTRs, whereas the remaining patients become affected after 1 year after the procedure.[26,27]

Also, there is no correlation between the type of immunosuppressive drugs used, age, or sex of the affected individuals. Many reports reveal that OMs in SORTs were not atypical or more severe or widespread compared with OMs in controls.[26] However, they may be persistent and treatment resistant.

The diagnosis is obtained based on direct analysis of nail clippings (KOH examination), fungal culture, histology, or molecular methods (PCR).[28] The most common dermatophytes isolated were *Trichophyton rubrum*, *T. interdigitale* (formerly *T. mentagrophytes* var. *interdigitale*), and *Epidermophyton floccosum* and were responsible for approximately 65% of isolates in SOTRs, which is about the same frequency as in otherwise healthy individuals.[5,26] The yeasts often affect not just the nail plate but also the paronychium and, apart from *Candida albicans*, *C. parapsilosis* and *C. guilliermondii* are also isolated.[28] Non-dermatophyte molds were the most commonly isolated species affecting the toenails and fingernails in SOTRs and did not differ significantly from those in healthy controls, i.e., included *Aspergillus fumigatus*, *A. flavus* and *A. niger*, *Scopulariopsis brevicaulis*, and *Fusarium* spp. Non-dermatophyte molds and yeast each contributed to 17.4% of isolates from OM in SOTRs. Among all superficial fungal infections reported in SORTs, approximately

30% were OM of the toenails and 5%–10% were OM of the fingernails.[26,28] The most common sources of infections were swimming pools, bathhouses, saunas, and sport facilities. Predisposing factors apart from immunosuppression comprised prior nail trauma, advanced age, vascular disease and poor limb circulation, lymphedema, diabetes, preexisting tinea pedis (20% in SOTRs), hyperhidrosis, and preexisting nail psoriasis.[26,28] In addition, occupational exposure is also worth considering, especially when dealing with rare fungal pathogens, particularly non-dermatophyte molds as a cause of OM both of the toenails and fingernails.[27] Environmental contact with soil, vegetation/plant material, contaminated and polluted water, sewage, wood, certain foods, and decaying fruit or residential exposure to the sites with mold habitation like attics, garages, crawlspaces, etc. could be a potential way of acquiring spores, conidia, or actual hyphal elements through minor trauma on the skin surrounding the nail apparatus or through the damaged nail plate itself, e.g., with preexisting nail dystrophy or psoriatic nail disease.[27] It should not be forgotten that these fungal infections have the potential to disseminate and can be fatal for immunosuppressed patients like SOTRs.[27] Therefore, the reports of rare nail involvement in SOTRs with pathogens like *Alternaria* spp., *Trichosporon mucoides*, or *Scytalidium dimidatum* could derive from such an exposure.[29–31]

Depending on the clinical presentation,[32] OM is classified as distal/lateral subungual onychomycosis (DLSMO); superficial (white or black) onychomycosis (SO); proximal subungual onychomycosis (PSO), total dystrophic onychomycosis (TDO), endonyx OM, mixed pattern OM and secondary OM (Figure 16.7a–d). Morphological characteristics of each clinical presentation as well as the most commonly

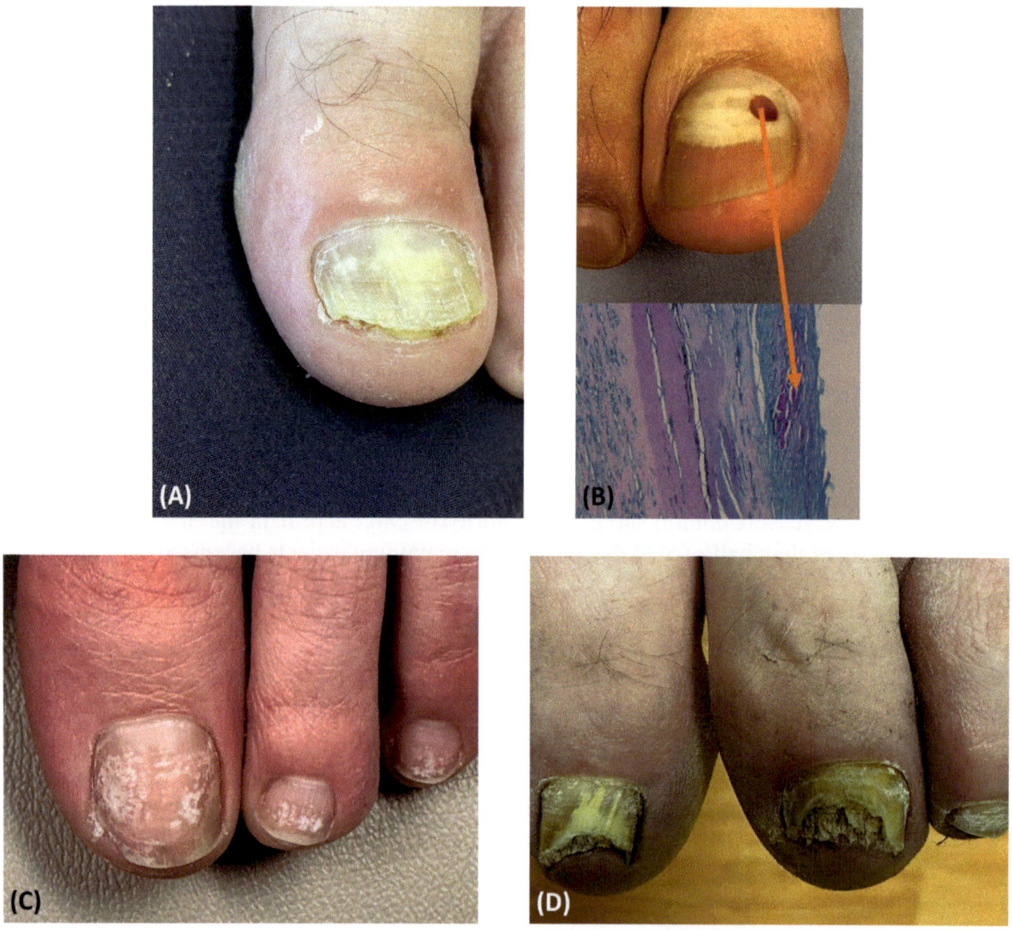

FIGURE 16.7 (**a**) Distal lateral onychomycosis; (**b**) proximal subungual onychomycosis with PAS stain showing purple hyphae in the nail plate; (**c**) white superficial onychomycosis; and (**d**) total dystrophic onychomycosis.

associated pathogens are presented in Table 16.3. PSO has been more often described in immunosuppressed patients, particularly those with HIV infection. However, it is not as frequently described in SOTRs compared with immunocompetent individuals.[33,34] In their case study, Abdelazziz et al.[5] found that the majority of OM presented as DLSO, i.e., in 85% of patients, with both TDO and PSO affecting two individuals each from their cohort. In PSO, the invasion of the nail plate occurs proximally from the cuticle or PNF. The involvement of the nail folds usually indicates the presence of non-dermatophyte mold (*Fusarium* spp., *Scytalidium* spp., *Aspergillus* spp.)[31,32] (Figure 16.8a and b) or *Candida* infection[28] (Figure 16.9) as a cause of OM. *Aspergillus* spp. involvement of the surrounding periungual skin was not common, but subungual hyperkeratosis was almost always present, sometimes forming subungual dermatophytoma ("fungal ball").[35] In conclusion, SOTRs have a similar distribution of OM morphological patterns as that in healthy controls, i.e., DLSO, SO (white or black), or TDO being the most common patterns observed. Endonyx OM[32] is characterized by lamellar splitting of the nail and white discoloration of the nail with the absence of nail bed invasion and onycholysis. This type has not been reported in SOTRs and is most commonly caused by *T. soudanense* and *T. violaceum*. Having in mind the fact that Mulvaney et al.[36] recently reported endonyx OM caused by *T. rubrum* (the most common pathogen in OM), we can speculate that more cases may be reported in the future, not just in immunocompetent individuals but also in SOTRs. In addition, endonyx OM has just recently been described and may not yet be well represented in the cohorts of nail studies in SOTRs. Another specific situation seen in SOTRs is the bacterial colonization and coinfection of the nail plates affected with OM, particularly *P. aeruginosa*

TABLE 16.3 Classification of Onychomycoses with the Most Common Isolates in SOTRs

TYPE	*CLINICAL CHARACTERISTICS*	*ASSOCIATED ORGANISMS*
Distal lateral subungual onychomycosis [DLSO]—Invasion from distal and lateral undersurface of the nail	White/yellow discoloration of the nail plate, onycholysis, hyperkeratosis, longitudinal streaking of mid/lateral nail plate	*T. rubrum*, *T. interdigitale*, *E. floccosum*, *C. albicans** (with paronychia); *Scytalidium* spp. (with paronychia). *Fusarium* spp.*.
Superficial (white or black) onychomycosis [SO]—Invasion of the superficial to deep aspects of the nail plate	White or black (*T. rubrum*, *Scytalidium*) patches or transverse dyschromia of the nail plate	*T. interdigitale*, *T rubrum*, *Fusarium* spp.*, *Scytalidium* spp.
Proximal subungual onychomycosis [PSO]—Invasion of the proximal nail plate under the proximal nail fold or from the paronychium	Patchy, striate transverse or longitudinal discoloration of the proximal nail plate extending distally	*T. rubrum*, *Fusarium* spp.*, *Candida* spp.*, *Aspergillus* spp.
Total dystrophic onychomycosis [TDO]—End stage nail plate invasion from DLSO and PSO	Hyperkeratotic, crumbled nail plate, with subungual debris, thick nail bed, ridged and hyperkeratotic	Dermatophytes, *Candida* spp.*, *Scytalidium* spp.
Endonyx OM [EO]—Total nail plate invasion without nail bed/paronychium involvement	Lamellar splitting of the nail, discoloration of the nail plate without nail bed invasion and without sunbungual hyperkeratosis	*T. soudanense*, *T. violaceum*, *T. rubrum*
Mixed pattern onychomycosis [MPO]	DLSO+PSO, DLSO+ SO SO+DLSO; SO+PSO	*T. rubrum* *T. rubrum* + *Fusarium* spp.*
Secondary OM	Secondary involvement of the nail plate affected by psoriasis or other nail dystrophy/disease	

Abbreviation: SOTRs, solid organ transplant recipients.

**Candida spp.* and *Fusarium spp.* may affect paronychium only without onychomycosis.

Source: modified from Hay RJ et al, 2011 J Am Acad Dermatol 2011; 65:1219–1227.

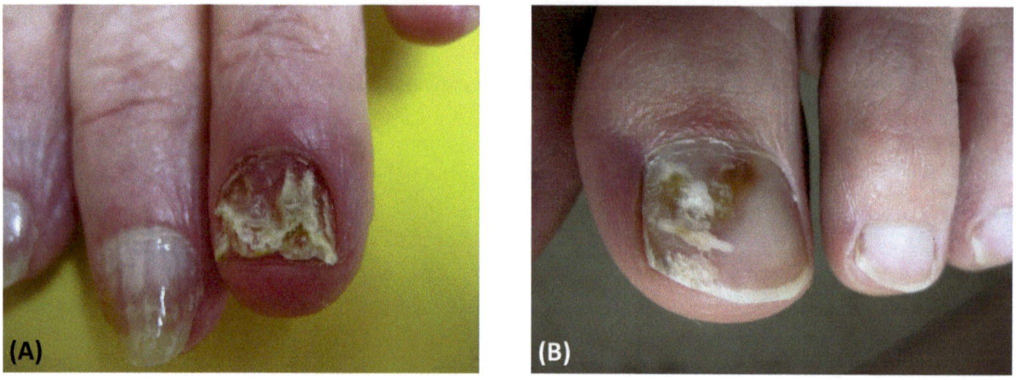

FIGURE 16.8 Non-dermatophyte mold onychomycosis cause by *Fusarium* spp. (**a**) and *Aspergillus* spp. (**b**). Note the simultaneous involvement of the nail plate and adjacent nail fold. (Phoebe Ritch, MD, Oregon Health Sciences University, Portland, OR, USA.)

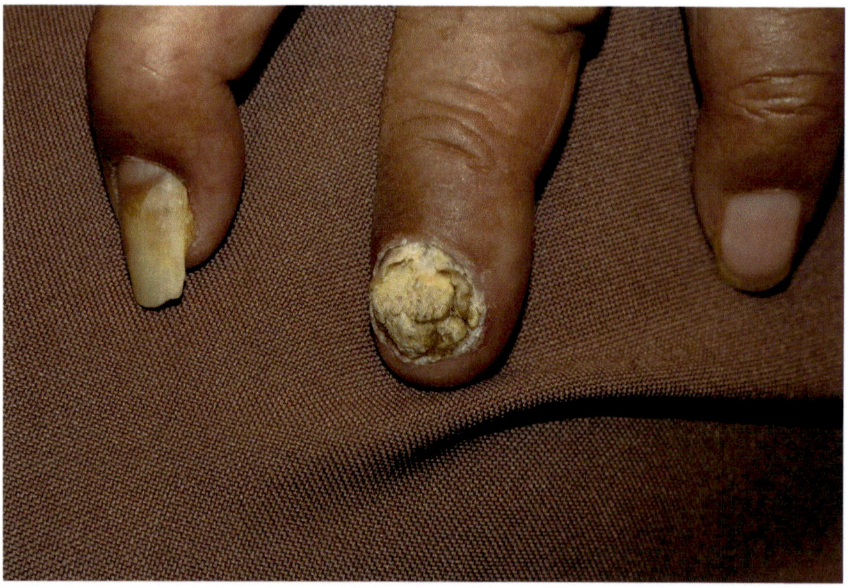

FIGURE 16.9 Candidal onychomycosis with the involvement of the paronychium and complete dystrophy of the nail plate. Note onycholysis of the adjacent fingernail, which is the more typical type of *Candida* involvement of the nail apparatus. (David Adam, MD, University of Toronto, Toronto, ON, Canada.)

with "green nail syndrome" as described previously.[14] One should bear in mind that the presence of *P. aeruginosa* can make isolation of the responsible fungal pathogen in the culture impossible because of the fungistatic/fungicidal properties of bacterial organisms. All common fungal isolates in OM (*T. rubrum*, *T. mentagrophytes*, *A. fumigatus*, *F. solani*, *C. albicans*) were shown to have their growth suppressed by *P. aeurigonsa*.[14,37] One of the helpful clinical hints in these coinfected cases is the presence of subungual hyperkeratosis with greenish discoloration and onycholysis of the nail plate.[37] All cases with coinfection require concomitant treatment of both bacterial infection (see prior) and OM (see following).

OMs in SOTRs are treated with topical antifungal nail solutions or gels, systemic oral antifungals combined with topical agents, or nail avulsion in resistant cases (chemical or surgical). The decision to consider systemic treatment is often based on the presence of the involvement of the nail matrix, often recognizable from the so-called yellow streaks.[28,32] In addition, the decision to consider oral antifungals could also be made based on the number of affected fingernails or toenails, extent of the nail involvement, multiple comorbidities, drug interactions with the current antirejection regimen in SOTRs, or the identified pathogen (non-dermatophytic molds or *Candida*).[28] The topical therapy with ciclopirox olamine, amorolfine, or the recently added tavaborole and efinaconazole is often combined with systemic terbinafine or azoles (itraconazole or fluconazole). Fluconazole is preferred for *Candida* OM, and itraconazole or terbinafine for tinea unguium or non-dermatophyte mold OM.[28,32] All systemic (oral) antifungals can be used for 3 months (fingernails OM) or up to 6 months (toenails OM), as intermittent or continuous therapy[32] (Table 16.4).

One of the emerging problems in the treatment of OM is the development of resistance to antifungal therapy.[38] The origin of this problem in SOTRs is multifactorial, i.e., caused by host resistance factors, fungal factors, and drug interactions. Fungal resistance could be further classified into microbiological (assessed by susceptibility testing) or clinical, which is characterized by the lack of response of OM to prescribed treatment. Fortunately, for OM caused by dermatophytes, the incidence of resistance to terbinafine is <1% and is usually caused by squalene oxidase mutation in *Trichophyton* spp.[39] Apart from depressed cellular immunity in SOTRs, other factors contributing to treatment failure of OM are the genetic alteration of the fungal organisms acquired during the treatment (aka, secondary or acquired microbiological resistance) or low treatment compliance.[38] The recommended approach to fight the increasing problem of fungal resistance in OM comprises the use of the antifungal drug in the proper

TABLE 16.4 Common Treatment Strategies for Onychomycosis in SOTRs

ANTIFUNGAL TREATMENT	*INDICATION*	*AGENT*	*DOSING SCHEDULE*	*COMMENT*
Topical	<50% of nail surface affected no more than 3 nails, no matrix involvement	Ciclopirox olamine, amorolfine, tavaborole, efinaconazole	Daily for 48 weeks	Low compliance
Systemic	>50% of nail surface affected, more than 3 nails, matrix involvement, PSO	Terbinafine	Daily: 250 mg for 6–12 weeks; Pulse: 500 mg for 1 week a month, for 3 months	Drug interactions with antirejection immunosuppressive medication; May need to extend treatment for 3 months (fingernails OM) or 6 months (toenail OM); Liver function tests monitoring;
		Itraconazole	Daily: 200 mg for 6–12 weeks; Pulse: 400 mg for 1 week a month, for 3 months	
		Fluconazole (preferred for *Candida* spp. infection)	Weekly: 150–300 mg for 3–12 months	
Nail avulsion—chemical	20%–40% urea with occlusion	Prior to specific nail treatment to soften the hyperkeratotic nail plate		
Nail avulsion—surgical	Nonresponse to oral/topical antifungal treatment	Surgical ablation of the nail plate—with digital block anesthesia		Consider postoperative antibiotics when doing nail surgery

Abbreviations: OM, onychomycosis; PSO, proximal subungual onychomycosis; SOTRs, solid organ transplant recipients.

dose and duration, combination of both topical and systemic antifungal agents, or even sequential use of two systemic agents with synergistic effect like itraconazole and terbinafine as described by Gupta et al.[40] Good nail and foot hygiene (see following) and treatment of the affected members of the household will also contribute to decrease the risk of reinfection.[38]

Combined systemic therapy, on the contrary, can lead to increased toxicity, drug interactions, increased cost, and is also poorly standardized for the testing efficacy of the combination. Itraconazole and voriconazole are potent inhibitors of cytochrome P450 3A4 and are associated with a greater risk of a broader range of potentially severe drug interactions and hepatotoxicity than that of fluconazole.[38] Recently published reports point out the combination of antifungal and non-fungal drugs expressing synergy in the treatment of dermatophytes like the use of terbinafine with statins for the treatment of *T. mentagrophytes* and *M. canis* infections. Furthermore, and especially interesting for the SOTR milieu, is the fact that calcineurin inhibitors (CNIs, cyclosporine and tacrolimus) increase fungal susceptibility to fluconazole because of fungal efflux pump deletion or alteration of their stress response caused by the CNI itself, hence increasing the efficacy of concomitant antifungal azole therapy.[38] Finally, consistent nonresponse or partial response of OM to antifungal treatment renders possible coinfection with molds (*Aspergillus*, *Fusarium*) and may require nail avulsion as a reasonable option as described previously.[39]

The prevention of recurrence of OM is of pivotal importance, because the published rates of recurrence vary from 30% to 50% within 36 months of the end of treatment.[28] All patients need to be educated about proper nail care during dermatology consultations. If someone comes with fingernail disease, toenails should always be examined and vice versa. Toenail infection rarely occurs without concomitant skin fungal infection either on the foot or between the digits, unless the patient visited a nail parlor or has used infected nail clippers. Keeping in mind that half of nail pathology seen in SOTRs is associated with fungal disease, measures to prevent reinfection and recurrence should be applied in every affected individual after clinical and mycological cure is achieved (Table 16.5).[28,41]

TABLE 16.5 Dermatological Consultation and Patient Care Recommendations in SOTRs with Onychomycosis (OM)

• Examine all fingernails and toenails in each patient.
• Half of abnormal nail findings are associated with onychomycosis.
• Evaluate and treat superficial fungal infection of the feet and interdigital area to avoid nail plate reinfection after completed therapy.
• Always investigate the cause of onycholysis, because if left untreated it may produce nail bed hyperkeratosis and permanent detachment of the nail plate from the nail bed.
• Examine and treat nail and foot fungal infections of the other family members of SOTRs.
• Advise patients to put antifungal powder in their shoes.
• Consider prescribing topical antifungals permanently in patient whose OM recurs.
• Recommend to the patients to protect the skin of the feet in gyms and swimming pool areas by wearing flip-flops or sport shoes and not to walk or exercise barefoot.
• Advise patients to use separate nail clipper to cut diseased and healthy toenails. Nail clippers are not be shared with family members and should be cleaned with alcohol before each use.
• Discourage patients from visiting pedicure salons, having footbaths, or wearing other people's shoes.
• Consider mixed bacterial/fungal infections in patients not responding to antibacterial or antifungal treatment and vice versa. Be aware of the suppressive effect of bacteria contaminating/coinfecting fungal cultures on the growth and isolation of fungal organisms.

Abbreviations: OM, onychomycosis ; SOTRs, solid organ transplant recipients.

Source: Modified from Elewski et al. Onychomycosis: an overview. J Drugs Dermatol 2013; 12: s96–s103.

Viral Infections of Nail Apparatus in Solid Organ Transplant Recipients

Viral infections of the nail apparatus are very common[42] with HPV affecting 50% or more SOTRs at 5 years posttransplantation. In the early months after transplantation, acute infections of the nail apparatus are most commonly caused by human herpesviruses (HHVs), herpes simplex viruses (HSV-1 and HSV-2 or HHV-1 and HHV-2) and cytomegalovirus (CMV, or HHV-5).[42]

Cytomegalovirus Infections of the Nail and Periungual Area

CMV is the most common viral infection in SOTRs, affecting 20%–60% of individuals, especially in the first year post transplantation.[19,42] Isolated infection of the periungual area is rare and usually presents as periungual erythema, with vesicles, which subsequently become necrotic and develop into chronic non-healing ulcers.[41] The virus has a propensity to infect the endothelium and hence produce direct cytotoxic effect or induce autoimmunity by molecular mimicry. Cutaneous manifestations occur in approximately 20% of individuals with disseminated infection and present with vasculitis, necrotic papules, vesiculobullous eruption, or purpura. Periungual involvement in these cases occurs as part of the disseminated infection and more commonly affects the toes than the fingers.[42,43] Isolated chronic ulceration with crusting and erythema in the perionychium of the digits (usually thumb or index finger) is a rare presentation,[44] often associated with ulcerations and erosions in the genital, perianal, or buttock areas, and occurs as a result of digito-anogenital contact. In 64.7% of cases, there is coinfection with HSVs, and SOTRs could have more than one lesion (see following).[42–44] Besides clinical findings, the diagnosis can also be obtained by skin biopsy showing cytopathic changes in the dermal vascular endothelium and by PCR studies, which can reveal coinfection with HSV.[44] Contrary to HSV-1 and HSV-2 infections, ungual/periungual CMV lesions have a much higher propensity to disseminate and have to be treated aggressively from the beginning with systemic ganciclovir or valganciclovir. The usual ganciclovir dosage is 5 mg/kg iv twice daily for 14 days, followed by oral ganciclovir 1 g three times a day for up to 6 weeks or until complete healing occurs.[44]

Herpes Simplex Virus Infections of the Nail and Periungual Area

Herpetic whitlow[28] (Figure 16.10) is rare; HSV viral infection of the fingers is caused by direct inoculation or direct spread of the virus to the periungual tissue from mucosal sites. In immunocompetent individuals, it is usually a self-limited disease with a reported incidence of 2.4 cases per 100,000 per year.[28] Mucosal

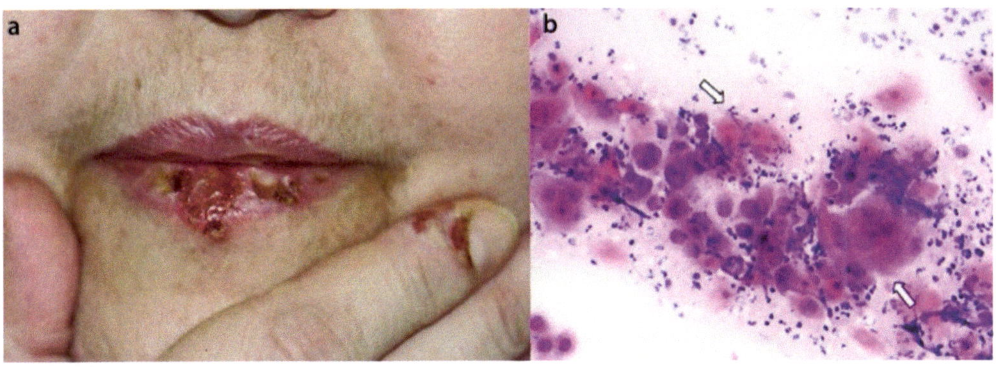

FIGURE 16.10 (**a**) Herpetic whitlow and inoculation from the herpes simplex infection from the lip; (**b**) positive Tzanck smear showing multinucleated cells. (From Solmaz D, Atalay E, Lebe B, et al. Herpetic whitlow during immunosuppressive therapy for Wegener's granulomatosis, Eur J Rheum 2014; 1: 46–7, with permission.)

oral/labial HSV infections were shown to reactivate immediately, i.e., in the first several weeks after transplantation, and Imko-Walczuk et al.[26] reported a 29.4% incidence in their cohort of SOTRs. Apart from digito-oral contact (e.g., nail biting), other potential sources for digital inoculation of HSV could be linear erosions in the intertriginous areas known as "knife-cut sign," which is a distinct presentation of HSV infection in immunocompromised patients[42] and should be sought and treated to control recurrence of herpetic whitlow in SOTRs. In addition, SOTRs were shown to have more common salivary shedding of HSV than that of healthy individuals, emphasizing the oral mucosa as in important source for skin inoculation after digit-oral contact.[45]

Clinical presentation of herpetic whitlow comprises sudden onset of edema, tenderness, and erythema in the periungual region with the subsequent development of classic coalescing vesicles, pustules, and hemorrhagic crusts.[28] The lesions may mimic or be associated with bacterial infection (staphylococcal paronychia) or candidal paronychia (see prior). Some immunosuppressive medications like sirolimus (see following) can also cause paronychia and should also be considered in the differential diagnosis of paronychia. The diagnosis may be confirmed with a Tzanck test, direct immunofluorescence, or PCR.[26] HSV infections in SOTRs last longer, may cover larger areas, and may be resistant to treatment. There is also the potential for dissemination.[42,45] Slow-healing mucocutaneous ulcerations and pseudotumoral vegetations are more often present at mucocutaneous junctions and are rarely seen in the ungual/periungual area.[46] The treatment of HSV infection of the nail apparatus should include topical and systemic regimens, i.e., 1% penciclovir cream every 2 hours with oral acyclovir 400 mg five times a day for 5–10 days or oral valacyclovir 1 g twice or thrice daily for 5–10 days.[45] The lack of response to the applied therapy should prompt one to consider coinfection with CMV or the presence of bacterial or candidal paronychia with appropriate modification of the treatment as discussed previously.[44]

Human Papillomavirus Infections of the Nail Apparatus

The vast majority of HPV infections of the skin occur via direct person-to-person transmission.[46] HPV infects basal epidermal cells by attaching to $\alpha6\beta4$ integrin via L1 capsid protein through skin microtrauma.[47] It replicates in the nucleus where it persists in the form of an episome. HPV evades the host immune response by various mechanisms[47]: 1) prolonged infection cycle; 2) relative lack of inflammatory response during viral replication (limited activation of Langerhans cells in such conditions); 3) downregulation of interferon (IFN) response (HPV E6 and E7 oncoproteins inhibition); 4) absence of cytolysis and subsequent viremia (infection localized to mucocutaneous surfaces away from the lymphatic or vascular system where innate/adoptive response initiates); 5) decreased activation and priming of CD8 cytotoxic HPV-specific T cells by promoting entrapment of peptide-loaded HLA and thus downregulation of HLA class I antigens expression on the cell surface; 6) inhibition of the p53 tumor suppressor gene (HPV E6) responsible for the arrest of the cell cycle for the repair of the DNA damage; and 7) inhibition of the retinoblastoma (Rb) protein tumor suppression gene responsible for inactivation of E2F-DP, which initiates cell replication. The last two mechanisms are crucial for malignant transformation of HPV-infected lesions and occur after long, persistent HPV infections and integration of the genome into the host nuclear DNA where HPV E6 and HPV E7 transcription becomes dysregulated because of the postintegration loss of the HPV E2 gene responsible for the control of HPV E6 and E7 transcription.[47,48] HPV types known to be mostly oncogenic and carcinogenic (HPV 16, 18, 31, 33, 45, 52, and 58) follow this scenario in the development of squamous cell carcinoma (SCC) in HPV-infected skin lesions.[48] HPVs present in common warts in the periungual area belong to types 1, 2, and 4, whereas the ones responsible for anogenital warts are types 6 and 11. These so-called "benign" HPV infections clear spontaneously over time and require successful cell-mediated response against viral proteins. Histologic analysis of regressing warts shows CD-4+ T cell dominated Th1 response.[46]

The prevalence of warts in SOTRs[12,19,42,45,46] increases with the duration of immunosuppressive therapy, with 50%–92% of SOTRs being affected after 4–5 years posttransplantation.[12,46] Apart from persistent HPV infection, immunosuppression caused by antirejection medications as well as ultraviolet (UV) damage is also a contributing factor because most lesions develop on sun-exposed areas (fingers rather than toes) where so-called beta HPVs like HPV-5, HPV-8 and HPV-9 are also involved.[48] Compared with immunocompetent individuals, SOTRs tend to have more persistent warts, multiple lesions, and take longer to clear. Sometimes, the verrucae tend to coalesce covering large confluent areas on the periungual skin[19] (Figure 16.11a and 11b). Progression to the nail bed and subungual area may lead to nail dystrophy and onycholysis. Eventually they may affect dexterity (fingernails), walking (toes/soles), become painful, and/or cause additional psychological stress because of the presence of visible, socially unacceptable lesions.[19,42] HPV-16 is the most common oncogenic type seen in periungual/digital warts associated with malignant transformation into Bowen's disease and subungual SCC.[19,42] Because of the lack of the antineoplastic effects of the competent immune system, SOTRs are ten-fold more likely to develop SCC caused by previous HPV infection.[19,49]

Treatment of ungual/periungual warts consists of patient or physician-applied modalities.[28] Commonly used methods include cryotherapy with liquid nitrogen (15–20 seconds, two freeze-thaw cycles), podophyllum, salicylic acid, trichloroacetic acid, topical retinoid, intralesional 5-fluorouracil 50 mg/mL, and intralesional bleomycin 1 mg (unit)/mL. Paring of the hyperkeratotic parts is of the utmost importance to facilitate the penetration of the cytotoxic (antiproliferative) agent or enable achievement of the optimal freezing temperature of −15°C to −20°C. The best response is achieved when multiple modalities are used in intervals of 2–4 weeks, with intermittent therapy with topical imiquimod 5% cream used three times weekly for 12–16 weeks.[50] Imiquimod efficacy has been shown to be approximately 36%. Regarding safety, as long as no more than 500 mg are used on areas <100 cm^2, there should be no concerns for transplant rejection because of the insignificant systemic absorption of 5% concentration.[50] Resistant warts could also be treated by intralesional cidofovir, and in any patient with incomplete or partial response, the resistant lesion should be biopsied to evaluate possible malignant transformation.[42]

Certain immunosuppressive medications are specifically associated with an increased incidence of warts, like cyclosporine A (CyA), prednisolone, and azathioprine.[26] Newly introduced mammalian target of rapamycin (mTOR) inhibitors (sirolimus, everolimus) have been associated with significant reduction of malignancy and regression of recalcitrant warts in SOTRs.[15] The antiproliferative activity and cytostatic properties of mTOR inhibitors are the probable reasons, among others, based on their property to inhibit the phosphatidylinositol-3-kinase (PI3k)/protein kinase B (Akt) pathway, which plays a key role in HPV replication.[15] After conversion of treatment to sirolimus, the warts become smaller and darker and finally regress completely, often through a period of several weeks, with significant cosmetic improvement.[15] One should also be aware of the potential of sirolimus to produce paronychia and overgrown granulation tissue in the periungual region after minimal trauma (see following) and differentiate this phenomenon from

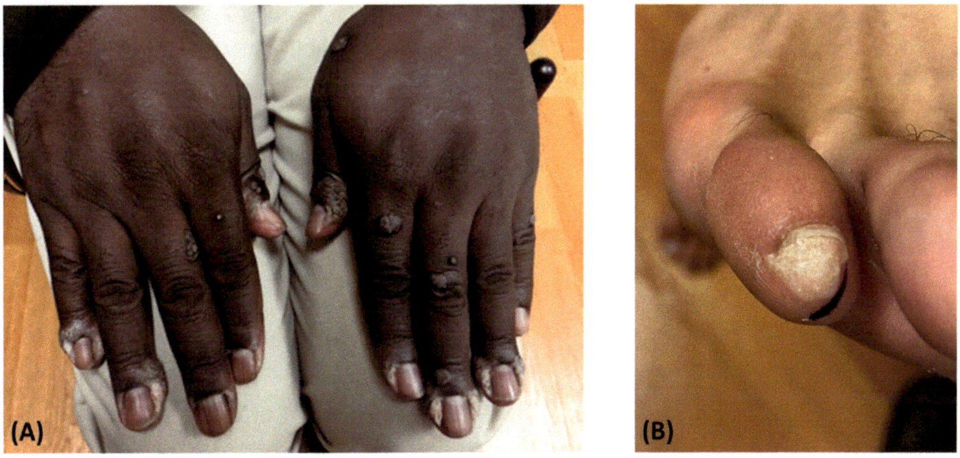

FIGURE 16.11 Periungual HPV infection with extensive multidactylous periungual involvement (**a**) and complete replacement of the nail bed and hyponychium with wart tissue (**b**).

other causes of subungual/periungual pathology. Another option is to consider systemic acitretin in doses of 25–50 mg daily combined with Candida antigen as it has been reported in small series.[16,17]

Human Papillomavirus Prophylactic Vaccination in SOTRs

Last but not least, it is worth discussing the use of HPV prophylactic vaccines in the SOTR population. Since December 2014, a nonavalent HPV vaccine was introduced and is slowly replacing previous versions of quadrivalent (HPV types 6, 11, 16, and 18) and bivalent (HPV types 16 and 18) HPV vaccines.[51] It consists of major L1 and L2 capsid proteins of HPV types 6, 11, 16, 18, 31, 33, 45, 52, and 58, which assemble into virus-like particles and induce the formation of neutralizing antibodies with 97% efficacy and 99% immunogenicity response in immunocompetent individuals. It is currently recommended for all children age 11–12 and recently was approved by the FDA in 2018 for individuals up to 45 years of age. The vaccine was also found to be safe and immunogenic in patients with HIV.[52] Because the vaccine does not contain the live virus but only its envelope, it is highly unlikely that its use would increase the risk of transplant rejection, and it could be used in the population of SOTRs in a similar manner as in immunocompetent individuals. Kumar et al.[53] found a 62% overall response (seropositivity—neutralizing antibodies) to at least one HPV type and 47% to all four HPV types in his cohort of 47 SOTRs when the quadrivalent vaccine was administered at least 5 months after transplantation. Response was higher after all 3 doses of the vaccine were received and less optimal in lung transplant recipients, ones who received the transplant after <1 year, or had lower tacrolimus levels.[53] The current recommendations[49] are to vaccinate all prospective SOTRs before the transplantation or wait at least 1 year after the procedure to vaccinate in order to obtain a better immunogenic response. Apart from measuring neutralizing antibody levels from the plasma, an elegant technique of assessing their level in saliva has also been introduced, making it possible to evaluate the response quickly and revaccinate when necessary in SOTR individuals.[54] At the present time, we do not have large controlled studies because most reports on HPV vaccine use in SOTRs are limited by the small sample size and younger age of the individuals, apart from the study by Kumaret al.,[53] whose patients were up to 35 years of age. Hopefully, in the forthcoming years, having in mind the fact that the population of SOTRs has increasingly longer life expectancy, we will learn more and have the HPV prophylactic vaccine become standard for pretransplant care in these patients,[51] the same way as it has already shown success in the nonimmunocompromised population.[49]

Ungual and Subungual Scabies

Scabies is one of the most common dermatologic conditions, affecting 130 million people worldwide at any given time. The risk of infestation is higher among immune compromised individuals, especially if living in crowded living conditions.[55] Isolated nail involvement without other dermatological manifestations is very rarely described in immunocompromised individuals.[56] More often, persistence of the sarcoptic parasite after apparently successful treatment of the skin disease was shown to provide a significant source for reinfection.[57] *Sarcoptes* can survive up to 96 hours outside of the human host, and nails and the subungual area present an excellent reservoir (Figure 16.12). Furthermore, if the nails are not cut short and treated aggressively with topical permethrin, the patient can easily get reinfected by scratching the skin to alleviate postscabietic pruritus occurring after topical treatment.[57] Finally, scabietic involvement of the nail apparatus with its thickened, yellowish, crumbly nail plates, subungual hyperkeratosis, and occasional erythema and edema of the paronychium can easily be misdiagnosed as OM, nail psoriasis, or other type of nail dystrophy.[28] Persistent skin infestation in SOTRs may eventually lead to the development of crusted scabies with hyperkeratotic plaques and thousands of parasites on the skin. Atypical presentation of crusted scabies with hyperkeratotic scaly plaques on the face and scalp has also been described in SOTRs and may further complicate the diagnosis and timely treatment.[58,59]

The diagnosis of nail scabies can be performed by KOH examination of the nail clippings or histopathological examination of the affected nail plate, which reveals *Sarcoptes* mites embedded in the nail keratin.[55] The treatment[58,59] of nail scabies comprises ivermectin 200 μg/kg two consecutive days a week for 2 weeks and once weekly for an additional 2–4 weeks at the same dosage. Topically the whole skin, as well as the

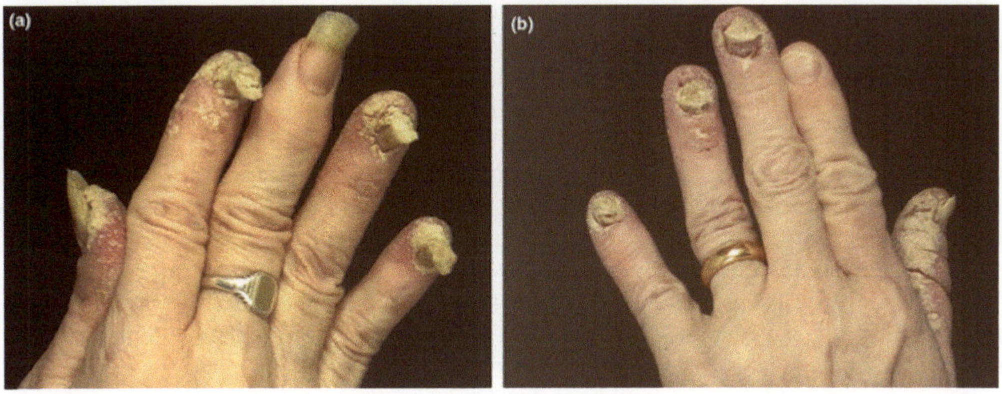

FIGURE 16.12 Ungual scabies with pronounced hyperkeratosis of all fingernails (an important source of reinfection). (From Goyal NN, Wong GA. Psoriasis or crusted scabies, Clinical and Experimental Dermatology, 2008;33: 211–212, with permission.)

nails (after being well trimmed) should be treated with 5% permethrin cream for 18–24 hours. After that, topical 10% sulfur ointment should be applied to the nail apparatus for 96 hours. Chemical ablation of the affected nail plates with 30% salicylic acid or 40% urea cream can also be an option in persistent cases.[60]

In conclusion, subungual/ungual scabies may be subclinical and difficult to diagnose and may serve as a reservoir for severe and persistent disease in SOTRs. Rigorous assessment and treatment of nail involvement in scabies may prevent the development of the crusted disseminated variant of the disease in SOTRs because of the continuously compromised immune status. Finally, one should have a high clinical suspicion to detect ungual/subungual reservoirs of scabies mite, because they are unlikely to respond to standard topical therapies.

NAIL APPARATUS CHANGES SECONDARY TO MEDICATIONS USED IN SOTRS

Nail changes secondary to antirejection medications depend on the type of medication, duration of its use, and the individual predisposition of each patient. Most of the nail changes due to medications may just be of cosmetic importance and as such do not require any treatment or modification of the antirejection regimen. Others may produce painful paronychia and hypergranulation response to minor trauma in the perionychium and require attention, especially if they become complicated by coinfection with bacteria and yeasts (see prior). Hence, any paronychia not responding to antibacterial or antifungal/anticandidal therapy and with negative cultures should prompt one to consider the possibility of drug-induced affliction of the nail apparatus in SOTRs.

Nail Changes Secondary to Acitretin Use in SOTRs

Acitretin is a second-generation retinoid that alters gene transcription by binding to RAR and RXR receptors in the nucleus of keratinocytes. The modulation of gene expression leads to normalization of epidermal growth and keratinization, contributing to its antiproliferative and antineoplastic properties.[17] Acitretin is used in SOTRs to decrease the rate of development and neoplastic transformation of precancerous lesions like actinic keratosis to Bowen's disease and invasive SCC. The initial dosage is 10 mg every other day, which is slowly increased to 25 mg daily over several weeks.[3,16,17] The majority of reported nail changes were of cosmetic importance like nail thinning, nail softening, increased nail fragility, and onychoschizia (splitting of the distal nails). Subungual hemorrhage, transverse LKN, trachyonychia, and paronychia were rarely described.[61] Trachyonychia comprises longitudinal ridging of the nail plate and is further classified as opaque if associated with sandpaper texture of the nail plate or shiny if multiple pits are present.[61] The most common approach in dealing with these changes is avoidance of nail trauma, use of topical emollients, nail polish, or biotin, and cysteine supplementation.[62] Acitretin-induced paronychia presents with erythema, edema, tenderness, and discharge on the lateral nail folds on the big toenails or, less commonly, the fingernails. It can also be associated with pyogenic granuloma (overgrown granulation tissue) (Figure 16.13), complicating the paronychia with bleeding and crusting worsening after minimal trauma. It affects multiple digits and usually develops 3–12 weeks into acitretin therapy.[63] Treatment possibilities are topical mupirocin, gentamicin, fusidic acid, 2% povidone iodine solution, or a combination of topical steroids and systemic antistaphylococcal antimicrobials.[21,28] Excessive granulation may be destroyed with electrocoagulation.[21] In case of recurrence, temporary reduction or complete cessation of acitretin is recommended.[63] This complication is very rarely reported with <30 cases described in the literature. The pathogenesis of the paronychia and pyogenic granuloma developing at the periungual tissue is explained by antiproliferative retinoid effects that affect wound healing and produce aberrant response to repetitive, minor, occult trauma of the paronychium.[6–17,63]

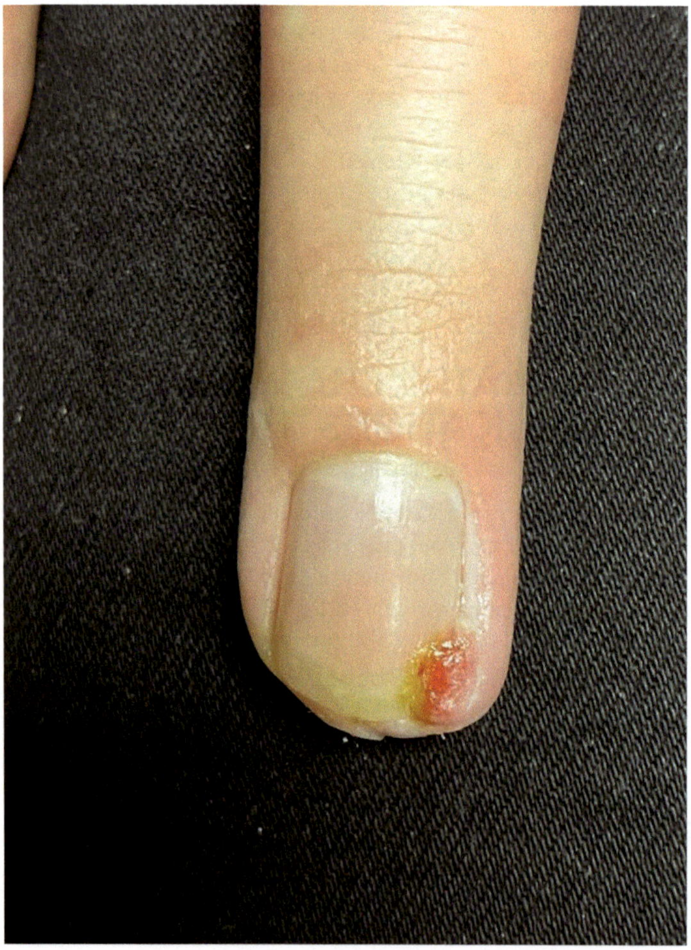

FIGURE 16.13 Pyogenic granuloma on the left middle finger in a patient on acitretin.

Nail Changes Secondary to Use of mTOR Inhibitors

Sirolimus, also known as rapamycin, is a macrolide antibiotic with powerful antiproliferative and immunosuppressive activity.[3] As previously described, it inhibits the activation of mTOR by binding the cytosolic FK-binding protein-12 (FKBP-12). The block of mTOR function results in suppressive effects of activation and proliferation of T cells and B cells by inhibiting their response to IL-2.[3,15] The same mechanism[15,64] is responsible for inhibition of other growth factors, mainly vascular endothelial growth factor (VEGF) and epidermal growth factor (EGF), which has profound effects on wound healing of the skin and adnexa.[64] Nail abnormalities with sirolimus are seen in >40% of patients but mostly comprise longitudinal ridging,[64] which is usually of cosmetic importance and does not require the cessation of immunosuppressive therapy. Other reports, though, challenge these findings,[65] suggesting that onychopathic changes with sirolimus are not statistically significant and can be found with a similar incidence in patients with different antirejection regimens. The development of chronic paronychia and sirolimus-associated pyogenic granuloma is uncommon[66] and rarely requires the cessation or modification of antirejection therapy (e.g., switch to mycophenolate mofetil). The pathogenesis is probably the aberrant response of the paronychial tissue to minor trauma because of suppressed wound healing and decreased concentration of VEGF.[66] The approach to therapy is the same as for acitretin-induced paronychia described prior.[21,28] The fact that abnormal wound healing[67] was found to be significantly higher (43.2%) among SOTRs on sirolimus in comparison with the rate in the control group (2.4%) in which mycophenolate mofetil was used is important when considering nail surgery procedures, because one can encounter more wound dehiscence, postoperative wound infection, or other complications.

TUMORS OF THE NAIL APPARATUS IN SOTRS

Nonmelanoma skin cancer (NMSC) is the most common malignancy in SOTRs[17] with an increased incidence of 60 to 250 times for SCC and 10 to 40 times for basal cell carcinoma (BCC), respectively. NMSC is responsible for 3% of cancer-specific deaths in SOTRs. Other solid skin malignancies that are overrepresented in SOTRs include KS and Merkel cell carcinoma, with risks increased by 100 and 24 times, respectively.[17] The incidence of melanoma in SOTRs is reported to be 2–8 times higher when compared with that in immunocompetent individuals[68] (Chapters 8, 11, and 12).

The involvement of the nail apparatus with BCC is extremely rare and usually presents with an erythematous pink nodule and plaque, in the periungual region, which bleeds easily and shows telangiectasia against a pink background on dermoscopy.[69] Involvement of the nail with Merkel cell carcinoma[70] and KS[71] is exceptional and is in a form of friable bluish red subungual nodule with onycholysis, whitish-yellow discoloration of the nail plate, and bleeding resembling pyogenic granuloma. The treatment of BCC of the nail apparatus comprises the use of Mohs micrographic surgery with maximal tissue preservation,[72] and for the other two, the approach complies with the same standard of care for identical tumors on different locations in SOTRs. The most important nail tumors in SOTRs are SCC and nail apparatus melanoma, which will be further discussed.

Squamous Cell Neoplasia of the Nail Apparatus in SOTRs

Squamous cell tumors of the nail apparatus[73] in SOTRs can be divided roughly in three groups: 1) subungual/periungual SCC in situ (SCCis) or Bowen's disease, 2) subungual/periungual invasive SCC, and 3) subungual keratoacanthoma (SUKA). Clinical presentation of the Bowen's disease[74] (Figure 16.14) is in a form of verrucous plaque, with fissures, hyperkeratosis, and erythema, especially when it involves

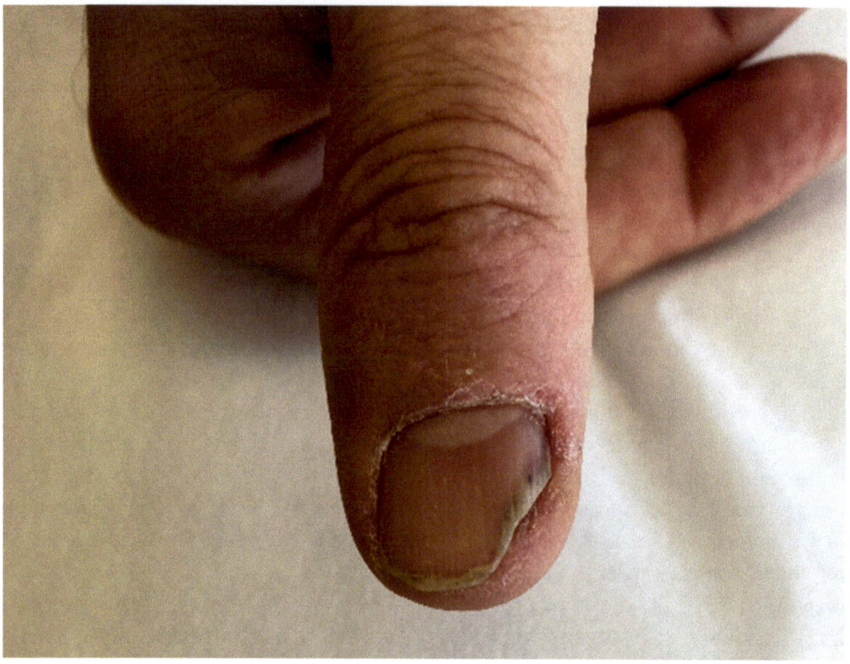

FIGURE 16.14 Bowen's disease (squamous cell carcinoma in situ) of the lateral nail fold; discrete hyperkeratotic plaque, slowly growing, with pinpoint bleeding and adjacent nail plate fragility.

the PNF. The plaque is usually painless, ill-defined, and may penetrate the nail matrix, resulting in nail plate dystrophy. Subungual presentation may also be in the form of the reddish pink streak, known as longitudinal erythronychia.[74] The presentation of the invasive SCC (Figure 16.15) is similar, but there is commonly oozing because of the fact that invasion goes into the dermis, and sometimes hemorrhage, erosion, edema, and secondary bacterial infection.[28] In individuals with dark skin, SCC of the nail unit can also present as laterally based striate melanonychia, sometimes associated with HPV type 56 infection as was recently been reported by Serret at al.[75] SUKA is the rarest presentation of squamous cell neoplasia of the nail apparatus and begins as a fast-growing subungual nodule, with central crater, onycholysis, and tenderness. Characteristic radiological presentation is bone erosion in comparison with the osteolysis seen with invasive SCC of the nail.[76] In immunocompetent individuals, SCC of the nail apparatus (SCCNA) is usually monodactylous, appears more commonly later in life (mean age is 67 years old), and has a male predominance.[28,73,74] SCCNA is more common on the fingers, affecting the thumbnails and index fingernails, as well as the third fingernail on the dominant hand. It is less common on the toenails and then it mainly affects the great toes.[77] The diagnostic delay is often several years, because early SCC of the nail apparatus may mimic OM, bacterial paronychia, nail dystrophy, or wart.[73,74] We have already emphasized that persistent, recalcitrant warts in SOTRs should be biopsied to rule out the presence of malignant transformation and development of SCCNA. Apart from immunosuppression, other risk factors for the development of SCC of the nail are radiation exposure (ionizing and UV), chemical toxicities (tar, arsenic), tobacco use, trauma (nail biting, burns) and HPV infection.[73] Approximately 60%–80% of cases of both SCC and SCCis of the nail apparatus are associated with HPV-16, the most common oncogenic subtype.[78,79] Other HPV subtypes isolated in the cases of periungual/subungual SCCis (HPV-18, HPV-36, HPV-56) and SCCNA (HPV-18, HPV-56, HPV-33, HPV-35, HPV-51, HPV-73, HPV-58) are less common.[78] Apart from the previously mentioned alpha HPV acquired by digito-anogenital contact, subtypes of beta HPV are also isolated (HPV-9, HPV-17, HPV-21, HPV-49).[45,78,79] The latter are more common on periungual skin, and are specifically associated with actinic keratoses and SCC outside the nail area with

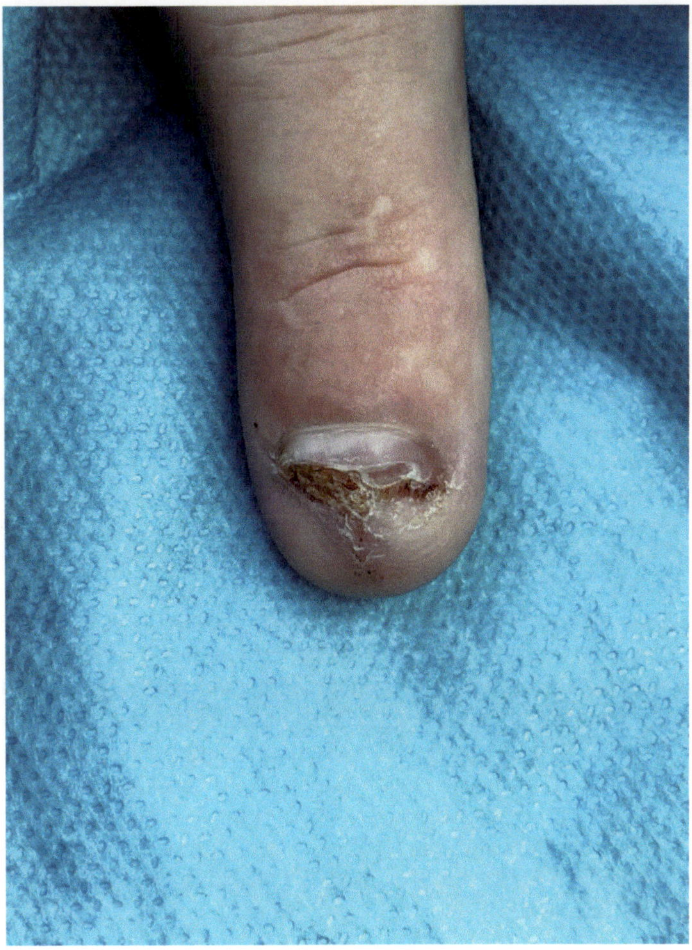

FIGURE 16.15 Invasive squamous cell carcinoma of the nail apparatus with destruction of the nail plate and subungual expansion.

UV radiation exposure as important co-carcinogen. Beta HPV subtypes usually produce asymptomatic infections in immunocompetent individuals.[48] In SOTRs who present with SCCNA, there is a 25% incidence of having HPV disease on other sites like the vulva, cervix, penis, or perianal area, and these areas should be examined during the initial consultation in order to recognize and treat these infections because they also carry the risk for neoplastic transformation and SCC development.[78] We have already discussed the pathogenesis of HPV infections and the modalities it uses to avoid recognition by the immune system (see prior). These mechanisms are much more pronounced in SOTRs in whom constant immunosuppression to prevent rejection creates an environment for the establishment of persistent infection. Ormerod and de Berker[80] compared the presentation of SCCNA in immunosuppressed vs. immunocompetent individuals and reported the following differences: 1) younger age at development (mean age 52 vs. 63 years); 2) earlier presentation (9 vs. 65 months); 3) higher frequency of polidactylous disease (57% vs. 6%) 4) same site relapse (29% vs. 0%), and 5) other site recurrence (57% vs. 0%). In SUKAs, apart from similar alpha and beta HPV types isolated in SCCNA,[78,79] HPV subtype 6 has also been described.[81]

The diagnosis of SCCNA is made by nail biopsy, and one should have a high index of suspicion to avoid treatment delays.[74,77,80] The immunohistochemical staining with $p16^{INK4a}$ and Ki-67 is a good marker for HPV-associated SCCNA[79] and is useful to indicate increased cellular proliferation and predict local aggressiveness. Imaging studies using X-ray and magnetic resonance imaging are worth doing before surgical treatment to evaluate possible invasion of the phalangeal bone, which may require a more extensive approach with distal phalanx amputation.[76,81] The treatment of choice for SCCNA without bone involvement is Mohs micrographic surgery, which provides the best tracing of the tumor including periosteal spread, and maximal presentation of the healthy tissue.[77] One should be aware of the "natural pockets" (Figure 16.16) where tumor cells may be hiding, e.g., cuticle/eponychium or lowest portions of the lateral nail folds, which should be removed during Mohs procedure to decrease the risk of tumor recurrence and avoid interference of this naturally folded anatomical structures with Mohs slides interpretation.[74,77] If skin graft is chosen as a repair option for the denuded phalanx after SCCNA, removal of the donor skin should always be harvested from areas nonexposed to the sun (e.g., flexural forearms) to alleviate the risk of de novo SCC developing on the grafted site.[83] Smaller defects, involving just the lateral part of the nail apparatus, could be repaired by using a lateral bipedicle flap aka "bridge flap" in which a relaxing incision is placed on the digital pulp, providing mobility of the volar skin to be transposed dorsally and cover the defect of the ipsilateral nail bed.[84] SUKA in SOTRs should always be treated surgically to avoid the risk of invasion and possible transformation to invasive SCC.[85]

As with recalcitrant warts, the modification of the antirejection regimen can be considered in SOTRs in whom SCCNAs develop frequently, become polydactylous, or demonstrate aggressive behavior with bone involvement. The risk of metastases after bone invasion is high with only 25% 5-year projected survival.[73,75,76,80,85] Thus, the dose reduction of medications with high oncogenicity like CNIs (e.g., cyclosporine A and tacrolimus), or to a lesser extent antimetabolite (azathioprine), may prove critical in these situations. CNIs have inhibitory effects on p53 and E-cadherin (tumor suppressors) and as such potentiate the oncogenic effect of other factors like UV damage, immunosuppression, and HPV persistent infection.[15,48] Future directions may be greater use of mTOR inhibitors in place of CNIs or tumor-lytic small molecule peptide of Notch pathway signaling.[3,15,48] The high frequency of HPV-16 association with subungual/periungual squamous cell neoplasia renders important the consideration of HPV vaccination in all individuals before transplantation or after the first year of the procedure as already emphasized.[49] Recent reports demonstrated the ability of nonavalent HPV vaccine to improve the activity of natural killer cells by upregulating their NKG2D, NKp30, NKp46, and ILT2 receptors, which are downregulated in unvaccinated SOTRs with HPV infection.[47]

Malignant Melanoma (MM) of the Nail Apparatus in SOTRs

Apart from a 2–8 times increased incidence, several studies on MM in SOTRs did not find clinical differences in its presentation compared with that in the immunocompetent population. Melanoma can present

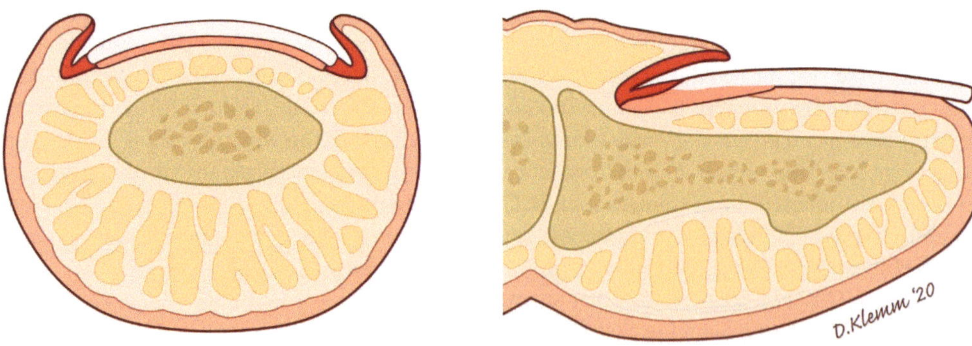

FIGURE 16.16 Natural pockets of the nail apparatus that can harbor foci of neoplastic proliferation in the lateral nail fold and subcuticular region.

before the transplantation or develop after the procedure.[68] For preexisting melanoma in situ, after successful removal, one may proceed without delay to the transplantation procedure. For invasive melanoma without sentinel lymph node involvement, standard guidelines recommend a waiting period of 2 years (for MMs with Breslow <1 mm, Breslow <2 mm) or 5 years (for MMs with Breslow >2 mm), respectively. Posttransplant acral melanomas probably have the same frequency (1%–7% of all melanomas) in Caucasian immunosuppressed as wells as immunocompetent individuals.[68,86]

However, in about 50% of Asian and 60%–70% of black patients, acral melanomas are more common. Nail apparatus melanoma (NAM) comprises about 25%–30% of acral melanomas.[83] The age of onset is from 59–63 years, and they develop within the range of 40–132 months after transplantation.[68,87]

The most common presentation of NAM (38%–76%) is a pigmented streak aka melanonychia striata (Figure 16.17 a, b, and c) where tumor melanocytes are derived from the nail matrix.[74,87] The streak is irregular, >3 mm in size, and often wider proximally than distally. Dermoscopically it is also irregular; the pigment lines are not parallel, and the area is asymmetric.[74] In benign melanonychia, the pigment is regular, lines are parallel, fine, either grayish (melanocytic activation) or light brown (matrical lentigo or matrical nevus). In dark-complexed individuals (Asians or Africans), melanonychia can also affect multiple digits and is usually of benign origin. In matrical nevus, there are often black dots, which

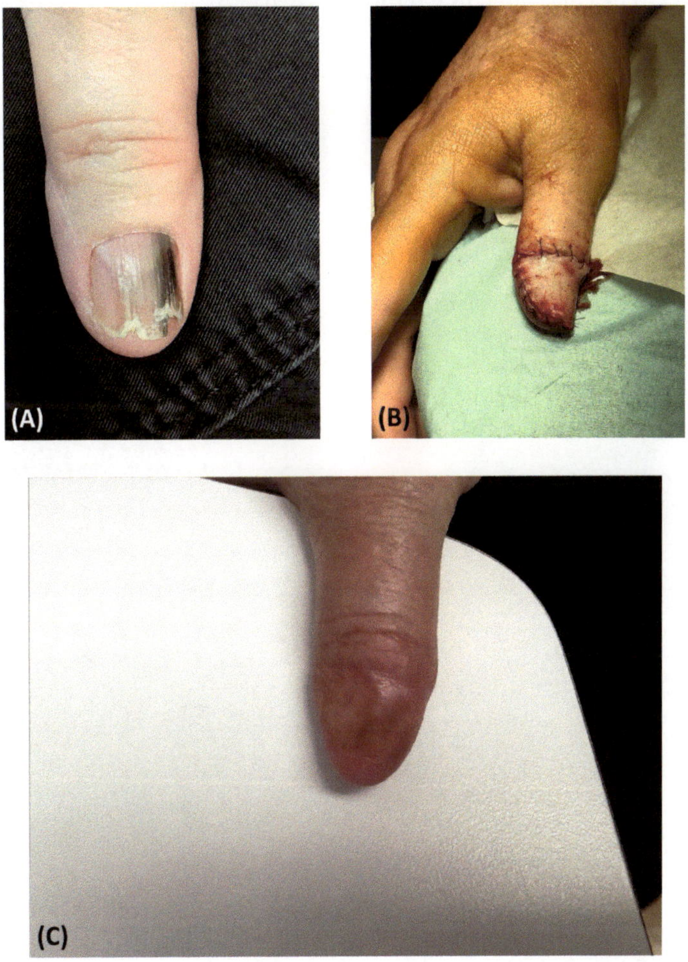

FIGURE 16.17 Melanonychia striata: (**a**) melanoma in situ of the great thumbnail, with (**b**) excellent cosmetic result after total en-bloc dissection of the nail apparatus and repair with full-thickness skin graft; (**c**) 3 years postoperatively.

correspond to transungual elimination of nevus nests. The appearance of black-brown pigmentation on the adjacent nail fold is known as Hutchinson's sign, is a bad prognostic sign, and usually corresponds to invasive melanoma of the adjacent nail fold.[74] The diffuse involvement of the nail matrix results in dystrophy of the nail plate and presents an ominous sign (Figure 16.18). In the late-stage total nail dystrophy, nodular change, ulceration, and bleeding may develop. Subungual melanomas (Figure 16.19), in comparison with matrical ones, are often amelanotic, because they start in the nail bed where the number of melanocytes is lower than in the nail matrix. They present as onycholysis, subungual nodule, erythema, erosion, and bleeding, and have much longer delay in diagnosis then the ones presenting as melanonychia striata.[74,87]

The diagnosis of NAM is obtained by performing a biopsy of the nail matrix with partial or total avulsion of the nail plate and/or reflection of the PNF to access the subungual tumor tissue. With the presence of pigment or invasion at the lateral nail fold, sampling can also be obtained from the periungual skin. However, the Breslow depth may not always correlate to matrical melanoma, where the tumor of origin has been present longer and could consequently be deeper.[68,74,87] The treatment of NAM in situ is total en-block resection of the nail apparatus, whereas the invasive NAM is usually treated by distal digital amputation. Proper staging, sentinel lymph node evaluation, and global assessment of the metastatic risk is mandatory, because modification, decrease, or complete cessation of immunosuppressive medications need to be considered to improve survival.[68] As has already been stated, a high index

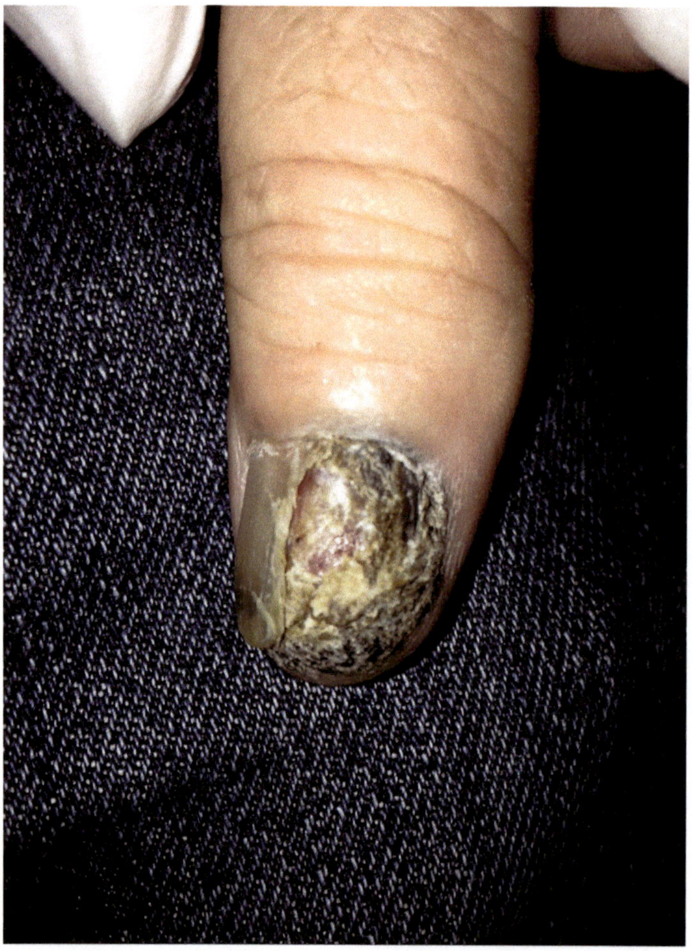

FIGURE 16.18 Complete destruction of the nail apparatus with invasive melanoma.

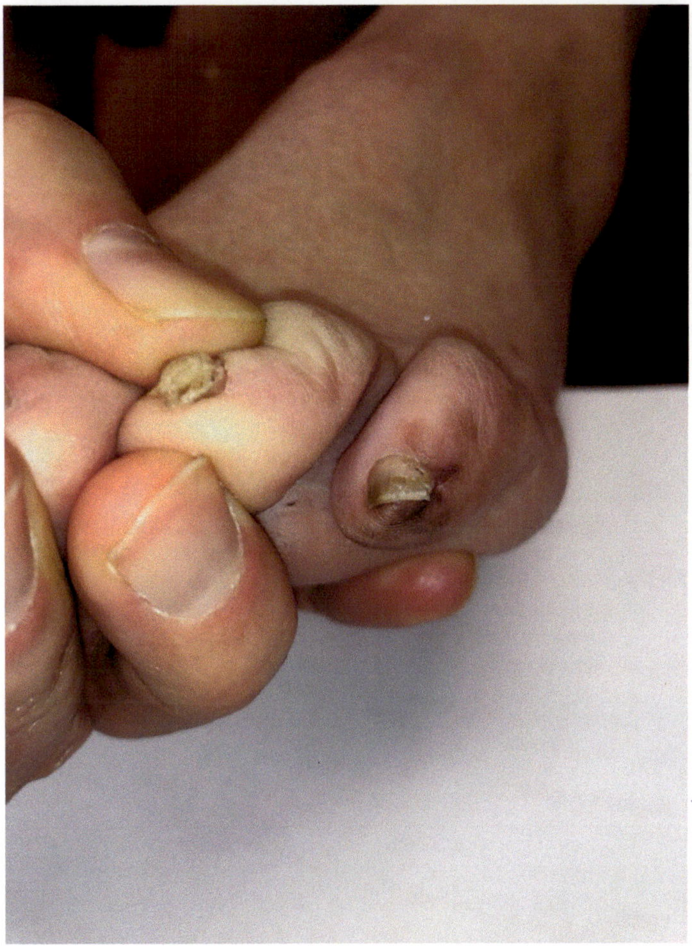

FIGURE 16.19 Subungual melanoma of the left small toe with no nail dystrophy but apparent periungual black discoloration (Hutchinson's sign).

of suspicion and decision for early biopsy will render prompt and successful treatment in affected individuals. One should bear in mind that NAM most often affects one nail, either the thumbnail or index fingernail or rarely a great toenail.[68,74] The differential is broad and includes among others subungual hematoma, pigmented OM, or green nails syndrome as described previously. Drug-induced nail pigmentation, on the contrary, is often polydactylous and almost never affects a single nail unit.[74] In conclusion, any monodactylous onychopathy not responding to antibacterial/antifungal therapy for several weeks should immediately prompt the clinician to perform histopathological analysis, especially if it presents in a streaky pattern.[74]

NAIL SURGERY IN SOTRS

Important factors to be considered when performing any type of nail surgery procedure in SOTRs is the presence of conditions or situations that may complicate the procedure itself or its postsurgical course. These include 1) aberrant wound healing (with the use of mTOR inhibitors)[65]; 2) risk of postoperative

TABLE 16.6 Nail Surgery Precautions and Guidelines in SOTRs

CONDITION	*RISK*	*RECOMMENDATIONS*	*REFERENCE*
Diabetes, advanced atherosclerosis in SOTRs	Ischemia, necrosis	Avoid epinephrine in digital blocks	4, 5, 6, 87
Nail biopsy	Postoperative infection—felon, matrix damage, nail dystrophy.	Preferably biopsy the nail fold, then the nail bed; avoid the matrix or distal subungual area when possible	2, 84
Nail plate avulsion	Nail bed infection, slow wound healing	Perform nail bed biopsy through partial avulsion of the nail plate, return the intact nail plate, if no pathology, to cover the nail bed until healing occurs	2, 21, 67
Benign nail conditions (paronychia, pyogenic granuloma, ingrown toenail, warts)	Paronychia, cellulitis, traumatic inoculation of HPV virus from vapor after electrosurgery	Perform excision only when necessary, rely on curettage and electrodessication whenever possible; Cryosurgery is preferable for the warts, avoid excision and laser ablation, because it may spread the HPV infection	21, 67
Toenail surgery vs. Fingernail surgery	Postoperative wound infection, cellulitis, osteomyelitis	Consider postoperative antibiotics, not just for the toenails, but also for the fingernails to decrease the risk of postoperative wound infection	12, 13, 18, 19, 20

Abbreviation: SOTRs, solid organ transplant recipients

infections because of immunosuppression[12,13,18–20]; 3) risk of skin necrosis with epinephrine digital block anesthesia because of compromised microcirculation (especially with toenail surgery) in preexisting atherosclerosis or diabetes in SOTRs[4–6,88]; and 4) risk of tumor recurrence after surgical removal because of the complex interplay of field cancerization (sun damage), immunosuppression, and HPV infection.[47,48,85] For benign nail tumors, conservative treatment is more reasonable. In contrast, for malignancies, even for in situ ones, aggressive surgical removal to alleviate the risk of early invasion and dissemination is preferable.[79,80,85] A summary of precautions and guidelines for nail surgery in SOTRs is presented in Table 16.6.

CONCLUSION

Nail changes in SOTRs include wide varieties of pathologies including but not limited to infections, tumors, nail plate abnormalities, and drug toxicities. They can vary in onset, presentation, severity, and prognosis when compared with those of similar conditions in immunocompetent individuals.

Comprehensive examination of all fingernails and toenails and familiarity with nail pathology would make SOTR providers successful in promptly identifying, diagnosing, and treating these conditions to obtain optimal control of nail-apparatus associated morbidity, and possible mortality, in affected individuals.

SUMMARY OF KEY POINTS

- Nail changes affect up to 60% of SOTR.
- Caused are metabolic, circulatory, inflammatory, infectious, and neoplastic factors.
- Nail problems should be diagnosed early and treated efficiently.
- Due to the proximity of nail apparatus to the phalangeal bone and immunocompromized milieu, any infection or neoplasia carries a risk of vascular invasion and dissemination.
- Patients should be educated about proper nail care and avoid trauma to decrease risk of nail apparatus morbidity.

REFERENCES

1. Ito T, Ito N, Saathoff M, Stamplachicacchiere B, Bettermann A, Bulfone-Paus S. Immunology of the human nail apparatus: the nail matrix is a site of relative immune privilege. J Invest Dermatol. 2005;125:1139–48.
2. Haneke E. Anatomy of the nail unit and the nail biopsy. Semin Cutan Med Surg. 2015;34:95–100.
3. Shafaeddin-Schreve B, Anliker M, Arnold A, Dziunycz P, Kempf W, Laffitte E. Skin care in solid organ transplant recipients: risk-adjusted follow-up. Expert Rev. Dermatol. 2012;7(3):227–33.
4. Saray Y, Seçkin D, Gülec AT, Akgün S, Haberal M. Nail disorders in hemodialysis patients and renal transplant recipients: a case control study. J Am Acad Dermatol. 2004;50:197–202.
5. Abdelaziz AM, Mahmoud KM, Elsawy EM, Bakr MA. Nail changes in kidney transplant recipients. Nephrol Dial Transplant. 2010;25:274–7.
6. Aqil N, Nassiri A, Gallouj S, Mernissi FZ. Nail disorders in patients with chronic renal failure. Dermatol Res Ther. 2019;5:065.
7. Grossman M, Scher RK. Leukonychia: review and classification. Int J Dermatol. 1990;29:535–41.
8. Canavan T, Tosti A, Mallory H, McKay K, Cantrell W, Elewski B. An idiopathic leukonychia totalis and leukonychia partialis case report and review of the literature. Skin Appendage Disord. 2015;1:38–42.
9. Cribier B, Mena ML, Rey D, Partisani M, Fabien V, Lang JM. Nail changes in patients infected with human immunodeficiency virus: a prospective controlled study. Arch Dermatol. 1998;134:1216–20.
10. Cohen PR. The nail flag sign in heart transplant recipients: case reports and review of the patients with the flag sign of the nail. Dermatol Online J. 2019;25(3):1–4.
11. Yadav DK, Bai XI, Liang T. Dermatological disorders following liver transplantation: an update. Can J Gastroenterol Hepatol. 2019:Article ID 9780952, 9 pages.
12. Seçkin D, Güleç TO, Demirag A, Bilgin N. Renal transplantation and skin disease. Transplant Proc. 1998;30(3):802–4.
13. Rerucha CM, Wing JT, Oppenlander KE, Cowan WC. Acute hand infections. Am Fam Physician. 2019;99(4):228–36.
14. Monteagudo B, Figueroa O, Suárez-Magdalena O, Méndez-Lagae S. Green nail caused by onychomycosis coinfected with pseudomonas aeruginosa. Eczema y urticaria en Portugal. 2019;110:783–5.
15. Dharancy S, Catteau B, Mortier L, Boleslawski E, Declerck N, Canva V, Piette F, Mathurin P, Pruvot FR. Conversion to sirolimus: a useful strategy for recalcitrant cutaneous viral warts in liver transplant recipient. Liver Transplant. 2006;12:1883–7.
16. Yuan ZF, Davis A, Macdonald K, Bailey RR. Use of acitretin for the skin complications in renal transplant recipients. N Z Med J. 1995;108: 255–6.

17. Herold M, Good AJ, Nielson CB, Longo MI. Use of topical and systemic retinoids in solid organ transplant recipients: update and review of the current literature. Dermatol Surg. 2019;45:1442–9.
18. Lima AM, Rocha SP, de Reis Filho EGM, Eid DRM, Reis CMS. Study of dermatoses in kidney transplant patients. An Bras Dermatol. 2013;88(3):361–7.
19. Pettit JC, Mazurek K, Kaffenberger B. Cutaneous manifestations of infections in solid organ transplant recipients. Curr Infect Dis Rep. 2018;20(16):1–10.
20. Ilyas M, Maganty N, Ginsberg Z, Sharma A. Skin infections due to bacteria in solid organ transplant recipients: a review. Dermatol. 2017;233:358–65.
21. Haneke E. Nail surgery. Clinics in Dermatol. 2013;31:516–25.
22. Bae Y, Lee GM, Sim JH, Lee S, Lee SY, Park YL. Green toenail syndrome treated with the application of tobramycin eye drop. Ann Dermatol. 2014;26(40):514–16.
23. Pettit JC, Stout JE, Gradkowski LB, Rath S, Alspaugh JA, Miller MB, Cox GM. Pedicure-associated rapidly growing mycobacterial infection: an endemic disease. Clin Infect Dis. 2011;53(8):787–92.
24. Cooksey CR, de Waard JH, Yakrus MA, Rivera I, Chopite M, Toney SR, Morlock GP, Butler RW. Mycobacterium cosmeticum sp. nov., a novel rapidly growing species isolated from a cosmetic infection and from a nail salon. Int J System Evolut Microbiol. 2004;54:2385–91.
25. Ilyas M, Sander A, Frank B. Paronychia caused by Bartonella henselae. Lancet. 1997;350(9804):1078.
26. Imko-Walczuk B, Okuniewska A, Prędota-Glowacka A, Jaśkiewicz J, Placek W, Włodarczyk Z, Dębska-Ślizien A, Rutkowski B. Benign cutaneous disease among Polish renal transplant recipients. Transplant Proc. 2016;48:1660–6.
27. Kubak BM, Huprikar SS. Emerging & rare fungal infections in solid organ transplant recipients. Am J Transplant. 2009;9(Suppl 4):S208–S226.
28. Wollina U, Nenoff P, Haroske G, Haenssle HA. The diagnosis and treatment of nail disorders. Dtsch Arztebl Int. 2016;113:509–18.
29. Rizzitelli G, Guanziroli E, Moschin A, Snagalli R, Veraldi S. Onychomycosis caused by trihosporon mucoides. Int J Infect Dis. 2016;42:61–3.
30. Baykal C, Kazancioglu R, Büyükbabani N, Çelik AV, Yegenoglu Y, Kayacan SM, Satana D, Sever MS. Simultaneous cutaneous and ungual alternariosis in a renal transplant recipient. Br J Dermatol. 2000;143:910–12.
31. Barua P, Barua S, Borkakoty B, Mahanta J. Onychomycosis by scytalidium dimidiatum in green tea leaf pluckers: report of two cases. Mycopathologia. 2007;164(4):193–5.
32. Hay RJ, Baran R. Onychomycosis: a proposed revision of the clinical classification. J Am Acad Dermatol. 2011;65:1219–7.
33. Weinberg JM, Koestenblatt EK, Don PC, White SM, Stein MN, Bamji MN. Proximal white subungual onychomycosis in the immunocompetent patient: report of two cases and review of the literature. Acta Dermatol Venereol (Stockh). 1999;79:81–2.
34. Liang SE, Cohen DE, Rieder EA. Proximal subungual onychomycosis in the immunocompetent: a case report and review of the literature. J Drugs Dermatol. 2018;17(4):475–8.
35. Bongomin F, Batac CR, Richardson MD, Denning DW. A review of onychomycosis due to aspergillus species. Mycopathologia. 2018;183:485–93.
36. Mulvaney PM, Telang GH, Jellinek N. Trichophytum rubrum endonyx onychomycosis resistant to standard oral and topical therapies. Dermatol Online J. 2015;21(9):8–10.
37. Yang YS, Ahn J, Shin MK, Lee MH. Fusarium solani onychomycosis of the thumbnail coinfected with pseudomonas aeruginosa: report of two cases. Mycoses. 2011;54:168–71.
38. Pai V, Ganavalli A, Kikkeri NN. Antifungal resistance in dermatology. Indian J Dermatol. 2018;63(5):361–8.
39. Monod M, Méhul B. Recend findings in onychomycosis and their application for appropriate treatment. J Fungi. 2019;5(20):1–10.
40. Gupta AK, Lynde CW, Konnikov N. Single-blind randomized, prospective study of sequential itraconazole and terbinafine pulse compared with terbinafine pulse for the treatment of toenail onychomycosis. J Am acad Dermatol. 2001;44:485–91.
41. Elewski BE, Rich P, Tosti A, Pariser DA, Scher R, Daniel RC, Gupta AK. Onychomycosis: an overview. J Drugs Dermatol. 2013;12(7 Suppl 2):s96–103.
42. Ilyas M, Maganty N, Sharma A. Cutaneous infections from viral sources in solid organ transplant recipients. J Clin Virol. 2017;97:33–7.
43. Arslan F, Batirel A, Mert A, Ozer S. Cytomegalovirus (CMV)-related cutaneous necrotizing vasculitis: case report and literature review. Braz J Infect Dis. 2012;16(5):482–5.
44. Choi YL, Kim JA, Jang KT, Kim DS, Kim WS, Lee JH, Yang JM, Lee ES, Lee DY. Characteristics of cutaneous cytomegalovirus infection in non-acquired immune deficiency syndrome, immunocompromised patients. Br J Dermatol. 2001;155:977–82.

45. Smith SR, Butterly DW, Aexander BD, Greenberg A. Viral infections after renal transplantation. Am J Kidney Dis. 2001;37:659–76.
46. Chin-Hong PV, Kwak EJ. Human papillomavirus in solid organ transplants. Am J Transplant. 2013;13:189–200.
47. Amador-Molina A, Hernández-Valencia JF, Lamoyi E, Contreras-Paredes A, Liziano M. Role of innate immunity against human papillomavirus (HPV) infections and effect of adjuvant in promoting specific immune response. Viruses. 2013;5:2624–42.
48. Reusser NM, Downing C, Guidry J, Tyring SK. HPV carcinomas in immunosuppressed patients. J Clin Med. 2015;4:260–81.
49. Chin-Hong PV, Reid EG. Human papillomavirus infection in solid organ transplant recipients: guidelines from the American society of transplantation infectious disease community of practice. Clinical Transplant. 2019;33:1–15.
50. Brown VL, Atkins CL, Ghali L, Cerio R, Harwood CA, Proby CM. Safety and efficacy of 5% imiquimod cream for the treatment of skin dysplasia in high-risk renal transplant recipients: randomized, double-blind placebo-controlled trial. Arch Dermatol. 2005;141:985–93.
51. Petrosky E, Bocchini JA, Hariri S, Chesson H, Robinette Curtis C, Saraiya M, Unger ER, Markowitz LE. Use of 9-valent human papillomavirus (HPV) vaccine: updated HPV vaccination recommendations of the advisory committee on immunization practices. MMWR Morb Mortal Wkly Rep. 2015;64(11):300–4.
52. Wilkin T, Lee JY, Lensing SY, Stier EA, Goldstone SE, Berry JM et al. Safety and immunogenicity of the quadrivalent human papillomavirus vaccine in HIV-1-infected men. J Infect Dis. 2010;202(8):1246–53.
53. Kumar D, Unger ER, Panicker G, Medvedev P, Wilson L, Humar A. Immunogenicity of quadrivalent human papillomavirus vaccine in organ transplant recipients. Am J Transplant. 2013;13(9): 2411–17.
54. Parker KH, Kemp TJ, Pan Y, Yang Z, Giuliano AR, Pinto LA. Evaluation of HPV-16 and HPV-18 specific antibody measurements in saliva collected in oral rinse and Merocel® sponges. Vaccine. 2018;36(19):2705–11.
55. Fuller LC. Current epidemiology of scabies. Curr Opin Infect Dis. 2013;26:123–6.
56. Zou Y, Hu W, Zheng J, Pan M. Nail infestation: an atypical presentation of typical scabies. Lancet. 2018;391:2272.
57. Scher RK. Subungual scabies. J Am Acad Dermatol. 1985;12(3):577–8.
58. Wang MK, Chin-Yee B, Lo CKL, Lee S, El-Helou P, Alowami S et al. Crusted scabies in a renal transplant recipient treated with daily ivermectin: a case report and literature review. Transpl Infect Dis. 2019;21:e13077.
59. Dondonis FP, Costa Jappur DM, Pires GC, Silva Cartell A, Bonamigo RR. Facial crusted scabies on renal transplant patient. Nefrologia. 2019;39(3):315–17.
60. Last O, Reckhow J, Bogen B, Rozenblat M. Subungual and ungual scabies: avoiding severe presentation in high-risk patients. BMJ Case Rep. 2018;11:e225623.
61. Thieman T, Clarey D, Jonson RA, Trowbridge RM. Trachyonychia secondary to acitretin usage. Cureus. 2020;12(1):e6703.
62. Chessa MA, Iorizzo M, Richert B, López-Estebaranz JL, Rigopoulos D, Tosti A et al. Pathogenesis, clinical signs and treatment recommendations in brittle nails: a review. Dermatol Ther (Heidelb). 2020;10:15–27.
63. Badri T, Hawilo AM, Benmously R, Feninche S, Mokhtar I. Acitretin-induced pyogenic granuloma. Acta Dermatoven APA. 2011;20(4):217–18.
64. Özcan D, Seçkin D, Ada S. Havberal M. Mucocutaneous disorders in renal transplant recipients receiving sirolimus-based immunosuppressive therapy: a prospective, case-control study. Clinic Transplant. 2013;27:742–8.
65. Ilyas M, Colegio OR, Kaplan B, Sharma A. Cutaneous toxicities from transplant medications. Am J Transplant. 2017;17:2782–9.
66. Raju DL, Bitzan M. Sirolimus-associated chronic pyogenic periungual infection. Kidney Int. 2007;71:476.
67. Valenta JF, Hricik D, Weigel K, Seaman D, Knauss T, Siegel CT et al. Comparison of sirolimus vs. mycophenolate mofetil on surgical complications and wound healing in adult kidney transplantation. Am J Transplant. 2003;3:1128–34.
68. Džambová M, Sečníková Z, Jiráková A, Juzlová K, Viklick O, Hoškova L et al. Malignant melanoma in organ transplant recipients: incidence, outcomes and management strategies: a review of the literature. Dermatol Therapy. 2016;29:64–8.
69. Tavares LL, Costa JCMD, Delcourt NC, Rodrigues NCDS. Periungual basal cell carcinoma. An Bras Dermatol. 2018;93(1):114–15.
70. Rebecca MA, Craft RO, Smith AA. Digital Merkel cell carcinoma. Can J Plast Surg. 2005;13(4):199–202.
71. Lee DY. Kaposi sarcoma mimicking pyogenic granuloma below the toenail. Int J Dermatol. 2014;53:e202–e204.
72. Boix-Vilanova J, Izquierdo-Herce N, Pozo LJ. A refractory periungual lesion. Actas Dermosifiliogr. 2019;110(2):e9–10.

73. Dijksterhuis A, Friedeman E, van der Heijden B. Squamous cell carcinoma of the nail unit: review of the literature. J Hand Surg Am. 2018;43(4):374–9.
74. Haneke E. Important malignant and new nail tumors. J Dtsch Dermatol Ges. 2017;15(4):367–86.
75. Serret CA, Wang S, Marsch A, Hernandez C. Pigmented squamous cell carcinoma presenting as longitudinal melanonychia in transplant recipient. Cutis. 2018;101(5):375–7.
76. Clark MA, Filitis D, Samie FH, Piliang M, Knackstedt TJ. Evaluating the utility of routine imaging in squamous cell carcinoma of the nail unit. Dermatol Surg. 2020:1–8.
77. Gou D, Nijhawan RI, Srivastava D. Mohs micrographic surgery as the standard of care for nail unit squamous cell carcinoma. Dermatol Surg. 2019:1–8.
78. Shimizu A, Kuriyama Y, Hasegawa M, Tamura A, Ishikawa O. Nail squamous cell carcinoma: a hidden high-risk human papilloma virus reservoir for sexually transmitted infections. J Am Acad Dermatol. 2019;81:1358–70.
79. Riddel C, Rashid R, Thomas V. Ungual and periungual human papilloma virus—associated squamous cell carcinoma: a review. J Am Acad Dermatol. 2011;64:1147, 1153.
80. Omerod E, de Berker D. Nail unit squamous cell carcinoma in people with immunosuppression. Br J Dermatol. 2015;173:701–12.
81. Göktay F, Kaynak E, Günes P, Yasar S, Küçükodaci Z, Aytekin S. Relationship between human papilloma virus and subungual keratoacanthoma: two case reports and the outcomes of surgical treatment. Skin Appendage Disord. 2016;2:92–6.
82. Mundada P, Becker M, Lenoir V, Stefanelli S, Rougemont AL, Beaulieu JY, Boudabbous S. High resolution MRI of nail tumors and tumor-like conditions. Eur J Radiol. 2019;112:93–105.
83. Lazar A, Abimelec P, Dumontier C. Full thickness skin graft for nail reconstruction. J Hand Surg. 2005;30B(2):194–8.
84. Haneke E. Advanced nail surgery. J Cut Aesthetic Surg. 2011;4(3):167–75.
85. Sung W, Sam H, Deleyiannis FWB. Subungual squamous cell carcinoma after organ transplantation. J Am Podiatr Med Assoc. 2010;100(4):304–8.
86. Zwald F, Leitenberger J, Zeitouni N, Soon S, Brewer J, Arron S et al. Recommendations for solid organ transplantation for transplant candidates with a pretransplant diagnosis of cutaneous squamous cell carcinoma, merkel cell carcinoma and melanoma: a consensus opinion from the international transplant skin cancer collaborative (ITSCC). Am J Transplant. 2016 Feb;16(2):407–13.
87. Lee WJ, Lee JH, Won CH, Chang SE, Choi JH, Moon KC, Lee MW. Nail apparatus melanoma: a comparative, clinical and morphological characteristics of 49 patients. J Am Acad Dermatol. 2015;73:213–20.
88. Krunic AL, Wang LC, Soltani K, Weizul S, Taylor RS. Digital anesthesia with epinephrine: an old myth revisited. J Am Acad Dermatol. 2004;51(5):755–9.

How to Build a Transplant Dermatology Clinic

17

Amarachi Eseonu, Kristin Bibee, and Manisha Loss

INTRODUCTION

Improvements in immunosuppressive medication regimens have increased the longevity of graft function and prolonged survival of solid organ transplant recipients (SOTRs); however, this longevity has also put SOTRs at increased risk for multiple skin-related complications as highlighted elsewhere in this book.[1] Dermatologic conditions also impact SOTRs beyond their medical burden. A questionnaire-based study showed that dermatologic complications significantly impaired quality of life measures in patients undergoing extensive posttransplant immunosuppressive therapy.[2] These patients warrant subspecialty care, which would provide surveillance, prompt diagnosis, treatment, and appropriate education to SOTRs.

Transplant medicine physicians often assume many of the primary care responsibilities for SOTRs; yet, the atypical presentation and location of skin cancers within SOTRs can make a prompt diagnosis quite difficult for physicians who do not regularly examine subtle skin lesions.[3] The existence of dermatologic input in the care of transplant patients therefore plays an essential role by facilitating the surveillance and prevention of skin diseases as well as the management of cancers as they arise.[2] Furthermore, consideration should be made to develop a subspecialty clinic within dermatology focused on the care of these patients. This recommendation is evident in a study that showed significantly lower photoprotective measures and level of skin cancer awareness in SOTRs who did not attend a specialty dermatology clinic.[4] The main missions of this subspecialty clinic include creating an accessible environment that provides opportunities for SOTRs to be seen in the dermatology clinic, including coordination amongst multiple subspecialties, providing pre- and posttransplant surveillance and treatment of a variety of cutaneous findings, such as medication-induced side effects, as well as thoroughly educating not only the patients, but also colleagues and the community, on skin cancer risk factors and preventative measures.

The purpose of this chapter is to outline vital steps in creating a specialized dermatology clinic for transplant patients. Overall, the care of SOTRs can occur in three major clinical settings as depicted in Figure 17.1: a multidisciplinary transplant clinic, a designated transplant dermatology specialty clinic, or an integration of transplant recipients into an existing medical or surgical dermatology clinic.[5] It is therefore important to apply key elements of this chapter into the clinical setting that is most appropriate for your practice.

DOI: 10.1201/9781003001461-17

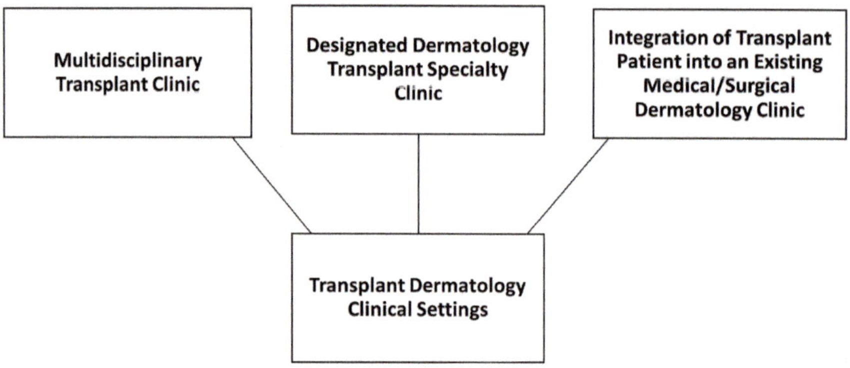

FIGURE 17.1 Various settings of transplant dermatology clinics.

STEPS TO BUILD A TRANSPLANT CLINIC

Initial Steps

Each practice model has the potential of providing the specialized care needed for this patient population. Which model is used, however, will depend on a multitude of factors. Regardless of the practice model, "buy in" from colleagues is essential. In the setting of the multidisciplinary transplant clinic and designated transplant specialty clinic in an academic setting, this may entail first speaking with other faculty members, including those within the dermatology department, such as the Chair, as well as the transplant team, to ensure support. It is important to recognize the rapport colleagues have established with these patients and assure them that this clinic is a resource. If SOTRs are being integrated into a general dermatology clinic, early recognition of dermatology physicians who feel comfortable seeing transplant patients is essential. Early recognition will allow for the prompt participation of these physicians in the set-up process, including clinic scheduling changes and patient recruitment. Communication with the transplant patients is also important to determine their comfort level with these changes. As previously noted, rapport is critical in the effective treatment of SOTRs; therefore, these patients must also be agreeable to shifts in practice models.

Clinic space will likely be variable depending on availability. It may be beneficial to use surgical units, which are larger and give more space to perform procedures, especially in a patient population that may require multiple biopsies. Co-location with other specialists may afford patients that travel long-distance convenience but is also dependent on your practice model.

Funding

In many practice models, no additional funding is necessary as clinical revenue generated from the evaluation and management of this patient population, even when fewer patients per session are seen than in a traditional general dermatology clinic, will likely cover the fixed costs of running the clinic given the higher incidence of diagnostic procedures performed compared with that of the general dermatology population. However, if the majority of patients are allotted additional time to enable more patient education, or an additional staff member is hired to provide more intensive patient education, that additional cost may need to be covered by the department. In developing a revenue model, one must consider the potential of this patient population to feed into additional services that the department oversees, such as dermatopathology and dermatologic surgery for appropriate tumors, as this patient population tends to have higher utilization of diagnostic and therapeutic services. By capturing these patients in a general dermatology clinic, additional service lines within the department will benefit.

Unless the subspecialty patient appointments are part of a general dermatology clinic session, there may not be enough patients to support an entire clinical session initially. If this issue is the case, consider seeing general dermatology patients in the open appointment slots initially to financially support the resources and gradually phase out those appointments as the specialty demand grows.

Key Support Staff

In considering the need for support staff, there are two main streams of the patient encounter: the staff needed for the actual visit and the pre- and post-appointment contact. During the visit, key support staff include front desk staff for check-in/out purposes and medical assistants to room patients and setup for procedures. For transplant clinics located in an academic institution, involvement of residents and/or medical students during the visit is a good learning opportunity, when permitted. Pre- and post-appointment patient contact will benefit from assigned support staff members, especially for patients who require frequent visits and telephone follow up. Assigned staff members assist with triaging biopsy results and coordination of care, i.e., referrals between providers, because SOTRs often require a multidisciplinary team. It is important to note that these duties can be performed by a skilled registered nurse (RN). If an RN is not available, a medical assistant or other clinical staff with appropriate training and review of scope of practice in your state can also be employed.

Access and Scheduling

One resounding benefit of a subspecialty clinic is streamlined access to dermatologic care for this high-risk group. Given the high demand for dermatology services in various regions, patients have to wait several months prior to receiving care. It is important to establish a system of easy access for both the patient and their transplant team to make appointments. Many patients travel a significant distance for their transplant care. By providing coordination of appointments on same or adjacent days to their transplant medicine appointments, access will be easier and patient volume will be higher. For example, some transplant specialties in academic institutions have dedicated clinic days at which time the majority of transplant visits occur. It may be beneficial to communicate with transplant clinics to determine the day(s) of the week that the majority of SOTRs are seen in order to establish your transplant dermatology clinic on these same day(s). If transplant clinics see SOTRs every single day of the week, and this is not feasible for your clinic, it is up to you to determine the most appropriate day(s) based on your clinical setting. In urgent situations, it may also be important to provide an available clinic phone number or teledermatology platform for communication.

The frequency of the subspecialty clinic or specialty appointment slots within a dermatology schedule will depend on the anticipated volume. Clinics may be held one to two times per month or as frequently as multiple times per week based on clinical need and departmental support. Leveraging scheduling logic and automatic scheduling tools can facilitate schedule utilization and conversion to non-specialty appointments to flex capacity as needed. Appointment slot times usually range from 15 to 30 minutes for both new and established patient visits. Variability in the needs of each patient make it difficult to differentiate appointment types. For example, a new transplant patient visit may take only 10 minutes for a routine skin evaluation whereas an established transplant patient, who has an extensive skin cancer history, may take up to 45 minutes. The number of patients per clinic is dependent on the amount of support staff available.

If transplant patients are integrated into a general dermatology clinic, the frequency of transplant clinics is dependent on the original existing general dermatology clinic schedule. This setup is beneficial in the beginning as transplant referrals can be slow at first, allowing for the rest of the slots to be filled by general dermatology visits.

Regardless of the practice model, accessibility is an important theme. Add-on slots should be available during clinic in case a transplant patient has an emergency for a new or changing dermatologic problem that needs to be taken care of.

The Referral System

One challenge in establishing a subspecialty clinic is creating a referral system for the clinic. In many institutions, there is not an established referral system for SOTRs to be seen by a dermatologist. There are five main types of patients that will be seen within the dermatology transplant subspecialty clinic:

1. Pretransplant evaluation.
2. SOTRs with an established skin cancer history.
3. SOTRs at high risk of posttransplant malignancy and need for regular dermatologic surveillance.
4. SOTRs at low risk of posttransplant malignancy needing periodic "spot checks"/skin surveillance.
5. Pre- or posttransplantation patients needing nonmalignancy-related dermatologic care, such as skin health education and evaluation of medication reactions, skin infections, inflammatory conditions, etc.

It is important to note that initial skin screening for SOTRs may vary based on your institutional guidelines; however, in 2019, Crow et al.[6] proposed a standardized approach based upon a multidisciplinary expert panel. Recommendations include initial screenings within 2 years of transplant for high-risk Caucasian SOTRs and within 5 years for low-risk Caucasian, Asian, Hispanic, and high-risk African American SOTRs. High-risk characteristics include a thoracic organ transplant, male sex, and age >50 years at the time of transplant.[6] For SOTRs without established dermatologic care pretransplant, not only should the transplant team be educated on the importance of referrals, but the SOTRs should also be educated on the significance of seeing a dermatologist. Education can be done through talks at grand rounds, transplant clinics, and SOTR support groups as well as the distribution of flyers to various transplant clinics both within and outside your institution. The media, i.e., use of society websites, can also be used to target a broader dermatology audience, especially those within the community. The transplant team can also be educated on the use of the Skin and Ultraviolet Neoplasia Transplant Risk Assessment Calculator (SUNTRAC), which is a simple tool used to help transplant providers assess the need for patient referrals for skin cancer screening.[7] It will also be important to determine whether a referral system can be created within the electronic medical record (EMR) at the institution that can be easily accessed by the transplant team and sent directly to the dermatology transplant clinic schedulers. This system should also include a space for the time frame of when the patient needs to be seen.

For SOTRs with already established dermatologic care pretransplant, it will be important to target the SOTRs, themselves, as well as their outside providers, whether it be in the local community or at another institution. Many of these transplant recipients, as well as SOTRs without a prior dermatologist, will prefer a local provider for their dermatologic surveillance because of better accessibility and availability. Communication and coordination should be established with the local dermatologists about when SOTRs should be seen at the institution, especially in times when conditions are worsening or changing. Examples include providing modes of communication, e.g., email, phone, or pager, which can be used by local providers to reach your clinic. SOTRs should also be educated to recognize the threshold of when to be referred to a dermatologist.

The Visit

As with any dermatology clinic, the type of appointment will vary. The majority of visits will likely be full skin evaluations given the potential complexity of SOTRs; however, this should be tailored to the individual patient. Additionally, follow-up appointments for evaluation of conditions that do not require a full skin check may be built into the schedule. For example, a patient may only warrant annual skin surveillance given his or her risk factors for skin cancer but may need to be seen in 6–8 weeks to follow up on treatment of tinea pedis. That same patient may also have a new lesion of concern and be scheduled for a spot check appointment in the interim.

Common procedures done during the visit include cryotherapy and skin biopsies. Other procedures, including electrodessication and curettage (ED&C), chemo wraps, and photodynamic therapy may require an additional visit. A streamlined system to expedite care provided by other dermatology specialists (e.g., Mohs surgery) is recommended given the higher risk of skin cancer in this patient population.

The transplant dermatology clinic visit is also an opportunity to advertise, recruit, and discuss available clinical trials with SOTRs, which can be beneficial to the SOTRs. A study by Hartman et al.[9] showed an increase in sun protective behaviors in SOTRs after participating in a skin cancer research study.

In conclusion, we found that use of multiple sun protection behaviors increased among organ transplant recipients after participation in a skin cancer research study.

The Clinic Note

Each visit should include an associated visit note. All notes, except for procedure-only visit notes, should include three main sections: history of present illness (HPI), physical examination, and assessment.

The following are essential points to include in the note:

- Transplanted organ(s), reason for transplant, and date of transplant.
- Immunosuppressive medication list, preferably with start and end dates.
- Prophylactic medications (e.g., trimethoprim-sulfamethoxazole [TMP-SMX], voriconazole, acyclovir).
- List of prior skin cancers, location, year diagnosed, and treatment used.
- List of other viral dermatologic conditions, e.g., warts, herpes simplex virus (HSV).

The Importance of Education

Patient education is an important aspect of the visit and should include information on the appearance of skin cancers, the patient's individual risk factors, and preventative measures, including daily use of sunscreens, hat use, midday sun avoidance, and chemopreventative methods, when appropriate. It is important to note that education should occur, in some format, at each visit. Work done by Skiveren et al.[8] showed that one of the main reasons for insufficient sun protective behavior within the renal transplant patient population was that skin cancers were considered minor health problems in comparison with the risk of rejecting their kidneys. Frequent conversations serve as a reminder of the importance of photoprotection on the prevention of skin cancers. Mudigonda et al.[2] showed that patients who received more intensive educational intervention were more adherent to recommendations for sun-protective behavior than those who received standard education.

The way in which education is provided, however, may vary. Methods include verbal discussions with the patient during the visit, educational pamphlets, or media, such as referral to the International Immunosuppression and Transplant Skin Cancer Collaborative (ITSCC) website. Conflicting data exist regarding which method of education is most effective and may have a generational divide.[10] A study by Traboulsi et al.[11] suggested that patients prefer to receive information verbally and through pamphlets, whereas Trinh et al.[12] showed that video education was more effective at increasing patient knowledge. The positive influence of educational videos was further supported by a study done by Patel et al.[13] that showed that the use of videos increased patient knowledge and positively influenced sun-protective behaviors. Sachse et al.[14] showed the use of text-messaging as a reminder to patients to use sunscreens doubled sunscreen application when compared with that of controls; however, this was only well accepted amongst young SOTRs, suggesting that multimedia methods may not be as effective among older patients, who are considered at higher risk of skin cancer development.[11]

Recognition that patients are receiving education about a number of health-related measures in the pre- and immediate postoperative period can influence the education provided at each visit. SOTRs have many other transplant-related worries to deal with, which makes it difficult for them to retain essential information about sun-protective behaviors.[3,8]

The Multidisciplinary Team

The transplant patient's multidisciplinary team is a vital part of care. Many of these patients have complex medical histories that need the attention of multiple subspecialties, many of whom have dealt with similar patients. The team can be divided into five main categories: oncology, surgery, transplant, dermatology, and primary care.

Oncology includes:

- Medical oncology
- Radiation oncology

Surgery includes:

- Mohs micrographic surgery
- Otolaryngology
- Surgical oncology
- Plastic and reconstructive surgery

The transplant team includes:

- Transplant Coordinator
- The medical specialty focusing on the transplanted organ (e.g., Pulmonology, Cardiology, Hepatology, Nephrology)
- Transplant Infectious Disease
- Primary Care (especially when involved in immunosuppression management)

Dermatology includes:

- General dermatology
- Dermatopathology
- Cutaneous oncology

The transplant coordinator is a key individual in the effective coordination and communication among all the above subspecialties, as this is the person who first manages questions and concerns about the patient, and it will therefore be important to exchange contact information between this coordinator and other subspecialties.

It is important to acknowledge that the frequency of communication among the various subspecialties may vary. For example, coordinated care with oncology subspecialties tends to occur mainly for the treatment of complex skin cancers. Despite this potentially limited interaction, avenues to communicate with oncology should be readily available because of the increased risk of recurrence and spread in this patient population. On the other hand, constant communication with transplant medicine teams, e.g., pulmonary or infectious disease, will likely occur because this is usually the primary care team for the patient that manages day-to-day transplant surveillance, including medication monitoring. For example, discussion about adjustments in immunosuppressive medications with the transplant team may occur after dermatology evaluation of SOTRs if they exhibit significant cutaneous medication-induced side effects.

The Tumor Board

Many academic institutions have a multidisciplinary consensus conference to allow for the discussion of cancer care. These "Tumor Boards" are often composed of medical oncologists, radiation oncologists, and surgical oncologists. We recommend participation in the local Tumor Board that has the best representation for treatment of skin malignancies. It is important to note that each institution may have different boards, so finding the one that will help guide high-risk squamous cell carcinomas, as well as melanomas, may be challenging.

CONCLUSION

In conclusion, regardless of whether SOTRs are integrated into an existing general dermatology clinic or seen within a multidisciplinary transplant center, it is important to incorporate the following key elements to ensure an overall successful transplant dermatology clinic as seen in Figure 17.2:

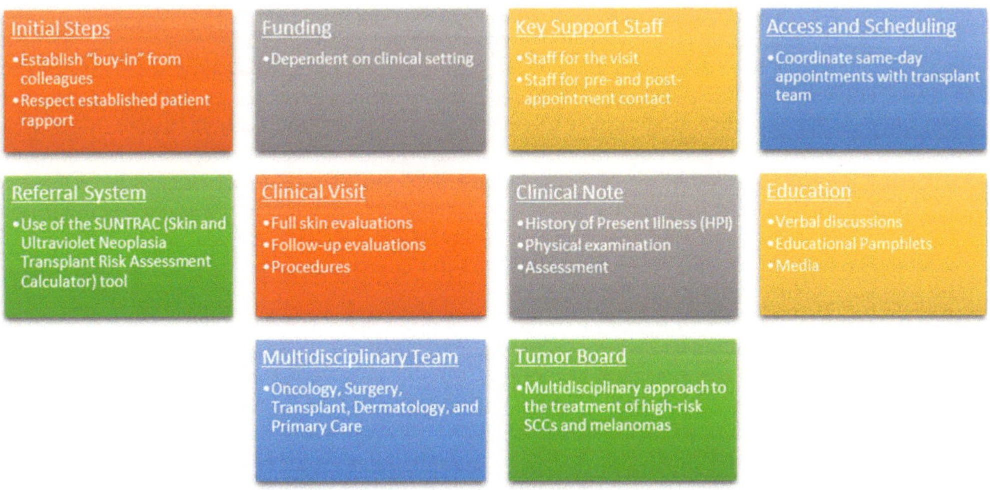
Initial Steps
•Establish "buy-in" from colleagues
•Respect established patient rapport
Funding
•Dependent on clinical setting
Key Support Staff
•Staff for the visit
•Staff for pre- and post-appointment contact
Access and Scheduling
•Coordinate same-day appointments with transplant team
Referral System
•Use of the SUNTRAC (Skin and Ultraviolet Neoplasia Transplant Risk Assessment Calculator) tool
Clinical Visit
•Full skin evaluations
•Follow-up evaluations
•Procedures
Clinical Note
•History of Present Illness (HPI)
•Physical examination
•Assessment
Education
•Verbal discussions
•Educational Pamphlets
•Media
Multidisciplinary Team
•Oncology, Surgery, Transplant, Dermatology, and Primary Care
Tumor Board
•Multidisciplinary approach to the treatment of high-risk SCCs and melanomas

FIGURE 17.2 Summary of key points in starting a transplant dermatology clinic.

SUMMARY OF KEY POINTS

- Provide pre- and posttransplant surveillance and treatment.
- Provide proper education to the patients, colleagues, and the community.
- Create an accessible environment that provides multiple opportunities for SOTRs to be seen in the clinic.
- Utilize the power of a multidisciplinary team to ensure a well-rounded treatment experience through coordination and communication.

REFERENCES

1. Euvrard S, Kanitakis J, Claudy A. Skin cancers after organ transplantation. N Engl J Med. 2003;348(17):1681–91.
2. Mudigonda T, Levender MM, O'Neill JL, West CE, Pearce DJ, Feldman SR. Incidence, risk factors, and preventative management of skin cancers in organ transplant recipients: a review of single- and multicenter retrospective studies from 2006 to 2010. Dermatol Surg. 2013;39(3 Pt 1):345–64.
3. Cowen EW, Billingsley EM. Awareness of skin cancer by kidney transplant patients. J Am Acad Dermatol. 1999;40(5 Pt 1):697–701.
4. Ismail F, Mitchell L, Casabonne D et al. Specialist dermatology clinics for organ transplant recipients significantly improve compliance with photoprotection and levels of skin cancer awareness. Br J Dermatol. 2006;155(5):916–25.
5. Christenson LJ, Geusau A, Ferrandiz C et al. Specialty clinics for the dermatologic care of solid-organ transplant recipients. Dermatol Surg. 2004;30(4 Pt 2):598–603.
6. Crow LD, Jambusaria-Pahlajani A, Chung CL et al. Initial skin cancer screening for solid organ transplant recipients in the United States: Delphi method development of expert consensus guidelines. Transpl Int. 2019;32(12):1268–76.
7. Jambusaria-Pahlajani A, Crow LD, Lowenstein S et al. Predicting skin cancer in organ transplant recipients: development of the SUNTRAC screening tool using data from a multicenter cohort study. Transpl Int. 2019;32(12):1259–67.
8. Skiveren J, Mortensen EL, Haedersdal M. Sun protective behaviour in renal transplant recipients: a qualitative study based on individual interviews and the health belief model. J Dermatolog Treat. 2010;21(6):331–6.
9. Hartman RI, Green AC, Gordon LG. Skin tumours and allograft recipients (STAR) study: sun protection among organ transplant recipients after participation in a skin cancer research study. JAMA Dermatol. 2018;154(7):842–4.
10. James LJ, Saglimbene V, Wong G et al. Behavioural and pharmaceutical interventions for the prevention of skin cancers in solid organ transplant recipients: a systematic review of randomised controlled trials. BMJ Open. 2020 May 17;10(5):e029265.
11. Traboulsi D, Potok OV, Ruzycki SM et al. Skin cancer knowledge and photoprotective practices of organ transplant recipients. Clin Transplant. 2019;33(5):e13524.
12. Trinh N, Novice K, Lekakh O, Means A, Tung R. Use of a brief educational video administered by a portable video device to improve skin cancer knowledge in the outpatient transplant population. Dermatol Surg. 2014;40(11):1233–9.
13. Patel PH, Bibee K, Lim G, Malik SM, Wu C, Pugliano-Mauro M. Evaluating retention of skin cancer education in kidney transplant recipients reveals a window of opportunity for re-education. Transplant Proc. 2017;49(6):1318–24.
14. Sachse MM, Böttcher S, Pape L et al. Face-to-face sun protection training and text messages improve sun protection behaviour in adolescent organ transplant recipients: hippolino feasibility study. Acta Derm Venereol. 2016;96(3):341–5.

Index

Note: Numbers in **bold** indicate a table. Numbers in *italics* indicate a figure on the corresponding page.

5-Fluorouracil (5-FU), 64
  intralesional, 72
  see also, chemowraps
5-year survival rate
  melanoma, 124
  Merkel cell carcinoma (MCC), 179–182
  squamous cell carcinoma (SCC) 10, 43, 156, 161
  SCC nail apparatus, 284

A

ablative fractional carbon dioxide laser (AFXL) 68, 85–87, **94**
acitretin
  as chemoprophylaxis, 53–54, 57, 70
  as chemoprevention, 53, 55, 144, 147
  nail changes secondary to use of, 281
  paronychia induced by, 281–282
acneiform eruption, 253
acquired immunodeficiency syndrome (AIDS), 173–174, 189, *222*
actinic keratoses (AKs)
  acitretin, 53
  identification, 38, **44**
  field cancerization, 63
  HPV associated with, 282
  hyperkeratotic, 64
  management of, 53–54
  nicotinamide, 54–55
  photodynamic therapy for, 82, 85–93, **94**
  sunscreens impact on, 52
  therapy, field-directed, 57
  topical treatment options for, *65*, **69**
Actinomycetales, 221
actinomycosis, 221
acyclovir, 238, 276, 297
  resistance to, 238
adnexal tumor, 193
adrenal insufficiency, 250
AFX, *see* atypical fibroxanthoma
AFXL, *see* ablative fractional carbon dioxide laser (AFXL)
AJCC, *see* American Joint Committee on Cancer (AJCC)
alemtuzumab (Campath), 26
allograft
  antibodies against, 31
  checkpoint inhibitor therapy, **132**
  and imiquimod, 54, 67
  and immune system of host, suppression of, 23, 118, 121, **126–127**
  and immunosuppression, risks of decreasing, 192, 200
  implantation, 27
  induction therapy for, 27
  and interferon (IFN), **73**, 76, 192
  and nephrotoxicity, 25
  and PDT, 93
  rejection, 24, 32, 56, 131, 209–210
  survival, 2, 31
  and T-cell activation, 205, 206
  and thrombotic microangiopathy, 25
  and viral skin infection, 235
Alternaria spp., **226**, 232, 234, 270
  A. infectoria, *233*
alternariosis *233*
alopecia
  azathioprine-induced, 266
  and immunosuppressant therapy, 252, 255–256
  tacrolimus, associated with, 107, 252, 257
  and Trichodysplasia spinulosa (TS), 104
  and transplant surgery, 106
American Joint Committee on Cancer (AJCC)
  cancer stage-based model, 124
  cancer staging manual, 6th edition, 129
  cancer staging manual, 7th edition (AJCC-7), 124, 152–153, 158
  cancer staging manual, 8th edition (AJCC-8), 154–155, 158, 160, 164, 178, 195
  immune status, inclusion of, 161
  TMN system, 128, 178
AMERK test, 182
antimetabolites, 26, **29**, 30
  see also, azathioprine
anti-thymocyte globulin (ATG), 247, 257
  rabbit, 26–27, 32
aphthous stomatitis, 253, 256
aspergillosis, *231*
Aspergillus spp., 217
  A. flavus, **226**, 269
  A. fumigatus, **226**, 228, 232, 231, 269, 272
  A. niger, **226**, 232, 269
  fungal infections due to, 225, **226**
  nail fold involvement, 271
  onychomycosis caused by, 272
ATG, *see* anti-thymocyte globulin (ATG)
atherosclerosis, 288, **288**
atopic dermatitis (AD), 106–108
atypical fibroxanthoma (AFX), 195–197, 200
azathioprine, 2, 6–7, **8**, **12**, **14**
  alopecia induced by, 255
  as cutaneous malignancy risk factor, 204
  for immunosuppression, **28**, 193, 195, 255
  and Merkel cell carcinoma (MCC), 182
  as melanoma risk factor, 123, 125–126, 129, 142, 173
  as nonmelanoma risk factor, 255, 257
  and MPA, compared to, 30
  photosensitizing effects of, 142

replaced by newer agents, 55, 129
and T-cells, effect on, 26
and warts, effect on, 277
azathioprine hypersensitivity syndrome, 255–256
azole antifungals, 225
C. krusei's resistance to, 229
efinaconazole, 273
fluconazole, 229, 273, 274
itraconazole, 9, **12**, 143, 273–275
posaconazole, **12**, 143, 234
sulfamethoxazole, 75
see also, voriconazole

B

B7, *208*
family receptors, 256
ligands, 206, 257
protein, 57
see also, belatacept
Bacillary angiomatosis (BA), 222, *222*
bacterial skin infections (BSIs), 219
Bartonella
B. henselae, **220**, 222, 269
B. quintana, 222
basal cell carcinoma (BCC), 4–6, 99–101, 139
belatacept, 57
bleomycin, 72
cure rate, 157
imaging modalities in detection of, **37**
imiquimod, 71
infiltrative (iBCC), 40, 71
intralesional therapies for, **72–73**
nail apparatus, involvement of, 281
nicotinamide, 55
nodular (nBCC), 40, 43, 71, 82, 86
nonpigmented, 38
optical coherence tomography (OCT) used to diagnose, 41
photodynamic therapy (PDT), 71, **86–87**, 88
pigmented, 39
reflectance confocal microscopy (RCM) used to diagnose, 40
risk factors, 9–10, **11–12**, **17**, 51
superficial (sBCC), 42, 54, 63, 67, 83, 84
basiliximab, 26, 27, 248, 257
basosquamous cell carcinoma (BSCC), 9–10
BCC, *see* basal cell carcinoma (BCC)
belatacept, 25, **29**, 31, 57, 256
Blastomyces dermatitidis, **227**, 234
bleomycin, 75
bone marrow
suppression, 26, **28–29**
transplantation, *234*
Bowen's disease 38, 85, 277, 279, 281, *282*
see also, squamous cell carcinoma in situ (SCCis)
BRAF, *121*, 129–130, **207**
Brigham and Women's Hospital (BWH) staging system, 153–155, 158, 160–164
BSCC, *see* basosquamous cell carcinoma (BSCC)
Buschke-Löwenstein tumor, *240*

C

calcineurin inhibitors (CNIs), 25–26, 250
cyclosporine, 2, **29**
early manifestations, 250
and gingival hyperplasia, 250–251
and hypertrichosis, 251
immunosuppression, used for, 28, **29**
mTOR inhibitors as replacement for, 30–31
and skin cancer, 7
sirolimus vs., 57
see also, tacrolimus
Candida spp., 217–218, 225, 228, 229, **271**
acute and chronic paronychia, cause of, 267
anticandidal therapy, 279
antigen, 287
and artificial nails, 269
C. albicans, **226**, 228, 229, 269, **271**, 273
C. balanitis, 226
C. glabrata, **226**, 229
C. guiellermoni, 232
C. krusei, **226**, 228
C. parapsilosis, **226**, 229
C. tropicalis, **226**
fluconazole as treatment for infection by, **273**
onychomycosis (OM), as cause of, 270, **273**, 286
Candidiasis, 228
capecitabine, 55, 144, 145
cat-scratch disease, *see* Bacillary angiomatosis (BA)
CAVATEK (coxsackievirus A21), 213
cellulitis, 217, 219–220, **226–227**
Cryptococcus spp. as cause of, 232, *232*
and fingernails, surgery on, **288**
necrotizing, **227**
P. aeruginosa responsible for, 221
chemoprophylaxis
acitretin, 53, 59, 71
chemoprevention, 53, 144
acitretin, 53, 57, 144, 147
nicotinamide, 54–55
and OTRs and pOTRS, literature on, 102
chemowraps, 66–67, **69**
chloronychia, *see* green nail syndrome
ciclopirox olamine, 273, **273**
cidofovir, 76
Coccidioides 217
C.immitis **227**, 234
Paracoccidioides brasiliensis, **228**
corticosteroids, 248
cellular rejection, used for treatment of, 31
commonly used, 26
Cushing syndrome as side effect of, 249
early manifestations, 248
late manifestation, 249
steroid acne, 248
prednisone, 26, **29**
systemic use of, 2
topical, 102, 108
cortisol, 249
cryotherapy, 63
Cryptococcus, 225
A. neoformans, 217, 228, 232
Curvularia spp., **226**

Cushing syndrome, 249–250, 257
cutaneous squamous cell carcinoma (cSCC), 119, 139–147, 181, **208**
 and antifungal agents, 142
 adjuvant radiation therapy for, 159–161
 BRAF inhibitor monotherapy to reduce incidence of, 131
 capecitabine to reduce, 55
 commonality of, 82, 139, 204
 epidemiology, 139–140
 hematopoietic cell transplant recipients, risk of, 142
 high risk, 45
 HPV associated with, 141
 and immunosuppression, 56, 142
 incidence of, 87
 Mohs micrographic surgery (MMS), treatment with, 152, 157–159
 NCCN guidelines for, 152
 oncogenic viruses, role of, 141
 pathogenesis, 141
 prevention of (in OTRCs) 143–145
 rapamycin (mTOR) inhibitor to treat, 152
 risk factors for, 146, 150–151
 risk of, 5, 6, 9, 51
 sentinel lymph node biopsy (SLNB) to diagnose, 161–163
 spindle cell, 196
 staging systems for, 153–157, 158, 160–164
 see also, squamous cell carcinoma (SCC); thoracic transplants
cyclin-dependent kinase inhibitor 2A (CDKN2A), 119
cyclooxygenase (COX) inhibitors, 63
cyclooxygenase-2, 68
cyclosporine (CyA), 2, 6–7, **8**, **15**
 AFX, 195
 belatacept compared to, 31
 changes induced by, 106
 and children, 108
 and dermato brosarcoma protuberans (DFSP), 199
 hirsutism associated with, 25, 30, 106
 and Kaposi's sarcoma, risk of, 191
 and melanoma, risk of, 125–126, 129
 and Merkel cell carcinoma (MCC), risk of, 173, 181
 neurotoxicity associated with, 25
 and pediatric organ transplant recipients, **104**
 survival rates associated with, 13
 and T-cells, effect on, 142
 usage and adverse effects of, **29**
cytomegalovirus (CMV), 235, 275–276
 and aphthous ulcers, 254, 256
 clinical criteria to diagnose, **221**
 cutaneous findings with, 237
 everolimus to treat, **29**
 human herpesvirus (HHV) as co-pathogen, 238, 275
 nail and periungual area, infections of, 275–276
 sirolimus to treat, **29**
 organ transplant, infection timeline following, *218*
 tissue-invasive, 30
cytotoxic T-lymphocyte-associated antigen 4 (CTLA-4), **29**, 57, 131
 blockade, 182, 206
 discovery and FDA approval of, 206, **207**

D

dabrafenib, 130–131
dapsone, 256
dematiaceous fungi, **226–227**, 232, 234
dermato brosarcoma protuberans (DFSP), 198–201
DFSP *see* dermato brosarcoma protuberans (DFSP)
diabetes mellitus, 263
 adult-onset, **266**
 chronic paronychia, risk factor, 267
 fungal infections of the nail apparatus, 269
 nail surgery, 287
 new onset, 30
diclofenac, 54, 68, **69**
 sodium, 85
dimorphic fungi, **227**, 229, 234
distal lateral subungual onychomycosis (DLSO), 270, **271**, 271
DLSO, *see* distal lateral subungual onychomycosis (DLSO)
dyslipidemia, 26, 31

E

ecthyma, 219, **220**
 gangrenosum, 219, 269
endonyx OM (EO), **271**, 271
endothelium, lymphatic,190
Epstein-Barr virus (EBV)
 infection, 25
 -naïve status, 102
 oral papulosis with, *239*
 seronegative, 57
 viral skin infection, 235
everolimus, 2, 30
 dosing schedule, 16
 drug interactions, 131
 immunosuppression maintenance and therapy, **29**, 56, 125, 253
 and Karposi's sarcoma, 191
 keratinocyte cancers, risk of, 57
 and skin malignancies, risk of, 205
 and warts, effect on, 277
 and wound healing, effect on, 255

F

FAT1, 174
felon (infection), 267, 269, **288**
field-based therapy, 53–54
fluconazole, 273–274
folliculitis, 219, **220**, **226**, 228
 bacterial, 219
 cutaneous candidiasis presenting as, 229
 pityrosporum, 229, 249
fungal skin infection, 225–234
 classical, 225
 opportunistic, 225–234
 rare, 234
furuncles, 219, **220**, 269
Fusarium spp., **227**, 234, 269–271, **271**, 274

G

gingival hyperplasia
 calcineurin inhibitors and, 251–252
 cyclosporine and, 25, 106, 257
gingivectomy, 251
graft-versus-host disease (GVHD), 109
graft rejection, 209

graft loss, 209
granulocyte-macrophage colony-stimulating factor (GM-CSF), 133, 212
granuloma, 222–225, **228**
 Majocci's, 229
 pyogenic, 269, *280*, 281, **288**
green nail syndrome, 267, 269, 272, 287

H

heart/lung transplants 7–8
 basil cell carcinoma (BCC), risk of **11**
 graft loss, 209, 211
 immunosuppression and malignancy risk, 125–126
 Kaposi's sarcoma, risk of, 188–189
 melanoma, risk of **14**, 122, 129, 130, 133
 squamous cell carcinoma (SCC), risk of, 140, 147, 159
 survival rates, 193
herpes simplex virus (HSV), *218*, 219, **220**, 235, 267
 acyclovir to treat, 236
 and aphthous ulcers, 256
 cytomegalovirus (CMV), coinfection with, 275
 nail apparatus, infections caused by, 275
 paronychia coinfected with, 267
herpes simplex virus-1 (HSV-1), 213, **220**, 235
herpes simplex virus-2 (HSV-2), 235, *237*
herpes vegetans, *237*
herpes zoster (HZ), 236
herpetic whitlow, 275–276
High-Risk Cutaneous cSCC Workgroup of the Association of Professors of Dermatology, 163
Histoplasma capsulatum 217, **227**, 234
Hormographiella aspergillata, 233
HPV, *see* human papilloma virus (HPV)
human herpesvirus (HHV), **220**, 235–238
human herpesvirus-8 (HHV-8), **220**
 and Kaposi's sarcoma, 16, **18**, 72, 188–190, *191*, 201
human immunodeficiency virus (HIV), 72
human papilloma virus (HPV), 76, 217–218, 238–239
 α-HPV strains, 141, 283
 β-HPV strains, 141, 283
 bacterial and skin lesions, critical criteria for, **221**
 HPV-6, *240*, 278, 283
 HPV-7, 101
 HPV-11, *240*, 278
 HPV-16, 239, 278
 HPV-17, 282
 HPV-18, 239, 278, 282
 HPV-21, 282
 HPV-31, 278
 HPV-33, 278, 282
 HPV-35, 282
 HPV-45, 278
 HPV-49, 282
 HPV-51, 282
 HPV-52, 278
 HPV-56, 282
 HPV-58, 278, 282
 HPV-73, 282
 lesions, 240
 nail apparatus, 275, 276–278, 288
 periungual and subungual, 267, *277*
 subclinical infection with, 235
 transplant associated, 205
 vaccination for, 101–103, 277–278, 284
Hutchinson's sign, 286, *287*
hyperlipidemia, 25
hypertension, 25
hyperthyroidism, 263
hypertrichosis, 30, 248
 suicidal ideation linked to, 106

I

immune checkpoint inhibitors (ICIs), 182, 206–212
impetigo contagiosa, 219, **220**
infection
 cutaneous, 101–106, 109
 lymphocutaneous, **220**, 221
Ingenol mebutate, 63, 68, **69**
interferon (IFN), 72
International immunosuppression and Transplant Skin Cancer Collaborative (ITSCC), 4–5, 101, 146
 American Joint Committee on Cancer (AJCC), creation of cancer staging model 124
 immunosuppression guidelines, 128
 wait times to transplantation, guidelines for 146, 183
 website, referring patients to, 297
ITSCC, *see* International immunosuppression and Transplant Skin Cancer Collaborative (ITSCC)

J

janus kinase, 109

K

Kaposi's sarcoma (KS), 13–16, 72, **73**, 189–193
 HHV-8, 102
keratinocyte carcinoma (KC), 41, 53, 62, **91**
 commonality and risk, of 4–7, 204
 lip, 100
 mTOR inhibitors, effect on, 210
 nerve, *159*
 skin infections, impact on 219
 see also, squamous cell carcinoma (SCC)
kidney
 carcinomas of, 4, 204
 SIR higher in, **11**
kidney transplant, 2, 16, **17**, 23, 27
 and atopic dermatitis, risk of, 106
 and CNIs, 25, 30
 first successful, 122, 247
 giant condylomata acuminata (Buschke-Löwenstein tumor), *240*
 graft loss, 32
 and graft-versus-host disease (GVHD), 109
 with heart, combined, 133
 and Kaposi's sarcoma, *239*
 and MCPyV, 173
 and melanoma risk, 122, **129**
 and Mollusca contagiosa, *241*
 and non-melanoma skin cancer (NMSC), 140
 rejection, **132**, 210

and sebaceous hyperplasia, *252*
sirolimus, impact on, 159
and skin diseases, 218
and squamous cell carcinoma, 43
and steroids, 30
and verrucae vulgares, *240*

L

leukemia, lymphoblastic, 104
leukocytoclastic vasculitis (LCV), 255
leukonychia, 263
classification of, **266**
total, *264*
leukonychia (LKN), 262–264, 265, 280
leukopenia, 26
Lichttheimia spp., **226**, 232
liver transplant recipient (LTR), 2, 6, **11**, 13, 219
early fungal infection, risk of, 225
S. aureus infection, risk of in, 219
lymphadenectomy, **207**
lymphadenitis, **223**, 223
tuberculous, *223*
lymphadenopathy, 161, 237, 269
lymphangitis, 267
lymphatic system, 276
lymphedema, **29**, 31, 254, 257
lymph nodes
basin, 133, 152, 163–164, 181
biopsy, 45
dissection, 146, 161
examination, 155
metastases, 10, 157, **179**, 212
monitoring, 47
sentinel, 45, 101, 128, 285, 286
ultrasonography to evaluate, 156
see also, Kaposi's sarcoma; sentinel lymph node biopsy (SLNB)
lymphatic endothelium, *see* endothelium
lymphedema, **29**, 31, 163, 254
lymphoblastic leukemia, *see* leukemia
lymphocutaneous infection, *see* infection
lymphocyte-depleting therapies, 28, **32**, 33
lymphocytes
allograft, 211
B, 25, 26
intra-tumoral, 183
and Kaposi's sarcoma, 190
and mycophenolate mofetil, 256, 257
T, 23, 126, **28**, **29**, 57, 210
tumor cells between, 43
tumor-infiltrating, 183
see also, cytotoxic T-lymphocyte-associated antigen 4 (CTLA-4)
lymphoma, 4, 53, 177, 204
agents that may cause, 108
lymphoproliferative disorders, 25, 31, 219, 256
see also, posttransplant lymphoproliferative disorders (PTLD)
lymphotropic polyomavirus, 174
lymphovascular invasion, 175
Lynch syndrome, 119, 193–194

M

malignant fibrous histiocytoma (MFH), 195
MAL-PDT, *see* methyl aminolevulinate photodynamic therapy (MAL-PDT)
mammalian target of rapamycin (mTOR)
acneiform eruption, 253
aphthous stomatitis, 253
early manifestations, 253
lymphedema, 254
and Merkel cell carcinoma (MCC), increased risk, 173
palmoplantar peeling, 254
and skin malignancies, 7, 205
mammalian target of rapamycin inhibitors (mTORi)
as immunosuppressant therapy, 125, 152, 191, 253–254
and Kaposi's sarcoma (KS), 16, **18**, 191
and non-malignant skin cancer (NMSC), effect on, 141
PI3K/Akt/mTOR signaling pathway, effect on, 141
and solid organ transplant, 2
and skin cancers, 7, 31, 56, 205
switching to, **9**, 16
warts, treatment of, 277
see also, sirolimus
Mayo Muir-Torre syndrome risk score, *see* Muir-Torre syndrome
MCPyV, *see* Merkel cell polyomavirus (MCPyV)
MEK inhibitors, *130*, 130–131
melanocortin-1 receptor gene, 119
melanocytes, 38–41
atypical, 43, *120*
tumor, 285
melanoma, 10–13
IIIB, IIIC, and IVM1a, 212
acral, 285
clinical features of, 119, 121
cutaneous, 172
deep dermal, 119
dermatological imaging for, 37–47
desmoplastic, 196
donor-derived, 124
epidemiology, 118–119
factors for, 119
and immunity, 121
and immunosuppression, 125–127
invasive, *286*
malignant (MM), 204, **207**, 284–287
markers, 177–178
matrical, 286
metastatic, 206
mucosal, 119
nail apparatus (NAM), 281, 284–287
and nevi, arising from, 119
pathogenesis, 121
pediatric, 99–101
primary, 123
rates of incidence, 281
risk factors for, posttransplant, **12**, **14–15**
and SLNB, recommendation for, 162–163
small cell, 177
in solid organ transplant recipients (SOTRs), 122–133, 211
spitzoid, 119
subungual, *287*
and transplantation, 183

treatment, 127–133
"tumor board" guidance for, 299
see also, nonmelanoma skin cancers (NMSC)
melanonychia, 262–263
striata, 282, 285–286
Merkel cell carcinoma (MCC), 4, 139, 172–183
immune checkpoint inhibitors, **208**
nail involvement with, 281
rate of occurrence, 204
Merkel cell polyomavirus (MCPyV), 173–175, 175–176, 180, 182–183
methicillin-resistant *S. aureus* (MRSA), 219, **220**, 267
methotrexate (MTX), 73–75, **104**
atypical fibroxanthoma (AFX), 196
nonmelanoma skin cancer, 72
pediatric use, 108
methyl aminolevulinate photodynamic therapy (MAL-PDT), 63–65, 68, 70, 85–90, 93
mismatch repair (MMR) protein, 195, 200
mitochondrial permeability transition (MPT), 142
mitogen-activated protein kinase (MAPK) pathway, 129–130
mixed pattern onychomycosis (MPO), **271**
Mohs micrographic surgery (MMS), 69, 297
on children, 100–101
for melanoma, 128
on nail apparatus, 281, 284
surgical defect, *140*
and squamous cell carcinoma, 152, 157–158
transplantation wait time, 146
and wide local incision, 180
Molluscum contagiosum, 104, **221**, **226–227**, 235, 240–241
MPA (antimetabolite), 30
MRSA, *see* methicillin-resistant *S. aureus* (MRSA)
mTOR inhibitor, *see* mammalian target of rapamycin inhibitor (mTORi)
Mucor spp., 232
Mucorales spp., 225, **226**
mucormycosis, **226**, 232
mucosa
buccal, 256
oral, 254, 267, 276
mucosal melanoma, *see* melanoma
mucous membranes, 217–219, **226**, 229
Muir-Torre Syndrome (MTS), 193–195
mycetoma, **220**, **226**
Mycobacterium
disease-causing, classification of, **223**
M. avescens, 224
M. cheloneae/abscessus **223**, 269
M. cosmeticum, 269
M. fortuitum **223**, 269
M. gordonae, 224
M. kansasii, 224
M. marinum, 224
M. szulgai, 224
M. tuberculosis (TB), 222
mycophenolate mofetil (MMF), 6–7, **104**, 256–257

N

nail apparatus melanoma (NAM), 285–286
nail disease in solid organ transplant recipients (SOTRs), 261–289
nail dystrophy, 255
nail surgery, 287–288
National Comprehensive Cancer Network (NCCN) guidelines
for cSCC, 43, 152, 153–157, 159
for dermatofibrosarcoma, 199
for melanoma, 128
for Merkel cell carcinoma (MCC), 179–183
on sun avoidance, 146
Nattrassia mangiferae, **226**, 232, *234*
necrotizing fasciitis, **220**, 219, 267, 269
necrosis
acute tubular, 54, 67
mitochondrial permeability transition (MPT), 142
Merkel cell carcinoma (MCC), 175
Mohs micrographic surgery (MMS), adverse event following, 158
mucormycosis leading to, 232
PV-10 as cause of, 132
skin, 288
tissue, 106
tumor, 196
neoadjuvant agents, 88
neoplasms
benign, 38
cervical, 239
cutaneous, 63, 157, 200, 213
HPV-associated, **221**
malignant, 119, 139, 147
melanocytic, 119
nail, 261, 281–284
sebaceous, 193
squamous cell, 281–284
neoplastic blood vessels, *190–191*
nevus, nevi
atypical, 119
basal cell, 158
benign, 38, **44**, 121
dermoscopically suspicious, 37–38
dysplastic, 13
malignant blue, 119
matrical, 285
melanoma-adjacent melanocytic, 13
melanomas arising from 119, 123
nicotinamide, 54–55, 144, 145, 147
nivolumab 131, **132**, 182
clinical trials involving, 211
for cutaneous malignancies, **207**
transplant rejection, risk of 210
NMSCs, *see* nonmelanoma skin cancers (NMSCs)
Nocardia spp., 217, **220**, 221
nocardiosis, 221
nonmelanoma skin cancers (NMSCs) 10, **11**, 25, 42, 62–66
5-FU cream for, 66
azathioprine, risks associated with, 255–256, 257
basal cell carcinoma (BCC), 71
diffuse, 63, *74*
inflammatory prostaglandins, increased activity of, 68
intralesional therapies for, 72–73
invasive squamous cell, 70–71
low-risk, 63
and Mohs micrographic surgery (MMS), indications for, 158
and Mycophenolate mofetil (MMF), risks associated with, 256
photodynamic therapy (PDT) as primarily modality for, 68, 85

rates of incidence, 139
solid organ transplant recipients (SOTRs), risk of developing, 62, 76
see also, squamous cell carcinoma in situ (SCCis)
nonsteroidal anti-inflammatory drugs (NSAIDs), 68, **69**, 75
nontuberculous mycobacteria (NTM), 222, **223**
NOTCH1, 174

O

oncogenes, 121, 129
oncogenics, 126, 129
and calcineurin inhibitors (CNIs), 284
antioncogenics, 9
oncogenesis, 141, 174
oncology
dermatological, 82
mTOR inhibitors as therapy, 56–57
as multidisciplinary team, 298–299
posttransplant cutaneous, 4
radiation, 150
oncolytic virus 133, 141–142, 205, 212
intralesional therapy, 212–213
talimogene laherparepvec (TVEC), 182
skin, 235
see also, HPV
oncoproteins, 180,182
large T-antigen (LT), 174
ST, 174
see also, MCPyV
onycholysis, **262**
dorsolateral, 269
subungual melanomas presenting as, 286
onychomycosis (OM), *230*, 267
candidal, *272*
common strategies for, **273**
dermatological consultation/recommendations, **274**
distal/lateral subungual (DLSMO), 270, **271**
endonyx, 270, **271**
mixed pattern (MPO), 270, **271**
proximal subungual onychomycosis (PSO), 270, **271**
Scopulariopsis brevicaulis as cause of, 228
superficial (white or black) (SO), 270, **271**
total dystrophic onychomycosis (TDO), 270, **271**
white, **228**
onychopathy, 255, 287
onychotillomania, 267
optical coherence tomography (OCT), 41–42, 45–46
organ transplant recipient (OTR), 2
see also, pediatric organ transplant recipients (pOTRs); solid organ transplant recipient (SOTR)
oropharyngeal
candidiasis, 229
infection, **226**
lesions, 141
oropharynx, 235
OTR, *see* organ transplant recipient (OTR)

P

p53
apoptic response, blocking, 141
induction, 88
mutations, 174
tumor-suppressing gene, 141
palmoplantar peeling, 254
Paracoccidioides brasiliensis, **227**
paronychia
acitretin-induced, 280
bacterial, 282
Bartonella henseale, presentation as, 269
benign, **288**
candidal, 276
chronic, 267, 281
proximal, 269
staphylococcal, 276
PD1, *see* programmed cell death protein-1 (PD1)
PD-L1, *see* programmed death-ligand 1 (PD-L1)
PD-L2, *see* programmed death-ligand 2 (PD-L2)
PDT, *see* photodynamic therapy (PDT)
pediatric organ transplant recipients (pOTRs), 99–109
penicillin, 269
Penicillium, **227**, 234
P. marneffei, **227–228**
Peptostreptococcus, 267
perionychium, 275
edema of, 279
occult trauma of, 280
peripheral artery disease (PAD), 67
phaeohyphomycosis, **226**, 232, *233*
photodynamic therapy (PDT), 54, **69**
actinic keratoses (AK), 54, *65*, 76, **86–57**, 87
BCC, 71
combination methods to enhance, 87–90
daylight (dPDT), 83–84
mechanism of action, 82
as preventive modality, 88–92
as primary modality, 84–88
squamous cell cancer in situ (SCCis), 70
see also, methyl aminolevulinate photodynamic therapy (MAL-PDT)
Piroxicam, 68, **69**
pityriasis, 105
versicolor, **226**, 228
pityrosporum folliculitis, *229*, 249
posttransplant lymphoproliferative disorders (PTLD), **29**, **220**
belatacept contraindicated for, 57
cutaneous, 101
in pediatric organ transplant recipients, 99, 108
prednisone
and allograft rejection, 211
and alopecia, 256
clinical trials administering, 211
and immunosuppression, 28, **29**, 125, **127**, **210**
and pediatric organ transplants, **104**, 108
and sebaceous hyperplasia (SH), eruptive, 253
and skin cancer risk, 6, **12**, 159, 193
oral, 26
and warts, 277
pOTRs, *see* pediatric organ transplant recipients (pOTRs)
programmed cell death protein 1 (PD-1), 131–133, 205–211
programmed death-ligand 1 (PD-L1), 128, 182, 206, **208**, *208*, 210–211
programmed death-ligand 2 (PD-L2), 206, 211
progression free survival (PFS), 173–174, 181–182
prophylactic use of drugs

acitretin, 53
antiviral regimens, 242
isotretinoin, 195
PDT, 54
radiation, 181
retinoids, 144
sirolimus, 56
vaccination, 278
Propionibacterium acnes, 249
proximal nail fold (PNF), 261–262, 267, 271, 282, 286
proximal subungual onychomycosis (PSO), 270–271, **271**, **273**
pruritus, 54, 248, 257, 278
Pseudomonas aeruginosa, **220**, 267–268, 271
antipseudomonal penicillin, 269
ecthyma gangrenosum, manifestation as, 219
sepsis, 269
see also, green nail syndrome
PSO, *see* proximal subungual onychomycosis (PSO)
psoralen plus ultraviolet A (PUVA), 108, 119
psoriasis, 265, **266**
nail, 267, 270–271, 278
PUVA, *see* psoralen plus ultraviolet A (PUVA)
pyogenic granuloma, 222, 255, 269, 280–281, **288**

R

rapamycin, 281
see also, mammalian target of rapamycin (mTOR)
RB1, 174, 178
RCM, *see* reflectance confocal microscopy (RCM)
reflectance confocal microscopy (RCM), 39–42, 45–46
renal transplant recipient (RTRs) 2–3
basal cell carcinoma (BCC), 9
belatacept, 65
Kaposi's sarcoma risk, 13
melanoma risk, 13, **14**
squamous cell cancer (SCC) in, 5–6
retinoids, **94**
acitretin 53, 57, 144, 147, 267, 278, 279–281
as chemoprophylaxis, 53, 57, 71
as chemoprevention, 144–145
isotretinoid, 144, 147, 195
PDT, in conjunction with, 88
topical, **69**, 88, 249, 253, 277
Rhizopus, **226**, 232
RTRs, *see* renal transplant recipients (RTRs)

S

scabies, ungual and subungual, 278–279
SCC, *see* squamous cell carcinoma (SCC)
Scopulariopsis spp. **226–227**, 234
S. brevicaulis, 228, 270
scrofuloderma, **220**, 223, *224*
sebaceous carcinoma, 193–195, 200
sebaceous glands, 42
sebaceous hyperplasia, 252, 257
sentinel lymph node biopsy (SLNB), 161–163, 181, 195
sequelae
cutaneous, 109
dermatologic, 247
surgical, 105–106
see also leukocytoclastic vasculitis (LCV)
sirolimus, 2, **8**
AFX tumors and, 195
antioncogenic effects, 9
carcinogenesis, risk of, 145
complication risks associated with, 159
dosing schedule, 26
and immunosuppression, **29**, 30, 56–57, **104**, 125
and Kaposi's sarcoma (KS), 192
lymphedema as side effect of, 254
and malignancy, risk of, 125–126, 142, 205
as melanoma risk factor, 123, 125
nail changes as a result of using, 291
palmoplantar peeling as side effect of, 254–255
paronychia caused by, 267, 276–277
sebaceous neoplasm formations, 195
survival outcomes, **13**. **15**
and warts, impact on, 277
and wound healing, effect on, 255
Skin and Ultraviolet Neoplasia Transplant Risk Assessment Calculator (SUNTRAC), 143, 296
skin cancer, posttransplant 5–16
see also, Kaposi's sarcoma; melanoma; Merkel cell carcinoma (MCC); non-melanoma skin cancer (NMSC)
Skin Care in Organ Transplant Patients, Europe (SCOPE), 4
solid organ transplantation (SOT)
advances in, 2
and cancer, 2–3
immunosuppressive therapies for, 23–33
photodynamic therapy for, 82–93
solid organ transplant recipients (SOTRs)
bacterial, fungal, and viral infections in, 217–242
immunosuppressive therapy side effects in, 247–257
immunotherapy in, 204–213
melanoma in, *see* melanoma
Merkel cell carcinoma in, *see* Merkel cell carcinoma (MCC)
nail disease and surgery in, 261–289
squamous cell carcinoma in, *see* squamous cell carcinoma
Sporothrix schenckii 234
squamous cell carcinoma (SCC), 3, 5–6, 40
cutaneous, 139–147
dermoscopy to identify, 38, 47
head and neck, 206
invasive, 63, 69
management of, 150–163
metastatic, **132**
recurrent, *140*
reflectance confocal microscopy (RCM) to identify, 40, 46
risk factors for, **7**
subungual/periungual invasive, 281
see also, cutaneous squamous cell carcinoma (cSCC); squamous cell carcinoma in situ (SCCis); squamous cell carcinoma of the nail apparatus (SCCNA)
squamous cell carcinoma in situ (SCCis), 63–67
combination therapies for, 70
of the nail apparatus, 281–282
surgical treatment options for, 70
topical treatments for, 70
photodynamic therapy (PDT) for, 82, 85, 87, **89**
squamous cell carcinoma of the nail apparatus (SCCNA), 282–284
SSSS, *see* staphylococcal scalded-skin syndrome (SSSS)

superficial (white or black) onychomycosis (SO), *270*, **271**
staphylococcal scalded-skin syndrome (SSSS), **220**
staphylococcal infection, 102, *103*, 108, 219, **220**
  anti-staphylococcal antimicrobials, 280
Staphylococcus aureus, 108, 217, 219, 267
streptococcal infection, 102, 217, 219, **220**
Streptomyces verticillus, 75
streptomycin, 225
subungual keratoacanthoma (SUKA), 281–284
sunscreens, 52, 57, 63, 297
  Piroxicam, 69, **69**
SUNTRAC, *see* Skin and Ultraviolet Neoplasia Transplant Risk Assessment Calculator (SUNTRAC)

T

tacrolimus, 2, 7, **8**
  and aphthous stomatitis, 256
  Astagraf XL, 25
  clinical trials, 211
  dermatologic side effects of, 250
  drug interactions, 131
  Envarsus XR, 25
  and fungal susceptibility to fluconazole, 274
  hair loss (alopecia) associated with, 25, 106, 252, 257
  and hypertrichosis, 252
  immunosuppression, benefits of using, 28, 55, **104**, 125, 210
  interleukin, suppression of, 108
  intolerance of, **29**
  and Kaposi's sarcoma (KS), higher risk of, 191
  and lymphoma, risk of, 108
  and Merkel cell carcinoma (MCC), lower risk of, 173
  Prograf, 25
  as pro-oncogenic immunosuppressant, 128
  risk factors associated with, 125, 159
  and sebaceous hyperplasia (SH), eruptive, 253
  and sebaceous neoplasms, development of, 195
  and Trichodysplasia spinulosa, **104**
talimogene laherparepvec (T-VEC), 133, 182, 212
T-antigen, 174
T-cell, **29**, 57
  disease, 101
  function, suppression or inhibition of, 128, 142, 157
  low regulatory levels of, 106
  lymphoma, 108
  regulatory (Tregs), 206
  response, altered, **107**
TDO, *see* total dystrophic onychomycosis (TDO)
terbinafine, 225, 273–274
thalidomide, *239*, 256
thoracic transplants, **7**, 9, 13
  risk factor, 143, **145**, 147, 205
thrombocytopenia, 26
thymic stromal lymphopoietin (TSLP), 65
TNM, *see* tumor, node, metastasis (TNM) staging system
total dystrophic onychomycosis (TDO), 271, **271**
TP53, 56, 121, 174
trachyonychia, 280
trametinib, *130*, 131
transplant dermatology
  clinic, how to build, 293–300
  history of, 3–5
Tregs, *see* T-cells
triamcinolone, 75
Trichophyton, spp., 225, 273
  T. interdigitale, **226**, 269
  T. mentagrophytes, **226**
  T. rubrum, **226**, 267, 269
  T. tonsurans, **226**
  T. verrucosum, **226**
tumor, node, metastasis (TNM) staging system, 178

U

ultrasound, 42–43
undifferentiated pleomorphic sarcoma (UPS), 195

V

varicella zoster virus (VZV), 102, **218**, 219, **220–221**
  skin disease due to, 235–236
vasculitis, *221*, 275
  see also, leukocytoclastic vasculitis (LCV)
vemurafenib, 130–131
verruca, verrucae
  cutaneous, 102
  external genital, 67
  periungual, 276
  vulgaris, *103*, *240*
verrucous plaques, 223, **227**, 281
voriconazole, 142–143, **205**, 225, 234
  as inhibitor of cytochrome, P450 3A4 274
  as prophylactic, 297
  and skin cancer, increased risk of, **8**, 9, 85, 100

W

wound healing, impaired, 26, 31, 255

X

xeroderma pigmentosum, 46, 119, 158

Z

zygomycosis, 232